Management of Multiple Drug-Resistant Infections

Infectious Disease

Series Editor: ***Vassil St. Georgiev, PhD***

National Institute of Allergy and Infectious Diseases
National Institutes of Health

Management of Multiple Drug-Resistant Infections, by ***Stephen H. Gillespie, MD,*** 2004

Microbial Genomes, by ***Claire M. Fraser, PhD, Timothy D. Read, PhD, and Karen E. Nelson, PhD,*** 2004

Aging, Immunity, and Infection, by ***Joseph F. Albright, PhD, and Julia W. Albright, PhD,*** 2003

Handbook of Cytokines and Chemokines in Infectious Diseases, edited by ***Malak Kotb, PhD, and Thierry Calandra, MD, PhD,*** 2003

Opportunistic Infections: *Treatment and Prophylaxis,* **Vassil St. Georgiev, PhD,** 2003

Innate Immunity, edited by ***R. Alan B. Ezekowitz, MBChB, DPhil, FAAP, and Jules A. Hoffmann, PhD,*** 2003

Pathogen Genomics: *Impact on Human Health,* edited by ***Karen Joy Shaw, PhD,*** 2002

Immunotherapy for Infectious Diseases, edited by ***Jeffrey M. Jacobson, MD***, 2002

Retroviral Immunology: *Immune Response and Restoration,* edited by ***Giuseppe Pantaleo, MD,*** and ***Bruce D. Walker, MD,*** 2001

Antimalarial Chemotherapy: *Mechanisms of Action, Resistance, and New Directions in Drug Discovery,* edited by ***Philip J. Rosenthal, MD***, 2001

Drug Interactions in Infectious Diseases, edited by ***Stephen C. Piscitelli, PharmD*** and ***Keith A. Rodvold, PharmD,*** 2001

Management of Antimicrobials in Infectious Diseases: *Impact of Antibiotic Resistance,* edited by ***Arch G. Mainous III, PhD,*** and ***Claire Pomeroy, MD***, 2001

Infectious Disease in the Aging: *A Clinical Handbook,* edited by ***Thomas T. Yoshikawa, MD*** and ***Dean C. Norman, MD***, 2001

Infectious Causes of Cancer: *Targets for Intervention,* edited by ***James J. Goedert, MD,*** 2000

Infectious Disease

Management of Multiple Drug-Resistant Infections

Edited by

Stephen H. Gillespie, MD

Department of Medical Microbiology,
Royal Free and University College Medical School,
London, England

Springer Science+Business Media, LLC

Softcover reprint of the hardcover 1st edition 2004

This publication is printed on acid-free paper. ∞

ANSI Z39.48-1984 (American Standards Institute) Permanence of Paper for Printed Library Materials.

Cover design by Patricia F. Cleary.

Production editor: Wendy S. Kopf

10 9 8 7 6 5 4 3 2 1

ISBN 978-1-61737-438-8 ISBN 978-1-59259-738-3 (eBook)

DOI 10.1007/978-1-59259-738-3

Library of Congress Cataloging in Publication Data

Management of multiple drug-resistant infections / edited by Stephen H. Gillespie.

p. ; cm. -- (Infectious disease)

Includes bibliographical references and index.

1. Multidrug resistance. 2. Drug resistance in microorganisms.

[DNLM: 1. Bacterial Infections--drug therapy. 2. Drug Resistance, Multiple. 3. Anti-Infective Agents--therapeutic use. 4. Communicable Diseases--drug therapy. 5. Infection Control. WC 200 M265 2004] I. Gillespie, S. H. II. Infectious disease (Totowa, N.J.)

QR177.M36 2004

616.9'041--dc22

2003014628

Preface

The past few years have seen dire predictions of the appearance of the post-antimicrobial era. There have been dramatic headlines in the lay and medical press with lurid accounts of the untreatable super-bugs that stalk our streets and hospitals. In the future, we are told, we will have to learn to live without antimicrobials. To cap it, all the doom-mongers place the blame on irresponsible doctors. It is said to be all our own fault! This version of the future of antimicrobial therapy is inaccurate. It marries deeply hidden folk memories of past epidemic diseases with a legitimate concern about antimicrobial prescribing and the means to preserve the longevity of current anti-infective therapies.

History

The concept of an antimicrobial is a recent one. Indeed the concept of a micro-organism as the cause of what we now describe as infectious diseases—the germ theory of disease—is only 150 years old. It is true that quinine had long been available for the treatment of malaria in Europe since the mid-17th century, but there was no coherent understanding of its mechanism of action or against what it acted. Rather, it was seen that in a universe balanced by God, where a threat, malaria, was present, a solution, chinchona bark, would be found. It was Paul Erhlich who made the first systematic account of the possibilities of specific antimicrobial medicines. His imaginative leap was to recognize that if his colleague, Robert Koch, could specifically stain *Mycobacterium tuberculosis* so that it could be identified in the sputum of patients with tuberculosis, then that specificity could be used to kill the organisms responsible for the disease. This led him to investigate specific dyes. There is a misunderstanding about his famous phrase "magic bullets"; it was not antimicrobial drugs that he described in that way but rather antibodies whose specificity he craved. Dyes active against trypanosomes, which were needed to curb the threat of sleeping sickness in Germany's new colony in East Africa, were developed. During his research, Ehrlich noted that trypanosomes could develop resistance to the dyes that they were treated with. These same organisms, however, could also be successfully treated with dyes different from those to which they had developed the resistance. Further research on dyes led to the discovery of salvarsan, the first specific treatment against syphilis—Ehrlich's crowning achievement.

Erhlich's approach to chemotherapy finally bore its full fruit with the development of Prontosil by Domagk. A whole series of synthetic compounds with activity against bacteria, most notably against *M. tuberculosis*, flowed from this research. But it was serendipity that brought about the most significant change. Fleming's chance finding led to the discovery of penicillin. Initially, the difficulties of producing enough pure substance hindered the development of the drug, but the pressure of war stimulated a concerted drive to produce large quantities. Over the next 15 years, most of the main classes of antimicrobials were discovered.

Resistance

The significance of the fact that the first description of resistance coincides with Erhlich's description of antimicrobial chemotherapy is often forgotten. In Fleming's original paper, he systematically describes the organisms that were intrinsically resistant to his new compound. The emergence of resistance is a natural consequence of the use of an antimicrobial agent. Improved living conditions in industrialized countries reduced the threat of infectious diseases, and year by year new drug discoveries overcame problem organisms as well as the resistance that was emerging. However, the significance of the threat posed by resistant organisms was recognized when one of the major pathogens tamed by penicillin became untreatable owing to resistance. The penicillinase-producing *Staphylococcus aureus* posed a significant threat to hospital patients. The solution was to modify the amido-penicillin nucleus, which resulted in ampicillin, and of more importance for the treatment of *S. aureus*, methicillin and its imitators. The subsequent decades saw an antimicrobial "arms race" as new agents were introduced to deal with increasing resistance among mainly Gram-negative pathogens. Falling research investment on the part of major pharmaceutical companies has reduced the number of new antimicrobials reaching the marketplace. Thus, with the appearance of glycopeptide-intermediate and later-resistant *S. aureus* (GISA, GRSA), glycopeptide-resistant *Enterococci*, and multiple drug-resistant *Acinetobacter*, *Stenotrophomonas*, *Klebsiella*, and *Pseudomonas*, the choice of antimicrobials to manage infections has become more difficult.

In the community, the first flush of antimicrobials remained for the most part effective. With the exception of *S. enteritidis* serovar Typhi, there were effective antimicrobials against the major community acquired bacterial infections. The first description of multiple drug-resistant *Streptococcus pneumoniae* and later intercontinental spread of resistant clones raised an alarm that was repeated with the explosive outbreaks of multiple drug-resistant *M. tuberculosis* in prisons and hospitals in the United States. A reduction in therapeutic choices has not been matched with new antimicrobial compounds for evaluation. The situation for both of these indications is bleak.

So have we reached the post-antimicrobial age? Not yet, for there are still therapeutic choices for most bacterial infections. It is true that clinicians managing infections in the hospital environment are now seeing with increasing regularity a small number of bacteria that are completely resistant to antimicrobials and these organisms occasionally cause infection. However, in most instances diligent application of sound clinical judgment allied with appropriate culture and susceptibility testing permits effective therapeutic regimens to be constructed. In the community, the antimicrobial treatment door has not yet closed, although we are all managing more cases where the therapeutic options are few, and in some cases none. Those of us who manage tuberculosis have had to revisit the old textbooks to relearn the natural history of untreated tuberculosis (untreated because it is untreatable) and to watch patients be slowly consumed by this inexorable disease.

We are not yet in the post-antimicrobial age, although we may fear that it is our final destination. It is a time when there are likely to be difficult therapeutic choices in every area of infectious disease practice. *Management of Multiple Drug-Resistant Infections* is intended to provide practical advice about the management of multiple drug-resistant infections. Consequently, the focus has been on major hospital and community-acquired pathogens, including *S. aureus*, *S. pneumoniae*, *Acinetobacter*, and *M. tuberculosis*. In some parts of infection practice, managing resistance has become so much part of the fabric of life that it is no longer noticed. Thus, chapters on the management of multiple drug-resistant urinary tract infection and gonorrhoea have been included.

As Fleming initially observed in his first penicillin paper, some organisms are naturally resistant to antimicrobials; therefore, chapters discussing the management of some of these infections (naturally amphotericin-resistant fungi, nontuberculosis mycobacteria, and melioidosis) are included. Partly unrecognized by microbiologists in industrialized countries is the growing problem of resistance in *Plasmodium falciparum* malaria for more than one billion people who are at risk of infection by this pathogen. The extent of resistance problems extends to helminths and there is evidence that schistosomes are becoming resistant to the only drug effective against all of the species that infect humans. Antiviral agents are relative late-comers to the field of antimicrobial chemotherapy. As was the case for antibacterials, resistance to the antiviral drugs emerged rapidly. Two chapters have been included that address resistance among some of the most important antiviral classes: antiretrovirals and drugs that act against cytomegalovirus.

It is impossible to manage multiple drug-resistant infections without considering measures necessary to prevent spreading to other patients. It is for this reason that two chapters, one dealing with the epidemiology of tuberculosis and another dealing with the evidence base that supports infection control procedures, are included.

Antimicrobial and multiple drug resistance is a multifaceted problem that applies to almost all microorganisms for which science has developed drugs. The chapters selected are intended to reflect this diversity. In addition to providing scientific and epidemiological background, *Management of Multiple Drug-Resistant Infections* is also intended to be a practical guide to managing some of the most difficult infection problems with multiple drug-resistant organisms. I hope that those who have to wrestle with resistance every day will find it useful.

Stephen H. Gillespie, MD

Contents

Preface ... *v*

Contributors ... *xi*

PART I: GRAM-POSITIVE BACTERIA

1 Management of Community-Acquired Pneumonia Caused by Drug-Resistant *Streptococcus pneumoniae*
Eric L. Nuermberger and William R. Bishai ... ***3***

2 Management of Meningitis Caused by Resistant *Streptococcus pneumoniae*
P. Fernández Viladrich ... ***31***

3 Emerging Resistance to Vancomycin, Rifampin, and Fluoroquinolones in *Streptococcus pneumoniae*
Joseph M. Blondeau ... ***49***

4 Management of Glycopeptide-Resistant *Staphylococcus aureus* Infections
A. Peter R. Wilson ... ***79***

5 Infections Caused by Glycopeptide-Resistant Gram-Positive Bacteria Excluding Staphylococci
Armine Sefton ... ***91***

6 Isolation Policies and the Hospital Management of Methicillin-Resistant *Staphylococcus aureus: A Case of Evidence-Free Medicine?*
Sheldon P. Stone ... ***101***

PART II: GRAM-NEGATIVE PATHOGENS

7 The Management of Resistant *Acinetobacter* Infections in the Intensive Therapy Unit
Nicola Baker and Peter Hawkey ... ***117***

8 Drug-Resistant *Helicobacter pylori*
Peter J. Jenks ... ***141***

9 The Management of Antibiotic-Resistant *Neisseria gonorrhoeae*
Catherine A. Ison and Jonathan Ross ... ***159***

10 Management of Urinary Tract Infections Caused by Multiresistant Organisms
Jeremy M. T. Hamilton-Miller ... ***173***

11 Management of Multiple Drug-Resistant *Salmonella* Infections
Christopher M. Parry *189*

12 Management of Melioidosis
Andrew J. H. Simpson *209*

PART III: MYCOBACTERIA

13 The Molecular Epidemiology of MDR-TB
Paul D. van Helden, Robin M. Warren, Pieter Uys, Gian D. van der Spuy, and Thomas C. Victor *225*

14 The Management of Multiple Drug-Resistant Tuberculosis
Sanjay Bhagani and Marc Lipman *243*

15 Management of Infection With Nontuberculosis Mycobacteria
Stephen H. Gillespie *257*

PART IV: FUNGAL AND PARASITIC INFECTIONS

16 Management of Resistant *Candida* Infections
Sanya Clements and Christopher C. Kibbler *271*

17 Management of Infection With Naturally Amphotericin B-Resistant Fungi
Thean Yen Tan and Rosemary A. Barnes *297*

18 Management of Multiple Drug-Resistant Malaria
Elizabeth Ashley and François Nosten *319*

19 Schistosome Drug Resistance: *Praziquantel*
Michael J. Doenhoff and Katherine Wheatcroft-Francklow *341*

PART V. VIRAL INFECTIONS

20 Management of HIV Drug-Resistant Infections
Deenan Pillay *355*

21 Multidrug Resistance in Human Cytomegalovirus
Vincent C. Emery, Mohammad Raza Naqvee, and Anuradha Chawla *379*

Index 393

Contributors

ELIZABETH ASHLEY, BSc, MBBS, MRCP • *Shoklo Malaria Research Unit, Mae Sot, Thailand and Faculty of Tropical Medicine, Mahidol University, Bangkok, Thailand*

NICOLA BAKER, MB, BCh, BSc, MRCPATH • *Public Health Laboratory, Birmingham Heartlands Hospital, Birmingham, UK*

ROSEMARY A. BARNES, MD • *Department of Medical Microbiology, University of Wales College of Medicine, Cardiff, UK*

SANJAY BHAGANI, BSc, MRCP • *Department of Thoracic and HIV Medicine, University College London, Royal Free Hospital, London, UK*

WILLIAM BISHAI, MD, PhD • *Division of Infectious Diseases, Department of Medicine, Johns Hopkins University of Medicine, Baltimore, MD*

JOSEPH M. BLONDEAU, MSc, PhD, RSM(CCM), SM(AAM), FCCP • *Department of Clinical Microbiology, Saskatoon Health Region and Department of Microbiology and Immunology, University of Saskatchewan, Saskatoon, Saskatchewan, Canada and Department of Pathology, University College London, Royal Free Hospital, London, UK*

ANURADHA CHAWLA • *Department of Virology, University College London, Royal Free Hospital, London, UK*

SANYA CLEMENTS, MB, MRCP • *Department of Medical Microbiology, University College London, Royal Free Hospital, London, UK*

MICHAEL J. DOENHOFF, BSc, PhD • *School of Biological Sciences, University of Wales, Bangor, Gwynedd, UK*

VINCENT C. EMERY, BSc, PhD • *Department of Virology, University College London, Royal Free Hospital and Royal Free NHS Trust, London, UK*

STEPHEN H. GILLESPIE, MD, FRCP, FRCPATH • *Department of Medical Microbiology, University College London, Royal FreeHospital, London, UK*

JEREMY M. T. HAMILTON-MILLER, DSc, FRCPATH • *Department of Medical Microbiology, University College London, Royal Free Hospital, London, UK*

PETER HAWKEY, BSc DSc, MBBS, MD, FRCPATH • *Public Health Laboratory, Birmingham Heartlands Hospital, Division of Immunity and Infection, The Medical School, University of Birmingham, Birmingham, UK*

CATHERINE A. ISON, PhD, FRCPATH • *Department of Infectious Diseases and Microbiology, Imperial College London, St. Mary's Campus, London, UK*

PETER J. JENKS, PhD, MRCP, MRCPATH • *Institute of Infections and Immunity, University Hospital, Queen's Medical Centre, Nottingham, UK*

CHRISTOPHER C. KIBBLER, MA, FRCP, FRCPATH • *Department of Medical Microbiology, University College London, Royal Free Hospital, London, UK*

MARC LIPMAN, MD, FRCP • *Department of Thoracic and HIV Medicine, University College London, Royal Free Hospital, London, UK*
MOHAMMAD RAZA NAQVEE • *Department of Virology, University College London, Royal Free Hospital, London, UK*
FRANÇOIS NOSTEN, MD, PhD • *Shoklo Malaria Research Unit, Mae Sot, Thailand and Mahidol University, Bangkok, Thailand and Nuffield Department of Clinical Medicine, Centre for Tropical Medicine, John Radcliffe Hospital, Oxford, UK*
ERIC L. NUERMBERGER, MD • *Division of Infectious Diseases, Department of Medicine, Johns Hopkins University, School of Medicine, Baltimore, MD*
CHRISTOPHER M. PARRY, BA, MB, FRCPATH, MRCP • *University Department of Medical Microbiology and Genitourinary Medicine, Royal Liverpool University Hospital, Liverpool, UK*
DEENAN PILLAY, PhD, FRCPATH • *Department of Virology, Royal Free and University College Medical School, University College London, UK*
JONATHAN ROSS, MD, FRCP • *Whittall Street Clinic, Department of Infectious Diseases and Microbiology, Faculty of Medicine, St. Mary's Campus, Imperial College London, London, UK*
ARMINE SEFTON, MD, FRCP(EDIN), FRCPATH • *Department of Medical Microbiology, St. Bartholomew's and London Medical School, London, UK*
ANDREW J. H. SIMPSON, MB, BSc, MSc, FRCPATH • *Department of Medical Microbiology, University College London, Royal Free Hospital, London, UK*
SHELDON P. STONE, BSc, MD, FRCP • *Academic Department of Geriatric Medicine, Royal Free and University College Medical School, London, UK*
THEAN YEN TAN • *Department of Medical Microbiology, University of Wales College of Medicine, Cardiff, UK*
PIETER UYS, PhD • *Center for Molecular and Cellular Biology, Department of Medical Biochemistry, Faculty of Health Science, Stellenbosch University, Tygerberg, South Africa*
GIAN D. VAN DER SPUY, MSc • *Center for Molecular and Cellular Biology, Department Medical Biochemistry, Stellenbosch University, Tygerberg, South Africa*
PAUL D. VAN HELDEN, PhD • *Center for Molecular and Cellular Biology, Department of Medical Biochemistry, Stellenbosch University, Tygerberg, South Africa*
THOMAS C. VICTOR, PhD • *Center for Molecular and Cellular Biology, Department Medical Biochemistry, Faculty of Health Science, Stellenbosch University, Tygerberg, South Africa*
P. FERNÁNDEZ VILADRICH, MD • *Infectious Disease Department, Hospital Universitario de Bellvitge, Barcelona, Spain*
ROBIN M. WARREN, PhD • *Center for Molecular and Cellular Biology, Department of Medical Biochemistry, Stellenbosch University, Tygerberg, South Africa*
KATHERINE WHEATCROFT-FRANCKLOW, BSc, PhD • *School of Biological Sciences, University of Wales Bangor, Bangor, Gwynedd, UK*
A. PETER R. WILSON, MA, MD, FRCP, FRCPATH • *Department of Clinical Microbiology, Royal Free and University College Medical School, London, UK*

I

Gram-Positive Bacteria

1

Management of Community-Acquired Pneumonia Caused by Drug-Resistant *Streptococcus pneumoniae*

Eric L. Nuermberger and William R. Bishai

1. INTRODUCTION

There are between 2 and 3 million cases of community-acquired pneumonia (CAP) annually in the United States alone, leading to 500,000 hospitalizations and 45,000 deaths each year *(1,2)*. *Streptococcus pneumoniae* is the most common pathogen that causes CAP *(3)*, even in cases in which the routine diagnostic evaluation fails to demonstrate the etiology *(4)*. Pneumococcal pneumonia has always exacted significant morbidity and mortality. In the preantibiotic era, this "Captain of the Men of Death" *(5)* carried a 25–35% case fatality rate, which increased to 80% if bacteremia was present *(6,7)*. The advent of penicillin reduced mortality to rates below 10% *(8)*. Mortality rates 60 yr later still hover around 12% for all hospitalized patients *(3,9)* and up to 25% for those with bacteremia *(3,10)*. This apparent stability, however, belies a dramatic rise in the resistance of *S. pneumoniae* to penicillin and other drugs.

Pneumococci resistant to penicillin were isolated as early as 1943 in an experimental animal model *(11)*, but the first clinical isolate with reduced susceptibility was not reported until 1967 *(12)*. The prevalence of resistance remained low until the early 1990s, when an alarming increase in resistance became apparent. Today, more than one-third of US isolates have reduced susceptibility to penicillin, and 15–20% are considered resistant *(13,14)*. In certain countries outside the United States, the majority of clinical isolates are not susceptible to penicillin.

The situation is made worse by the concurrent rise of resistance to other drugs, particularly in isolates that are already penicillin-resistant. Multidrug-resistant *S. pneumoniae* (MDRSP), defined by resistance to penicillin and at least two other antibiotic classes, was first reported from South Africa in 1978 *(15)*, but has now spread to every continent. In the United States, among isolates of *S. pneumoniae* with a penicillin MIC (minimum inhibitory concentration) of 2 μg/mL or higher, 48% are resistant to tetracyclines, 78% are resistant to macrolides, and fully 94% are resistant to trimethoprim-sulfamethoxazole (Table 1) *(13)*. MDRSP now comprise nearly one-quarter of pneumococcal isolates in the United States *(13)*.

The explosive global emergence of MDRSP is not the result of a common mechanism of resistance, but rather clonal spread of a limited number of pneumococcal strains

From: *Management of Multiple Drug-Resistant Infections*
Edited by: S. H. Gillespie © Humana Press Inc., Totowa, NJ

Table 1
US Antimicrobial Resistance Rates for *S. pneumoniae*

	% Resistant			
Antimicrobial	All strains	Pen-S	Pen-I	Pen-R
Macrolides	25.7	5.6	42.3	77.8
Clindamycin	8.9	1.3	19.6	25.8
Tetracycline	16.3	3.1	31.4	48.0
Trimethoprim–sulfamethoxazole	30.3	7.6	39.2	94.5
Chloramphenicol	8.3	1.0	13.4	27.7

Source: Adapted from ref. *13.*
Pen-S, MIC ≤ 0.06 μg/mL; Pen-I, MIC = 0.12–1 μg/mL; Pen-R, MIC ≥ 2 μg/mL.

that have acquired multiple resistance determinants *(16)*. Indeed, the majority of MDRSP in the United States belong to one of six clones that have disseminated throughout the country under the selective pressure of antibiotic use *(17)*. The rapidity with which such an MDRSP clone can become established in a community and drive up resistance rates is illustrated by the situation in a Hong Kong hospital, in which the rates of drug-resistant *S. pneumoniae* (DRSP) infection rose from 6.6 to 55.8% over 18 mo, with an MDRSP serotype 23F clone accounting for the majority of isolates *(18)*.

In the last decade, the specter of DRSP has dramatically altered the way in which antibiotics are prescribed for CAP and threatens to reverse the progress of the last six decades since the introduction of penicillin. This chapter reviews the current state of resistance of *S. pneumoniae* to each of the three major antibiotic classes (β-lactams, macrolides, and fluoroquinolones) recommended for therapy of CAP and critically examines the clinical utility of agents from each class in the upcoming era of drug resistance.

2. RESISTANCE TO β-LACTAMS

2.1. Epidemiology

Recently published surveillance data suggest that up to 34% of *S. pneumoniae* isolates in the United States have reduced susceptibility to penicillin (MIC ≥ 0.12 μg/mL), and 16–21.5% of all isolates have high-level resistance (MIC ≥ 2 μg/mL) *(13,14)*. The corresponding prevalence rates were 23.6 and 9.5%, respectively, in 1994–1995 *(13)*. Certain areas of the world, such as Spain, Hungary, and South Africa, have reported reduced susceptibility to penicillin in up to 40–70% of isolates *(19–21)*.

2.2. Risk Factors

The risk factors for infection with DRSP center on the two factors most important to the spread of DRSP: antibiotic selection pressure and exposure to carriers. Not surprisingly, recent β-lactam therapy (within 3 mo) has been identified in multiple studies as a major risk factor for both carriage of and infection with β-lactam-resistant *S. pneumoniae (22)*. Recent hospitalization, institutional residence, immunosuppressive illness such as human immunodeficiency virus (HIV) infection, extremes of age, day

Table 2
Cross-Resistance to β-Lactams Among US Isolate of *S. pneumoniae*

	MIC$_{90}$[a] (μg/mL)		
Antimicrobial	Pen-S	Pen-I	Pen-R
Amoxicillin/clavulanate	0.03	1	4
Cefixime	0.5	16	64
Cefuroxime	0.12	4	16
Ceftriaxone	0.06	1	4

[a] MIC$_{90}$, minimum concentration that inhibits growth of 90% of the strains tested.
Source: Adapted from ref. *13*.
Pen-S, MIC ≤ 0.06μg/mL; Pen-I, MIC = 0.12–1 μg/mL; Pen-R, MIC ≥ 2 μg/mL.

care attendance (for children), or exposure to children in day care are markers for recent antibiotic usage or exposure to carriers of DRSP *(23–26)*.

2.3. Mechanism

Resistance to β-lactams in *S. pneumoniae* results from stepwise mutations in one or more of the five major penicillin-binding proteins (PBPs) in the bacterial cell wall that serve as targets for β-lactam action. In general, alterations of more than one PBP are necessary for reduced susceptibility to penicillin, whereas strains with MICs above 1 μg/mL typically have reductions in binding affinity that affect all major PBPs *(27)*. Because all β-lactams utilize the same targets to some extent, resistance to cephalosporins and carbapenems has emerged with penicillin resistance (Table 2).

2.4. Impact of Resistance

Streptococcus pneumoniae is a virulent human pathogen, and the benefits of antimicrobial therapy on mortality from bacteremic disease are well known *(6)*. Meehan et al. showed that a delay in the initiation of antibiotic therapy for CAP was also associated with an increase in mortality *(28)*. Despite the obvious concerns regarding the emergence of DRSP and the risk that initial empiric regimens may include drugs to which the infecting organism is resistant, the real clinical impact of pneumococcal resistance has been difficult to measure. Specifically, although treatment failures during β-lactam therapy for meningitis and otitis media caused by β-lactam-resistant *S. pneumoniae* have been well described *(29–31)*, there is little convincing evidence that the emergence of DRSP has resulted in increased clinical failures in patients with pneumonia.

A number of observational studies have been conducted to determine the effect of DRSP versus drug-susceptible *S. pneumoniae* on pneumonia outcomes (Table 3). When taken as a whole, these studies have yet to demonstrate clearly an impact of drug resistance on mortality. As depicted in Table 3, only one study demonstrated greater mortality for patients with pneumonia caused by penicillin-resistant *S. pneumoniae (32)*.

In summarizing the available clinical data, Bishai described a paradox in which the interpretation of in vitro resistance profiles does not appear to predict the in vivo outcome of pneumococcal pneumonia *(33)*. Several possible reasons for such a paradox exist, including the fact that accepted susceptibility breakpoints are not appropriate for

Table 3
Observational Studies of Mortality From Invasive Pneumococcal Pneumonia Caused by Drug-Susceptible and Drug-Resistant Strains

Location	Year	Fraction of patients with DRSP	Mortality (%) Pen-S	Mortality (%) Pen-I + Pen-R	*p* value	Reference
Barcelona	1984–1993	145/504 (29%)	24	38	NS	*40*
Israel	1987–1992	67/293 (23%)	11	16	NS	*38*
Ohio	1991–1994	39/499 (8%)	19	21	NS	*10*
New York[a]	1992–1996	30/421, Pen-I + Pen-R (7%)	14	27	NS	*32*
		19/421, Pen-R (5%)	16	42	0.02	
S. Africa (children)	1993–1994	35/108 (32%)	16	24	NS	*39*
Atlanta	1994	44/192 (23%)	11	23	NS	*37*
N. America	1995–1997	741/4193 (18%)	11	14	NS	*9*
Barcelona	1996–1998	49/101, penicillin (49%)	6	16	NS	*23*
		12/101, macrolide (12%)	14[b]	7[c]	NS	

[a]70% of patients with penicillin-nonsusceptible strains were HIV-infected.
[b]Macrolide susceptible.
[c]Macrolide nonsusceptible (MIC ≥ 1 μg/mL).
NS, not statistically significant; Pen-S, susceptible to penicillin (MIC ≤ 0.06 μg/mL); Pen-I, intermediate resistance to penicillin (MIC = 0.12–1 μg/mL); Pen-R, high-level resistance to penicillin (MIC ≥ 2 μg/mL).

pneumococcal pneumonia. The stepwise accumulation of PBP mutations means that susceptibility to β-lactams is not an all-or-none phenomenon, but rather is concentration dependent. Therapeutic efficacy is therefore determined by the concentration of drug at the site of infection in addition to the organism's susceptibility. The incremental nature of β-lactam resistance requires arbitrary breakpoints for establishing susceptibility in vitro. Until recently, the National Committee for Clinical Laboratory Standards (NCCLS) recommended that isolates with penicillin MICs less than 0.06 μg/mL be considered susceptible, isolates with MICs of 0.12–1 μg/mL be considered intermediate, and isolates with MICs of 2 μg/mL or above be considered resistant to penicillin *(34)*. These guidelines were based on achievable concentrations of penicillin in the cerebrospinal fluid (CSF) and were intended to prevent clinical failures in the treatment of meningitis caused by penicillin-intermediate isolates *(34,35)*. Because the levels of penicillin obtained in the lung parenchyma are higher than those in CSF and are similar to those in serum, the designations of susceptibility based on these guidelines may not be appropriate for pneumococcal pneumonia and may have overstated the problem as it relates to pneumonia caused by DRSP *(36)*.

Few patients with highly resistant isolates (penicillin MIC ≥ 4 μg/mL) have been included in studies to determine the impact of DRSP. The study by Turett et al. *(32)* is important as the first study in which penicillin nonsusceptibility was divided into higher (MIC ≥ 2 μg/mL) and lower (MIC = 0.12–1.0 μg/mL) levels of resistance for the mortality analysis. Although less than 5% of all isolates had MICs of 2 μg/mL or above, the authors were able to detect a higher mortality for patients harboring these more resistant organisms, whereas all patients infected with isolates with MICs between 0.12 and 1.0 µg/mL survived.

An additional caveat in these studies concerns the sensitivity of the outcome variables used to detect clinical failures. Previous work suggested that mortality from bacteremic pneumococcal pneumonia within the first 5 d of presentation is independent of the administration of antibiotics *(6)*. Therefore, a true association between drug resistance and mortality may only become apparent five or more days from presentation. In an analysis of nearly 6000 patients with pneumococcal pneumonia, Feikin et al. *(9)* failed to link penicillin resistance to mortality. However, if deaths in the first 4 d were excluded as likely refractory to any effective antimicrobial therapy, mortality was significantly associated with penicillin MICs ≥ 4 µg/mL or higher or cefotaxime MICs ≥ 2 µg/mL or higher. This study was limited, however, because information about the severity of illness on presentation and whether the specific antimicrobial agents received were active in vitro was not included in the analysis.

It is also possible that outcomes other than mortality are more sensitive to the influence of drug resistance. Indeed, although a retrospective cohort study by Metlay et al. *(37)* demonstrated only a trend toward increased mortality that was not statistically significant, patients infected with penicillin-nonsusceptible isolates (penicillin MIC≥ 0.1 µg/mL) did have a significantly higher rate of suppurative complications such as empyema, abscess, and osteomyelitis despite most patients receiving at least one antimicrobial to which the isolate was fully susceptible. Other markers of severity (shock, respiratory failure, intensive care unit [ICU] admission) were no different. Two studies found that patients infected with penicillin-nonsusceptible isolates had a longer stay, although patients in both studies were not stratified by severity of illness on presentation or comorbidity *(10,38)*. Other studies have not found associations between resistance and length of stay or pneumonia-related complications *(23,37,39)*.

A final limitation of the studies assessing the impact of resistance on outcomes is that the in vitro activity of the actual antibiotic regimen the patients received has not been correlated with outcomes. It would be expected that clinical failures could only be ascribed to drug resistance for patients receiving discordant therapy (i.e., the infecting organism is resistant to all drugs used) rather than concordant therapy. The studies listed in Table 3 either did not find an association between discordant therapy and an increased risk of clinical failure *(23,32,37,40)* or did not have the pertinent data available for analysis *(9,10,38)*.

2.5. Pharmacodynamic Approach to β-Lactam Use

Large, randomized, controlled clinical trials of β-lactam therapy for DRSP pneumonia are unlikely to be performed. The number of patients with resistant infections needed for statistical power is prohibitive, and under the current resistance breakpoints, obvious ethical concerns exist about using antibiotics of questionable activity for potentially fatal infections. With the difficulty of obtaining pertinent clinical information on the impact of antimicrobial resistance on treatment outcomes, the results of pharmacodynamic studies using in vitro systems and in vivo animal models are receiving greater attention.

Pharmacodynamics describe the relationship between the in vitro potency of an antibiotic (e.g., the MIC) and the time course of its activity. The latter aspect is determined by the rate of bacterial killing, the effect of changing concentrations of drug on this rate, and the presence of persistent effects on bacterial growth after antibiotic removal. Specific pharmacodynamic parameters that correlate with antibacterial activity include the time above the MIC (expressed as the proportion of the dosing interval that serum concentrations exceed the MIC), the maximal serum concentration divided by the MIC (C_{max}/MIC), and the area under the 24-h serum concentration–time curve divided by the MIC (AUC/MIC). For a given antibiotic class, specific pharmacodynamic parameters have the ability to predict antimicrobial efficacy in animal models and in human infections *(41)*. As a result, the information gained from animal models is helpful in determining dosing regimens for humans with DRSP infections.

Pharmacodynamic considerations suggest therapy with a number of β-lactams would be effective for pneumonia caused by pneumococcal strains that appear nonsusceptible in vitro. Based on mouse model studies, most commonly in the neutropenic thigh infection model, the pharmacodynamic parameter that best correlates with the efficacy of β-lactams is time above MIC *(41)*. For these drugs, the maximal bactericidal effect is achieved at concentrations that are four times the MIC. Higher concentrations do not enhance killing. Dosing regimens should therefore aim to maximize the time that serum concentrations exceed the MIC of the infecting organism.

Fortunately, antibiotic levels do not need to exceed the MIC for 100% of the dosing interval. The optimal bactericidal activity and clinical efficacy are achieved when free drug concentrations exceed the MIC for more than 40% of the dosing interval for the penicillins and more than 50% of the dosing interval for cephalosporins *(41)*. A bacteriostatic effect may be achieved at shorter times above the MIC: 30% for penicillins, 40% for cephalosporins. Carbapenems have the most rapid bactericidal activity. Concentrations may exceed the MIC for only 25 to 30% of the dosing interval for optimal bactericidal activity, and times above the MIC of 5 to 10% are associated with bacteriostatic activity *(42,43)*. Table 4 depicts the time above MIC achieved with standard dosing of β-lactams commonly used for community-acquired lower respiratory tract infections (RTIs).

Currently, all parenteral β-lactams recommended for the treatment of pneumococcal pneumonia can achieve a time above MIC of 40 to 50% against organisms with an MIC ≤ 2 μg/mL using standard dosing, although some, such as cefuroxime, barely reach this critical value *(36)*. Amoxicillin is the most active oral β-lactam against *S. pneumoniae*, whereas many oral cephalosporins do not achieve adequate concentrations against penicillin-nonsusceptible isolates *(44–46)*. The most active oral cephalosporins include (in no particular order) cefprozil, cefpodoxime, cefuroxime, and cefditoren, but even these agents must be used with caution when the penicillin MIC is above 1 μg/mL.

Largely based on the clinical and pharmacodynamic data presented, the NCCLS has changed the interpretive breakpoints for amoxicillin, cefotaxime, and ceftriaxone against isolates from nonmeningeal infections such as CAP (Table 5) *(34,47)*. Under the new standards, an isolate with an amoxicillin MIC of 2 μg/mL or lower is susceptible, with 4 μg/mL is intermediate, and with 8 μg/mL or higher is resistant. An isolate with a cefotaxime or ceftriaxone MIC of 1 μg/mL or lower is susceptible, with 2 μg/mL is intermediate, and with 4 μg/mL or higher is resistant. Using these new definitions, over 90% of all pneumococci are now considered susceptible to amoxicillin *(13)*, and more than 95% are susceptible to ceftriaxone *(14)*, making amoxicillin/clavulanate, ceftriaxone, and cefotaxime the preferred β-lactams for empiric CAP treatment. Parenteral agents to avoid based on pharmacodynamic considerations include ceftazidime, ceftizoxime, and ticarcillin.

From a pharmacodynamic standpoint, intravenous penicillin G is still a viable option for DRSP infections with a penicillin MIC up to 4 μg/mL. Optimal dosing for intravenous penicillin is 18 to 24 million units (MU) per day, divided every 4 to 6 h. As seen in Table 4, the highest dose of intravenous penicillin (5 MU) should provide serum concentrations above 4 μg/mL for 55% of the 6-h dosing interval *(48)*. When using cefotaxime, ceftriaxone, ampicillin, or amoxicillin against DRSP isolates with penicillin MICs of 4 μg/mL or higher, the amoxicillin 500 mg tid dose and the other doses depicted in Table 4 may be doubled to increase the probability of a favorable response.

3. RESISTANCE TO MACROLIDES

Whether used alone or with a β-lactam for more seriously ill patients, macrolides remain first-line agents for CAP. The rapid escalation of microbiological resistance in the last decade, however, has raised questions regarding their efficacy for serious infections, particularly for bacteremic pneumococcal pneumonia. Although reports of treatment failure in association with resistant isolates have heightened concerns, the clinical experience to date is not consistent with widespread treatment failures because of resistant organisms. It remains uncertain whether the reported treatment failures reveal the tip of the iceberg representing the clinical impact of macrolide resistance or mere anecdotes?

3.1. *Epidemiology*

The prevalence of macrolide resistance increased markedly among *S. pneumoniae* isolates in the last decade, concomitant with penicillin resistance. Surveillance studies have demonstrated resistance rates of 26% in the United States *(13,14)*, although for penicillin-resistant isolates, macrolide resistance rates now exceed 75% *(13)*. Similarly, alarming rates are reported from countries in Europe, Asia, and South America *(49)*.

3.2. *Risk Factors*

Previous antibiotic use is the major risk factor for macrolide resistance *(50)*. As a result, the prevalence of resistance is higher in children (particularly those with recurrent otitis media or in day care), recently hospitalized patients, and patients with penicillin-resistant isolates *(49)*. Resistance is more common in insured or affluent adults or those who receive repeated courses of antibiotics for exacerbations of chronic bronchitis *(49)*.

Increasing usage of new, longer-acting macrolides has been strongly correlated with increasing resistance rates *(51,52)*. Some have suggested that long-acting macrolides are more likely to lead to resistance because of lower peak serum concentrations and longer periods with sub-MIC levels *(49,51)*. Azithromycin use has repeatedly been associated with pharyngeal carriage of resistant pneumococci *(53–55)*.

3.3. *Mechanisms*

According to current NCCLS guidelines, isolates of *S. pneumoniae* are considered intermediately resistant to erythromycin and clarithromycin at an MIC of 0.5 μg/mL,

Table 4
Time Above MIC for Parenteral and Oral β-Lactam Antibiotics Against *S. pneumoniae* With Differing Susceptibility to Penicillin

		Penicillin susceptible		Penicillin intermediate		Penicillin resistant	
Drug	Regimen	MIC	Time > MIC (%)	MIC	Time > MIC (%)	MIC	Time > MIC (%)
Parenteral							
Penicillin G	2 MU q6h	< 0.1	100	0.5–1	58–66	2–4	41–50
Penicillin G	5 MU q6h	< 0.1	100	0.5–1	85–100	2–4	55–75
Ampicillin	1 g q6h	< 0.1	100	0.5–2	71–100	2–4	54–71
Cefuroxime	750 mg q8h	0.12	100	0.5–2	58–88	4–8	28–42
Cefotaxime	1 g q8h	< 0.1	100	0.25–1	63–87	1–2	52–63
Ceftriaxone	1 g q24	< 0.1	100	0.25–1	76–100	1–2	48–76
Oral							
Amoxicillin	500 mg tid	< 0.1	100	0.25–1	55–80	1–2	43–55
Amoxicillin	1 g tid	< 0.1	100	0.25–1	100	1–2	88–100
Ceftibuten	400 mg qd	4	29	8–64	0–17	64+	0
Cefixime	400 mg qd	0.5	59	4–16	0	32–64	0
Cefaclor	500 mg tid	0.5	60	8–16	0–20	32–64	0
Loracarbef	400 mg bid	0.5	50	2–16	0–33	16+	0
Cefprozil	500 mg bid	0.25	75	0.5–4	32–64	4–16	0–32
Cefpodoxime	200 mg bid	0.25	83	0.25–2	21–83	2–4	0–21
Cefdinir	300 mg bid	0.12	77	0.5–4	0–43	4–16	0
Cefuroxime	500 mg bid	0.12	75	0.5–2	35–55	4–8	0–25
Cefditoren	400 mg bid	< 0.1	85	0.12–0.5	33–54	0.5–2	11–33

Source: Data are from refs. *41* and *45*, except for data pertaining to parenteral cefuroxime, penicillin 5 MU, amoxicillin 1 g tid, ceftibutin, cefdinir, and cefditoren. These data were adapted from refs. *13*, *48*, and *136–141*.

and resistant at MICs above this value. The breakpoint for azithromycin is one dilution higher at 1 μg/mL *(34)*.

Macrolides exert their activity by binding to specific domains in the ribosomal RNA (rRNA) of the 50S ribosomal subunit and blocking the extension of the nascent polypeptide chain through the exit tunnel in the ribosome. Resistance to macrolides occurs by one of two mechanisms in over 97% of resistant isolates (Table 6). The first mechanism elucidated was modification of the ribosomal target site. This mode of resistance is conferred by the *erm*B gene, which may be constitutively or inducibly expressed in *S. pneumoniae*. The *erm*B gene codes for a ribosomal methylase that methylates a single adenine residue in the 23S rRNA, markedly reducing the affinity of macrolides for the target site. This mechanism results in high-level macrolide resistance (i.e., erythromycin MICs ≥ 64 μg/mL) and cross-resistance with lincosamides such as clindamycin and streptogramins (so-called MLS resistance) because of overlapping binding sites. Rarely, mutations in the 23S rRNA or the ribosomal proteins L4 or L22 may also alter the target site and result in MLS resistance.

The second common mechanism of macrolide resistance in pneumococci is active drug efflux, mediated by an efflux pump encoded by the *mef*A gene. This pump confers

Table 5
Recent Changes on Susceptibility Breakpoints for Selected β-Lactams Against Nonmeningeal Infections Caused by *S. pneumoniae*

	Old breakpoints (μg/mL)			New breakpoints (μg/mL)		
	S	I	R	S	I	R
Amoxicillin ± clavulanate	< 1	1	> 1	< 4	4	> 4
Cefuroxime	< 1	1	> 1	< 2	2	> 2
Cefotaxime, ceftriaxone	< 1	1	> 1	< 2	2	> 2

Source: Breakpoints established by the National Committee for Clinical Laboratory Standards, refs. *34* and *47*.

Abbr: S, susceptible; I, intermediate; R, resistant.

resistance to 14- and 15-member macrolides, but not to 16-member macrolides (e.g., spiramycin and josamycin), clindamycin, or streptogramins. This mechanism results in low- to midlevel resistance, with MICs for erythromycin between 1 and 32 μg/mL, although the MICs of efflux strains appear to be increasing over time *(56)*.

Interestingly, the prevalence of the respective macrolide resistance mechanisms varies by geography. The efflux mechanism accounts for more than two-thirds of resistant isolates in North America. In Europe and South Africa, however, ribosomal methylation appears to be the predominant form of macrolide resistance *(49)*. Most of the dramatic rise in macrolide resistance in the United States during the last decade is attributable to the efflux mechanism *(52,56)*.

The new ketolide telithromycin is a derivative of clarithromycin. Ketolides are generally active against pneumococci expressing *erm*B because of greater affinity for the ribosomal binding site and weaker induction of inducible *erm*B expression. Ketolide activity is compromised, however, when *erm*B expression is constitutive. Telithromycin is also a weak inducer and poor substrate for the *mef*A efflux pump *(57)*. A recent report described an isolate with only moderate resistance to macrolides but high-grade resistance to telithromycin because of a mutation in the ribosomal protein L4 *(58)*.

3.4. Pharmacodynamic Approach to Macrolide Use

The most important pharmacodynamic parameters for macrolide activity are not conclusively established. As with β-lactams, the time above MIC correlates best with efficacy for erythromycin and clarithromycin, and optimal efficacy is obtained when the time above MIC is more than 40% of the dosing interval *(41)*. For azithromycin, however, AUC/MIC appears to be the most important parameter, and the ratio should exceed 25 for optimal efficacy *(59)*.

Clarithromycin and azithromycin differ substantially in their pharmacokinetic profiles. For clarithromycin, a 500-mg oral dose produces a C_{max} of about 2.5 μg/mL, with a half-life of 6 h *(60)*. Therefore, serum levels would be expected to exceed 1 μg/mL (the NCCLS breakpoint for intermediate [I] to full [R] resistance) for more than 50% of the 12-h dosing interval. Azithromycin, on the other hand, achieves a C_{max} of only 0.4 μg/mL and an AUC of 4.5 μg-h/mL after a 500-mg dose *(60)*. Therefore, the target

Table 6
Macrolide Resistance Genes in *S. pneumoniae*

	*erm*B	*mef*A
Mechanism	Methylation of 23S rRNA target site	Efflux pump
Macrolide MICs	≥ 64 μg/mL	1–32 μg/mL
Cross-resistance with clindamycin	Yes	No
Proportion of US resistant strains	Approximately one-third	Two-thirds

AUC/MIC ratio for optimal efficacy is obtainable in serum only if the MIC of the infecting isolate is less than 0.25 μg/mL, notably less than the current NCCLS I-to-R breakpoint.

Through exceptional tissue penetration and long tissue elimination half-lives, macrolides may achieve concentrations at the site of infection substantially greater than serum levels. In the case of pneumonia caused by extracellular pathogens such as *S. pneumoniae*, antimicrobial levels in the alveolar epithelial lining fluid (ELF) (and to a lesser extent, within leukocytes and alveolar macrophages) are thought to be more important in determining therapeutic efficacy than serum levels *(61–63)*. Steady-state concentrations of both clarithromycin and azithromycin in the ELF of normal volunteers are significantly higher than in serum *(64,65)*. After repeated doses, mean clarithromycin concentrations may exceed 32 μg/mL in the ELF and may be another 10-fold higher inside alveolar macrophages (AMs) 6 h postdose. At 24 h postdose, levels in ELF and AMs are approx 4.5 and 100 μg/mL, respectively. Azithromycin does not concentrate as well in the ELF, in which achievable levels are 1–2 μg/mL in normal volunteers, but it is heavily concentrated intracellularly *(64)*. A variety of studies suggests, however, that azithromycin concentrations are higher in the presence of inflammation, with the drug delivered to the site of infection by leukocytes *(66–68)*. Amsden and coworkers demonstrated azithromycin concentrations exceeding 10 μg/mL in peripheral blood neutrophils and monocytes during conventional dosing and prolonged elevation of tissue levels following even a single dose *(61)*, but the drug concentrations in contact with an extracellular pathogen such as *S. pneumoniae* remain uncertain.

3.5. Impact of Resistance

The preceding pharmacodynamic argument suggests that pneumonia caused by *S. pneumoniae* with lower levels of resistance (i.e., MICs < 32 μg/mL) may be treatable with clarithromycin and possibly azithromycin. Indeed, several authors have questioned whether an in vitro–in vivo paradox similar to that described for β-lactams exists for macrolides *(33,61,69)*. The existing clinical data are inadequate to determine whether in vitro macrolide resistance predicts adverse treatment outcomes. In the only prospective study in which outcomes for pneumococcal pneumonia were analyzed by macrolide susceptibility, Ewig et al. were unable to show increased mortality for macrolide-nonsusceptible versus susceptible infections and for discordant versus concordant therapy for these infections. In fact, mortality was higher for those with macrolide-susceptible infections, but the number of patients studied was small, and the differences were not statistically significant *(23)*.

It seems probable that the mechanism of macrolide resistance will determine the clinical impact. The MICs associated with *erm*B-mediated resistance are often 128 μg/mL or higher, far greater than the drug levels routinely achieved in serum or ELF. As a result, the resistance conferred by this mechanism would be expected to be clinically relevant. For a majority of isolates with *mef*A-mediated resistance, however, the MICs are within a range of drug concentrations achievable in the ELF by routine dosing of clarithromycin or possibly azithromycin. If true, the rates of clinically significant macrolide resistance in North America, where the efflux mechanism predominates, may well be less than 10% rather than 16–22% *(49)*.

3.6. Failures in Bacteremia

The preceding pharmacodynamic argument predicts that macrolides would have limited efficacy for bacteremic pneumonia caused by resistant *S. pneumoniae*, for which outcomes are more dependent on serum drug levels. Indeed, a multitude of case reports and small case series have described breakthrough bacteremia with resistant isolates during or immediately following macrolide therapy *(70–76)*. To date, these clinical failures have generally occurred in outpatients receiving oral macrolide therapy for infections caused by isolates with MICs of 8 μg/mL or higher, although failures of parenteral macrolide therapy have also recently been reported *(72,75,76)*; in two cases, the macrolide MICs were 4 μg/mL or less *(72,76)*.

Erythromycin, azithromycin, and clarithromycin have each been represented among the clinical failures. The most compelling cases for clinical failure as a result of macrolide resistance are those in which bacteremia persists after more than 48 h of macrolide therapy and for which therapeutic success follows a switch to another antimicrobial class. For example, Waterer et al. *(75)* reported a previously healthy 49-yr-old woman admitted with bilobar pneumonia but a low score on the Pneumonia Severity Index who developed septic shock after more than 72 h of intravenous azithromycin therapy and died with pneumococcal bacteremia. The bloodstream isolate had an MIC of 16 μg/mL.

Whether such cases reflect the tip of the iceberg *(77)* of the clinical impact of macrolide resistance is difficult to judge. For example, it has long been known that, in bacteremic pneumococcal pneumonia, about 12% of patients will fail antimicrobial therapy, independent of the in vitro susceptibility, because of intrinsic pathogenicity *(6)*. Given the large denominator of patients who develop pneumonia and receive treatment with macrolides, we are not witnessing wholesale clinical failures at the current levels of resistance. Clearly, more information is needed from clinical studies and pharmacodynamic models.

The treatment of uncomplicated pneumonia caused by isolates with MICs as high as 4 μg/mL or even 8–16 μg/mL may be possible because of the exceptional tissue penetration of the macrolides. Based on drug levels achievable in serum and the ELF of healthy volunteers and lower MICs among *S. pneumoniae*, clarithromycin appears to offer a pharmacodynamic advantage over azithromycin, although the delivery of the latter drug to the site of infection via leukocytes and release from intracellular compartments requires further study. For now, macrolide monotherapy remains a reasonable alternative for outpatients and the least severely affected inpatients without risk factors for drug resistance suggested by recent guidelines *(78)*. For bacteremic disease or more severe infections requiring hospitalization, however, caution is warranted when the MIC is above the currently accepted NCCLS breakpoints. Combination therapy with a β-lactam is recommended when macrolides are used in these scenarios. Continued monitoring of the clinical efficacy of the macrolides will be important particularly if the prevalence and the magnitude of macrolide resistance continue to increase.

4. RESISTANCE TO FLUOROQUINOLONES

The introduction of new fluoroquinolones with enhanced activity against *S. pneumoniae* (e.g., levofloxacin, gatifloxacin, moxifloxacin), coupled with rising rates of resistance to other antimicrobial classes, has led to a dramatic upsurge in the use of this class for RTIs. In an oft-repeated theme, resistance has followed heavy usage in some geographic areas and may soon compromise the use of these potent agents. Recognizing the potential for abuse of these potent, broad-spectrum agents and rapid emergence of resistance, a working group convened by the Centers for Disease Control and Prevention (CDC) recommended that fluoroquinolones be reserved for selected patients with CAP *(36)*. Patients for whom a fluoroquinolone may be appropriate include those who have failed another first-line agent, who are allergic to alternative agents, or who have a documented infection with a pneumococcus highly resistant to penicillin (i.e., MIC ≥ 4 μg/mL) *(36)*. The American Thoracic Society (ATS) and Canadian Infectious Diseases Society have been less stringent in their recommendations for fluoroquinolone use by restricting use in outpatients to high-risk patients with pre-existing chronic obstructive pulmonary disease (COPD), immunosuppression, recent hospitalization, nursing home residence, or recent antibiotic use *(78,79)*.

4.1. Epidemiology

The first alarm for rising fluoroquinolone resistance among pneumococci came from Canada, where the prevalence of resistant isolates (ciprofloxacin MIC ≥ 4 μg/mL) among adults increased from 0 to 2.9% between 1988 and 1998 *(80)*. This emergence of resistance was associated with a marked increase in the use of fluoroquinolones, mainly ciprofloxacin and ofloxacin, over the same period. Adults older than 65 yr received 18 prescriptions per 100 patient-years and had higher rates of resistance than did younger adults. Resistance rates were also highest in Ontario, the province with the highest per capita fluoroquinolone usage.

Published surveillance studies have not revealed such an alarming trend in U.S. isolates, most likely because of limited use of older, less-potent fluoroquinolones for RTIs *(81)*. Nevertheless, the number of fluoroquinolone prescriptions for RTIs has increased dramatically in the last 5 yr, and resistance rates are likely to rise in kind even for the more potent agents. The published data reflecting the 1999–2000 and the 2000–2001 respiratory seasons showed levofloxacin resistance rates of 0.7%, up from 0.2% in 1997–1998; rates of gatifloxacin and moxifloxacin resistance were 0.4 and 0.3%, respectively *(13)*.

Other countries have already experienced more dramatic increases in levofloxacin resistance *(82,83)*. For example, in Hong Kong, levofloxacin resistance has risen from less than 0.5% in 1995, to 5.5% in 1998, and to 13.3% in 2000. In 2000, the prevalence of levofloxacin resistance was 27.3% among isolates resistant to penicillin (up from 9.2% 2 yr prior) *(82,84)*. Remarkably, all levofloxacin-resistant isolates were also resistant to penicillin, cefotaxime, erythromycin, and trimethoprim–sulfamethoxazole. Molecular typing confirmed that this dramatic rise in resistance was because of a fluoroquinolone-resistant variant of the global Spain^{23F}-1 clone.

Authors in the United States have confirmed the appearance of fluoroquinolone resistance in isolates that are genetically indistinguishable from two highly prevalent multidrug-resistant clones *(85)*. If these clones were to become established in the community, selection by a number of unrelated antibiotics could fuel a dramatic rise in fluoroquinolone resistance similar to that seen for macrolides and β-lactams. The appearance of fluoroquinolone resistance in MDRSP is particularly worrisome because the fluoroquinolones are currently the most active agents against MDRSP among first-line therapies recommended for CAP.

4.2. Risk Factors

Because fluoroquinolones are not commonly used for pediatric infections, the vast majority of resistant isolates come from adults. Risk factors for resistance in pneumococci include old age, prior fluoroquinolone exposure, COPD, nursing home residence, and nosocomial infection *(80,86,87)*. Ironically, many of these risk factors are also risk factors for RTI caused by Gram-negative rods and are frequently cited as indications for empiric fluoroquinolone therapy *(78)*.

4.3. Mechanisms

According to current NCCLS guidelines, the susceptibility breakpoints (for susceptible, intermediate, and resistant isolates of *S. pneumoniae*) are, respectively, ≤ 2, 4, and ≥ 8 μg/mL for levofloxacin and ≤ 1, 2, and ≥ 4 μg/mL for moxifloxacin and gatifloxacin *(34)*.

Fluoroquinolones exert their activity through the inhibition of two enzymes necessary for the replication of bacterial DNA, DNA gyrase (encoded by *gyr*A and *gyr*B) and topoisomerase IV (encoded by *par*C and *par*E). All fluoroquinolones inhibit both enzymes to some degree, but the majority target one preferentially. Ciprofloxacin and levofloxacin preferentially target topoisomerase IV; moxifloxacin and gatifloxacin preferentially target DNA gyrase *(88)*.

The development of resistance to fluoroquinolones arises chiefly by one of two mechanisms: (1) stepwise accumulation of chromosomal mutations in the quinolone-resistance-determining regions (QRDRs) of *gyr*A or *par*C or (2) active drug efflux mediated by the multidrug transporter PmrA.

Spontaneous mutations that confer resistance occur in the QRDRs of *gyr*A and *par*C of *S. pneumoniae* with frequencies varying from 1 in 10^6 to 1 in 10^9 organisms *(89)*. The first mutation to confer a survival advantage over the wild type during fluoroquinolone exposure occurs predictably in the preferred enzymatic target (i.e., *gyr*A or *par*C) for the particular fluoroquinolone providing the selection pressure. These first-step mutations are generally associated with a four- to eightfold elevation in the MIC for all fluoroquinolones that preferentially target the mutated enzyme, but have little impact on the activity of fluoroquinolones that prefer the other enzyme as a target.

When a population of such first-step mutants again reaches a density of 10^6–10^9 organisms, it becomes probable that a second mutation in the other enzyme will occur. The double mutant will now display more complete resistance to any fluoroquinolone and cross-resistance to all fluoroquinolones. If, as suggested by some investigators, more than 10^9 organisms may be present in the lungs of patients with acute exacerbations of chronic bronchitis (AECB) or pneumonia, then there is ample opportunity to select for mutants that occur with a frequency of 1 in 10^6 to 10^9 *(90)*. Continued or repetitive fluoroquinolone exposure may then select increasingly resistant isolates. A fluoroquinolone with comparable potency for both enzymes should be less likely to select drug-resistant mutants because spontaneous mutations in both enzymes are necessary to become resistant, an event that occurs with a frequency less than 1 in 10^{12}. However, no clinically available agent has been clearly demonstrated to have such dual activity *(88)*.

Alternatively, a fluoroquinolone that is able to achieve concentrations at the site of infection sufficient to inhibit the growth of all first-step mutants should severely restrict the stepwise selection of double mutants. Assuming that first-step mutants are usually four to eight times less susceptible than wild-type cells, the fluoroquinolone of choice should achieve a concentration at the site of infection that is at least eightfold higher than the wild-type MIC to restrict mutant selection *(91)*. On the other hand, overreliance on less-potent fluoroquinolones may well facilitate the stepwise selection of fluoroquinolone-resistant pneumococci.

Active efflux of hydrophilic quinolones such as norfloxacin and ciprofloxacin is mediated by the membrane-associated protein PmrA (pneumococcal multidrug resistance), which may be expressed by up to half of norfloxacin-resistant isolates *(92)*. Other efflux mechanisms are evident, but have yet to be characterized *(93)*. Efflux mechanisms alone appear to contribute to low-level ciprofloxacin resistance (MIC 4–8 μg/mL), but may confer additive resistance when combined with mutations in *par*C *(94)*. Further study is necessary to define better the role of efflux mechanisms in resistance to levofloxacin, gatifloxacin, and moxifloxacin.

4.4. Pharmacodynamic Approach to Fluoroquinolone Use

Fluoroquinolones have concentration-dependent bactericidal activity against *S. pneumoniae*. In vitro and in vivo models show that AUC/MIC and, to a lesser extent, C_{max}/MIC correlate best with antimicrobial activity and treatment efficacy *(41)*. Although the magnitude of each parameter that correlates with optimal activity against *S. pneumoniae* is still a matter of some debate, the preponderance of data from experimental models suggests that AUC/MIC ratios of more than 25 to 40 predict bactericidal activity and treatment efficacy *(95–99)*. Data from experimental models are supported by a clinical study that found AUC/MIC ratios above 33.7 were associated with a positive microbiological response in patients with community-acquired RTIs *(100)*.

In the only prospective human study to examine the issue, Preston et al. *(101)* found that a C_{max}/MIC ratio of 12.2 for levofloxacin correlated with successful clinical and microbiological outcomes for a variety of infections. However, because there were few failures in patients with CAP and the outcomes were not broken down by etiology (*S. pneumoniae* was only 16% of all isolates), it is not clear whether this threshold applies directly to pneumococcal pneumonia. AUC/MIC was also significantly correlated with outcomes in this study.

As seen in Table 7, moxifloxacin and gatifloxacin have better pharmacodynamic profiles than levofloxacin and therefore should more reliably achieve important pharmacodynamic targets with standard dosing. Nicolau and Ambrose *(102)* estimated the

Table 7
Pharmacokinetic and Pharmacodynamic Parameters for Fluoroquinolones Against *S. pneumoniae*

Drug	Dose (mg)	$T_{1/2}$ (h)	MIC_{90} (μg/mL)	C_{max} (μg/mL)	C_{max}/MIC	AUC_{24} (μg-h/mL)	AUC/MIC
Ciprofloxacin	500	5.4	1	3.0	3	11.5	11.5
Levofloxacin	500	7.0	1	6.2	6.2	44.8	44.8
Gatifloxacin	400	6.5	0.25	3.4	13.6	30.0	120
Moxifloxacin	400	9.2	0.12	4.3	34.4	39.3	314.4

Source: Adapted from ref. *142*.

probability of achieving various target AUC/MIC ratios using gatifloxacin and levofloxacin in a simulated population of 5000 patients infected with 881 clinical isolates of *S. pneumoniae*. The probabilities of achieving an AUC/MIC ratio of 35 were 97 and 72% for gatifloxacin and levofloxacin, respectively. It is evident, therefore, that levofloxacin may not enjoy the same margin of efficacy as gatifloxacin as MICs rise.

A 750-mg formulation of levofloxacin is now approved for complicated skin and soft tissue structure infections and is under investigation for nosocomial pneumonia. It appears to be well tolerated and gives significantly higher serum levels (C_{max} = 7–9 μg/mL and AUC = 61–82 mg-h/L) *(103–105)* than does the 500-mg dose (C_{max} = 5–6 μg/mL and AUC = 48–58 mg-h/L) *(106,107)*. This dosing regimen would more closely approximate the pharmacodynamic profiles of moxifloxacin and gatifloxacin and increase the probability that important pharmacodynamic targets are met when using levofloxacin.

With fewer genetic barriers to the development of resistance, occurrence of fluoroquinolone resistance in *S. pneumoniae* is likely to occur more rapidly under conditions of expanded use than the occurrence witnessed with β-lactams. The evolution of clinically relevant resistance to a fluoroquinolone is determined by the drug's intrinsic potency, the additive effects of resistance mechanisms on its antimicrobial activity, and the concentrations of drug achievable at the site of infection. The greater the intrinsic potency and the higher the achievable levels, the greater the number of mutations required for clinically significant resistance.

The newer fluoroquinolones moxifloxacin and gatifloxacin combine the highest in vitro potency and the best pharmacokinetic profiles. These drugs require two spontaneous mutations (typically, one in *gyr*A, one in *par*C) before a wild-type pneumococcus develops clinically significant resistance. Thus, these agents should not only be more effective, but should also be less likely to select for resistance. Peak levels for these drugs in serum exceed the MIC for first-step *gyr*A mutants *(108)*. This rationale for preferential use of moxifloxacin and gatifloxacin is undermined if the infecting isolate already harbors a mutation in *par*C, as might occur after ciprofloxacin exposure. Such an isolate, although still susceptible to gatifloxacin and moxifloxacin, then requires only a single mutation in *gyr* to acquire resistance to these agents, an event that occurs at a frequency of 1 in 10^6 to10^9 *(89)*. For reasons already discussed, such an event is probable during the treatment of CAP and may set the stage for selective amplification of the double mutant under continued fluoroquinolone pressure.

4.5. Impact of Resistance

Microbiological failures and the selection of resistant organisms during therapy for CAP and AECB with ciprofloxacin and ofloxacin have been well described *(109)*. More recently, clinical failures have been reported for patients receiving levofloxacin for AECB or pneumonia in the setting of fluoroquinolone resistance *(110–113)*. Most failures have occurred in older adults with underlying lung disease and recent exposure to fluoroquinolones. Failure has occurred despite intravenous administration, and most patients responded to agents of another antibiotic class, suggesting that failure was related to fluoroquinolone resistance.

Two illustrative reports came from Canada. Davidson et al. reported four clinical failures with levofloxacin *(90)*. Two patients had no prior history of fluoroquinolone usage, although use of other antibiotics was not reported. One patient presented with pneumonia and a susceptible isolate from sputum before a double mutant (*gyr*A + *par*C) emerged during levofloxacin therapy. The second patient's initial isolate from sputum had a *par*C mutation (MIC = 4 μg/mL; intermediately susceptible to levofloxacin) before a double mutant was selected during therapy. The two other patients in the report may have been infected primarily with a highly resistant double mutant before failing therapy. These two patients had recently been treated with ciprofloxacin for exacerbations of chronic bronchitis, and at least one had a history of heavy fluoroquinolone usage.

Weiss et al. reported a nosocomial outbreak of pneumococcal RTIs in 16 patients on a respiratory ward in which ciprofloxacin was heavily used *(110)*. Initially, the infecting strain harbored a *par*C mutation and had a ciprofloxacin MIC of 4 μg/mL. Over the course of the outbreak, under heavy ciprofloxacin pressure, the strain acquired a second mutation in *gyr*A, raising the ciprofloxacin MIC to 16 μg/mL. Overall, 10 of 10 patients with AECB treated with ceftriaxone or erythromycin were cured, whereas all 5 patients (4 with AECB, 1 with pneumonia) treated with ciprofloxacin failed therapy. The patient with pneumonia was infected with the double mutant, failed a 14-d course of ciprofloxacin, and died while receiving cefuroxime.

These two reports suggest thinking twice when choosing a fluoroquinolone for empiric treatment of CAP for patients with a history of recent or prior heavy use of less-potent fluoroquinolones for RTI. Although treatment failures have not been described for gatifloxacin or moxifloxacin, prior selection of resistant double mutants with less-potent fluoroquinolones may compromise the activity of these newer, more potent agents. Even prior selection of an isolated *par*C mutation increases the probability of selecting a double mutant with high-level resistance during treatment with gatifloxacin or moxifloxacin. Unfortunately, current methods for susceptibility testing are not sufficiently sensitive to detect such isolates harboring *par*C mutations *(114)*. Consideration should be given to revising current treatment guidelines for CAP to recommend avoiding empiric fluoroquinolone use in patients with a recent history of fluoroquinolone exposure.

The same logic may be used to argue that the most potent agents should not be saved under the premise that patients who fail a less-potent fluoroquinolone should still respond to moxifloxacin or gatifloxacin. It will be difficult to preserve the efficacy of the last agents if resistant mutations enriched by less-potent fluoroquinolones continue to increase in prevalence.

The clinical impact of efflux-mediated resistance remains unclear, particularly for moxifloxacin and gatifloxacin. This mechanism appears to contribute to low-level ciprofloxacin and levofloxacin resistance (i.e., MIC ≤ 4 μg/mL) and may complement mutations in *par*C, raising the MICs further *(94)*.

5. ANTIBIOTIC THERAPY OF CAP IN THE ERA OF DRSP

5.1. Recommendations for Therapy

Currently, three sets of practice guidelines exist in the United States for the management of CAP. Although generally unified in recommendations for antibiotic therapy, the guidelines differ on the role of fluoroquinolones in the treatment of outpatients and less severely ill inpatients with CAP. Guidelines from the ATS and, particularly, from the CDC have attempted to restrict the usage of these important drugs when the likelihood of DRSP or clinical failure is low. Guidelines from the Infectious Diseases Society of America (IDSA) are less restrictive.

Table 8 presents a summary of the recommendations for empiric antibiotic therapy in these three sets of guidelines. One caveat we add is to recommend caution when considering fluoroquinolones for patients with recent or repeated exposure to fluoroquinolones, particularly the less-potent agents. This recommendation is made based on emerging evidence that prior treatment is a risk factor for fluoroquinolone resistance and may result in treatment failure *(80,86)*.

When DRSP is isolated from a patient with CAP, antibiotic choices should be made based on susceptibility testing. Table 8 also provides our recommendations for pathogen-directed therapy.

5.2. Prevention of Resistance

The clinical impact of antimicrobial resistance is already evident in pneumococcal meningitis and otitis media, for which restricted drug penetration to the site of infection has resulted in failures because of β-lactam and macrolide resistance. The widespread emergence of DRSP now threatens the traditional therapy of pneumococcal pneumonia. Some experts believe the state of drug resistance in *S. pneumoniae* is approaching a point of no return *(115,116)*. Others have presaged a "postantimicrobial era" *(117)*. Although the results of clinical trials have yet to demonstrate convincingly an association between resistance and treatment failure in pneumonia, there is growing concern over the rising pneumococcal MICs for the current antibiotic arsenal and an expanding literature documenting anecdotal reports of poor outcomes in the setting of resistance. If resistance levels to each of the major classes of antimicrobials continue to increase, it is possible that the clinical impact of resistance will become more evident. Active measures must be taken now to reduce the factors leading to the emergence and spread of DRSP. These measures should focus chiefly on reducing antibiotic selective pressure and preventing DRSP transmission.

The chief factor contributing to the spread of DRSP is the selective pressure of oral antibiotics prescribed for outpatient RTIs. It is clear that the antibiotic arsenal is widely abused for upper respiratory tract infections for which no indication for antibiotics exists *(118–122)*. A "trickle-down effect" *(123)*, in which the most potent agents rec-

Table 8
American Guideline Treatment Recommendations for Community-Acquired Pneumonia

	Preferred agents	Alternative agents
Empiric therapy		
Outpatients		
Without modifying factors[a]	Macrolide[b,c,d] Doxycycline[b,c,d]	Fluoroquinolone[b,e] β-lactam[d]
With modifying factors[a]	Fluoroquinolone[b,c,e,f] β-lactam + (macrolide or doxycycline)[c]	
Inpatients, non-ICU setting		
Without modifying factors[a]	β-lactam + (macrolide[b,d] or doxycycline[c]) Fluoroquinolone[b,c,e]	Azithromycin[c,g]
With modifying factors[a]	β-lactam + (macrolide or doxycycline)[c] Fluoroquinolone[c,e,f]	
Inpatients, ICU setting		
All patients	β-lactam + (macrolide or fluoroquinolone)[b,c,d]	
Pathogen-directed therapy		
Penicillin MIC < 2 μg/mL	Penicillin G or amoxicillin/ampicillin	Cephalosporin, macrolide, doxycycline, fluoroquinolone, clindamycin
Penicillin MIC ≥ 2 μg/mL	Cefotaxime or ceftriaxone[h] Fluoroquinolone	Clindamycin, vancomycin[i]

Note: Macrolides include azithromycin, clarithromycin, and erythromycin. Fluoroquinolones include gatifloxacin, levofloxacin, and moxifloxacin. Parenteral β-lactams include cefotaxime, ceftriaxone, ampicillin ± sulbactam. Oral β-lactams include amoxicillin (≥ 3 g/d if concern for DRSP) ± clavulanate, cefpodoxime, cefprozil, cefuroxime.

[a]Modifying factors defined by ATS include risk factors for DRSP: age older than 65 yr, β-lactam therapy within 3 mo, alcoholism, immunosuppression, multiple medical comorbidities, exposure to a child in day care *(78)*.

[b]Recommended as preferred agent by IDSA *(124)*.

[c]Recommended as preferred agent by ATS *(78)*.

[d]Recommended as preferred agent by CDC *(36)*.

[e]Fluoroquinolone recommended by CDC for failure of another first-line regimen, allergy to first-line agents *(36)*.

[f]Use caution if patient has received a fluoroquinolone recently or repeatedly.

[g]Intravenous azithromycin recommended by ATS for patients without concomitant cardiopulmonary disease or risk factors for DRSP, enteric Gram-negative rods *(78)*.

[h]Cefotaxime or ceftriaxone alone recommended only if MIC for either drug is less than 2 μg/mL.

[i]Vancomycin use is discouraged unless it is for an ICU patient with β-lactam allergy, suspected meningitis, or failure of other agents.

ommended for treatment of CAP are also assumed to be the optimal choices for all RTIs, creates needless selective pressure and carries great risk for the development of resistance to the most vital agents. Acquisition of fluoroquinolone resistance by a dominant circulating MDRSP clone or clones could result in rapid dissemination and have drastic consequences for the management of patients with CAP and AECB. Guidelines for the clinical evaluation of RTIs and the decision to use antimicrobials have been published *(121)*.

Proper diagnosis of bacterial infection, isolation of the causative agent, and antimicrobial susceptibility testing will help limit excessive antibiotic use, although it must do so without increasing costs excessively. Knowing the susceptibility profile of infecting organisms allows for use of agents with a narrower spectrum, such as amoxicillin, and avoidance of antimicrobials to which the organism is already nonsusceptible. These measures may simultaneously improve outcomes and prevent further resistance. For this reason, sputum culture is recommended for all patients with CAP *(124)* or for those with risk factors for resistant organisms *(78)*.

It is also important for providers to be familiar with local resistance profiles to reduce the potential for clinical failures and continued selection pressure from certain antimicrobial classes. Studies from Finland and Iceland have demonstrated reversion of resistance to specific classes of antimicrobials after reductions in use *(125,126)*.

Optimal use of antimicrobials begins by selecting the most potent agents as the first choices for therapy. Pharmacodynamic data from experimental models and clinical studies allow comparisons among members of each antibiotic class to predict the agents that are most likely to effect the greatest bacterial eradication and result in the least selection of resistant mutants *(41,127)*. Suboptimal exposure to any antimicrobial may occur through inadequate dosing, duration of administration, failure to consider the antimicrobial concentrations at the site of infection, and patient nonadherence. Inadequate antibiotic therapy contributes to carriage of DRSP, which in turn promotes spread of resistant clones *(128–130)*.

Avoidance of potent new antimicrobials based on their expense may not make for cost-effective practice. In CAP, the attendant costs of treatment failure, especially hospitalization costs, far exceed drug acquisition costs *(131)*.

Last, appropriate immunization against pneumococcal pneumonia and influenza should reduce the need for antimicrobials to treat these RTIs. Immunization against *S. pneumoniae*, with Pneumovax® for adults or Prevnar® for children, can reduce the incidence of invasive infections as well as reduce nasopharyngeal carriage *(132–134)*. Because more than 80% of resistant pneumococci and all six of the predominant MDRSP clones in the United States are covered by the vaccines *(135)*, more appropriate use of both vaccines could play a very valuable role in reducing the spread of DRSP.

REFERENCES

1. Marston BJ, Plouffe JF, File TM Jr, et al. Incidence of community-acquired pneumonia requiring hospitalization. Results of a population-based active surveillance study in Ohio. The Community-Based Pneumonia Incidence Study Group. Arch Intern Med 1997; 157:1709–1718.
2. Premature deaths, monthly mortality and monthly physician contacts—United States. Centers for Disease Control and Prevention. MMWR Morb Mortal Wkly Rep 1997; 46: 556–561.

3. Fine MJ, Smith MA, Carson CA, et al. Prognosis and outcomes of patients with community-acquired pneumonia: a meta-analysis. JAMA 1996; 275:134–141.
4. Ruiz-Gonzalez A, Falguera M, Nogues A, Rubio-Caballero M. Is *Streptococcus pneumoniae* the leading cause of pneumonia of unknown etiology? A microbiologic study of lung aspirates in consecutive patients with community-acquired pneumonia. Am J Med 1999; 106:385–390.
5. Osler W. The Principles and Practice of Medicine. 4th ed. New York: Appleton, 1901.
6. Austrian R, Gold J. Pneumococcal bacteremia with especial reference to bacteremic pneumococcal pneumonia. Ann Intern Med 1964;60:759–776.
7. Evans G, Gainsford W. Treatment of pneumonia with 2-(*p*-aminobenzenesulfonamido)pyridine. Lancet 1938; 2:14–19.
8. Austrian R. Confronting drug-resistant pneumococci. Ann Intern Med 1994; 121:807–808.
9. Feikin DR, Schuchat A, Kolczak M, et al. Mortality from invasive pneumococcal pneumonia in the era of antibiotic resistance, 1995–1997. Am J Public Health 2000; 90:223–229.
10. Plouffe JF, Breiman RF, Facklam RR. Bacteremia with *Streptococcus pneumoniae*. Implications for therapy and prevention. Franklin County Pneumonia Study Group. JAMA 1996; 275:194–198.
11. Schmidt LH, Sesler CL. Development of resistance to penicillin by pneumococci. Proc Soc Exp Biol Med 1943; 52:353–357.
12. Hansman D, Bullen M. A resistant pneumococcus. Lancet 1967; 2:264–265.
13. Doern GV, Heilmann KP, Huynh HK, Rhomberg PR, Coffman SL, Brueggemann AB. Antimicrobial resistance among clinical isolates of *Streptococcus pneumoniae* in the United States during 1999–2000, including a comparison of resistance rates since 1994–1995. Antimicrob Agents Chemother 2001; 45:1721–1729.
14. Thornsberry C, Sahm DF, Kelly LJ, et al. Regional trends in antimicrobial resistance among clinical isolates of *Streptococcus pneumoniae*, *Haemophilus influenzae*, and *Moraxella catarrhalis* in the United States: results from the TRUST Surveillance Program, 1999–2000. Clin Infect Dis 2002; 34(suppl. 1):S4–S16.
15. Jacobs MR, Koornhof HJ, Robins-Browne RM, et al. Emergence of multiply resistant pneumococci. N Engl J Med 1978; 299:735–740.
16. Munoz R, Coffey TJ, Daniels M, et al. Intercontinental spread of a multiresistant clone of serotype 23F *Streptococcus pneumoniae*. J Infect Dis 1991; 164:302–306.
17. Doern GV, Brueggemann AB, Blocker M, et al. Clonal relationships among high-level penicillin-resistant *Streptococcus pneumoniae* in the United States. Clin Infect Dis 1998; 27:757–761.
18. Lyon DJ, Scheel O, Fung KS, Cheng AF, Henrichsen J. Rapid emergence of penicillin-resistant pneumococci in Hong Kong. Scand J Infect Dis 1996; 28:375–376.
19. Fenoll A, Martin BC, Munoz R, Vicioso D, Casal J. Serotype distribution and antimicrobial resistance of *Streptococcus pneumoniae* isolates causing systemic infections in Spain, 1979–1989. Rev Infect Dis 1991; 13:56–60.
20. Marton A, Gulyas M, Munoz R, Tomasz A. Extremely high incidence of antibiotic resistance in clinical isolates of *Streptococcus pneumoniae* in Hungary. J Infect Dis 1991; 163:542–548.
21. Friedland IR, Klugman KP. Antibiotic-resistant pneumococcal disease in South African children. Am J Dis Child 1992; 146:920–923.
22. Dowell SF, Schwartz B. Resistant pneumococci: protecting patients through judicious use of antibiotics. Am Fam Physician 1997; 55:1647–1648.
23. Ewig S, Ruiz M, Torres A, et al. Pneumonia acquired in the community through drug-resistant *Streptococcus pneumoniae*. Am J Respir Crit Care Med 1999; 159:1835–1842.
24. Clavo-Sanchez AJ, Giron-Gonzalez JA, Lopez-Prieto D, et al. Multivariate analysis of risk factors for infection due to penicillin-resistant and multidrug-resistant *Streptococcus pneumoniae*: a multicenter study. Clin Infect Dis 1997; 24:1052–1059.

25. Nava JM, Bella F, Garau J, et al. Predictive factors for invasive disease due to penicillin-resistant *Streptococcus pneumoniae*: a population-based study. Clin Infect Dis 1994; 19:884–890.
26. Campbell GD, Silberman R. Drug-resistant *Streptococcus pneumoniae*. Clin Infect Dis 1998; 26:1188–1195.
27. Chambers HF. Penicillin-binding protein-mediated resistance in pneumococci and staphylococci. J Infect Dis 1999; 179(suppl. 2):S353–S359.
28. Meehan TP, Fine MJ, Krumholz HM, et al. Quality of care, process, and outcomes in elderly patients with pneumonia. JAMA 1997; 278:2080–2084.
29. John CC. Treatment failure with use of a third-generation cephalosporin for penicillin-resistant pneumococcal meningitis: case report and review. Clin Infect Dis 1994; 18: 188–193.
30. Dagan R, Abramson O, Leibovitz E, et al. Impaired bacteriologic response to oral cephalosporins in acute otitis media caused by pneumococci with intermediate resistance to penicillin. Pediatr Infect Dis J 1996; 15:980–985.
31. Dagan R, Abramson O, Leibovitz E, et al. Bacteriologic response to oral cephalosporins: are established susceptibility breakpoints appropriate in the case of acute otitis media? J Infect Dis 1997; 176:1253–1259.
32. Turett GS, Blum S, Fazal BA, Justman JE, Telzak EE. Penicillin resistance and other predictors of mortality in pneumococcal bacteremia in a population with high human immunodeficiency virus seroprevalence. Clin Infect Dis 1999; 29:321–327.
33. Bishai W. The in vivo–in vitro paradox in pneumococcal respiratory tract infections. J Antimicrob Chemother 2002; 49:433–436.
34. National Committee for Clinical Laboratory Standards. Performance Standards for Antimicrobial Susceptibility Testing. 11th Informational Supplement, M100-S13. Wayne, PA: National Committee for Clinical Laboratory Standards, 2001.
35. Musher DM, Bartlett JG, Doern GV. A fresh look at the definition of susceptibility of *Streptococcus pneumoniae* to β-lactam antibiotics. Arch Intern Med 2001; 161:2538–2544.
36. Heffelfinger JD, Dowell SF, Jorgensen JH, et al. Management of community acquired pneumonia in the era of pneumococcal resistance: a report from the Drug-Resistant *Streptococcus pneumoniae* Therapeutic Working Group. Arch Intern Med 2000; 160:1399–1408.
37. Metlay JP, Hofmann J, Cetron MS, et al. Impact of penicillin susceptibility on medical outcomes for adult patients with bacteremic pneumococcal pneumonia. Clin Infect Dis 2000; 30:520–528.
38. Rahav G, Toledano Y, Engelhard D, et al. Invasive pneumococcal infections. A comparison between adults and children. Medicine (Baltimore) 1997; 76:295–303.
39. Friedland IR. Comparison of the response to antimicrobial therapy of penicillin-resistant and penicillin-susceptible pneumococcal disease. Pediatr Infect Dis J 1995; 14:885–890.
40. Pallares R, Linares J, Vadillo M, et al. Resistance to penicillin and cephalosporin and mortality from severe pneumococcal pneumonia in Barcelona, Spain. N Engl J Med 1995; 333:474–480.
41. Craig WA. Pharmacokinetic/pharmacodynamic parameters: rationale for antibacterial dosing of mice and men. Clin Infect Dis 1998; 26:1–10.
42. Van Ogtrop ML, Andes D, Craig WA. In vivo antimicrobial activity of MK-0826, a new carbapenem, against various penicillin-resistant pneumococci. In: Program and Abstracts of the 38th Interscience Conference on Antimicrobial Agents and Chemotherapy, San Diego, CA; September 24–27, 1998. Abstract F-48.
43. Xuan D, Banevicius M, Capitano B, Kim MK, Nightingale C, Nicolau D. Pharmacodynamic assessment of ertapenem (MK-0826) against *Streptococcus pneumoniae* in a murine neutropenic thigh infection model. Antimicrob Agents Chemother 2002; 46:2990–2995.
44. Goldstein FW. Choice of an oral β-lactam antibiotic for infections due to penicillin-resistant *Streptococcus pneumoniae*. Scand J Infect Dis 1997; 29:255–257.

45. Craig WA, Andes D. Pharmacokinetics and pharmacodynamics of antibiotics in otitis media. Pediatr Infect Dis J 1996; 15:255–259.
46. Appelbaum PC. Microbiological and pharmacodynamic considerations in the treatment of infection due to antimicrobial-resistant *Streptococcus pneumoniae*. Clin Infect Dis 2000; 31(suppl. 2):S29–S34.
47. National Committee for Clinical Laboratory Standards. Performance Standards for Antimicrobial Susceptibility Testing. 10th Informational Supplement, M100-S11. Wayne, PA: National Committee for Clinical Laboratory Standards, 2001.
48. Bryan CS, Talwani R, Stinson MS. Penicillin dosing for pneumococcal pneumonia. Chest 1997; 112:1657–1664.
49. Lynch JP, Martinez FJ. Clinical relevance of macrolide-resistant *Streptococcus pneumoniae* for community-acquired pneumonia. Clin Infect Dis 2002; 34(suppl. 1):S27–S46.
50. Moreno S, Garcia-Leoni ME, Cercenado E, Diaz MD, Bernaldo de Quiros JC, Bouza E. Infections caused by erythromycin-resistant *Streptococcus pneumoniae*: incidence, risk factors, and response to therapy in a prospective study. Clin Infect Dis 1995; 20:1195–1200.
51. Baquero F. Evolving resistance patterns of *Streptococcus pneumoniae*: a link with long-acting macrolide consumption? J Chemother 1999; 11(suppl. 1):35–43.
52. Hyde TB, Gay K, Stephens DS, et al. Macrolide resistance among invasive *Streptococcus pneumoniae* isolates. JAMA 2001; 286:1857–1862.
53. Leach AJ, Shelby-James TM, Mayo M, et al. A prospective study of the impact of community-based azithromycin treatment of trachoma on carriage and resistance of *Streptococcus pneumoniae*. Clin Infect Dis 1997; 24:356–362.
54. Ghaffar F, Friedland IR, Katz K, et al. Increased carriage of resistant non-pneumococcal α-hemolytic streptococci after antibiotic therapy. J Pediatr 1999; 135:618–623.
55. Morita JY, Kahn E, Thompson T, et al. Impact of azithromycin on oropharyngeal carriage of group A streptococcus and nasopharyngeal carriage of macrolide-resistant *Streptococcus pneumoniae*. Pediatr Infect Dis J 2000; 19:41–46.
56. Gay K, Baughman W, Miller Y, et al. The emergence of *Streptococcus pneumoniae* resistant to macrolide antimicrobial agents: a 6-year population-based assessment. J Infect Dis 2000; 182:1417–1424.
57. Leclercq R, Courvalin P. Resistance to macrolides and related antibiotics in *Streptococcus pneumoniae*. Antimicrob Agents Chemother 2002; 46:2727–2734.
58. Tait-Kamradt A, Davies T, Appelbaum PC, et al. Two new mechanisms of macrolide resistance in clinical strains of *Streptococcus pneumoniae* from eastern Europe and North America. Antimicrob Agents Chemother 2000; 44:3395–3401.
59. Craig WA. The hidden impact of antibacterial resistance in respiratory tract infection. Re-evaluating current antibiotic therapy. Respir Med 2001; 95(suppl. A):S12–S19.
60. Carbon C. Pharmacodynamics of macrolides, azalides, and streptogramins: effect on extracellular pathogens. Clin Infect Dis 1998; 27:28–32.
61. Amsden GW. Pneumococcal macrolide resistance—myth or reality? J Antimicrob Chemother 1999; 44:1–6.
62. Baldwin DR, Honeybourne D, Wise R. Pulmonary disposition of antimicrobial agents: in vivo observations and clinical relevance. Antimicrob Agents Chemother 1992; 36:1176–1180.
63. Baldwin DR, Honeybourne D, Wise R. Pulmonary disposition of antimicrobial agents: methodological considerations. Antimicrob Agents Chemother 1992; 36:1171–1175.
64. Rodvold KA, Gotfried MH, Danziger LH, Servi RJ. Intrapulmonary steady-state concentrations of clarithromycin and azithromycin in healthy adult volunteers. Antimicrob Agents Chemother 1997; 41:1399–1402.
65. Patel KB, Xuan D, Tessier PR, Russomanno JH, Quintiliani R, Nightingale CH. Compari-

son of bronchopulmonary pharmacokinetics of clarithromycin and azithromycin. Antimicrob Agents Chemother 1996; 40:2375–2379.
66. Girard AE, Cimochowski CR, Faiella JA. Correlation of increased azithromycin concentrations with phagocyte infiltration into sites of localized infection. J Antimicrob Chemother 1996; 37(suppl. C):9–19.
67. Ballow CH, Amsden GW, Highet VS, Forrest A. Healthy volunteer pharmacokinetics of oral azithromycin in serum, urine, polymorphonuclear leukocytes and inflammatory versus non-inflammatory skin blisters. Clin Drug Invest 1998; 15:159–167.
68. Freeman CD, Nightingale CH, Nicolau DP, Belliveau PP, Banevicius MA, Quintiliani R. Intracellular and extracellular penetration of azithromycin into inflammatory and noninflammatory blister fluid. Antimicrob Agents Chemother 1994; 38:2449–2451.
69. Gotfried MH. Comparison of bacteriologic eradication of *Streptococcus pneumoniae* by clarithromycin and reports of increased antimicrobial resistance. Clin Ther 2000; 22:2–14.
70. Sanchez C, Armengol R, Lite J, Mir I, Garau J. Penicillin-resistant pneumococci and community-acquired pneumonia. Lancet 1992; 339:988.
71. Lonks JR, Medeiros AA. Emergence of erythromycin-resistant *Streptococcus pneumoniae.* Infect Med 1994; 11:415–424.
72. Lonks JR, Garau J, Gomez L, et al. Failure of macrolide antibiotic treatment in patients with bacteremia due to erythromycin-resistant *Streptococcus pneumoniae.* Clin Infect Dis 2002; 35:556–564.
73. Fogarty C, Goldschmidt R, Bush K. Bacteremic pneumonia due to multidrug-resistant pneumococci in three patients treated unsuccessfully with azithromycin and successfully with levofloxacin. Clin Infect Dis 2000; 31:613–615.
74. Kelley MA, Weber DJ, Gilligan P, Cohen MS. Breakthrough pneumococcal bacteremia in patients being treated with azithromycin and clarithromycin. Clin Infect Dis 2000; 31:1008–1011.
75. Waterer GW, Wunderink RG, Jones CB. Fatal pneumococcal pneumonia attributed to macrolide resistance and azithromycin monotherapy. Chest 2000; 118:1839–1840.
76. Musher DM, Dowell ME, Shortridge VD, et al. Emergence of macrolide resistance during treatment of pneumococcal pneumonia. N Engl J Med 2002; 346:630–631.
77. Garau J. The hidden impact of antibacterial resistance in respiratory tract infection. Clinical failures: the tip of the iceberg? Respir Med 2001; 95(suppl. A):S5–S11.
78. Niederman MS, Mandell LA, Anzueto A, et al. Guidelines for the management of adults with community-acquired pneumonia. Diagnosis, assessment of severity, antimicrobial therapy, and prevention. Am J Respir Crit Care Med 2001; 163:1730–1754.
79. Mandell LA, Marrie TJ, Grossman RF, Chow AW, Hyland RH. Canadian guidelines for the initial management of community-acquired pneumonia: an evidence-based update by the Canadian Infectious Diseases Society and the Canadian Thoracic Society. The Canadian Community-Acquired Pneumonia Working Group. Clin Infect Dis 2000; 31:383–421.
80. Chen DK, McGeer A, de Azavedo JC, Low DE. Decreased susceptibility of *Streptococcus pneumoniae* to fluoroquinolones in Canada. Canadian Bacterial Surveillance Network. N Engl J Med 1999; 341:233–239.
81. Brueggemann AB, Coffman SL, Rhomberg P, et al. Fluoroquinolone resistance in *Streptococcus pneumoniae* in the United States since 1994–1995. Antimicrob Agents Chemother 2002; 46:680–688.
82. Ho PL, Yung RW, Tsang DN, et al. Increasing resistance of *Streptococcus pneumoniae* to fluoroquinolones: results of a Hong Kong multicentre study in 2000. J Antimicrob Chemother 2001; 48:659–665.
83. Glatz K, Szabo D, Szabo G, Boriszova D, Rozgonyi F. Emergence of extremely high peni-

cillin and cefotaxime resistance and high-level levofloxacin resistance in clinical isolates of *Streptococcus pneumoniae* in Hungary. J Antimicrob Chemother 2001; 48:731–734.
84. Ho PL, Que TL, Tsang DN, Ng TK, Chow KH, Seto WH. Emergence of fluoroquinolone resistance among multiply resistant strains of *Streptococcus pneumoniae* in Hong Kong. Antimicrob Agents Chemother 1999; 43:1310–1313.
85. Doern GV. Antimicrobial use and the emergence of antimicrobial resistance with *Streptococcus pneumoniae* in the United States. Clin Infect Dis 2001; 33(suppl. 3):S187–S192.
86. Ho PL, Tse WS, Tsang KW, et al. Risk factors for acquisition of levofloxacin-resistant *Streptococcus pneumoniae*: a case-control study. Clin Infect Dis 2001; 32:701–707.
87. Linares J, de la Campa AG, Pallares R. Fluoroquinolone resistance in *Streptococcus pneumoniae*. N Engl J Med 1999; 341:1546–1548.
88. Smith HJ, Nichol KA, Hoban DJ, Zhanel GG. Dual activity of fluoroquinolones against *Streptococcus pneumoniae*: the facts behind the claims. J Antimicrob Chemother 2002; 49:893–895.
89. Fukuda H, Hiramatsu K. Primary targets of fluoroquinolones in *Streptococcus pneumoniae*. Antimicrob Agents Chemother 1999; 43:410–412.
90. Davidson R, Cavalcanti R, Brunton JL, et al. Resistance to levofloxacin and failure of treatment of pneumococcal pneumonia. N Engl J Med 2002; 346:747–750.
91. Sanders CC. Mechanisms responsible for cross-resistance and dichotomous resistance among the quinolones. Clin Infect Dis 2001; 32(suppl. 1):S1–S8.
92. Brenwald NP, Gill MJ, Wise R. Prevalence of a putative efflux mechanism among fluoroquinolone-resistant clinical isolates of *Streptococcus pneumoniae*. Antimicrob Agents Chemother 1998; 42:2032–2035.
93. Piddock LJ, Johnson MM, Simjee S, Pumbwe L. Expression of efflux pump gene *pmr*A in fluoroquinolone-resistant and -susceptible clinical isolates of *Streptococcus pneumoniae*. Antimicrob Agents Chemother 2002; 46:808–812.
94. Bast DJ, Low DE, Duncan CL, et al. Fluoroquinolone resistance in clinical isolates of *Streptococcus pneumoniae*: contributions of type II topoisomerase mutations and efflux to levels of resistance. Antimicrob Agents Chemother 2000; 44:3049–3054.
95. Lacy MK, Lu W, Xu X, et al. Pharmacodynamic comparisons of levofloxacin, ciprofloxacin, and ampicillin against *Streptococcus pneumoniae* in an in vitro model of infection. Antimicrob Agents Chemother 1999; 43:672–677.
96. Lister PD, Sanders CC. Pharmacodynamics of levofloxacin and ciprofloxacin against *Streptococcus pneumoniae*. J Antimicrob Chemother 1999; 43:79–86.
97. Zhanel GG, Roberts D, Waltky A, et al. Pharmacodynamic activity of fluoroquinolones against ciprofloxacin-resistant *Streptococcus pneumoniae*. J Antimicrob Chemother 2002; 49:807–812.
98. Mattoes HM, Banevicius M, Li D, et al. Pharmacodynamic assessment of gatifloxacin against *Streptococcus pneumoniae*. Antimicrob Agents Chemother 2001; 45:2092–2097.
99. Wright DH, Brown GH, Peterson ML, Rotschafer JC. Application of fluoroquinolone pharmacodynamics. J Antimicrob Chemother 2000; 46:669–683.
100. Ambrose PG, Grasela DM, Grasela TH, Passarell J, Mayer HB, Pierce PF. Pharmacodynamics of fluoroquinolones against *Streptococcus pneumoniae* in patients with community-acquired respiratory tract infections. Antimicrob Agents Chemother 2001; 45:2793–2797.
101. Preston SL, Drusano GL, Berman AL, et al. Pharmacodynamics of levofloxacin: a new paradigm for early clinical trials. JAMA 1998; 279:125–129.
102. Nicolau DP, Ambrose PG. Pharmacodynamic profiling of levofloxacin and gatifloxacin using Monte Carlo simulation for community-acquired isolates of *Streptococcus pneumoniae*. Am J Med 2001; 111(suppl. 9A):13S–18S.
103. Chien SC, Wong FA, Fowler CL, et al. Double-blind evaluation of the safety and phar-

macokinetics of multiple oral once-daily 750-milligram and 1-gram doses of levofloxacin in healthy volunteers. Antimicrob Agents Chemother 1998; 42:885–888.
104. Chow AT, Fowler C, Williams RR, Morgan N, Kaminski S, Natarajan J. Safety and pharmacokinetics of multiple 750-milligram doses of intravenous levofloxacin in healthy volunteers. Antimicrob Agents Chemother 2001; 45:2122–2125.
105. Piscitelli SC, Spooner K, Baird B, et al. Pharmacokinetics and safety of high-dose and extended-interval regimens of levofloxacin in human immunodeficiency virus-infected patients. Antimicrob Agents Chemother 1999; 43:2323–2327.
106. O'Donnell JA, Gelone SP. Fluoroquinolones. Infect Dis Clin North Am 2000; 14: 489–513.
107. Schentag JJ, Scully BE. Quinolones. In: Yu VL, Merigan TC, Barriere SL (eds.). Antimicrobial Therapy and Vaccines. Baltimore, MD: Williams and Wilkens, 1999, pp. 875–900.
108. Blondeau JM, Zhao X, Hansen G, Drlica K. Mutant prevention concentrations of fluoroquinolones for clinical isolates of *Streptococcus pneumoniae*. Antimicrob Agents Chemother 2001; 45:433–438.
109. Chodosh S, Schreurs A, Siami G, et al. Efficacy of oral ciprofloxacin versus clarithromycin for treatment of acute bacterial exacerbations of chronic bronchitis. The Bronchitis Study Group. Clin Infect Dis 1998; 27:730–738.
110. Weiss K, Restieri C, Gauthier R, et al. A nosocomial outbreak of fluoroquinolone-resistant *Streptococcus pneumoniae*. Clin Infect Dis 2001; 33:517–522.
111. Urban C, Rahman N, Zhao X, et al. Fluoroquinolone-resistant *Streptococcus pneumoniae* associated with levofloxacin therapy. J Infect Dis 2001; 184:794–798.
112. Fishman NO, Suh B, Weigel LM, et al. Three levofloxacin treatment failures of pneumococcal respiratory tract isolates. In: Program and Abstracts of the 39th Interscience Conference on Antimicrobial Agents and Chemotherapy, San Francisco, CA; September 26–29, 1999. Abstract C1-825.
113. Kuehnert MJ, Nolte FS, Perlino CA. Fluoroquinolone resistance in *Streptococcus pneumoniae*. Ann Intern Med 1999; 131:312–313.
114. Richardson DC, Bast D, McGeer A, Low DE. Evaluation of susceptibility testing to detect fluoroquinolone resistance mechanisms in *Streptococcus pneumoniae*. Antimicrob Agents Chemother 2001; 45:1911–1914.
115. Craig WA. Have we reached the point of no return? The hidden impact of antibacterial resistance in respiratory tract infection. Introduction. Respir Med 2001; 95(suppl. A):S2–S4.
116. Ball P, Baquero F, Cars O, File T, et al. Antibiotic therapy of community respiratory tract infections: strategies for optimal outcomes and minimized resistance emergence. J Antimicrob Chemother 2002; 49:31–40.
117. Cohen ML. Epidemiology of drug resistance: implications for a post-antimicrobial era. Science 1992; 257:1050–1055.
118. McCaig LF, Hughes JM. Trends in antimicrobial drug prescribing among office-based physicians in the United States. JAMA 1995; 273:214–219.
119. Metlay JP, Stafford RS, Singer DE. National trends in the use of antibiotics by primary care physicians for adult patients with cough. Arch Intern Med 1998; 158:1813–1818.
120. Nyquist AC, Gonzales R, Steiner JF, Sande MA. Antibiotic prescribing for children with colds, upper respiratory tract infections, and bronchitis. JAMA 1998; 279:875–877.
121. Gonzales R, Bartlett JG, Besser RE, et al. Principles of appropriate antibiotic use for treatment of acute respiratory tract infections in adults: background, specific aims, and methods. Ann Intern Med 2001; 134:479–486.
122. Gonzales R, Steiner JF, Sande MA. Antibiotic prescribing for adults with colds, upper respiratory tract infections, and bronchitis by ambulatory care physicians. JAMA 1997; 278:901–904.

123. Bishai W. Current issues on resistance, treatment guidelines, and the appropriate use of fluoroquinolones for respiratory tract infections. Clin Ther 2002; 24:838–850.
124. Bartlett JG, Dowell SF, Mandell LA, File TM Jr, Musher DM, Fine MJ. Practice guidelines for the management of community-acquired pneumonia in adults. Infectious Diseases Society of America. Clin Infect Dis 2000; 31:347–382.
125. Seppala H, Klaukka T, Vuopio-Varkila J, et al. The effect of changes in the consumption of macrolide antibiotics on erythromycin resistance in group A streptococci in Finland. Finnish Study Group for Antimicrobial Resistance. N Engl J Med 1997; 337:441–446.
126. Kristinsson KG, Hjalmarsdottir MA, Gudnason TH. Continued decline in the incidence of penicillin non-susceptible pneumococci in Iceland. In: Program and Abstracts of the 38 Interscience Conference on Antimicrobial Agents and Chemotherapy, San Diego, CA; 1998. Abstract C-22.
127. Schentag JJ, Gilliland KK, Paladino JA. What have we learned from pharmacokinetic and pharmacodynamic theories? Clin Infect Dis 2001; 32(suppl. 1):S39–S46.
128. Dagan R, Klugman KP, Craig WA, Baquero F. Evidence to support the rationale that bacterial eradication in respiratory tract infection is an important aim of antimicrobial therapy. J Antimicrob Chemother 2001; 47:129–140.
129. Yagupsky P, Porat N, Fraser D, et al. Acquisition, carriage, and transmission of pneumococci with decreased antibiotic susceptibility in young children attending a day care facility in southern Israel. J Infect Dis 1998; 177:1003–1012.
130. Dabernat H, Geslin P, Megraud F, et al. Effects of cefixime or co-amoxiclav treatment on nasopharyngeal carriage of *Streptococcus pneumoniae* and *Haemophilus influenzae* in children with acute otitis media. J Antimicrob Chemother 1998; 41:253–258.
131. Nicolau DP. The challenge of prescribing treatment for respiratory tract infections. Am J Manag Care 2000; 6(8 suppl.):S419–S426.
132. Black S, Shinefield H, Fireman B, et al. Efficacy, safety and immunogenicity of heptavalent pneumococcal conjugate vaccine in children. Northern California Kaiser Permanente Vaccine Study Center Group. Pediatr Infect Dis J 2000; 19:187–195.
133. Shinefield H, Black S, Elvin L, et al. Impact of the introduction of pneumococcal conjugate vaccine on the epidemiology of invasive pneumococcal disease in children less than 5 years of age within Northern California Kaiser Permanente (NCKP). In: Program and Abstracts of the 39th Annual Meeting of the Infectious Diseases Society of America; San Francisco, CA; October 25–28, 2001. Abstract 28.
134. Dagan R, Melamed R, Muallem M, et al. Reduction of nasopharyngeal carriage of pneumococci during the second year of life by a heptavalent conjugate pneumococcal vaccine. J Infect Dis 1996; 174:1271–1278.
135. Whitney CG, Farley MM, Hadler J, et al. Increasing prevalence of multidrug-resistant *Streptococcus pneumoniae* in the United States. N Engl J Med 2000; 343:1917–1924.
136. Foord RD. Cefuroxime: human pharmacokinetics. Antimicrob Agents Chemother 1976; 9:741–747.
137. Grisetti M, Brundusino A, Vasconcellos-Lopes H, Lai HJ, Oliani C. Pharmacokinetic profile of three different daily dosages of amoxicillin. Eur Bull Drug Resist 1999; 7:15–20.
138. Guay DRP. Ceftibuten: a new expanded-spectrum oral cephalosporin. Ann Pharmacother 1997; 31:1022–1033.
139. Nix DE, Symonds WT, Hyatt JM, et al. Comparative pharmacokinetics of oral ceftibuten, cefixime, cefaclor, and cefuroxime axetil in healthy volunteers. Pharmacotherapy 1997; 17:121–125.
140. Richer M, Allard S, Manseau L, Vallee F, Pak R, LeBel M. Suction-induced blister fluid penetration of cefdinir in healthy volunteers following ascending oral doses. Antimicrob Agents Chemother 1995; 39:1082–1086.
141. Johnson DM, Biedenbach DJ, Beach ML, Pfaller MA, Jones RN. Antimicrobial activity

and in vitro susceptibility test development for cefditoren against *Haemophilus influenzae*, *Moraxella catarrhalis*, and *Streptococcus* species. Diagn Microbiol Infect Dis 2000; 37:99–105.
142. Lubasch A, Keller I, Borner K, Koeppe P, Lode H. Comparative pharmacokinetics of ciprofloxacin, gatifloxacin, grepafloxacin, levofloxacin, trovafloxacin, and moxifloxacin after single oral administration in healthy volunteers. Antimicrob Agents Chemother 2000; 44:2600–2603.

2

Management of Meningitis Caused by Resistant *Streptococcus pneumoniae*

P. Fernández Viladrich

1. INTRODUCTION

Pneumococcal infections are very prevalent worldwide, and *Streptococcus pneumoniae* is a major cause of bacteremia, pneumonia, meningitis, acute otitis media, and acute sinusitis *(1)*. Overall, invasive pneumococcal infections are associated with high morbidity and mortality. Pneumococcal meningitis is a particularly severe form of the disease that accounts for about 10% of invasive pneumococcal infections; its overall annual incidence in industrialized countries is about 1.5 per 100,000 inhabitants *(2,3)*. In children younger than 5 yr, an incidence of 8 per 100,000 was found *(3)*.

Except for epidemics or hyperendemic situations of meningococcal disease, *S. pneumoniae* has long been and continues to be the most frequent cause of community-acquired bacterial meningitis in adults older than 30 yr. In developed countries, the same may be true for children, a population in which *Haemophilus influenzae* type b meningitis has practically disappeared because of the systematic vaccination of infants with the *H. influenzae* conjugated vaccine. Estimates showed that *S. pneumoniae* causes about 50% of community-acquired meningitis, excluding those of the neonatal period *(2–4)*.

Among community-acquired bacterial meningitis, pneumococcal meningitis causes the most morbidity and mortality. In industrialized countries, mortality due to pneumococcal meningitis in adults ranges from 25 to 30%, and these figures have remained constant throughout the antibiotic era in spite of improved critical care medicine. This emphasizes the need to develop new adjunctive therapy *(4,5)*. Serious neurological sequelae are also frequent, especially in children *(6,7)*. To date, the high mortality and morbidity of pneumococcal meningitis has not been caused by failure of antibiotic treatment. However, in view of the current loss of susceptibility of many *S. pneumoniae* strains to β-lactam agents, that situation could become even worse. The prognosis of pneumococcal meningitis, especially in adults, depends more on early diagnosis and early preventive treatment of neurological complications than on antibiotic failure.

From: *Management of Multiple Drug-Resistant Infections*
Edited by: S. H. Gillespie © Humana Press Inc., Totowa, NJ

2. PATHOGENESIS OF PNEUMOCOCCAL MENINGITIS

Pneumococci reach the central nervous system (CNS) either by a hematogenous route from a distant focus of infection, usually the lower airways with or without pneumonia, or, even more frequently, by direct cerebrospinal fluid (CSF) entrance of bacteria from an infectious focus near the CNS, such as acute otitis media, acute sinusitis, or a cranial fistula. Once organisms have reached the CSF, they quickly multiply, leading to the release of several cytokines. This creates an inflammatory process that increases blood–brain barrier permeability and produces cytotoxic and vasogenic brain edema, intracranial hypertension, ischemia, and neuronal damage. The inflammatory process and consequences may be greatly increased when cell wall fragments are released after bacteriolytic antibiotics are administered. On the other hand, bacterial growth in the meningeal spaces frequently leads to secondary bacteremia, which may contribute to morbidity. Hemodynamic instability or shock, if not properly treated, will worsen the neurological function by lowering the cerebral perfusion pressure and increasing brain ischemia *(8–10)*.

3. CLINICAL MANIFESTATIONS

As in other types of bacterial meningitis, clinical manifestations of pneumococcal meningitis are because of the meningeal inflammation and its neurological consequences, the original source of infection, and possible concurrent primary or secondary septicemia.

Although symptoms and signs of meningismus do not differ from those of other bacterial meningitis, neurological complications are more frequent, especially those related to intracranial hypertension and seizures. Seizures are a complication of bacterial meningitis that have repeatedly been associated with higher mortality and neurological sequelae *(4,11–13)*. In adults, they occur much more frequently in pneumococcal meningitis than in meningitis caused by other pathogens.

About 30% of adults with pneumococcal meningitis convulse *(4,14)*. Moreover, the majority of these seizures occur early in the natural history. In my experience, about 10% of adults with pneumococcal meningitis have already convulsed when first visited, and another 20% convulse after antibiotic treatment has been initiated, usually during the first 24 or 48 h of therapy. Some patients go on to status epilepticus. Additional impairment of consciousness level and signs of brain herniation also often occur after the initiation of antibiotic treatment.

Other neurological complications, such as brain infarcts because of cortical thrombophlebitis or arteritis, occur in about 15% of adults with bacterial meningitis *(15)*. In fact, early death related to the occurrence of one of these complications after CSF has been sterilized by appropriate antibiotic therapy has been a common experience when treating patients with pneumococcal meningitis (and occasionally other types of bacterial meningitis) and may be explained in part by the CSF inflammation described in Section 2. That is why, for more than a decade, to prevent these neurological complications very early adjunctive therapy (*see* Section 5.1.) has been administered to all adult patients with suspected pneumococcal meningitis and to those individuals with bacterial meningitis of any other etiology who show signs of high intracranial hypertension *(16)*.

Of paramount importance when approaching a patient with bacterial meningitis are symptoms and signs caused by a primary focus of infection because they are valuable not only for discovery of the etiologic agent, but also for indication of the most appropriate approach. Thus, when bacterial meningitis is preceded by respiratory symptoms, a classical meningeal pathogen such as meningococcus or pneumococcus is probably the cause *(17)*. Meningitis caused by *Listeria monocytogenes* will not usually be preceded by respiratory symptoms.

Acute bacterial meningitis is the most frequent intracranial complication of acute otitis media at all ages. In adults, this process is almost exclusively caused by *S. pneumoniae*; conversely, about 35% of adult pneumococcal meningitis cases are a complication of an attack of acute otitis media *(14,17)*. On the other hand, a brain abscess is the most frequent intracranial complication of cholesteatomatous chronic otitis media, in which the classical meningeal pathogens are usually not implicated *(18)*.

Thus, in patients with both meningeal signs and otitis, ascertaining the type of otitis has diagnostic and therapeutic implications. A lumbar puncture should be performed without delay if the otitis media is acute, whereas a computed tomographic (CT) brain scan should be performed first if the otitis media is chronic to rule out a suppurative intracranial collection clinically presenting as bacterial meningitis. A pericranial fistula is likely if the patient has suffered, even many years before, cranial or facial trauma, an operation involving either the ethmoid or sphenoid sinuses or the otic cavities, or CSF rhinorrhea or recurrent episodes of bacterial meningitis. *Streptococcus pneumoniae* is also the most frequent cause of bacterial meningitis in this setting, although such other respiratory pathogens as *H. influenzae*, *Neisseria meningitidis*, or streptococci of the *viridans* group may also be the cause *(17)*.

Septicemia may be both the cause and the consequence of the meningeal infection and may cause distant infection, such as arthritis or endocarditis, or shock. Patients with meningitis secondary to pneumococcal septicemia with or without pneumonia or endocarditis have a higher mortality rate (about 50%) than those whose pneumococcal meningitis is secondary to a parameningeal focus. A maculopetechial or purpuric skin rash is characteristic of meningococcal septicemia, although it may also be caused by other microorganisms, including overwhelming pneumococcal infection.

4. DIAGNOSIS

When a diagnosis of community-acquired bacterial meningitis is suspected, a lumbar puncture should be performed immediately, and the CSF opening pressure must be recorded and its aspect observed. For patients with a nonacute clinical course, especially if coma, hemiparesis, or papilledema are found, and in patients who present with a primary focus of infection (e.g., chronic cholesteatomatous otitis media, chronic sinusitis, or dental or anaerobic lung infection) that characteristically complicates with a brain abscess, a CT brain scan should be performed before lumbar puncture *(19,20)*. In these cases, a loading dose of dexamethasone must be immediately administered. Moreover, if acute bacterial meningitis is suspected, empirical antibiotic therapy must be given (after obtaining blood samples for cultures) before performing a CT scan.

As stated in the section on clinical manifestations, seizures are quite frequent in bacterial meningitis, so they do not constitute an indication for brain scanning prior to lumbar puncture if the illness runs an acute course. Because pneumococcal meningitis usually runs an acute course and rarely coexists with a brain abscess, a cranial CT prior to lumbar puncture is not usually indicated, especially considering that the early administration of dexamethasone is necessary in almost all circumstances (*see* Section 5.1.).

In many cases of community-acquired bacterial meningitis, a pneumococcal etiology can usually be suspected, especially in the adult population, for whom acute otitis media, the presence of a posttraumatic or postsurgical pericranial fistula, or an acute lower respiratory disease (frequently, lobar pneumonia) are the primary infection foci in about 80% of cases. All these entities can easily be diagnosed or strongly suspected based on clinical antecedents and clinical data. In addition, CSF Gram stain is clearly positive in around 80% of patients with pneumococcal meningitis who have not received previous antibiotic therapy. If pneumococcal meningitis is suspected and the Gram stain is negative, a CSF determination of pneumococcal antigen must be performed *(21)*.

5. TREATMENT

Like bacterial meningitis caused by other etiologies, pneumococcal meningitis constitutes a medical emergency that must be rapidly treated to minimize both mortality and neurological sequelae. Cognitive defects have been detected in adults surviving a bout of pneumococcal meningitis without apparent sequelae *(6)*. As mentioned in the introduction, in developed countries the overall mortality from pneumococcal meningitis in adults has remained around 30% *(4,14,15,22)*. This mortality is mainly caused by early neurological complications. When these complications, especially brain herniation, do occur, brain damage is frequently irreversible, and measures aimed at lowering inflammation and cranial hypertension are usually ineffective. Although a general rule for the treatment of bacterial meningitis is not to delay antibiotic treatment because significant delays will certainly increase mortality and neurological sequelae, precocious antibiotic treatment not only may be insufficient to avoid neurological complications, especially those associated with pneumococcal meningitis, but also may favor occurrence of these complications through their bacteriolytic effect. Therefore, because the administration of appropriate adjunctive therapy in these cases may be even more urgent than administration of the antibiotic, I begin with this aspect of therapy.

5.1. Early Adjunctive Therapy

An initial perfusion of mannitol may occasionally be lifesaving by rapidly lowering cranial hypertension *(23,24)*. In deeply comatose patients, consciousness level frequently improves rapidly after mannitol administration. This improvement may be manifested by progression from coma to an agitated state. Moreover, improvement of bradycardia and the respiratory rhythm irregularities that these patients sometimes present may also be observed. Although the routine use of mannitol in acute bacterial meningitis is not usually recommended, I think that there might be some rationale for using it in every case of suspected pneumococcal meningitis.

As reported, the practice of cranial CT does not discriminate which patients will have cerebral herniation after a lumbar puncture, so some patients with a normal cranial CT will suffer this life-threatening complication *(25)*. On the other hand, routine cranial CT in suspected meningitis may significantly delay antibiotic therapy, thereby increasing the probability of neurological or cognitive sequelae *(19)*. For more than a decade, it has been my usual practice to administer adjunctive therapy with mannitol (a bolus of 0.5–1 g per kilogram body weight) and dexamethasone (a loading dose of 8–16 mg followed by doses of 4 mg every 6 h for 48 h) immediately after lumbar puncture of adults with bacterial meningitis who show clinical signs of severe intracranial hypertension or a CSF opening pressure higher than 30 cm water, as well as to all suspected cases of pneumococcal meningitis regardless of CSF opening pressure. Such treatment has been administered to many patients with bacterial meningitis without significant adverse events.

With regard to anti-inflammatory treatment, there is general agreement as to the convenience of administering dexamethasone to children with bacterial meningitis *(26)*. Dexamethasone has been shown to reduce neurological and audiologic sequelae in children with meningitis caused by *H. influenzae* type b *(27)*. The same may be true for pneumococcal meningitis in children provided the dexamethasone is given before or at the same time as antibiotic therapy. The administration of dexamethasone during the first 48 h of therapy has not been associated with significant adverse events in this population *(28)*. On the other hand, early dexamethasone therapy has been proved to reduce mortality of adult patients with pneumococcal meningitis to 14% *(29)*. A study published by Girgis et al. in 1989 showed that early dexamethasone therapy reduced mortality, but because of several deficiencies, it was not seriously considered *(30)*. Since 1987, I have been treating pneumococcal meningitis in adults with the early administration of mannitol and dexamethasone and with intravenous sodium phenytoin to prevent seizures (a loading dose of 18 mg per kilogram body weight followed by standard doses every 8 h), with an attributable mortality of 12% *(16)*.

Regarding the administration of dexamethasone in bacterial meningitis, and especially in pneumococcal meningitis, there are several considerations. First, early administration of corticosteroids constitutes an excellent symptomatic therapy, contributing to accelerate improvement of such cranial hypertension symptoms as headache, which is frequently very intense and difficult to control with analgesic treatment, as well as improvement of consciousness level. Fever is also more quickly abated by using these drugs. These beneficial effects of corticosteroids have never been considered as end points in comparative studies, but I think they are worthy of consideration in view of the intense suffering of patients in the initial phases of meningeal inflammation. Second, side effects of corticosteroids, especially clinically significant gastrointestinal hemorrhage, are infrequent, especially if the corticosteroids are administered for only 48 h *(28,29)*. Third, corticosteroids impair the passage of several antibiotics, such as β-lactam agents and vancomycin, through the blood–brain barrier. This effect may have negative consequences in cases of bacterial meningitis in which there is a low therapeutic index because of the class of antibiotic used (e.g., vancomycin) or to the susceptibility of the causal organism (e.g., moderate resistance to β-lactam agents). However, this problem will probably be minimized if dexamethasone use is limited to the first 48 h of treatment, when the permeability of the blood–brain barrier is expected to be clearly increased by the inflammatory process. Although a dosage of 10 mg every 6 h for 4 d has recently been recommended for bacterial meningitis in adults *(29)*, based on experience, I believe that both lower dosage and shorter treatment are probably sufficient for this population.

If adjunctive therapy is appropriately conducted, many patients with severe neurological disease will improve rapidly, and the need for more aggressive measures may be avoided. However, hospitalization in an intensive care unit is mandatory for those patients who convulse in spite of adjunctive therapy; for those with other severe neurological complications that require mechanical support, hyperventilation, and monitoring of cranial hypertension; and, obviously, for those patients who have hemodynamic instability or shock *(31)*.

5.2. Antibiotic Treatment

5.2.1. Historical Perspective

It is well known that, over the past 30 years or more, pneumococci have developed resistance to several antimicrobial agents, including penicillin, cephalosporins, chloramphenicol, trimethoprim-sulfamethoxazole, erythromycin, and other drugs. But, in terms of therapy and especially for the treatment of meningitis, the most important problem has been the development of resistance to penicillin. This is because penicillin was the time-honored treatment for decades for pneumococcal infections, and alternative drugs were only necessary in penicillin-allergic patients.

An interesting fact is that, shortly after the introduction of penicillin in 1940, the first strain with decreased susceptibility to penicillin was produced in the laboratory *(32)*. However, the first clinical isolate did not appear until more than 20 yr later in Boston *(33)*. In the late 1960s, pneumococcal strains with moderate penicillin resistance (defined as those pneumococci with minimum inhibitory concentrations [MICs] of penicillin G of 0.1 to 1 μg/mL) were isolated in Australia and New Guinea *(34–36)*. Some cases of meningitis caused by pneumococci with those levels of resistance responded to high dosages of penicillin, but others failed to respond *(37)*. This happened because attainable peak CSF levels of penicillin—around 1 μg/mL *(38)*—are close to the MICs of those partially penicillin-resistant pneumococci. So, penicillin G had to be discarded for empirical treatment of suspected pneumococcal meningitis.

In the 1970s, an epidemic of high-level penicillin-resistant pneumococci (with MICs of penicillin G > 1 μg/mL) that were also resistant to chloramphenicol and other antibiotics was reported in pediatric wards in South Africa *(39,40)*. The patients with meningitis caused by those strains who received penicillin or chloramphenicol died. At present, most penicillin-resistant pneumococci are also resistant to chloramphenicol, and even when they show susceptibility to this antibiotic by usual methods of susceptibility, they are tolerant, and the clinical response to treatment with this antibiotic has been poor *(41)*. So, chloramphenicol, once the elective alternative for pneumococcal meningitis in patients allergic to penicillin, must not be used as either empirical treatment of suspected pneumococcal meningitis or treatment of cases caused by pneumococci with any degree of penicillin resistance.

The solution to this problem seemed to be the third-generation cephalosporins—cefotaxime and ceftriaxone, which remained active against moderately penicillin-resistant pneumococci. However, penicillin-resistant pneumococci show diminished sensitivity to all β-lactam agents, including cefotaxime and ceftriaxone *(42)*, and failures with the standard doses of these antibiotics soon occurred when the illnesses were caused by pneumococcal strains with MICs of cefotaxime greater than or even equal to 0.5 μg/mL *(37,43–57)*.

At present, pneumococci with MICs of cefotaxime of 1 μg/mL are defined as partially cefotaxime resistant, and those with MICs greater than 1 μg/mL are defined as highly cefotaxime resistant *(58)*. However, a pneumococcus showing an MIC of cefotaxime of 0.5 μg/mL might have a minimal bactericidal concentration of 1 or even 2 μg/mL. Therefore, I consider that, for therapeutic purposes, it should be classified as cefotaxime nonsusceptible. After one of my patients with penicillin-resistant pneumococcal meningitis showed a rapid response to high-dose cefotaxime therapy *(37)*, such treatment was considered suitable for penicillin-resistant and partially cefotaxime-resistant pneumococcal meningitis in adults *(37,59)*.

Other authors also obtained good results in such cases with even lower doses of cefotaxime *(60)*. However, high-dose cefotaxime therapy has not reached initial general acceptance, probably because there is concern about the administration of higher-than-conventional doses and, especially, because a few cases of meningitis caused by pneumococci with a high level of cefotaxime resistance (MICs of cefotaxime from 4 to 32 μg/mL) occurred in the United States *(47–49)*.

Initially, the solution to the problem of resistance to β-lactam agents seemed to be the use of vancomycin, an antibiotic to which all pneumococci remained (and still remain) susceptible, with MICs ranging between 0.25 and 1 μg/mL. However, surprisingly for the medical community, several clinical failures were documented when vancomycin was used in conjunction with dexamethasone *(61)*. Those failures were mainly because of insufficient antibiotic penetration into CSF, due both to individual variability in its passing through the blood–brain barrier and to the effect of dexamethasone, which was shown to reduce CSF vancomycin penetration *(62,63)*. Since this experience, the recommendation is that vancomycin not be used alone for treatment of pneumococcal meningitis; based on a few studies performed both in vitro and in the rabbit model of meningitis, combined antibiotic regimens have been recommended for both empirical treatment and treatment of those cases caused by β-lactam-resistant pneumococcal strains *(64–67)*.

5.2.2. *Initial Empirical Therapy*

Initial empirical therapy refers to the initial treatment for a patient with either suspected or diagnosed pneumococcal meningitis (e.g., compatible clinical features plus one of the following: CSF Gram stain showing typical Gram-positive diplococci, CSF-positive pneumococcal antigen, or CSF culture yielding pneumococci with unknown antibiotic susceptibility). Empirical therapy must also be given to patients with suspected pneumococcal meningitis based on clinical grounds only in cases when urgent CSF Gram stain could not be performed or there is a contraindication for performing an immediate lumbar puncture.

Although antibiotic treatment must be immediately instituted in those patients with skin lesions suggestive of meningococcal sepsis, in cases of pneumococcal meningitis, it can probably be delayed for some minutes to perform a CSF Gram stain and to institute preantibiotic adjunctive therapy. I review some possibilities for the empirical antibiotic therapy.

5.2.2.1. High-Dose Cefotaxime Therapy

If the patient is not allergic to β-lactam agents, the empirical therapy for pneumococcal meningitis should always include a third-generation cephalosporin such as cefotaxime or ceftriaxone. As mentioned in the historical perspective, neither penicillin nor chloramphenicol must be administered for empirical therapy. These cephalosporins will also cover the other respiratory pathogens usually causing community-acquired bacterial meningitis. Treatment with either standard intravenous dose of cefotaxime (150–200 mg/kg body weight per day with a maximum of 12 g) or ceftriaxone (100 mg/kg body weight per day with a maximum of 4 g; higher doses of ceftriaxone are not recommended because of potential side effects, especially biliary precipitation stones) has sometimes failed to cure some cases of meningitis caused by pneumococci partially resistant to cefotaxime (MICs = 1 μg/mL) and even with some diminution of sensitivity (MIC = 0.5 μg/mL) *(37,56,57)*. For almost two decades, I have used high doses of cefotaxime (300–350 mg/kg body weight per day to a maximum of 24 g) as sole therapy for the empirical treatment of pneumococcal meningitis in adults, and this therapy was safe and effective for cefotaxime-resistant cases (MICs of cefotaxime up to 2 μg/mL), with all experiencing a good response with sterile CSF cultures.

In Spain, the percentage of pneumococcal strains that were resistant to cefotaxime was 21% in 2000 *(68)*. Of these, 17% were partially resistant (MICs of cefotaxime of 1 μg/mL), and 6% were highly resistant (MICs of cefotaxime equal to or higher than 2 μg/mL). The majority of these resistant strains showed MICs of cefotaxime of 2 μg/mL. Pneumococci with MICs of cefotaxime higher than 2 μg/mL have been not found in adults, and in more than 20 years in the era of pneumococcal resistance, not one case of meningitis caused by such a strain has been found in Spain. However, in 2000, a few pneumococcal strains with MICs of cefotaxime equal to or even higher than 4 μg/mL were isolated from invasive pneumococcal disease in children younger than 5 yr *(68,69)*.

At present, these limits in levels of cefotaxime resistance are probably found in the majority of areas in the world. It is very improbable that cases with the aforementioned levels of cefotaxime resistance cannot be controlled with such high doses of cefotaxime during the first 24 to 48 h of treatment, when the blood–brain barrier must remain quite permeable, and the results of susceptibility tests can be obtained.

In spite of the above considerations, high-dose cefotaxime therapy might occasionally fail when CSF levels do not sufficiently exceed the MIC of the causal strain *(70)* because of individual variability of CSF levels or when there is an MIC of cefotaxime equal to or greater than 4 μg/mL. Therefore, although this is my present approach for empirical treatment in the adult population in my area, use a combination of cefotaxime and vancomycin (*see* Section 5.2.2.2.) for empirical treatment while awaiting the results of cultures and susceptibility tests. However, combined empirical therapy must only be given in those cases that I defined in this section as either practically certain or really probable pneumococcal meningitis.

5.2.2.2. Third-Generation Cephalosporin Plus Vancomycin

The combination of standard doses of cefotaxime or ceftriaxone plus vancomycin for empirical therapy of pneumococcal meningitis was recommended for the first time in 1994 *(64)*. This antibiotic combination was synergistic in studies in vitro *(71)*, in the rabbit model of meningitis *(72)*, and in an in vitro study using CSF of children treated with this antibiotic combination *(73)*. However, these experiences have been limited.

In another in vitro study, the combination of cefotaxime plus vancomycin was found to be indifferent against 26 pneumococcal strains *(74)*; in work with colleagues, I found this combination to be bactericidal, but not synergic *(75)*. In any case, this antibiotic combination has been increasingly used over the last years, and it constitutes the current standard recommendation for empirical treatment of suspected pneumococcal meningitis, especially in children *(67)*. However, I believe it is important to keep in mind some considerations regarding this antibiotic combination:

1. Little clinical experience with this therapy has been published *(76,77)*.
2. It does not seem to be synergistic against all strains of pneumococci.
3. It is possible that neither of the two antibiotics reach the necessary CSF levels for rapid bactericidal activity. Vancomycin at the recommended dosage for adult patients (30 mg/kg body weight per day) does not reach reliable CSF levels, especially if dexamethasone is administered concurrently *(61)*, and CSF cefotaxime levels might also be insufficient for some cephalosporin-resistant pneumococcal strains *(70)*. That is why I recommend that high-dose cefotaxime (e.g., around 350 mg/kg body weight per day, with a maximum dose of 24 g per day) always be administered initially to adults with suspected pneumococcal meningitis.
4. In contrast, standard doses of cefotaxime or ceftriaxone are sufficient for empirical treatment in children because the standard dosage of vancomycin they are receiving for treatment of meningitis (60 mg/kg body weight per day, double that of adults) is sufficient to cure the infection even if dexamethasone is given concurrently *(73)*.

5.2.2.3. Third-Generation Cephalosporin Plus Rifampin

The combination of cefotaxime or ceftriaxone with rifampin has been recommended in lieu of therapy with cephalosporin plus vancomycin for empirical treatment of pneumococcal meningitis when dexamethasone was given concurrently *(64–66)*, especially because CSF penetration of rifampin, unlike that of vancomycin, is unaffected by dexamethasone administration *(62)*. At present, when it is known that adjunctive dexamethasone therapy is obligatory *(29)*, this therapeutic recommendation could even be reinforced. Rifampin is bactericidal against *S. pneumoniae*, and around 99% of pneumococci remain susceptible, with MICs equal to or less than 0.12 μg/mL *(69,78–80)*. CSF levels of rifampin, when administered at maximum dosage (about 900 mg/d for adults, 20 mg/kg body weight per day for children), are around 1 μg/mL *(73,81)*, which is sufficient for reaching appropriate activity against *S. pneumoniae*.

On the other hand, rifampin reduced early mortality when compared with ceftriaxone in experimental pneumococcal meningitis in mice by reducing the release of inflammatory cytokines *(82)*. In another experiment in rabbits, it reduced the release of reactive oxygen species in CSF *(83)*. However, rifampin cannot be used as monotherapy because of rapid development of resistance, and it must be administered in combination with another antibiotic.

Nevertheless, in vitro studies with the combination of rifampin with β-lactams or vancomycin have led to conflicting results. In an in vitro study using antibiotic combinations at clinically achievable concentrations in CSF, rifampin frequently reduced the killing activity of ceftriaxone, vancomycin, and imipenem against 15 penicillin-resistant pneumococcal strains with MICs of ceftriaxone of 0.5–1 μg/mL *(74)*. In a study with colleagues, we found the combination ceftriaxone-rifampin antagonistic in vitro *(75)*. However, in another study using much lower concentrations of rifampin, Barakett et al. reported that rifampin combined with vancomycin or cefotaxime usually had synergistic or indifferent activity *(84)*; in another study, CSF concentrations above those observed in humans with usual dosage regimens led to a decrease in bacterial killing *(85)*.

In a report of vancomycin-rifampin therapy in the animal model of meningitis, rifampin activity was reduced during the first few hours of therapy, showed moderately bactericidal activity compared with that of ceftriaxone or vancomycin, and killing rates comparable to those of β-lactam antibiotics could not be obtained by increasing the dose of rifampin *(72)*. In contrast, in an in vitro study using CSF of children treated with various antibiotic combinations, the combination of ceftriaxone plus rifampin was synergistic, with treatment with rifampin significantly increasing the bactericidal activity of ceftriaxone against two cefotaxime-resistant strains of *S. pneumoniae* (either partially ceftriaxone resistant or highly ceftriaxone resistant) *(73)*.

To my knowledge, clinical experience with the combination of cephalosporins with rifampin for empirical therapy of suspected pneumococcal meningitis is lacking. At present, it is generally not recommended for empirical therapy because clinical experience is lacking, concerns exist as to whether it might reduce the bactericidal activity of β-lactam agents, and the possibility of selection for rifampin resistance exists. However, if chosen for empirical treatment in combination with a third-generation cephalosporin, I also would advise that a high dose of cefotaxime be administered because if insufficient levels of cephalosporin were reached in CSF, it could constitute real monotherapy with rifampin, possibly leading to the rapid development of rifampin resistance during treatment.

In spite of the above-mentioned negative considerations, I believe that, if a rifampin-susceptible pneumococcus is the cause and high-dose cefotaxime therapy was used, this antibiotic combination may be effective for cefotaxime-resistant pneumococcal meningitis, provided the MICs of cefotaxime were no higher than 4 μg/mL.

5.2.2.4. Vancomycin Plus Rifampin

For patients allergic to β-lactams, I favor the combination of vancomycin and rifampin for empirical therapy. In the rabbit model of experimental meningitis, my group found that this combination was bactericidal—although not synergic—and effective against cefotaxime-resistant pneumococci, and that CSF vancomycin levels were not reduced by dexamethasone *(86)*. Moreover, it cured some children who had experienced therapeutic failure when treated with other antibiotics *(49,52,55,87)*; my group has administered this antibiotic combination with good results to several adults with pneumococcal meningitis *(88)*. However, because failures can occur in the case of low CSF vancomycin levels, strict monitoring of both CSF microbiological parameters and serum vancomycin levels is necessary. My impression is that the regimen of vancomycin plus rifampicin is somewhat better than that of vancomycin alone, especially concomitant with dexamethasone therapy. CSF bactericidal titers achieved with this combination appear moderately higher than those achieved with vancomycin alone *(61,88)*.

5.2.3. Therapy for Pneumococcal Meningitis if Susceptibility Is Known

Appropriate antibiotic treatment of pneumococcal meningitis requires knowledge of the causal strain's susceptibility to penicillin and to broad-spectrum cephalosporins. If a pneumococcus is growing on CSF culture, it is possible to obtain preliminary information about its susceptibility to β-lactam agents in less than 24 h by performing an Etest® (AB Biodisk, Solna, Sweden) directly on seeded culture plates. After results of susceptibility tests are known, empirical antibiotic therapy can be modified.

If vancomycin or rifampin is given in conjunction with a third-generation cephalosporin, they must be discontinued if the causal strain is sensitive to penicillin or third-generation cephalosporins. They must also be discontinued if CSF and blood cultures are sterile at 48–72 h of incubation whether or not the patient has received prior antibiotic therapy. If the patient received prior treatment with a β-lactam antibiotic (penicillin or cephalosporin), it can be assumed that, if a bacterial agent is the cause, it will be sensitive to β-lactams; if not, it is very improbable that the patient has pneumococcal meningitis.

5.2.3.1. Penicillin-Sensitive Pneumococcal Meningitis

Penicillin remains the therapy of choice for susceptible strains of pneumococci, and alternative drugs are only necessary in penicillin-allergic patients. Penicillin should be given at doses of 300,000 U/kg body weight (2 to 4 MU in adults) scheduled every 4 h intravenously. As an alternative, treatment with a standard dose of ceftriaxone may occasionally be convenient for the patient's comfort (especially to avoid catheter phlebitis); this dose may be given once a day intramuscularly if necessary. This is my usual practice for adult patients, and this therapy has proved safe and effective.

Chloramphenicol constitutes the therapy of choice for penicillin-allergic patients with penicillin-susceptible pneumococcal meningitis because the majority (if not all) of penicillin-sensitive pneumococci are also chloramphenicol sensitive, and chloramphenicol must replace empirical vancomycin therapy. As mentioned in the historical perspective section, chloramphenicol must not be given in penicillin-resistant cases even if the causal strain appeared susceptible by the Kirby-Bauer method *(41)*. In this case, determinations of minimal bactericidal concentrations of this antibiotic should be performed before it is selected as an alternative therapy.

5.2.3.2. Penicillin-Resistant and Cefotaxime-Sensitive Pneumococcal Meningitis

As mentioned in Section 5.2.1., patients infected with strains with decreased susceptibility to penicillin (MICs of penicillin equal to or higher than 0.12 μg/mL) should not be treated with this antibiotic. In such cases, standard-dose cefotaxime or ceftriaxone is the therapy of choice for those with MICs of cefotaxime equal to or less than 0.25 μg/mL. Cases with MIC of cefotaxime of 0.5 μg/mL, although defined as sensitive, have a significant loss of susceptibility, and I recommend they be treated with high-dose cefotaxime (*see* Section 5.2.1.).

5.2.3.3. Penicillin-Resistant and Cefotaxime-Resistant Pneumococcal Meningitis

If the causal strain shows any degree of penicillin and cephalosporin resistance, the empirical treatment that was initially administrated must be continued until completion of treatment if the patient does well. However, a control lumbar puncture should always be performed at 24–48 h after the start of antibiotic therapy to document the sterility of CSF culture and to test CSF antibiotic levels or bactericidal titers if possible. A repeated lumbar puncture is also recommended if signs of clinical recrudescence occur at any time during the treatment.

In cefotaxime-resistant pneumococcal meningitis in adults, it has been my usual practice to continue with the high doses of cefotaxime initially administered if clinical evolution is good and to add vancomycin if there is some doubt about a satisfactory response. High-dose cefotaxime therapy has been effective in curing several of my patients with meningitis caused by pneumococci with MICs to cefotaxime of 1 and 2 µg/mL *(37)*. However, in one recent case with MICs of cefotaxime of 2 µg/mL, vancomycin was added on d 5 in response to persistent fever, meningeal signs, and inflammatory CSF parameters despite negative CSF Gram stain and culture. That patient experienced an immediate response to the addition of vancomycin.

If the combination of cephalosporin plus vancomycin was initially given to an adult patient, it is mandatory to determine serum vancomycin levels at 36–48 h of therapy to ensure trough serum vancomycin levels of about 10 µg/mL and to modify the dosage if necessary. This is important because there is quite individual variability in vancomycin pharmacokinetics, so occasionally a patient receiving the appropriate standard vancomycin dosage (15 mg/kg body weight every 12 h) could possibly have either insufficient or excessive serum levels. Determination of vancomycin levels is less important in the pediatric population.

In case of suspected therapeutic failure (e.g., reappearance of fever and recrudescence of meningeal signs or, especially, if positive CSF culture persists at 24–48 h of treatment), one of the following alternative therapies may be considered.

5.3. *Alternative Therapies for Penicillin- and Cefotaxime-Resistant Pneumococcal Meningitis*

For therapeutic failure in a case of penicillin- and cefotaxime-resistant pneumococcal meningitis, some possible alternatives are as follows: If the patient is not receiving vancomycin, add this antibiotic to the regimen initially administrated. If the patient is already receiving an appropriate dosage of vancomycin (appropriate serum levels documented), any of the following therapeutic regimens could be effective:

1. Change to high-dose cefotaxime therapy if the patient was receiving a standard dosage of cefotaxime or ceftriaxone.
2. Add rifampin to the regimen of high-dose cefotaxime plus vancomycin.
3. Add intrathecal vancomycin (10–20 mg every 24 or 48 h) to the systemic regimen *(49,53,55,89)*.
4. Change to imipenem with or without rifampin. Imipenem MICs tend to be lower than those of cefotaxime against penicillin-resistant pneumococci, but because the dosage of imipenem is lower (maximum 4 g/24 h), it does not seem to me that it would be able to significantly ameliorate the CSF activity obtained with high-dose cefotaxime. However, some children with cefotaxime-resistant pneumococcal meningitis have been cured with imipenem alone *(43)* or combined with rifampin *(54)*. On the other hand, the potential risk of seizures should be taken into account when treating bacterial meningitis with imipenem *(50)*.
5. Meropenem could be considered. Dosage of meropenem is somewhat higher (maximum 6–8 g/24 h) than that of imipenem, and CSF levels of around 3 µg/mL can be reached *(90)*. However, meropenem MICs tend to be two- to fourfold higher than those of imipenem *(91)*, so I do not believe it is a good alternative for cefotaxime-resistant pneumococcal meningitis. The same might be said about fourth-generation cephalosporins such as cefpirome or cefepime.
6. Some of the new quinolones could perhaps be tested for a desperate case. Some of the newer quinolones have been very effective in the animal model of β-lactam-resistant pneumococcal meningitis *(92–97)*, and trovafloxacin was found safe and similar to ceftriaxone with or without vancomycin in a series of bacterial meningitis in children *(98)*. However, great concern exists about its tendency to develop antibiotic resistance *(99)*. Resistance to

levofloxacin has developed during treatment for pneumococcal pneumonia *(100,101)*; information on a case of fatal meningitis caused by levofloxacin-resistant *S. pneumoniae* has been published *(102)*; and at present, almost 1.5% of *S. pneumoniae* strains from Spain are resistant to this antibiotic *(68,103)*.

7. Some new antibiotics, such as linezolid *(104)*, against Gram-positive bacteria could perhaps be useful for β-lactam-resistant pneumococcal meningitis in the future.

5.4. *Duration of Treatment*

The recommended length of therapy for pneumococcal meningitis is 10 to 14 d of effective antibiotic therapy. If the patient does well, I treat this illness for 10 d regardless of the susceptibility characteristics of the causal strain. My group and others have demonstrated that β-lactam-resistant pneumococcal meningitis is not more severe than penicillin-susceptible pneumococcal meningitis *(37,105)*.

6. PREVENTION

Bacterial meningitis will continue to be a serious disease. The best efforts must be directed toward prevention. Thus, pneumococcal vaccines must be given. The routine administration of heptavalent conjugate pneumococcal vaccine to infants will probably lower the incidence of pneumococcal meningitis in this population *(106–108)*. Moreover, the 23-serotype polysaccharide pneumococcal vaccine must be administered to all adult patients who have the known indications. If the patient has a CSF pericranial fistula, he or she must promptly receive surgery to avoid new episodes of bacterial meningitis. In such a circumstance, pneumococcal vaccination has been inefficient in preventing recurrent episodes of pneumococcal meningitis, even when caused by pneumococcal strains of the serotypes included in the vaccine *(109)*.

REFERENCES

1. Musher DM. *Streptococcus pneumoniae*. In: Mandell GM, Bennet JE, Dolin R (eds.). Principles and Practice of Infectious Diseases. 4th ed. New York: Churchill Livingstone, 1995, pp. 1811–1826.
2. Schuchat A, Robinson K, Wenger JD, et al. Bacterial meningitis in the United States in 1995. N Engl J Med 1997; 337:970–976.
3. Spanjaard L, van der Ende A, Rumke H, Dankert J, van Alphen L. Epidemiology of meningitis and bacteraemia due to *Streptococcus pneumoniae* in The Netherlands. Acta Pediatr Suppl 2000; 89:22–26.
4. Durand ML, Calderwood SB, Weber DJ, et al. Acute bacterial meningitis in adults. A review of 493 episodes. N Engl J Med 1993; 328:21–28.
5. Aronin SI, Peduzzi P, Quagliarello VJ. Community-acquired bacterial meningitis: risk stratification for adverse clinical outcome and effect of antibiotic timing. Ann Intern Med 1998; 129:862–869.
6. van de Beek D, Schmand B, de Gans J, et al. Cognitive impairment in adults with good recovery after bacterial meningitis. J Infect Dis 2002; 186:1047–1052.
7. Kornelisse RF, Westerbeek CML, Spoor AB, et al. Pneumococcal meningitis in children: prognostic indicators and outcome. Clin Infect Dis 1995; 21:1390–1397.
8. Saez-Llorens X, Ramilo O, Mustafa MM, Mertsola J, McCracken GH Jr. Molecular pathophysiology of bacterial meningitis: current concepts and therapeutic implications. J Pediatr 1990; 116:671.
9. Quagliarello V, Scheld WM. Bacterial meningitis: pathogenesis, pathophysiology, and progress. N Engl J Med 1992; 327:864–872.

10. Pfister HW, Fontana A, Täuber MG, Tomasz A, Sheld WM. Mechanisms of brain injury in bacterial meningitis: workshop summary. Clin Infect Dis 1994; 19:463–479.
11. Viladrich PF. Enfermedad Meningocócica en Adolescentes y Adultos (Hospital de Bellvitge, 1977–1990) [doctoral thesis]. Universidad de Barcelona, Spain, 1993.
12. Lacroix J, Deal C, Gauthier M, Rousseau E, Farrell FA. Admissions to a pediatric intensive care unit for status epilepticus: a 10-year experience. Crit Care Med 1994; 22: 827–832.
13. Casado Flores J, García Teresa MA, Cambra F, et al. Estudio prospectivo multicéntrico de la meningitis bacteriana grave pediátrica. An Esp Pediatr 1997; 47:466–472.
14. Viladrich PF, Buenaventura I, Gudiol F, et al. Meningitis neumocócica del adulto. Estudio de 141 episodios. Med Clin (Barc) 1986; 87:569–574.
15. Pfister HW, Feiden W, Einhäupl KM. Spectrum of complications during bacterial meningitis in adults. Arch Neurol 1993; 50:575–581.
16. Viladrich PF, Gudiol F. Avances en las infecciones del sistema nervioso central producidas por bacterias grampositivas. Rev Clin Esp 1994; 194:847–852.
17. Viladrich PF, Gudiol F, Rufí G, et al. Meningitis bacteriana. Etiología y focos de origen de 482 episodios. Med Clin (Barc) 1986; 86:615–620.
18. Ariza J, Casanova A, Viladrich PF, et al. Etiological agent and primary source of infection in 42 cases of focal intracranial suppuration. J Clin Microbiol 1986; 24:899–902.
19. Hasbun R, Abrahams J, Jekel J, Quagliarello VJ. Computed tomography of the head before lumbar puncture in adults with suspected meningitis. N Engl J Med 2001; 345:1727–1733.
20. van Crevel H, Hijdra A, de Gans J. Lumbar puncture and the risk of herniation: when should we first perform CT? J Neurol 2002; 249:129–137.
21. Marcos MA, Martínez E, Almela M, Mensa J, Jiménez de Anta MT. New rapid antigen test for diagnosis of pneumococcal meningitis. Lancet 2001; 357:1499–1500.
22. Milhaud D, Bernardin G, Rastello M, Mattei M, Blard JM. Meningites bacteriennes de l'adulte en reanimation medicale. Analyse clinique et etude des facteurs pronostiques. Presse Med 1996; 25:353–359.
23. Horwitz SJ, Boxerbaum B, O'Bell J. Cerebral herniation in bacterial meningitis in childhood. Ann Neurol 1980; 7:524–528.
24. McDonald JT, Uden DL. Intravenous glycerol and mannitol therapy in children with intracranial hypertension. Neurology 1982; 32:437–440.
25. Kastenbauer S, Winkler F, Pfister HW. Cranial CT before lumbar puncture in suspected meningitis. N Engl J Med 2002; 346:1248–1251.
26. Coyle PK. Glucocorticoids in central nervous system bacterial infection. Arch Neurol 1999; 56:796–801.
27. Odio CM, Faingezicht I, Paris M, et al. The beneficial effects of early dexamethasone administration in infants and children with bacterial meningitis. N Engl J Med 1991; 324:1525–1531.
28. McIntyre PB, Berkey CS, King SM, et al. Dexamethasone as adjunctive therapy in bacterial meningitis. A meta-analysis of randomized clinical trials since 1988. JAMA 1997; 278:925–931.
29. de Gans J, van de Beek D. Dexamethasone in adults with bacterial meningitis. N Engl J Med 2002; 347:1549–1556.
30. Girgis NI, Farid Z, Mikhail IA, et al. Dexamethasone treatment for bacterial meningitis in children and adults. Pediatr Infect Dis J 1989; 8:848–851.
31. Alvarez Lerma F, Cisneros JM, Viladrich PF, et al. Indications for admission to the intensive care service of adult patients with severe infections. Enferm Infecc Microbiol Clin 1998; 16:423–430.
32. Eriksen KR. Studies on induced resistance to penicillin in a pneumococcus type 1. Acta Pathol Microbiol Scand 1945; 22:398–405.

33. Kislac JV, Razavi LMB, Daly AK, Finland M. Susceptibility of pneumococci to nine antibiotics. Am J Med Sci 1965; 250:262–268.
34. Hansman D, Bullen MM. A resistant pneumococcus. Lancet 1967; 2:264–265.
35. Hansman D, Glasgow H, Surt J, Devitt HL, Douglas R. Increased resistance to penicillin of pneumococci isolated from man. N Engl J Med 1971; 284:175–177.
36. Hansman D, Devitt HL, Miles H, Riley I. Pneumococci relatively resistant to penicillin in Australia and New Guinea. Med J Aust 1974; 2:353–356.
37. Viladrich PF, Gudiol F, Liñares J, Rufí G, Ariza J, Pallarés R. Characteristics and antibiotic therapy of adult meningitis due to penicillin-resistant pneumococci. Am J Med 1988; 84:839–846.
38. Hieber JP, Nelson JD. A pharmacologic evaluation of penicillin in children with purulent meningitis. N Engl J Med 1977; 297:410–413.
39. Appelbaum PC, Scragg JN, Bowen AJ, Bhamjee A, Hallet AF, Cooper RC. *Streptococcus pneumoniae* resistant to penicillin and chloramphenicol. Lancet 1977; 2:995–997.
40. Jacobs MR, Koornhof HJ, Robins-Browne RM, et al. Emergence of multiply resistant pneumococci. N Engl J Med 1978; 299:735–740.
41. Frieland IR, Klugman KP. Failure of chloramphenicol therapy in penicillin-resistant pneumococcal meningitis. Lancet 1992; 339:405–408.
42. Liñares J, Alonso T, Perez JL, et al. Decreased susceptibility of penicillin-resistant pneumococci to 24 β-lactam antibiotics. J Antimicrob Chemother 1992; 30:279–288.
43. Asensi F, Pérez-Tamarit D, Otero MC, et al. Imipenem-cilastin therapy in a child with meningitis caused by a multiply resistant pneumococcus. Pediatr Infect Dis J 1989; 8:895.
44. Alonso J, Madrigal V, García-Fuentes M. Recurrent meningitis from a multiply resistant *Streptococcus pneumoniae* strain treated with erythromycin. Pediatr Infect Dis J 1991; 10:256.
45. Bradley JS, Connor JD. Ceftriaxone failure in meningitis caused by *Streptococcus pneumoniae* with reduced susceptibility to β-lactam antibiotics. Pediatr Infect Dis J 1991; 10:871–873.
46. Gellert G, Bock BV, Meyers H, Robertson C, Ehling LR. Penicillin resistant pneumococcal meningitis in an HIV-infected man. N Engl J Med 1991; 325:1047–1048.
47. Sloas MM, Barrett FF, Chesney PJ, et al. Cephalosporin treatment failure in penicillin- and cephalosporin-resistant *Streptococcus pneumoniae* meningitis. Pediatr Infect Dis J 1991; 1:662–666.
48. Friedland IR, Shelton S, Paris M, et al. Dilemmas in diagnosis and management of cephalosporin-resistant *Streptococcus pneumoniae* meningitis. Pediatr Infect Dis J 1993; 12:196–200.
49. Leggiadro RJ, Barret FF, Chesney PJ, Davis Y, Tenover FC. Invasive pneumococci with high level penicillin and cephalosporin resistance at a Mid-South Childrens Hospital. Pediatr Infect Dis J 1994; 13:320–322.
50. Asensi F, Otero MC, Pérez-Tamarit D, et al. Risk/benefit in the treatment of children with imipenem-cilastatin for meningitis caused by penicillin-resistant pneumococcus. J Chemother 1993; 5:133–134.
51. Kleiman MB, Weinberg GA, Reynolds JK, Allen SD. Meningitis with β-lactam-resistant *Streptococcus pneumoniae*: the need for early repeat lumbar puncture. Pediatr Infect Dis J 1993; 12:782–784.
52. John CC. Treatment failure with use of a third-generation cephalosporin for penicillin-resistant pneumococcal meningitis: case report and review. Clin Infect Dis 1994; 18:188–193.
53. Catalán MJ, Fernández JM, Vázquez A, Varela de Seijas E, Suárez A, Bernaldos de Quirós JCL. Failure of cefotaxime in the treatment of meningitis due to relatively resistant *Streptococcus pneumoniae*. Clin Infect Dis 1994; 18:766–769.

54. Guibert M, Chahime H, Petit J, Odievre M, Labrune P. Failure of cefotaxime treatment in two children with meningitis caused by highly penicillin-resistant *Streptococcus pneumoniae*. Acta Paediatr 1995; 84:831–833.
55. Lonks JR, Durkin MR, Meyerhoff AN, Medeiros AA. Meningitis due to ceftriaxone-resistant *Streptococcus pneumoniae*. N Engl J Med 1995; 332:893–894.
56. Flórez C, Silva G, Martín E. Cefotaxime failure in pneumococcal meningitis caused by a susceptible isolate. Pediatr Infect Dis J 1996; 15:723.
57. Michaus ML, Pérez-Díaz L, de Pablos M, Lezaun MJ, López-Bayón J. Fallo terapéutico con cefotaxima en dosis altas en meningitis neumocócica. Enferm Infecc Microbiol Clín 1997; 15:276–277.
58. National Committee for Clinical Laboratory Standards. Performance Standards for Antimicrobial Susceptibility Testing; Ninth Informational Supplement. Wayne, PA: National Committee for Clinical Laboratory Standards, 1999. M100-S9.
59. Viladrich PF, Cabellos C, Pallarés R, et al. High doses of cefotaxime in treatment of adult meningitis due to *Streptococcus pneumoniae* with decreased susceptibilities to broad-spectrum cephalosporins. Antimicrob Agents Chemother 1996; 40:218–220.
60. Tan TQ, Schutze GE, Mason EO, Kaplan SL. Antibiotic therapy and acute outcome of meningitis due to *Streptococcus pneumoniae* considered intermediately susceptible to broad-spectrum cephalosporins. Antimicrob Agents Chemother 1994; 38:918–923.
61. Viladrich P, Gudiol F, Liñares J, Rufí G, Ariza X, Pallarés R. Evaluation of vancomycin in the therapy of adult pneumococcal meningitis. Antimicrob Agents Chemother 1991; 35:2467–2472.
62. Paris M, Hickey SM, Uscher MI, Shelton S, Olsen KD, McCracken GH Jr. Effect of dexamethasone on therapy of experimental penicillin- and cephalosporin-resistant pneumococcal meningitis. Antimicrob Agents Chemother 1994; 38:1320–1324.
63. Cabellos C, Martínez-Lacasa J, Martos A, et al. Influence of dexamethasone on efficacy of ceftriaxone and vancomycin therapy in experimental pneumococcal meningitis. Antimicrob Agents Chemother 1995; 39:2158–2160.
64. Friedland IR, McCracken GH. Management of infections caused by antibiotic-resistant *Streptococcus pneumoniae*. N Engl J Med 1994; 331:377–382.
65. Paris MM, Ramilo O, McCracken GH. Management of meningitis caused by penicillin-resistant *Streptococcus pneumoniae*. Antimicrob Agents Chemother 1995; 39:2171–2175.
66. Quagliarello VJ, Scheld WM. Treatment of bacterial meningitis. N Engl J Med 1997; 336:708–716.
67. Kaplan SL. Management of pneumococcal meningitis. Pediatr Infect Dis J 2002; 21: 589–591.
68. Fenoll A, Asensio G, Jado I, et al. Antimicrobial susceptibility and pneumococcal serotypes. J Antimicrob Chemother 2002; 50(suppl. C):13–20.
69. Oteo J, Cruchaga S, Campos J, et al. Resistencia a antibióticos en 622 *Streptococcus pneumoniae* aislados de líquido cefalorraquídeo y sangre en 33 hospitales españoles de la Red Europea de Vigilancia de Resistencia de Antibióticos (2000). Enferm Infecc Microbiol Clín 2003; 21:12–19.
70. Friedland IR, Klugman KP. Cerebrospinal fluid bactericidal activity against cephalosporin-resistant *Streptococcus pneumoniae* in children with meningitis treated with high-dosage cefotaxime. Antimicrob Agents Chemother 1997; 41:1888–1891.
71. Friedland IR, Paris M, Shelton S, McCracken Jr. Time-kill studies of antibiotic combinations against penicillin-resistant and -susceptible *Streptococcus pneumoniae*. J Antimicrob Chemother 1994; 43:231–237.
72. Friedland IR, Paris M, Ehrett S, Hickey S, Olsen KD, McCracken GH. Evaluation of antimicrobial regimens for treatment of experimental penicillin and cephalosporin resistant pneumococcal meningitis. Antimicrob Agents Chemother 1993; 37:1630–1636.

73. Klugman KP, Friedland IR, Bradley JS. Bactericidal activity against cephalosporin-resistant *Streptococcus pneumoniae* in cerebrospinal fluid of children with acute bacterial meningitis. Antimicrob Agents Chemother 1995; 39:1989–1992.
74. Doit CP, Bonacorsi SP, Fremaux AJ, et al. In vitro killing activities of antibiotics at clinically achievable concentrations in cerebrospinal fluid against penicillin-resistant *Streptococcus pneumoniae* isolated from children with meningitis. Antimicrob Agents Chemother 1994; 38:2655–2659.
75. Tubau F, Liñares J, Ardanuy C, et al. Actividad bactericida in vitro de diferentes combinaciones de antibióticos frente a *Streptococcus pneumoniae* resistente a penicilina y cefotaxima. Enferm Infecc Microbiol Clin 1996; 14:590–595.
76. Fiore AE, Moroney JF, Farley MM, et al. Clinical outcomes of meningitis caused by *Streptococcus pneumoniae* in the era of antibiotic resistance. Clin Infect Dis 2000; 30:71–77.
77. Kellner JD, Scheifele DW, Halperin SA, et al. Outcome of penicillin-nonsusceptible *Streptococcus pneumoniae* meningitis: a nested case-control study. Pediatr Infect Dis J 2002; 21:903–910.
78. Liñares J, Pérez JL, Garau J, Murgui L, Martin R. Comparative susceptibilities of penicillin-resistant pneumococci to co-trimozazole, vancomyin, rifampin, and 14 β-lactam antibiotics. J Antimicrob Chemother 1984; 13:353–359.
79. Fenoll A, Jado I, Vicioso D, Pérez A, Casal J. Evolution of *Streptococcus pneumoniae* serotypes and antibiotic resistance in Spain: update (1990–1996). J Clin Microbiol 1998; 36:3447–3454.
80. Whitney CG, Farley MM, Hadler J, et al. Increasing prevalence of multidrug-resistant *Streptococcus pneumoniae* in United States. N Engl J Med 2000; 343:1917–1924.
81. Nahata MC, Fan-Havard P, Barson WJ, Bartkowski HM, Kosnic EJ. Pharmacokinetics, cerebrospinal fluid concentration, and safety of intravenous rifampin in pediatric patients undergoing shunt replacements. Eur J Clin Pharmacol 1990; 38:515–517.
82. Nau R, Wellmer A, Soto A, et al. Rifampin reduces early mortality in experimental *Streptococcus pneumoniae* meningitis. J Infect Dis 1999; 179:1557–1560.
83. Böttcher T, Gerber J, Wellmer A, et al. Rifampin reduces production of reactive oxygen species of cerebrospinal fluid phagocytes and hippocampal neuronal apoptosis in experimental *Streptococcus pneumoniae* meningitis. J Infect Dis 2000; 181:2095–2098.
84. Barakett V, Lesage D, Delisle F, Vergaz P, Petit JC. Killing kinetics of vancomycin and rifampin tested alone and in combination against penicillin-resistant *Streptococcus pneumoniae*. Eur J Clin Microbiol Infect Dis 1993; 12:69–71.
85. Nau R, Kaye K, Sachdeva M, Sande ER, Täuber MG. Rifampin for therapy of experimental pneumococcal meningitis in rabbits. Antimicrob Agents Chemother 1994; 38:1186–1189.
86. Martínez-Lacasa J, Cabellos C, Martos A, et al. Experimental study of the efficacy of vancomycin, rifampin and dexamethasone in the therapy of pneumococcal meningitis. J Antimicrob Chemother 2002; 49:507–513.
87. Radetsky MS, Johansen TL, Lauer BA, et al. Multiply resistant pneumococcus causing meningitis: its epidemiology within a day-care center. Lancet 1981; 2:771–773.
88. Viladrich PF, Tubau F, Cabellos C, et al. Vancomycin plus rifampin for therapy of adult pneumococcal meningitis. Ninth European Congress of Clinical Microbiology and Infectious Diseases; Berlin, Germany; March 21–24, 1999. Abstract P616.
89. Buzón LM, Guerrero A, Romero J, Santamaría JM, Bouza E. Penicillin-resistant *Streptococcus pneumoniae* meningitis treated with vancomycin. Eur J Clin Microbiol 1984; 3:442.
90. Dagan R, Velghe L, Rodda JL, Klugman KP. Penetration of meropenem into the cerebrospinal fluid of patients with inflamed meninges. J Antimicrob Chemother 1994; 34:497–498.
91. Fuchs PC, Barry AL, Brown SD. Pneumococcal susceptibility to meropenem. J Antimicrob Chemother 1996; 37:1036–1037.

92. Nau R, Schmidt T, Kaye K, Froula JL, Täuber MG. Quinolone antibiotics in therapy of experimental pneumococcal meningitis in rabbits. Antimicrob Agents Chemother 1995; 39:593–597.
93. Ostergaard C, Klitmoller Sorensen T, Dahl Knudsen J, Frimodt-Moller N. Evaluation of moxifloxacin, a new 8-methoxyquinlone, for treatment of meningitis caused by a penicillin-resistant pneumococcus in rabbits. Antimicrob Agents Chemother 1998; 42:1706–1712.
94. Shapiro M, Donovan KD, Gage JW. 2000. Comparative therapeutic efficacy of clinafloxacin in a pneumococcal meningitis mouse model. J Antimicrob Chemother 2000; 45:489–492.
95. Smirnov A, Wellmer A, Gerber J, Maier K, Henne S, Nau R. Gemifloxacin is effective in experimental pneumococcal meningitis. Antimicrob Agents Chemother 2000; 44: 767–770.
96. Cottagnoud P, Acosta F, Cottagnoud M, Tauber MG. Gemifloxacin is efficacious against penicillin-resistant and quinolone-resistant pneumococci in experimental meningitis. Antimicrob Agents Chemother 2002; 46:1607–1609.
97. Cottagnoud P, Acosta F, Cottagnoud M, Pfister M, Tauber MG. Efficacies of BMS284756 against penicillin-sensitive, penicillin-resistant, and quinolone-resistant pneumococci in experimental meningitis. Antimicrob Agents Chemother 2002; 46:184–187.
98. Sáez-Llorens X, McCoig C, Feris J, et al. Quinolone treatment for pediatric bacterial meningitis: a comparative study of trovafloxacin and ceftriaxone with or without vancomycin. Pediatr Infect Dis J 2002; 21:14–22.
99. Chen DK, McGeer A, de Azavedo JC, Low DE. Decreased susceptibility of *Streptococcus pneumoniae* to fluoroquinolones in Canada. N Engl J Med 1999; 341:233–239.
100. Empey PE, Jenning HR, Thornton AC, Rapp RP, Evans ME. Levofloxacin failure in a patient with pneumococcal pneumonia. Ann Pharmacother 2001; 35:687–690.
101. Davidson R, Cavalcanti R, Brunton JL, et al. Resistance to levofloxacin and failure of treatment of pneumococcal pneumonia. N Engl J Med 2002; 346:747–750.
102. Wortmann GW, Bennett SP. Fatal meningitis due to levofloxacin-resistant *Streptococcus pneumoniae*. Clin Infect Dis 1999; 29:1599–1560.
103. Liñares J, De la Campa AG, Pallares R. Fluoroquinolone resistance in *Streptococcus pneumoniae*. N Engl J Med 2001; 341:1546–1547.
104. Cottagnoud P, Gerber CM, Acosta F, Cottagnoud M, Neftel K, Tauber MG. Linezolid against penicillin-sensitive and -resistant pneumococci in the rabbit meningitis model. J Antimicrob Chemother 2000; 36:1403–1413.
105. Gomez-Barreto D, Calderon-Jaimes E, Rodríguez RS, de los Monteros LE. Clinical outcome of invasive infections in children caused by highly penicillin-resistant *Streptococcus pneumoniae* compared with infections caused by penicillin-susceptible strains. Arch Med Res 2000; 31:592–598.
106. Black S, Shinefield H, Fireman B, et al. Efficacy, safety and immunogenicity of heptavalent pneumococcal conjugate vaccine in children. Northern California Kaiser Permanent Vaccine Study Center Group. Pediatr Infect Dis J 2000; 19:187–195.
107. Dagan R, Fraser D. Conjugate pneumococcal vaccine and antibiotic-resistant *Streptococcus pneumoniae*: herd immunity and reduction of otitis morbidity. Pediatr Infect Dis J 2000; 19:S79–S88.
108. Pai VB, Heyneman CA, Erramouspe J. Conjugated heptavalent pneumococcal vaccine. Ann Pharmacother 2002; 36:1403–1413.
109. Viladrich PF, Cabellos C, Martos A, Martinez Lacasa JT, Gudiol F. Lack of efficacy of pneumococcal vaccine in preventing pneumococcal meningitis due to cerebrospinal fluid leaks. 32nd Interscience Conference on Antimicrobial Agents and Chemotherapy (ICAAC); Anaheim, CA; October 11–14, 1992. Abstract 1282.

3

Emerging Resistance to Vancomycin, Rifampin, and Fluoroquinolones in *Streptococcus pneumoniae*

Joseph M. Blondeau

1. INTRODUCTION

Antimicrobial resistance is a common global problem. During the 1970–1980s, resistance was considered a hospital-based problem mainly related to nosocomially acquired resistant organisms. Throughout the 1990s, there was recognition that many community-acquired pathogens were resistant to first-line antibiotics, thereby prompting the use (in some clinical situations) of broader spectrum agents. Toward the late 1990s and currently, the realization is that community-acquired pathogens may be multiresistant. Some patients may require hospitalization for therapy; others may be treated as outpatients. Regardless, the complexity of resistance is dictating a necessary change in the approach to therapy in patients with multiresistant pathogens. These developments have forced a reevaluation of the approach to empiric therapy—changes that have appeared in various expert working group guidelines.

The scope of resistance is broad and impossible to cover in one chapter. Rather, this summary focuses on *Streptococcus pneumoniae*; first, a broad overview on resistance is given, and then resistance to rifampin, vancomycin, and the quinolones is discussed more specifically. First, however, a brief summary on what is meant by antimicrobial resistance is presented.

A schematic representation of the mechanism of antimicrobial resistance is shown in Fig. 1. Resistance may be broadly categorized as intrinsic, acquired, or *de novo*. For intrinsic resistance, the organism either lacks the specific target to which the antimicrobial agent must bind to exert a biological effect or the target is present, but not readily accessible by the drug. For acquired resistance, an organism becomes less susceptible to the drug than it initially was. Acquisition of resistance may occur by transmissible genetic elements such as plasmids or transposons. Finally, *de novo* resistance arises from the bacterial population and results from mutation in the host chromosome that affects genes encoding for proteins targeted by various antimicrobial agents.

The major mechanisms of resistance described include the following:

- Decreased uptake/altered membrane permeability
- Efflux

From: *Management of Multiple Drug-Resistant Infections*
Edited by: S. H. Gillespie © Humana Press Inc., Totowa, NJ

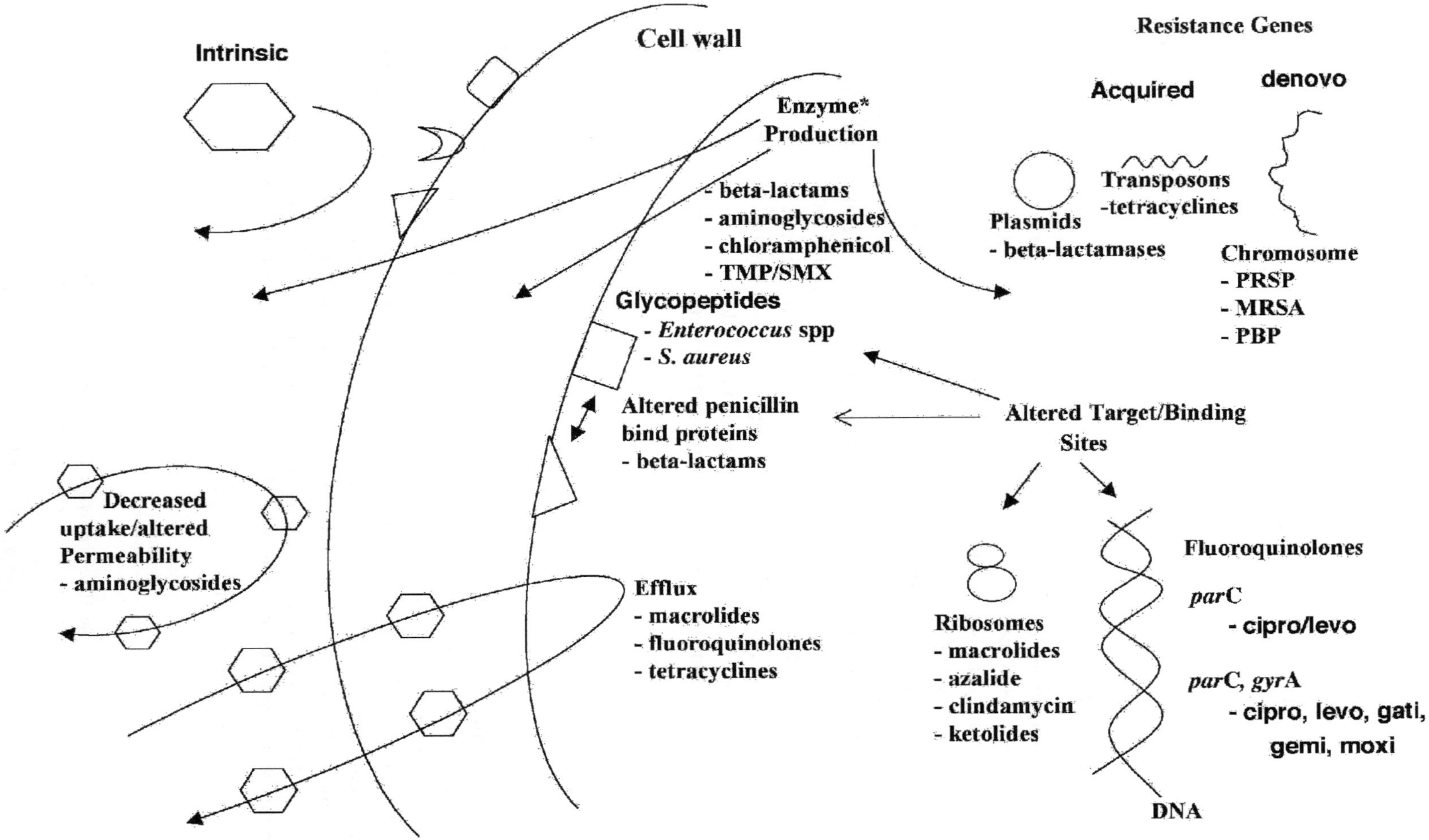

Fig. 1. Schematic representation of the mechanisms of antimicrobial resistance (cipro, ciprofloxacin; gati, gatifloxacin; gemi, gemifloxacin; levo, levofloxacin; moxi, moxifloxacin). (Adapted from ref. *1a*.)

- Enzymatic modification of the antimicrobial compound
- Altered target/binding sites

A single bacterium may have only one mechanism of resistance or may simultaneously possess multiple mechanisms, thereby conferring multidrug resistance.

2. *STREPTOCOCCUS PNEUMONIAE*

Streptococcus pneumoniae continues to be among the most common bacterial pathogens associated with community-acquired pneumonia and is a significant cause of sinusitis, acute bacterial exacerbations of chronic bronchitis, and otitis media. From data I summarized *(1)*, *S. pneumoniae* is associated with 30 to75% of cases of community-acquired pneumonia and is associated with the majority of the most severe cases, including those that caused death. For decades, *S. pneumoniae* was considered predictably susceptible to penicillin, which remained the drug of choice for therapy in infected patients. Erythromycin and tetracycline were alternatives for therapy in patients with β-lactam-related allergies. The rapid emergence of penicillin-resistant *S. pneumoniae* (particularly in the 1990s) and the concomitant cross-resistance to many other antimicrobial agents has demanded that routine susceptibility testing be performed on each isolate deemed clinically significant.

2.1. *Emergence of Resistance*

Penicillin-nonsusceptible pneumococci date back more than half a century, when an isolate with decreased susceptibility to sulfapyridine was recovered from a patient treated with that compound. During the 1940s, *S. pneumoniae* isolates demonstrating intermediate penicillin resistance were shown in laboratory strains. The era of clinically significant problems experienced with resistant pneumococci occurred in the 1960s, when Australian investigators *(2)* described pneumococci demonstrating intermediate levels of penicillin resistance. South African investigators *(3,4)* subsequently characterized pneumococcal isolates demonstrating full resistance to penicillin. Concurrently, a number of investigators reported pneumococci resistant to tetracycline in 1963 *(5)*, erythromycin in 1963 *(6)*, and clindamycin in 1967 *(7)*. Resistance to quinolones *(7a)* and third-generation cephalosporins was reported in the 1980s *(8)* and throughout the 1990s. As of yet, vancomycin resistance has not yet appeared; however, strains showing tolerance have been described *(9)*.

2.2. *Mechanism of Resistance*

β-Lactamase enzyme has not yet been associated with pneumococcal resistance, and no other enzymatic mechanism has been described. Pneumococci are naturally transformable *(10)*, a property that appears essential to the evolution of antimicrobial resistance *(11,12)*. Resistance occurs following mutations in native DNA as a result of incorporation of externally acquired naked DNA. Naked DNA may come from sources such as other strains of pneumococci, α-hemolytic *Streptococci*, or other organisms colonizing oral-pharyngeal surfaces. Alterations in native DNA result in changes of the penicillin-binding proteins (PBPs). The high molecular weight proteins 1A, 2B, and 2X are modified.

PBPs are important structural proteins found in the peptidoglycan layer of the bacterial cell wall and are essential for cell wall formation as they mediate the crosslinking of peptidoglycan. Peptidoglycan provides structured integrity and rigidity to the cell wall. PBPs are the targets for β-lactam antimicrobial agents. The binding of β-lactam agents to PBPs prevents cross-linking of the peptidoglycan layer. Instability of the bacterial cell wall because of interference with peptidoglycan formation leads to autolysis and death of the organism.

Clinical isolates of *S. pneumoniae* have also been shown resistant to other antimicrobial agents. Pneumococci resistant to macrolides, clindamycin, and lincosamides are the results of either constitutive or inducible methylation of the 23SrRNA *(13)*. Organisms demonstrating multiple resistant phenotypes, including erythromycin, streptomycin, kanamycin, tetracycline, and chloramphenicol, are likely because of the transposable element Tn1545 *(14)*. Resistance to chloramphenicol is often linked to other agents, such as penicillin or tetracycline. Unfortunately, there is a coincidental cross-resistance that correlates with the level of penicillin resistance among pneumococci. It has been reported repeatedly *(15–17)* that penicillin-susceptible pneumococci (minimum inhibitory concentration [MIC] ≤ 0.06 μg/mL) remain susceptible to a broad range of antimicrobial agents, including β-lactams, macrolides, cephalosporins, trimethoprim-sulfamethoxazole, tetracyclines, and quinolones. For pneumococci that demonstrate high-level (MIC ≥ 2 μg/mL) resistance to penicillin, resistance to all of the above agents, with the exception of quinolones, is found. The exact mechanisms of resistance have not been fully elucidated, but clearly involve the acquisition or development of one or more of the resistance determinants summarized in Fig. 1.

2.3. Epidemiology of Resistance

The dramatic increase in penicillin-nonsusceptible clinical isolates in the 1990s remains largely unexplained. Although antimicrobial use and misuse seems the most suitable target for a cause, it may not be the only explanation. Considerable emphasis has been placed on increasing antimicrobial resistance of respiratory pathogens. Clearly, the intensity of characterizing penicillin-resistant pneumococci was noticeable in the 1990s and continues today. This is undoubtedly because of the rapid increase in both intermediate and high-level penicillin-resistant pneumococci.

Data summarized to 1990 indicated that the incidence of penicillin-resistant *S. pneumoniae* fluctuated between 5 and 10% in North America *(18)*. Almost all isolates demonstrated intermediate resistance to penicillin. Since then, the numbers have climbed dramatically. For example, Canadian data summarized to 1996 indicated that 11.7% of pneumococcal isolates were penicillin resistant, with 8.4% having intermediate resistance and 3.3% high-level resistance. In the United States, Doern et al. *(19)* tested over 1500 clinical isolates of *S. pneumoniae* from 30 US medical centers and found that the overall incidence of penicillin resistance was 23.6%, with 14.1% intermediate and 9.5% high-level resistance. Subsequently, Thornsberry et al. *(20)* reported that 33.5% of over 9000 pneumococcal isolates demonstrated reduced susceptibility to penicillin, with 19.9% showing intermediate and 13.6% high-level resistance.

The studies of both Doern et al. *(19)* and Thornsberry et al. *(20)* demonstrated important regional or institutional differences in the percentage of isolates showing reduced susceptibility. As a consequence, these findings strengthen the argument that local susceptibility data are important for appropriate use of antimicrobial agents specific to a geographical area. An important difference in pneumococcal resistance data from the early 1990s to today is the dramatic increase in the incidence of pneumococci with a high level of resistance. As indicated, isolates from the late 1980s to early 1990s demonstrated intermediate resistance only, whereas 10 to 15% of isolates in the late 1990s demonstrated high-level resistance. Therapeutic failures are more likely to occur with organisms with a high level of resistance.

Critchley et al. *(17)* reported on pneumococcal susceptibility in the United States from the 1997–1998 respiratory season. Of more than 5600 pneumococcal isolates, 22% showed intermediate resistance to penicillin, and 14% were high-level resistant. The importance of geographical variability was demonstrated in this study as data from nine regions in the United States showed that the percentage of intermediate resistant isolates varied from 14 to 28% and from 11 to 24% for high-level resistant organisms. Combined nonsusceptibity varied from 26 to 49%. The data of Critchley et al. clearly emphasize the importance of defining local or geographical resistance rates as a guide to the appropriate use of antimicrobial agents. Both intermediate and high-level resistant pneumococci were more likely to be recovered from respiratory tract infections than from blood or other sources.

From another US-based study, Jacobs et al. *(23)* tested 1476 pneumococcal isolates from outpatients in six geographical regions of the United States. Some of the highest pneumococcal resistance rates in the United States were reported because 50.4% of isolates demonstrated some level of penicillin resistance (17.9% intermediate, 32.5% high level). Variability ranged from 35.8 to 60.7% overall from different regions (14.6 to 20.6% intermediate, 21.2 to 40.1% high level). Pfaller et al. *(21)* also reported that 36.1% of 341 pneumococcal bloodstream isolates were penicillin resistant.

Resistance to other antimicrobial agents is disturbing and problematic for both intermediate and high-level penicillin-resistant pneumococci. Data reported in studies by Doern et al. *(19)*, Simor et al. *(22)*, Jacobs et al. *(23)*, and work from my laboratory *(16)* reported, based on recommended breakpoints from the National Committee for Clinical Laboratory Standards (NCCLS) *(24)*, 36 to 38.3% of isolates with intermediate susceptibility to penicillin were also resistant to second-generation cephalosporins (i.e., cefuroxime), 1 to 9.5% were resistant to third-generation cephalosporins (cefotaxime/ceftriaxone), 8 to 34.5% were resistant to azalide/macrolide agents, 17 to 21% were resistant to tetracycline, and 40 to 54% were resistant to trimethoprim-sulfamethoxazole. Isolates fully resistant to penicillin showed the following levels of resistance: 99–100% were resistant to cefuroxime, 32 to 93.3% to cefotaxime/ceftriaxone, 17 to 66.7% to azalide/macrolide compound, 25 to 43% to tetracycline, and 80 to 97% to trimethoprim-sulfamethoxazole. Similar data were also reported by Critchley et al. *(17)*. For pneumococcal isolates demonstrating high-level resistance to penicillin, 96% were resistant to amoxicillin/clavulanic acid, 86% to ceftriaxone, and 99% to cefuroxime. Data from the same study showed that 93% of high-level resistant pneumococci were resistant to trimethoprim-sulfamethoxazole, and 72% were resistant to azalide/macrolide (azithromycin, clarithromycin, erythromycin) compounds. Recent changes to NCCLS susceptibility breakpoint for β-lactam agents will change (lower) percentage resistance to some compounds. The important point remains, however, that clinical isolates with *S. pnemoniae* are no longer as susceptible to antimicrobial agents as they once were and this has important clinical implications.

3. RIFAMPIN

Rifampin is a bactericidal, semisynthetic derivative of rifamycin B. Rifamycin B is a macrocyclic antimicrobial compound from the mold *Streptomyces mediterranei* and was first isolated in 1957. Rifampin is the 3-4-methyl-piperazinyl-iminomethyl derivative of rifamycin SV.

The bactericidal effect of rifamycin occurs by inhibition of DNA-dependent RNA polymerase at the level of the β-subunit *(25,26)*. This effect prevents chain initiation, but not chain elongation. According to Zillig et al. *(27)*, the RNA polymerase molecule consists of five subunits designated at α_2 BB^1 σ, and rifampin binds directly to the β-subunit. Bacterial resistance to rifampin occurs following mutation occurring in the *rpo*B gene, with the result being alteration in rifampin binding. Such alterations result in highly resistant organisms.

There are limited data on rifampin-resistant *S. pneumoniae*. Rifampin resistance has been studied with the following genus and species of bacteria: *Escherichia coli (28), Mycobacterium tuberculosis (29–32), Mycobacterium smegmatis (33,34), Mycobacterium leprae (35)*, and *Neisseria meningitidis (28)*.

To date, the designations for mutation within the *rpo*B gene are based on the protein coordinates for *E. coli*. Three distinct clusters of mutations in the *rpo*B gene have been characterized. These include cluster I, which spans amino acids 502 to 532; cluster II, which spans amino acids 560 to 572; and cluster III, which defines a single mutation at position 687 *(27,36–38)*. Although these regions and mutations have accounted for most of the rifampin resistance reported in most species of bacteria, the presence of other mutations has made mapping of the central rifampin resistance region more difficult *(39)*.

Rifampin resistance in *S. pneumoniae* was recently studied by Padayachee and Klugman *(40)* using clinical isolates collected from South Africa. They studied 32 isolates: 24 rifampin resistant and 8 rifampin susceptible. Sequence analysis of the 24 resistant strains revealed cluster I mutations in 18 isolates as well as some novel mutations that occurred in an area designated as pneumococcus cluster III. Cluster I mapped to *S. pneumoniae* amino acid position 406 to 434, and cluster II mapped to amino acids 462 to 472. Of the 18 isolates with mutations in cluster I, 11 displayed Asp_{415}-Glu as well as His_{425}-Asn substitutions. Isolates with the His_{425}-Asn substitutions had MICs between 32 and 128 μg/mL. For strains with both substitutions, the MICs were not elevated further. For the remaining 7 resistant isolates, 6 contained His_{425}-Asn mutations, and the remaining strain had a His_{425}-Asn mutation plus several novel downstream mutations (Arg_{523}-Lys, Glu_{526}-Ala, Iso_{534}-Val, Asn_{549}-Ser, Iso_{550}-Ser, Asn_{595}-Glu, Gln_{597}-Lys, Tyr_{600}-Phe). The isolate with the highest MIC (256 μg/mL) to rifampin contained a His_{425}-Asn (cluster I) plus all of the other novel mutations mentioned.

Several observations from the report of Padayachee and Klugman *(40)* are worthy of summary:

- Rifampin resistance with *S. pneumoniae* isolates appeared to be in the β-subunit of the *rpo*B gene.
- Most isolates (75%) had mutations in cluster I.
- This was the first report in *S. pneumoniae* of an Asp_{415}-Glu substitution, a mutation previously shown in *M. tuberculosis* and conferring resistance *(30,31)*.
- The His_{425}-Asn substitution has been reported for *S. pneumoniae (41), N. meningitids (28)*, and *M. tuberculosis (31,32)*.

- His_{425}-Asn mutations are sufficient to confer high-level resistance, and the addition of a second (Asp_{415}-Glu) or more mutations contributes to higher MICs.

The molecular evolution of rifampin resistance in *S. pneumoniae* was studied by Enright et al. *(41)*. Nucleotide sequence analysis was made of a 270-basepair (bp) fragment of the *rpo*B gene from 16 pneumococcal isolates that were rifampin susceptible and from 8 rifampin-resistant strains. Three spontaneous rifampin-resistant mutants were also studied. The isolates studied were collected from 1930 (1 isolate), 1944 (1 isolate), 1970 (1 isolate), the 1980s (6 isolates), and the 1990s (13 isolates); for 6 isolates, the year of collection was unknown. The isolates were collected from Spain, the United Kingdom, the United States, Poland, Kenya, South Africa, the Czech Republic, and Papua New Guinea.

The 270-bp fragment sequenced was homologous to part of the *rpo*B gene from *E. coli (38,41)*, and this included *rpo*B cluster I. Of the 22 clinical isolates, 8 were rifampin resistant, with MICs ranging from 6 to more than 256 µg/mL. Sequence analysis revealed that rifampin resistance in pneumococcal strains was similar to that reported for *E. coli*, *M. tuberculosis*, *N. meningitidis*, and *M. leprae* and involved amino acid alterations to the β-subunit of RNA polymerase, with the mutations usually found in the cluster I region. There were two rifampin-resistant pneumococcal strains from Poland that lacked cluster I amino acid substitution, but these isolates possessed cluster II mutations. This observation was consistent with a similar finding in *E. coli* reported by Severinov et al. *(42)*.

When numbering based on *E. coli* was used, the cluster I amino acid substitutions in rifampin resistant *S. pneumoniae* isolates mapped to two sites: Asp_{516} and His_{526}. In *E. coli*, the Asp_{516}-Asn and His_{526}-Tyr conferred rifampin resistance, and in the same was true for *S. pneumoniae*.

Several important observations were noted in Enright et al.'s *(41)* study:

- The 270-bp nucleotide sequence of all pneumococcal strains tested (susceptible and resistant) differed by 3% or more when compared to each other.
- No relationship appeared present between serogroup/serotype and DNA sequence.
- The DNA sequences of the eight naturally rifampin-resistant strains were not markedly distinct from rifampin-sensitive isolates.

Table 1 is a summary of select susceptibility surveillance data collected from numerous studies and representing a broad geographical distribution. Overall, the incidence of rifampin nonsusceptibility remains low, less than 3%, with the exception of the Ivory Coast, where a rate of 5.8% nonsusceptibility was reported. Whether these rates are linked to rifampin usage would be interesting to explore.

4. VANCOMYCIN

Vancomycin is a narrow-spectrum (Gram-positive) bactericidal antimicrobial agent isolated from *Streptomyces orientales*. Vancomycin was released in the mid-1950s and was effective against penicillin-resistant *Staphylococcus* species. Its activity against methicillin-resistant *Staphylococcus* species and penicillin-resistant *S. pneumoniae* has made this compound necessary when these resistant pathogens are suspected and alternative agents are not available.

Vancomycin is a soluble complex glycopolypeptide. Its method of action involves the inhibition of synthesis of the second stage of cell wall peptidoglycan polymers by

Table 1
Summary of Select Studies on Rifampin Susceptibility and Resistance for *Streptococcus pneumoniae*

Year/Country	Isolates (*n*)	Penicillin[a] susceptibility (%)	MIC_{90}	Rifampin susceptibility (%) S	I	R	Reference
1996–1997							
United States	820	S	0.03	99.8	—	0.2	*42a*
	218	I	0.03	100	—	0.2	
	238	R	0.03	99.6	—	0.4	
Ivory Coast	138	18.1 I, 4.3 R		94.2		5.8 (I & R)	*42b*
Morocco	98	8.2 I, 1 R		100	0	0	
Senegal	81	53.1 I, 8.6 R		100	0	0	
Tunisia	58	34.5 I, 6.9 R		100	0	0	
1997–1999							
United States	4193	86 S & I, 14 R	≤1	99.7		0.3	*45*
Canada	887	93.2 S & I, 6.8 R	≤1	99.8		0.2	*45*
Latin America	948	88.3 S & I, 11.7 R	≤1	97.5		2.5	*45*
Europe	1478	89.6 S & I, 10.4 R	≤1	99.2		0.8	*45*
Asia-Pacific	567	82.2 S & I, 17.8 R	≤1	99.4		0.6	*45*
Taiwan	200	28 I, 33 R	0.12	100		0	*46*

[a]Penicillin susceptible (S) ≤ 0.06 μg/mL; intermediate (I) = 0.1–1 μg/mL; resistant (R) ≥ 2 μg/mL.

binding with the D-alanyl-D-alanine precursor. A second mechanism of action involves damage to protoplasts by altering cytoplasmic membrane permeability. Vancomycin may also impair RNA synthesis.

Resistance became obvious in 1989 when vancomycin-resistant enterococci (VRE) emerged in the United States as an important and difficult-to-control nosocomial pathogen. Subsequent to this was the 1997 recognition of *S. aureus* from Japanese hospitals that was intermediately resistant to vancomycin.

The most significant recent development occurred in the United States in 2002 when a 40-yr-old male patient with diabetes, peripheral vascular disease, and chronic renal failure had vancomycin-resistant *S. aureus* (VRSA) isolated from a swab collected from a catheter exit site. The patient had previously been treated with multiple courses of antibiotics, including vancomycin. The patient had previously had infections related to methicillin-resistant *S. aureus* (MRSA), *Klebsiella oxytoca*, and vancomycin-resistant *Enterococcus faecalis*. From VRE, the vancomycin-resistant determinants *van*A, *van*B, *van*D, *van*E, *van*F, and *van*G have been reported, but none of these were reported from *S. aureus* isolates *(43)*. However, conjugative transfer of the *van*A gene from enterococci to *S. aureus* was demonstrated in vitro *(44)*.

A *van*A determinant was found in the VRSA isolate described in the preceding paragraph, and it was suggested that it was acquired by exchange of genetic material from the VRE isolate also present at the catheter site—it also was recovered with the VRSA from the swab of the site.

These observations have served notice that emerging vancomycin resistance may further compromise the use of this compound for serious multiresistant, Gram-positive infections.

Pneumococcal resistance to vancomycin remains rare or nonexistent. Some surveillance studies reported susceptibility rates of more than 99%; as such, some isolates must not be fully susceptible at breakpoint. This may not necessarily mean resistance as MICs may indicate intermediate levels of resistance. For example, Hoban et al. *(45)* reported that 0.1% of pneumococcal isolates from Europe and 0.3% from Asia-Pacific had MICs to vancomycin of more than 1 μg/mL. How likely is the occurrence of vancomycin resistance in *S. pneumoniae*? Novak et al. *(9)* reported on the emergence of vancomycin tolerance in *S. pneumoniae*.

Hsueh et al. *(46)* reported that the MIC_{90} values were not different for either rifampin or vancomycin and neither compound was affected by susceptibility to penicillin, macrolides, and trimethoprim-sulfamethoxazole. Song et al. *(47)* reported that 100% of 996 pneumococcal isolates collected from 11 Asian countries (Korea, $n = 177$; Japan, $n = 84$; Thailand, $n = 126$; Vietnam, $n = 46$; Sri Lanka, $n = 41$; Taiwan, $n = 137$; Indonesia, $n = 33$; Singapore, $n = 84$; Malaysia, $n = 34$; India, $n = 183$; China, $n = 51$) were susceptible to vancomycin. Penicillin susceptibility rates from the countries ranged from 3.8 to 79.7%.

Novak et al. *(9)* wrote that "the emergence of vancomycin resistance in this community-acquired bacterium (i.e., *S. pneumoniae*) would be catastrophic." Adding to their concern was the fact that multiresistant strains were widespread, and that vancomycin is the antibiotic of last resort. Tomasz et al. *(48)* indicated that antibiotic tolerance was the ability of bacteria to survive but not grow (replicate) in the presence of the drug, and that tolerance was a precursor phenotype to resistance.

Based on data provided by Tomasz et al. *(48)*, Moreillon et al. *(49)*, and Holtje and Tuomanen *(50)*, Novak et al. *(9)* summarized that activation of bacterially encoded death effectors was necessary for the bactericidal activity of antimicrobial agents that block cell wall synthesis. Tomasz et al. *(48)* had previously shown the autolysin protein (LytA) of *S. pneumoniae* digested the cell wall exoskeletons of the organisms following some form of stimulation by antibiotics. Moreillon et al. reported that penicillin kills pneumococci by two distinct mechanisms. The first involves amidase, which results in a 1-log killing every 6 h, and the second is an amidase-independent mechanism that results in a 3- to 4-log killing every 6 h. The mutation affecting amidase resulted in a reduction in killing potential.

From their report on vancomycin-tolerant *S. pneumoniae*, Novak et al. *(9)* showed that loss of function of the *vnc*S histidine kinase resulted in tolerance to vancomycin, β-lactams, cephalosporins, aminoglycosides, and quinolones. From their investigations of a penicillin- and vancomycin-tolerant mutant, they identified *vnc*S as an operon encoding a histidine kinase and *vnc*R as a contiguous response regulator. Insertion–duplication mutagenesis of either the *vnc*S or the *vns*R gene to create a loss of function was performed to determine what role, if any, either of these genes or gene products had in promoting tolerance to vancomycin.

Analysis of tolerance was determined by time-consuming kill experiments, and vancomycin tolerance was defined as killing of 2 ± 0.6 log or fewer bacteria in 4 h. Following exposure to 10 times the MIC of vancomycin, tolerance was not demonstrated

(4 log loss in viability by 4 h) for the parental strain or for a *vnc*R mutant. In contrast, a *vnc*S mutant stopped replicating, but had almost no loss in viability. The MIC values to both penicillin and vancomycin remained unchanged, and Novak et al. *(9)* suggested that this meant the compounds still had access to their respective targets. This unfortunate observation suggests that such tolerant strains cannot be detected by routine antimicrobial susceptibility testing. The observation that the vancomycin-tolerant strain also showed tolerance to other compounds suggests that signal transduction through *vnc*S is required for bacterial death in response to a broad range of components with very different mechanisms of action.

Further data from Novak et al. *(9)* on tolerant strains were also intriguing. These researchers compared deduced amino acid sequences of *vnc*S and *vnc*R to the *van*S_B-*van*R_B regulatory system encoded on plasmids or conjugative chromosomal elements of vancomycin-resistant *Enterococcus faecalis (51)* and found 38% homology. The mechanism of resistance in *Enterococci* may be different from the tolerance described for vancomycin with the pneumococci. As summarized by Novak et al. *(9)*, *van*R_B activates the transduction of *van*H_B, *van*B and *van*X_B genes were not found in the *S. pneumoniae* genome, suggesting that resistance and tolerance may be mediated by changes to different gene products.

In extending the role of the autolysin LytA and the bactericidal action of penicillin against *S. pneumoniae*, Novak et al. *(9)* reported that an alteration in the control of the autolytic pathway seemed more responsible for the lack of autolysis in the presence of vancomycin than the actual amount of inherent activity of the autolysis itself. This was concluded from Western blot experiments that showed the amount of LytA in *vnc*S mutants was not different from that of the wild type.

Several concerns relating to the observations summarized above arise. Liu and Tomasz *(52)* indicated that tolerance may accelerate the development of drug resistance as it allows for survivors in the presence of the drug; as such, tolerant strains may favor the acquisition of resistant mutations. Clearly, an increase in the prevalence of tolerant strains and the subsequent conversion to resistance would greatly compromise the clinical value of vancomycin for therapy of pneumococcal infections. Do vancomycin-tolerant strains exist in unselected clinical isolates? Unfortunately, the answer appears to be yes.

Novak et al. *(9)* screened 116 clinical isolates for vancomycin tolerance. Isolates were tested for killing of *S. pneumoniae* in the presence of 10 times the MIC of vancomycin. Vancomycin tolerance was found in 3/116 strains, and all tolerant strains were serotype 9V and were resistant to penicillin. Sequence analysis confirmed mutations in the *vnc*S gene at position 440 of the tolerant strains and was characterized as a valine-for-alanine substitution. Nontolerant strains did not have this substitution.

Are the organisms highlighted by Novak et al. *(9)* clinically important? Human data are not available; however, a series of experiments conducted in rabbits suggested vancomycin-tolerant strains may have profound clinical consequences. Using a rabbit meningitis model *(53)*, rabbits were inoculated intrathecally with 10^5 bacteria that were vancomycin sensitive, vancomycin tolerant, or an equal mixture of the two. Acute bacterial meningitis was present by 24 h in untreated animals. No difference in growth was seen between the vancomycin-sensitive and vancomycin-tolerant strains. Treatment was administered intravenously at 6 and 12 h at a vancomycin dose of 30 mg/kg body weight. The vancomycin-susceptible strain was killed, but the tolerant strain remained constant at 10^5 colony-forming units per milliliter (CFU/mL) following both the first and the second doses. At 12 h after the last dose of vancomycin, organism numbers increased to 10^7 CFU/mL; from this, the authors concluded therapeutic failure.

Anton et al. *(54)* were concerned about the possible emergence of vancomycin-tolerant *S. pneumoniae* in Spain as the incidence of penicillin-nonsusceptible strains is high. The discovery of vancomycin-tolerant strains could be a clinical concern, especially for patients with pneumococcal central nervous system (CNS) infection and as such tolerance may lead to relapse or persistent bacterial meningitis in treated patients. Anton et al. *(54)* studied 120 pneumococcal strains isolated in Madrid in 1999. Tolerance was considered to exist if death of 2 ± 0.6 log of the initial inoculum (5×10^7 CFU/mL) occurred at 6 h. Vancomycin tolerance was not detected in any strain of the 120 strains, and there was no report of elevated MICs. The observation that elevated MICs were not detected in fact may be explained by the initial work of Novak et al. *(9)*.

Several important observations stem from this work *(9)*:

- Tolerance may be a mechanism of resistance as significant as other mechanisms, such as enzymatic destruction, efflux, altered target sites, and so on that have a net result of not reducing the number of viable cells. Clinical failure would result from this form of resistance.
- Although different from traditional mechanisms of resistance, the vancomycin-tolerant strains were because of a reduction in the autolytic activity (or control of autolytic activity) in the presence of the drug.
- Tolerant strains were found among clinical isolates.
- Detection of tolerance is cumbersome and time consuming and may depend on sequence analysis for detection of relevant amino acid substitutions as routine susceptibility testing will not detect these strains.
- Tolerant strains persisted in the presence of the drug, suggesting the possibility of therapeutic failure in patients with meningitis (or other infectious conditions) and treated with a drug to which the organism is tolerant.

Table 2 summarizes vancomycin susceptibility data from various studies in numerous countries worldwide. Overall, 99.7 to 100% of pneumococcal isolates were susceptible to the drug. Unfortunately, characterization of the isolates that were nonsusceptible at breakpoint was not done. Characterization of nonsusceptible isolates is likely as essential as monitoring changing or increasing rates of antimicrobial resistance.

5. QUINOLONES

The development of quinolone antimicrobial agents can be traced to nalidixic acid, a naphthyridine compound *(55)*. Quinolones evolved along two major pathways. Some quinolone structural features remain constant throughout the class, such as a bicyclic aromatic core. The addition of a carbon at the 8-position yields a true quinolone, whereas the addition of a nitrogen results in a naphthyridine. Both quinolones and naphthyridines are commonly referred to as quinolones.

Antibacterial activity requires the presence of the pyridine ring on the right side of the molecule, a carboxylic acid at the 3-position, a ketone at the C-4 position, and the R^1-substituted nitrogen at the 1-position *(56,57)*. The addition of a fluorine at the C-6 position results in the designation fluoroquinolone. Substitutions at the C-5 and C-8

Table 2
Summary of Select Studies of Vancomycin Susceptibility for *Streptococcus pneumoniae*

				Vancomycin susceptibility (%)			
Year/Country	Isolates (*n*)	Penicillin[a] susceptibility (%)	MIC_{90}	S	I	R	Reference
1996–1997							
United States	820	S	0.25	100			*42a*
	217	I	0.25	100			*42a*
	238	R	0.25	100			*42a*
1998							
United States	195	23.2 I & R	0.5	99.5			*57a*
1997–1999							
United States	4193	86 S & I, 14 R	0.5	100		0	*45*
Canada	887	93.2 S & I, 6.8 R	0.5	100		0	*45*
Latin America	948	88.3 S & I, 11.7 R	0.5	100		0	*45*
Europe	1478	89.6 S & I, 10.4 R	0.5	99.9		0.1	*45*
Asia-Pacific	569	82.2 S & I, 17.8 R	0.5	99.7		0.3	*45*
1997–1998							
Japan	218	44 I, 10 R		100		0	*59*
China	124	14 I, 3.2 R	NR	100		0	*59*
United Kingdom	343	5.5 I, 5.2 R	NR	100		0	*59*
Germany	283	7.1 I, <1 R	NR	100		0	*59*
Spain	320	41 I, 25 R	NR	100		0	*59*
France	221	32.5 I, 34 R	NR	100		0	*59*
Italy	370	11.9 I, 4.9 R	NR	100		0	*59*
1991–1993							
Korea	131	37 I, 33 R	0.5	100		0	*57b*
1995							
Europe	289		0.5 (mode)	100		0	*57c*
1998							
Hong Kong	56	S	0.75	100		0	*83*
	27	I	0.75	100		0	*83*
	98	R	0.75	100		0	*83*
1996–1997							
Taiwan	200	28 I, 33 R	0.5	100		0	*46*
1995–1996							
Taiwan	1611	39.7–54.7 (I & R)		100		0	*57d*

NR, not reported.
[a]Penicillin susceptible (S) ≤ 0.06 mg/mL; intermediate (I) = 0.1–1 mg/mL; resistant (R) ≥ 2 mg/mL.

position can be made, and some substitutes in the C-8 position—such as fluorine and chlorine—have improved potency, but with increased toxicity. The addition of a methoxy group has enhanced potency, including Gram positives, and did not significantly increase toxicity *(56)*. The in vitro potency of the quinolone molecules is linked to certain side groups or substitutions. These were summarized in an extensive review by Ball *(58)*:

Although the relationship between penicillin resistance and other classes of antimicrobial agents was recognized early, the same was not true for penicillin resistance and the quinolones. Indications that such an association may exist was seen for data reported by Sahm et al. *(59)*, who found that none of 100 penicillin-susceptible strains were levofloxacin resistant as compared to 1% resistance for 96 organisms with intermediate resistance to penicillin and 45% of 22 penicillin-resistant strains collected from Japan. Similar trends were not seen for isolates collected from China, the United Kingdom, Germany, Spain, France, and Italy (Table 3).

Jones et al. *(60)* reported that quinolone-resistant pneumococcal isolates may not be uniformly resistant to all quinolones. Five quinolone-resistant strains (one also penicillin resistant) were collected from a European surveillance study; of these five isolates, all were resistant or intermediate in resistance to grepafloxacin, sparfloxacin, and levofloxacin, four remained fully susceptible to trovafloxacin, and three remained fully susceptible to moxifloxacin. The clinical significance of these observations was unknown.

5.1. Mechanisms of Action

Although DNA gyrase (topoisomerase type II) has been classically considered the target of the quinolones *(56)*, a second target—referred to as topoisomerase IV and reported by Kato et al. *(61)*—is also recognized as an important fluoroquinolone target. DNA gyrase is essential for DNA replication. It is responsible for negative supercoiling, thereby relieving the positive supercoils created ahead of the replication fork *(62)*. In contrast, topoisomerases are critical enzymes that maintain cellular DNA of both replicating and nonreplicating regions of the chromosome in its appropriate supercoiled state. Topoisomerase IV conducts separation of the linked daughter DNA molecules after replication is complete *(62)*. Two other topoisomerases have also been discovered. These include topoisomerase type I, which relaxes negatively supercoiled DNA, and topoisomerase III, which is responsible for decatenation of the replication intermediate.

Studies by Gellert et al. *(63)* and Sugino et al. *(64)* showed DNA gyrase to be the principal target of nalidixic acid. Although initial studies characterizing DNA gyrase were with *E. coli*, Hooper and Wolfson *(65)* summarized numerous other species that contain the enzyme. Structurally, DNA gyrase has a tetrameric A_2B_2 structure; in *E. coli*, it consists of two *gyr*A and *gyr*B subunits that are encoded, respectively, by *gyr*A and *gyr*B genes *(56)*. Topoisomerase IV also has a tetrameric structure with A and B subunits encoded by the *par*C and *par*E genes respectively *(56)*.

What is the target for fluoroquinolones in bacterial cells—DNA gyrase or topoisomerase IV? Early investigations with *E. coli* suggested that DNA gyrase was the principal target as resistance mutations were mapped to DNA gyrase *(66–68)*. In addition, Peng and Marians *(69)* and Kato et al. *(70)* reported that inhibition of DNA gyrase supercoiling was more sensitive than was inhibition of topoisomerase type IV; however, Khodursky et al. *(71)* and Hoshino et al. *(72)* subsequently reported that this difference in sensitivity was in the range of two- to threefold. For *E. coli* and *Neisseria gonorrhoeae*, DNA gyrase was more sensitive to quinolones than was topoisomerase type IV, and first-step resistant mutants appeared mostly in *gyr*A. Resistance mutations

Table 3
Summary of Select Studies of Fluoroquinolone Susceptibility and Resistance for *Streptococcus pneumoniae*

Fluoroquinolone	Country	Year	Isolates (*n*)	Penicillin[a] susceptibility	MIC_{90} (μg/mL)	Susceptibility resistance (%) S	I	R	Reference
Levofloxacin	United States	1996–1997	880	S	1	100	—	—	*42a*
			218	I	1	99.5	0.2	0.5	
			238	R	1	99.2	0.4	0.5	
Ciprofloxacin	United States	1996–1997	820	S	1	NA			*42a*
			218	I	1	NA			
			238	R	1	NA			
Levofloxacin	[b]	1996–1997	8252		1–2	99–99.6		0.4–1	*45*
Ciprofloxacin	[b]	1996–1997	8252		1–2	NA			*45*
Gatifloxacin	[b]	1996–1997	8252		0.5	≥99.6		≤0.4	*45*
Ciprofloxacin	Korea	1991–1993	131	37 I, 33 R	2	85	15		*57b*
Levofloxacin	Japan	1997–1998	218	44 I, 10 R	NR	95.5–100		0–4.5	*59*
	China	1997–1998	124	14 I, 3.2 R	NR	99–100		0–1	*59*
	United Kingdom	1997–1998	343	5.5 I, 5.2 R	NR	100			*59*
	Germany	1997–1998	283	7.1 I, <1 R	NR	100			*59*
	Spain	1997–1998	320	41 I, 25 R	NR	100			*59*
	France	1997–1998	221	32.5 I, 34 R	NR	100			*59*
	Italy	1997–1998	370	11.9 I, 4.9 R	NR	100			*59*
Levofloxacin	Europe	1998	938	S	1	99.7			*59a*
			139	I	1	100			*59a*
			174	R	1	98.3			*59a*
Ciprofloxacin	Europe	1998	938	S	2	66			*59a*
			139	I	2	69.1			*59a*
			174	R	2	68.4			*59a*
Levofloxacin	Europe	1998	766	S	1	99.5	0.2	0.3	*60*
			85	I	1	98.8		1.2	*60*
			49	R	1	100			*60*

Table 3 *(continued)*
Summary of Select Studies of Fluoroquinolone Susceptibility and Resistance for *Streptococcus pneumoniae*

Fluoroquinolone	Country	Year	Isolates (*n*)	Penicillin[a] susceptibility	MIC_{90} (μg/mL)	Susceptibility resistance (%) S	I	R	Reference
Moxifloxacin	Europe	1998	766	S	0.12	99.7	0.1	0.1	*60*
			85	I	0.12	100			*60*
			49	R	0.12	100			*60*
Ciprofloxacin	Great Britain	1997–1998	663	3.5 I, 5.6 R	2	64	31.1	4.9	*59a*
Levofloxacin	Great Britain	1997–1998	663	3.5 I, 5.6 R	1	99.4	0.3	0.3	*59a*
Ciprofloxacin	Ireland	1997–1998	154	4.5 I, 23.4 R	2	63.6	27.9	8.5	*59a*
Levofloxacin	Ireland	1997–1998	154	4.5 I, 23.4 R	2	100			*59a*
Ciprofloxacin	Hong Kong	1998	56	S	2	NA			*83*
			27	I	4	NA			*83*
			98	R	12	NA			*83*
Levofloxacin	Hong Kong	1998	56	S	1	100			*83*
			27	I	1.5	96.3		3.7	*83*
			98	R	3	90.8		9.2	*83*

Abbr: NA, no NCCLS breakpoint; NR, not reported.
[a]Penicillin susceptible (S) ≤ 0.06 μg/mL; intermediate (I) = 01–1 μg/mL; resistant (R) ≥ 2 μg/mL.
[b]United States (*n* = 4193); Canada (*n* = 887); Latin America (*n* = 948); Europe (*n* = 1478); Asia-Pacific (*n* = 746).

appearing in *par*C or *par*E and in the absence of *gyr*A provided little, if any, survival advantage for the organism in the presence of the drug *(73)*.

Studies with ciprofloxacin and *S. aureus* suggested that DNA gyrase may not be the principal target with Gram-positive organisms, but rather topoisomerase type IV is the target. Studies by Ferrero et al. *(74,75)* reported that the stepwise selections of mutants from *S. aureus* in the presence of ciprofloxacin resulted in resistance mutations first in the *par*C gene as opposed to the *gyr*A gene. Similar findings were also reported from studies involving ciprofloxacin and *S. pneumoniae (76,77)*, with selected mutants found to have substitutions at Ser79 in the *par*C gene.

These data suggest that, in Gram-negative bacteria, the principal target is DNA gyrase, whereas in Gram-positive organisms, the principal target is topoisomerase type IV. This designation is not completely uniform as Pan and Fisher *(78)* reported that the stepwise selection of mutants from *S. pneumoniae* in the presence of sparfloxacin resulted in mutants in *gyr*A first as opposed to *par*C. According to Gootz and Brighty *(79)*, the interactions of fluoroquinolones with either DNA gyrase or topoisomerase IV are complex, and the most sensitive topoisomerase target may vary between species and with respect to the particular quinolone. Although genetic and biochemical data may not always agree whether the primary target in *S. pneumoniae* is DNA gyrase or topoisomerase IV, genetic studies may be more revealing *(73)*.

Fluoroquinolone resistance among pneumococci arises *de novo (76,80)*, with the gradual accumulation of spontaneous mutations either affecting the target site of the molecule or reducing the intracellular drug concentration. Over time and perhaps under selective pressures, these mutants predominate and convert a once-susceptible population to a resistant one.

The quinolone-resistance-determining region (QRDR) defines a segment of amino acids that contains the genes that encode DNA gyrase and topoisomerase IV. In *E. coli*, the *gyr*A QRDR extends from amino acids 51 to 106 *(81)*, and it is from amino acids 49 to 105 in *S. pneumoniae*. Amino acid substitution frequently occurs at Ser81 and Glu85. For *par*C, the QRDR extends from amino acids 47 to 102, and substitutions are more frequent at Ser79 and Asp83. The impact of various amino acid changes at the sites listed most likely affect drug binding. Similarly, mutation in the genes encoding *gyr*B and *par*E mostly affect drug binding *(82)*.

Efflux is the only other type of fluoroquinolone resistance described for *S. pneumoniae*.

5.2. Resistance to Fluoroquinolones

A summary of quinolone susceptibility data against *S. pneumoniae* isolates is shown in Table 3. In most instances, susceptibility rates remained in excess of 90%. Studies with ciprofloxacin in Europe, Great Britain, and Ireland reported susceptibility rates of less than 70%, presumably based on a breakpoint of 1 μg/mL. The majority of the nonsusceptible isolates had intermediate levels of resistance. An interesting observation from the study of Ho et al. *(83)* from Hong Kong reported that 3.7% of 27 pneumococcal isolates with intermediate resistance to penicillin were levofloxacin resistant, and that 9.2% of 98 penicillin-resistant isolates were levofloxacin resistant.

To date, three main mechanisms conferring resistance to fluoroquinolones have been described. These include chromosomal mutations encoding for modifications in the target subunits of either DNA gyrase or topoisomerase IV *(79)*, alterations in expression of outer membrane proteins (i.e., *omp*F) *(79,84,85)*, and the uptake/efflux process, primarily with staphylococci *(86,87)*. Plasmid-mediated resistance has not been established *(88)*, and quinolones have not been shown to be inactivated by enzymes known to confer resistance to other compounds.

Although fluoroquinolone resistance among all organisms within their spectrum is interesting, more emphasis has been on quinolone resistance with *S. pneumoniae*. Part of the interest relates in part to the dramatic increase in the incidence of penicillin-resistant pneumococci globally and the concomitant co- or cross-resistance seen to many other classes of antimicrobial agents (summarized in Section 2.3.).

Although not a uniform observation, a mutation conferring resistance to one quinolone may also alter the susceptibility to other quinolones. Some examples are given in Table 4. Several quinolones were tested by the mutant prevention concentration (MPC) (described in detail in Section 5.3.). Organisms demonstrating elevated MPC values to levofloxacin (MPC value ≥ 4 μg/mL) were selected for sequencing of the QRDR region. Also, MPC values to other quinolones were compared for the same isolates. Mutants were found in *gyr*A and *par*C genes or both. Some of the mutants had previously conferred quinolone resistance, whereas others had not.

It appears clear from the data that some mutants result in organisms with reduced susceptibility to most compounds, whereas others may differentially affect the compounds summarized. For *S. pneumoniae*, it seems that cross-resistance may be low when the primary target differs for different compounds. According to the data summarized by Drlica and Malik *(73)*, the principal target in *S. pneumoniae* for ciprofloxacin, norfloxacin, trovafloxacin, and levofloxacin is topoisomerase IV, whereas it is DNA gyrase for sparfloxacin, moxifloxacin, gemifloxacin, garenoxacin, grepafloxacin, and gatifloxacin. As such, resistance mutations in *gyr*A would have less of an affect on compounds with topoisomerase IV as the principal target and vice versa.

5.3. Prevention of Pneumococcal Resistance to Fluoroquinolones

The majority, if not all, of novel bacterial targets have been exploited by the current antimicrobial agents marketed. Unless new targets are discovered, we must face the possibility that antimicrobial agents are a nonrenewable or nonsustainable resource. With the prospects of returning to the preantibiotic era, an attempt to develop strategies to preserve the utility of existing compounds seems essential. With fluoroquinolones at least (and perhaps other antimicrobial classes), one recent strategy provides a possible explanation for the emergence of fluoroquinolone resistance and the possible prevention or slowing of the rate at which it occurs. This section attempts to explain this concept.

In essence, the MPC defines the antimicrobial drug concentration that would require an organism to simultaneously possess two concurrent mutations to grow in the presence of the drug. Another definition is that the MPC represents the MIC of the most resistant first-step resistant bacterial cell present in a heterogeneous bacterial population. The MPC concept only applies to those bacterial populations that have been deemed susceptible to the antimicrobial agent by traditional antimicrobial susceptibility testing. In most clinical microbiology laboratories, the guidelines of the NCCLS are followed and as such utilize a standardized inoculum of 10^5 CFU/mL for routine susceptibility testing.

Table 4
Quinolone-Resistant Alleles Associated With High Values of Mutant Prevention Concentration (MPC)

	MPC (μg/mL)				Changes in QRDR[a]	
Isolate no.	Gati	Gemi	Levo	Moxi	*par*C	*gyr*A
Wt[b]	2		4	1		
10	4	0.5	32	4	D83N (GAT → AAT)	S81F (TTC → TTC)
12	8	0.5	32	4	S79F (TCT → TTT)	S81Y (TTC → TAC)
13	32	≥2	128	32	S79F (TCT → TT) S52G (AGC → GGC) N91D (AAC → GAC)	S114G (AGT → GGT)
15	8	0.25	32	1	S79F (TCT → TTT)	None
16	32	???	32	>128	S79F (GAT → TTT)	S81F (TTC → TTC)
18	8	0.25	64	2	S79F (TCT → TTT)	None
27	8	8	16	>128	S52G (AGC → GGC) N91D (AAC → GAC)	S114G (AGT → GGT)
33	2	0.063	8	1	K137N (AAG → AAT)	None
35	4	???	8	4	K137N (AAG → AAT)	None
36		0.25	4	8	K137N (AAG → AAT)	None
37	1	0.125	>512	4	K137N (AAG → AAT)	None
42	1	0.5	32	1	K137N (AAG → AAT)	None
43	0.5	0.5	8	2	None	None
48	1	0.5	8	1	K137N (AAG → AAT)	None
51	1	0.25	8	0.5	K137N (AAG → AAT)	None
64	1	0.25	8	2	None	None
74	8	32	8	16	S52G (AGC → GGC)	None
78	0.5	0.125	8	0.5	None	None
87	1	0.25	8	0.5	None	None
89	4	1	8	1	S52G (AGC → GGC)	S114G (AGT → GGT)
91	1	2	32	1	S52G (AGC → GGC) N91D (AAC → GAC)	S114G (AGT → GGT)
103	4	0.125	8	2	None	None

Abbr: Gati, gatifloxacin; Gemi, gemifloxacin; Levo, levofloxacin; Moxi, moxifloxacin.

[a]QRDR, quinolone-resistance-determining region *(17)*. Amino acid in wild-type protein is indicated before its number in the protein, followed by the amino acid change. D, aspartic acid; F, phenylalanine; G, glycine; K, lysine; N, asparagine; S, serine; Y, tyrosine.

[b]Wild-type strain ATCC 49619.

Although this approach for determining susceptibility has been valuable, it may not accurately portray the full dynamics of a bacterial population at a higher inoculum. In human infectious diseases, the organism load at the site of infection may exceed 10^8 bacterial cells. Indeed, Firsch et al. (1942) reported, that in pneumococcal pneumonia, the total organism load may be between 10^{10} and 10^{12} bacterial cells. Clearly, susceptibility testing utilizing inoculums substantially less than those observed at the site of infection may not truly be representative of the total bacterial population.

The frequency with which *S. pneumoniae* may acquire a first-step resistant mutant is approx 10^{-7} *(88a)*. As such, the likelihood that a dense bacterial population at the site of infection could contain a bacterial cell with a first-step resistant mutant is high based on natural genetic selection. Susceptibility testing utilizing a lower inoculum level is unlikely to detect the presence of the mutant cell because the number of organisms sampled is too low.

For MPC testing *(88a)*, approx 10^{10} cells are applied to agar plates containing antimicrobial agent; the plates are incubated and then read for the presence or absence of growth. Subculture of organisms with elevated MPC values to agar plates containing drug at the same concentrations as the plate from which the organisms were initially recovered confirms the elevated value and eliminates the likelihood of an inoculum effect. The lowest drug concentration that prevents growth is referred to as the MPC. As stated, the MPC represents the drug concentration that prevents the growth of first-step resistant cells.

My group *(89)* applied the MPC concept to clinical isolates of *S. pneumoniae* tested against gatifloxacin, grepafloxacin, levofloxacin, moxifloxacin, and trovafloxacin. Subsequent testing extended to gemifloxacin *(89a)*. The testing of *S. pneumoniae* resulted in the generation of a provisional value shown to be an overestimation of the actual MPC value by approximately one doubling dilution. The following values represent the corrected (one dilution below provisional value) MPC results for 150 clinical isolates and are summarized as the modal value (μg/mL) and the MPC_{90} (the antimicrobial drug concentration preventing growth for 90% of strains tested) (μg/mL), respectively: gatifloxacin 1, 2; gemifloxacin 0.25, 0.5; grepafloxacin 2, 4; levofloxacin 2, 4; moxifloxacin 0.5, 1; and trovafloxacin 1, 2. To appreciate fully the potential importance of these data, these values need to be viewed in light of the pharmacodynamic features of these drugs in vitro.

The mutant selection window defines the drug concentration between the MIC and the MPC values. This window is predicted as the "danger zone" for the drug concentration in as much as when the drug concentration falls or remains within this window, the selective amplification of first-step resistant mutants may occur as wild-type susceptible cells are inhibited, but first-step resistant mutants may not be inhibited based on the level of resistance in relationship to the drug concentrations. Drug concentrations in excess of the MPC prevent the growth of both wild-type susceptible and first-step resistant mutants; therefore, there is no selective amplification of resistant subpopulations. Drug concentrations that fall below the MIC value do not inhibit either wild-type susceptible or first-step resistant mutants; therefore, there is no selective amplification of resistant subpopulations. Based on MPC measurements completed to date, the ideal drug dosing would exceed the MPC, remain above the MPC to effect a significant reduction in the percentage of viable cells, and at the same time remain below the maximum safe drug concentration, above which unacceptable toxicities or side effects may occur.

The MPC concept in its current format may not have a direct impact on acute patient management—that is, whether the patient gets better. Rather, it alludes to potential societal consequences of continuing to use antimicrobial agents incorrectly and the ensuing rise in antimicrobial resistance, a trend that will ultimately impact acute patient management.

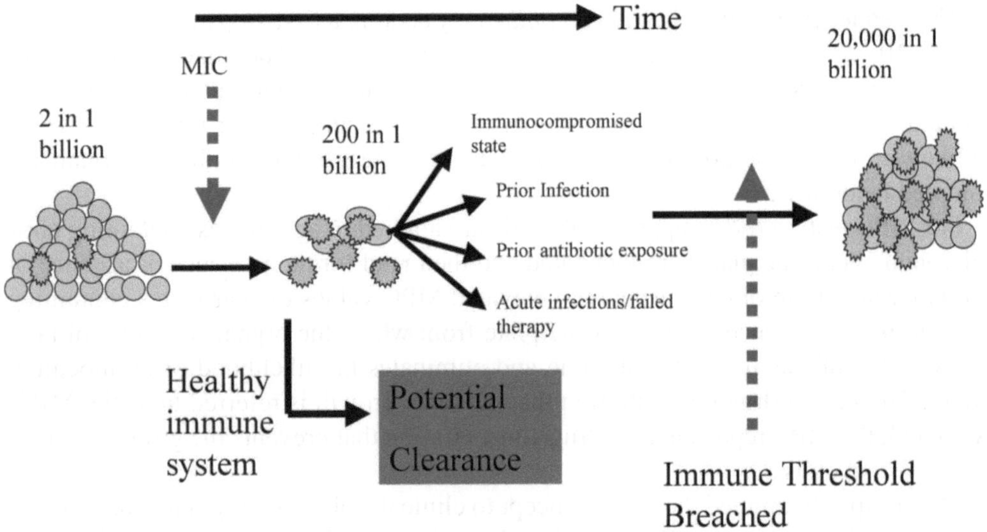

Fig. 2. Selective amplification of resistant mutants. (Adapted from ref. *89b*.)

A schematic representation of the selective amplification of resistance is presented in Fig. 2. Based on the normal mutational frequencies, a few resistant cells would be expected among a high inoculum of organisms. In the dosing of an antimicrobial agent, many variables are considered; one is the MIC. It is now known that the MIC may be insufficient to inhibit any first-step resistant mutants present in the bacterial population; as such, proliferation of these mutants can occur against a background of declining susceptible cells. In most individuals, these organisms are likely cleared by a healthy and functioning immune system. However, in some patients, such as those who are immunocompromised, with prior infection, or with prior antibiotic exposure or those who appear to be failing therapy for acute infection, you may have continued proliferation of the resistant subpopulation to the level at which they breach the immune threshold. Now, the patient is colonized or infected with this resistant subpopulation. The time line for this to occur may range from a couple to several days or perhaps longer.

Is there any proof that this scenario is possible? Davidson et al. *(90)* described the clinical failure of four patients with pneumococcal community-acquired pneumonia who were being treated with levofloxacin. One case involved a 64-yr-old male who presented with community-acquired pneumonia, but was otherwise well. He had had no history of fluoroquinolone use and was treated with 500 mg levofloxacin once daily for 10 d; the pretreatment sputum grew *S. pneumoniae*. At 1 wk following the completion of therapy, this patient was diagnosed with recurrent pneumonia, and the sputum again grew *S. pneumoniae*. Comparison of the pretreatment and post-treatment organisms by pulse field gel electrophoresis revealed an identical pulse field pattern. The levofloxacin MIC went from 1 μg/mL for the pretreatment organism and 8 μg/mL for the post-treatment organism. Susceptibility to penicillin and erythromycin remained unchanged. Sequence analysis of the *par*C and *gyr*A genes did not identify any mutations in the pretreatment organism, but did identify a single mutation in each of the two genes in the post-treatment organism.

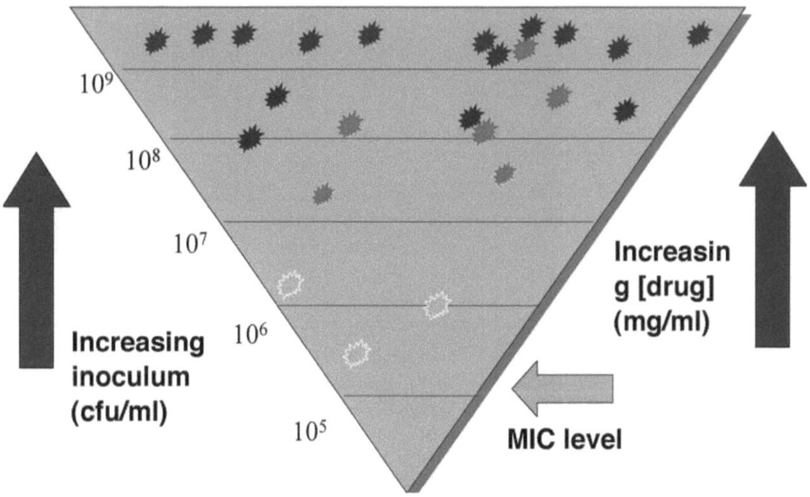

Fig. 3. Mutant prevention concentration (MPC) dynamics. (Adapted from ref. *90a*.)

For the second case, a 37-yr-old female with X-ray-proven community-acquired pneumonia and no prior fluoroquinolone therapy was treated with 500 mg levofloxacin once daily orally for 10 d. The pretreatment sputum culture grew *S. pneumoniae*; 3 d into therapy, the patient was admitted to the hospital because clinically there was no improvement. She did respond to therapy after she was switched to treatment with ceftriaxone and erythromycin. The pretreatment organism and the organism collected during therapy showed identical pulse field patterns, and the levofloxacin MIC went from 4 μg/mL for the pretreatment organism to 16 μg/mL for the organism collected during treatment. As with the first case, the susceptibilities to penicillin and erythromycin remained unchanged. Sequence analysis of the *par*C gene revealed a single mutation in the organism collected prior to the initiation of therapy, and no mutation was seen in the *gyr*A gene. For the organism collected during therapy, a single mutation was found in both the *par*C and the *gyr*A genes. Although this evidence is indirect, the model in Fig. 2 appears to explain it.

Figure 3 is a schematic of the proposed dynamics associated with the MPC concept. For routine susceptibility testing, an inoculum of 10^5 CFU/mL is used. At such an inoculum, detection of resistant subpopulations would be unlikely given that the mutational frequencies at which they occur are much lower. Quite simply, enough cells are not being sampled during routine susceptibility testing to find a resistant organism only present at much higher inoculums. As the organism inoculum increases, so does the likelihood of having first-step resistant mutants. To overcome these resistant cells or prevent them from growing in the presence of antimicrobial selective pressure, the drug concentration may need to be increased both to achieve and to maintain a drug concentration in excess of the most resistant first-step resistant mutant to prevent the selective amplification of any resistant subpopulations.

The MPC is a measurement of the inhibition of first-step resistant mutants, and it is not a measurement of kill. My group was interested in determining relationships that may exist among the MIC, MPC, and other drug concentrations for the killing of *S. pneumoniae*. Figure 4 is a schematic representation of the bacterial population dynam-

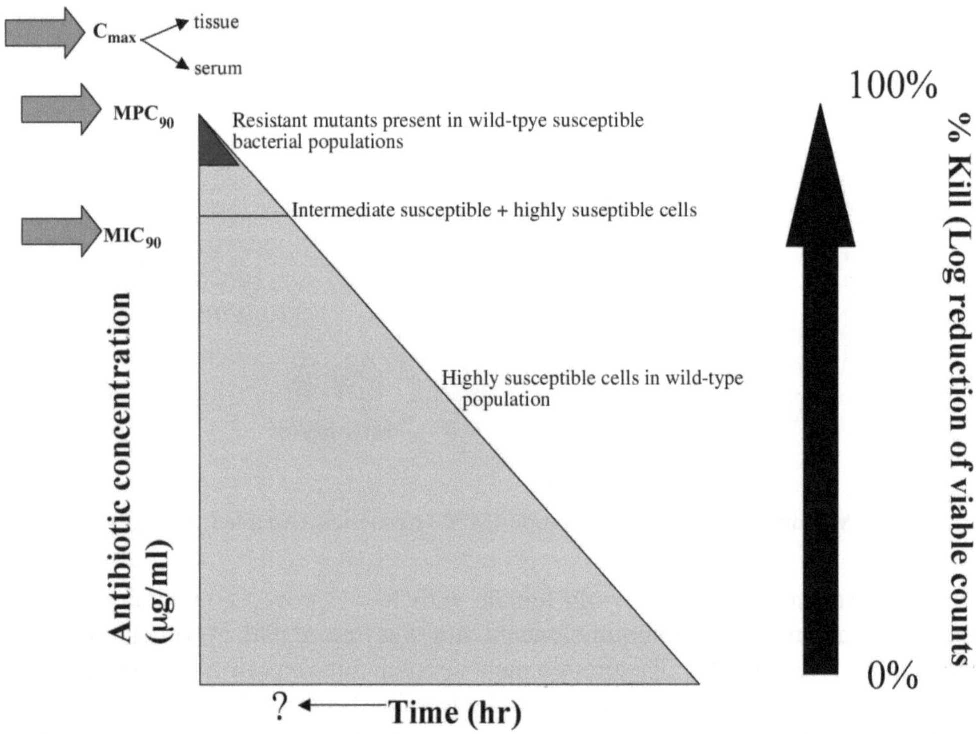

Fig. 4. Relationship between the mutant prevention concentration and fluoroquinolone killing of *S. pneumoniae*. Adapted from ref. *96*.

ics and its potential relationship to the killing of *S. pneumoniae* by various drug concentrations. It now appears that, beyond a reasonable doubt, resistant subpopulations may exist in a bacterial population that appears susceptible to an antimicrobial agent by traditional antimicrobial susceptibility testing. In these populations, the majority of organisms are likely killed by the MIC drug concentration in the presence of bactericidal drugs. Between the MIC and the MPC drug concentrations, resistant subpopulations may occur with MICs that may span the drug concentrations between the MIC and MPC values.

In kill experiments performed by my laboratory, an attempt was made to kill *S. pneumoniae* using the MIC, MPC, and C_{max} serum drug concentrations against a range of inoculum of bacteria extending from 10^6 to 10^9 CFU/mL *(91)*. Gemifloxacin, levofloxacin, and moxifloxacin were compared in the kill studies. Following 4 h of exposure at the MIC drug concentration to 10^9 CFU/mL of *S. pneumoniae*, there was a 76% reduction of viable cells in the moxifloxacin group compared to 39% for levofloxacin and 68% for gemifloxacin. There was a 99.99% reduction of viable cells for all agents by 24 h. Exposure of 10^9 CFU/mL of *S. pneumoniae* at the MPC drug concentration resulted in a 70% reduction in viable cells by 4 h in the presence of gemifloxacin compared to 97% with levofloxacin and 94% with moxifloxacin. By 24 h, there was 99.99% reduction in viable cells for all agents. Finally, when 10^9 CFU/mL were exposed to the C_{max} serum drug concentrations, there was a 72% reduction in viable cells in the presence of gemifloxacin, 76% for levofloxacin, and 94% with

Table 5
Fluoroquinolone Potency Based on MPC_{pr}

	MPC_{pr50}[a] (μg/mL)	MPC_{pr90}[a] (μg/mL)	MIC_{90}[b] (μg/mL)	MPC_{pr90}/MIC_{90} (μg/mL)
Moxifloxacin	0.5	2	0.25	8
Trovafloxacin	1	4	0.25	16
Gatifloxacin	1	4	0.5	8
Grepafloxacin	2	8	0.5	16
Levofloxacin	4	8	1	8
Gemifloxacin	0.25	1	0.03	33

[a]Data taken as MPC were designated in previous work (MPC_{pr}) because a twofold overestimate arises from the high inoculum used (> 10^{10} cells per plate). MPC_{pr} is a conservative estimate of MPC. MPC_{pr} in which 50% (MPC_{pr50}) or 90% (MPC_{pr90}) of the isolates were inhibited from growth.
[b]MIC_{90} drug concentration in which 90% of the strains were inhibited.

moxifloxacin. Again, by 24 h of exposure, a reduction of more than 99.78% in viable cells was seen against all three agents.

What might be a useful interpretation of these data? First, a test tube is a static environment when it comes to drug concentrations. Drug elimination does not occur in a test tube and, as such, may not accurately reflect the true dynamic interactions of an antimicrobial agent with a bacterial population in a living system. Table 5 is a summary of published data comparing in vitro susceptibility data (MIC, MPC) and various pharmacological parameters. Based on published data on peak serum drug concentrations and the subsequent elimination over time, my group calculated the time above either MIC or MPC the drug concentrations are expected to remain *(91a)*.

From these measurements, we were able to estimate that gemifloxacin drug concentrations would remain in excess of the MPC_{90} values for approx 12 h, for levofloxacin for approx 3 to 3.5 h, and for moxifloxacin for longer than 24 h. Based on our kill data, we were able to show that there was not a 100% reduction in viable cells by 4 h, which therefore provided an opportunity for regrowth of resistant subpopulations in the presence of various drug concentrations. These data seem to suggest that the longer the drug concentration remains in excess of the MPC_{90} values, then the less the likelihood for the selective amplification of resistant subpopulations. Clearly, these data are just one component, and ongoing work in both in vitro and in vivo systems will help further elucidate the various parameters of the MPC model.

Gillespie et al. *(92)* wrote that it was assumed that bacteria always pay a significant physiological price for the acquisition of resistance to antimicrobial agents. Then, it must be asked: Does the selection of a resistant mutant matter if mutants are disadvantaged in comparison with wild-type cells? Gillespie et al. sought to test if, indeed, antimicrobial-resistant mutants were as fit as the wild-type strains. A wild-type strain of *S. pneumoniae* and mutants to fluoroquinolones (selected from the wild-type strain) were tested for their fitness in comparative growth experiments. The growth rate of a *par*C (serine 79 to tyrosine, selected on ciprofloxacin) mutant showed no significant deficit with its susceptible isogenic parent. A *par*C (serine 79 to tyrosine), *gyr*A (serine 81 to tyrosine) double mutant had a relative fitness of 0.81 compared to the wild type.

For three double-mutant strains (*par*C serine 79 to tyrosine *gyr*A serine 81 to phenylamine, *par*C serine 79 to tyrosine and asparagine 83 to phenylalanine), the growth rates were similar to the isogenic susceptible parents (1.16, 0.99, and 0.95, respectively). From this work, Gillespie et al. indicated that the data suggested that *par*C and *gyr*A mutants, on some occasions, may not be associated with a physiological deficit.

Gillespie et al. *(92)* commented on the MPC concept: "There are no grounds for complacency about the development of resistance to quinolones in *S. pneumoniae*." The in vitro work that has defined mutation prevention concentration for new quinolones should confirm our thinking. Similarly, Dubreuil *(93)* wrote that "despite their limits, the MPC are of major interest for the prevention of mutants, which are always dangerous, since their underlying resistance mechanism is eventually unknown."

Of the fluoroquinolone compounds tested by MPC, the 8-methoxy-containing agents (gatifloxacin, moxifloxacin) had low MPC values. Kishii et al. *(94)* reported on the contribution of the 8-methoxy group to the activity of gatifloxacin (and moxifloxacin) against type II topoisomerase (DNA gyrase) of *S. pneumoniae*. In this study, the 50% inhibitory concentrations (IC_{50}) of several quinolones were measured against DNA gyrase and topoisomerase IV of the wild-type pneumococcal strains IID 553. The IC_{50} values ranged from 4.28 to 582 μg/mL against DNA gyrase for the 10 compounds tested (25.9 μg/mL for gatifloxacin, 21.8 μg/mL for moxifloxacin, 138 μg/mL for ciprofloxacin, and 83.3 μg/mL for levofloxacin). For topoisomerase IV, the IC_{50} values ranged from 1.90 to 35.2 μg/mL (gatifloxacin 72.7 μg/mL, moxifloxacin 6.04 μg/mL, ciprofloxacin 6.85 μg/mL, levofloxacin 15.9 μg/mL). The IC_{50} ratios (IC_{50} DNA gyrase/IC_{50} topoisomerase IV) for the four compounds were 3.56 μg/mL, 3.61 μg/mL, 20.1 μg/mL, and 5.62 μg/mL respectively, for gatifloxacin, moxifloxacin, ciprofloxacin, and levofloxacin. Testing by MPC resulted in MPC values of 1, 1, 8, and 4, respectively, for the same compounds.

Kishii et al. *(94)* further identified that the target that performed with *S. pneumoniae* was DNA gyrase for gatifloxacin and moxifloxacin and topoisomerase IV for ciprofloxacin and levofloxacin. Gatifloxacin and moxifloxacin showed less mutant selectivity than other quinolones, and it appeared that they inhibit both DNA gyrase and topoisomerase IV—a dual-targeting property—despite the fact that DNA gyrase was the preferred target.

Additional data from Kishii et al. *(94)* suggested that the 8-methoxy group of quinolones contributed to enhancement of the inhibition of DNA gyrase, leading to the dual-targeting properties. Finally, it was reported that the MPC values for gatifloxacin and moxifloxacin were the same or lower than for some of the other quinolones tested (i.e., ciprofloxacin, levofloxacin), and that these results were consistent with those reported by my group *(89)*, suggesting that both the dual-targeting property and potent antipneumococcal activity of the 8-methoxy quinolones contribute to the low MPCs.

6. CONCLUSION

Moreillon et al. *(95)* suggested the following four points for fighting the explosion of drug-resistant pneumococci:

1. Strict utilization of antibiotics.
2. The practice of microbiological sampling of infected foci before treatment.
3. The systematic surveillance of resistance profiles of pneumococci against antibiotics.
4. The adequate vaccination of the populations at risks.

The pneumococcus remains a significant cause of community-acquired respiratory tract infections in both adults and children. It is also associated with significant morbidity and mortality. Antimicrobial resistance has evolved to the multidrug resistance level and globally has had an impact on β-lactams, macrolides, tetracycline, and trimethoprim-sulfamethoxazole, reducing the confidence in these agents for treating *S. pneumoniae* infections.

Resistance to agents such as rifampin, vancomycin, and the fluoroquinolones remains low or nonexistent; however, complacency may result in an escalation of resistance to these agents. Some data summarized in this chapter highlight historical data on resistance rates to rifampin, vancomycin, and fluoroquinolones from several countries around the world. Data and arguments also were presented showing the mechanisms by which tolerance or resistance may develop to these agents.

Finally, a concept of mutation prevention is essential, as is the potential impact that such an approach may offer in terms of preserving the longevity of these compounds by slowing the rate at which resistance occurs. With the fluoroquinolones, data were also summarized to show the impact (cross-resistance) that some mutants have on various agents within the class. Understanding resistance and developing strategies that preserve the longevity of existing compounds or classes of compounds seems essential at a time when relatively few new agents appear in development.

REFERENCES

1. Blondeau JM. A review of the comparative in vitro activity of 12 antimicrobial agents with a focus on four new "respiratory quinolones." J Antimicrob Chemother 1999; 43:1–11.
1a. Blondeau JM. Community-aquired respiratory tract pathogens and increasing antimicrobial resistance. J Infect Dis Pharm 2000; 4(2):1–28.
2. Hansman D, Bullen MM. A resistant pneumococcus. Lancet 1967; 2:264–265.
3. Appelbaum PC, Bhamjee A, Scragg JN, Hallett AF, Bowen AJ, Cooper RC. *Streptococcus pneumoniae* resistant to penicillin and chloramphenicol. Lancet 1977; 2:995–997.
4. Jacobs MR, Koornhof HJ, Robins-Browne RM, et al. Emergence of multiply resistant pneumococci. N Engl J Med 1978; 299:735–740.
5. Evans W, Hansman D. Tetracycline-resistant pneumococcus. Lancet 1963; 1:451.
6. Francis RS, May J, Spicer CC. Influence of daily penicillin, tetracycline, erythromycin and sulphamethoxypyridazine on exacerbations of bronchitis: a report to the Research Committee of the British Tuberculosis Association. BMJ 1964; 1:728–732.
7. Kislak JW. Type 6 pneumococcus resistant to erythromycin and lincomycin. N Engl J Med 1967; 276:852.
7a. Klugmam KP. Pneumococcal resistance to antibiotics. Clin Microbiol Rev 1990; 3(2): 171–196.
8. Aseni F, Perez-Tamarit D, Otero MC, et al. Imipenem-cilastatin therapy in a child with meningitis caused by a multiply resistant pneumococcus. Pediatr Infect Dis 1989; 8:895.
9. Novak R, Henriquies B, Charpentier E, Normark S, Tuomanen E. Emergence of vancomycin tolerance in *Streptococcus pneumoniae*. Nature 1999; 399:590–593.
10. Tomasz A, Hotchkiss RD. Regulation of the transformability of pneumococcal cultures by macromolecular cell products. Proc Natl Acad Sci 1964; 51:480–487.

11. Shockley TE, Hotchkiss RD. Stepwise introduction of transformable penicillin resistance in pneumococcus. Genetics 1970; 64:397–408.
12. Dowson CG, Barcus V, King S, Pickerill P, Whatmore A, Yeo M. Horizontal gene transfer and the evolution of resistance and virulence determinants in *Streptococcus*. Soc Appl Bacteriol 1997; 26:42S–51S.
13. Leclercq R, Courvalin P. Bacterial resistance to macrolide, lincosamide and streptogramin antibiotics by target modification. Antimicrob Agents Chemother 1991; 35:1267–1272.
14. Courvalin P, Carlier C. Transposable multiple antibiotic resistance in *Streptococcus pneumoniae*. Mol Gen Genet 1986; 205:291–297.
15. Felmingham D, Washington JA, Group TAP. Trends in the antimicrobial susceptibility of bacterial respiratory tract pathogens—findings of the Alexander Project 1992–1996. J Chemother 1999; 11:5–21.
16. Blondeau JM, Vaughan D, Group. The Canadian Antimicrobial Resistance Study Group. Surveillance of antimicrobial resistance in *Streptococcus pneumoniae* (SP), *Haemophilus influenzae* (H) and *Moraxella catarrhalis* (MC) in Canada: results of a multicenter study (Abstract P210). J Antimicrob Chemother 1999; 44:86.
17. Nakamura S. Mechanisms of quinolone resistance. J Infect Chemother 1997; 3:128–138.
18. Klugman KP, Feldman C. Penicillin- and cephalosporin-resistant *Streptococcus pneumoniae*: emerging treatment for an emerging problem. Drugs 1999; 58:1–4.
19. Doern GV, Brueggemann AB, Holley HP, et al. Antimicrobial resistance of *S. pneumoniae* recovered from outpatients in the US during the winter months of 1994 to 1995: results of a 30-center national surveillance study. Antimicrob Agents Chemother 1996; 40:1208–1213.
20. Thornsberry C, Ogilvie P, Kahn J, Mauriz Y, Group TLI. Surveillance of antimicrobial resistant in *Streptococcus pneumoniae*, *Haemophilus influenzae* and *Moraxella catarrhalis* in the United States in 1996–1997 respiratory season. Diag Microbiol Infect Dis 1997; 29:249–257.
21. Pfaller MA, Jones RN, Doern GV, et al. Survey of blood stream infections attributable to Gram-positive cocci: frequency of occurrence and antimicrobial susceptibility of isolates collected in 1997 in the United States, Canada and Latin America from the SENTRY Surveillance Program. Diag Microbiol Infect Dis 1999; 33:283–297.
22. Simor AE, Louie M, Low DE. Canadian national survey of prevalence of antimicrobial resistance among clinical isolates of *Streptococcus pneumoniae*. Antimicrob Agents Chemother 1996; 40:2190–2193.
23. Jacobs MR, Bajaksouzian S, Zilles A, Lin G, Pankuch GA, Appelbaum PC. Susceptibilities of *Streptococcus pneumoniae* and *Haemophilus influenzae* to 10 oral antimicrobial agents based on pharmacodynamic parameters: 1997 U.S. Surveillance Study. Antimicrob Agents Chemother 1999; 43:1901–1908.
24. National Committee for Clinical Laboratory Standards (NCCLS). Performance Standards for Antimicrobial Susceptibility Tests for Bacteria that Grow Aerobically (M7-A4). Wayne, PA: National Committee for Clinical Laboratory Standards, 1997.
25. Hartmann G, Honikel KO, Knusel F, Nuesch J. The specific inhibition of the DNA-directed RNA synthesis by rifamycin. Biochim Biophys Acta 1967; 145:843–844.
26. Wehrli W. Rifampin: mechanisms of action and resistance. Rev Infect Dis 1983; 5:S407–S411.
27. Zillig W, Zechel K, Rabussay D, et al. On the role of different subunits of DNA-dependent RNA polymerase from *E. coli* in the transcription process. Cold Spring Harb Symp Quant Biol 1970; 35:47–58.
28. Carter PE, Abadi FJR, Yakubu DE, Pennington TH. Molecular characterization of rifampin-resistant *Neisseria meningitidis*. Antimicrob Agents Chemother 1994; 38:1256–1261.
29. Bodmer T, Zurcher G, Imboden P, Telenti A. Mutation position and type of substitution in the *B*-subunit of the RNA polymerase influence in vitro activity of rifamycins in rifampin-resistant *Mycobacterium tuberculosis*. J Antimicrob Chemother 1995; 35:345–348.
30. Kapur V, Ling-Ling L, Iordanescu S, et al. Characterization by automated DNA sequencing of mutations in the gene (*rpo*B) encoding the RNA polymerase *B*-subunit in rifampin-

resistant *Mycobacterium tuberculosis* strains from New York City and Texas. J Clin Microbiol 1994; 32:1095–1098.
31. Telenti A, Imboden P, Marchesi F, et al. Detection of rifampin-resistance mutations in *Mycobacterium tuberculosis*. Lancet 1993; 341:647–650.
32. Telenti A, Imboden P, Marchesi F, Schmidheini T, Bodmer T. Direct, automated detection of rifampin-resistant *Mycobacterium tuberculosis* by polymerase chain reaction and single-strand conformation polymorphism analysis. Antimicrob Agents Chemother 1993; 37:2054–2058.
33. Hetherington SV, Watson AS, Patrick CC. Sequence and analysis of the *rpo*B gene of *Mycobacterium smegmatis*. Antimicrob Agents Chemother 1995; 39:2164–2166.
34. Levin ME, Hatfull GF. *Mycobacterium smegmatis* RNA polymerase: DNA supercoiling, action of rifampin and mechanism of rifampin resistance. Mol Microbiol 1993; 8:277–285.
35. Honore N, Cole ST. Molecular basis of rifampin resistance in *Mycobacterium leprae*. Antimicrob Agents Chemother 1993; 37:414–418.
36. Heil A, Zillig W. Reconstruction of bacterial DNA dependent RNA polymerase from isolated subunits as a tool for the elucidation of the subunits in transcription. FEBS Lett 1970; 11:165–168.
37. Iwakura Y, Ishihama A, Yura T. RNA polymerase mutants of *Escherichia coli, H. streptolydigin* resistance and its relation to rifampin resistance. Mol Gen Genet 1973; 121:181–196.
38. Jin DJ, Gross CA. Mapping and sequencing of mutations in the *Escherichia coli rpo*B gene that lead to rifampin resistance. J Mol Biol 1988; 202:45–58.
39. Lisitsyn NA, Sverdlov ED, Moiseyera EP, Danilesvskaya ON, Nikiforov VG. Mutation of rifampin resistance at the beginning of the RNA polymerase *B* subunit gene in *Escherichia coli.* Mol Gen Genet 1984; 196:173–174.
40. Padayachee T, Klugman KP. Molecular basis of rifampin resistance in *Streptococcus pneumoniae*. Antimicrob Agents Chemother 1999; 43:2361–2365.
41. Enright M, Zawadski P, Pickerill P, Dowson CG. Molecular evolution of rifampin resistance in *Streptococcus pneumoniae*. Microb Drug Resist 1998; 4:65–70.
42. Severinov K, Soushko M, Goldfarb A, Nikiforov VG. New rifampicin-resistant and streptolydigin-resistant mutants in the subunit of *Escherichia coli* RNA polymerase. J Biol Chem 1993; 268:14–16.
42a. Thornsberry C, Ogilvia PT, Holley HP Jr., and Sahm DF. Survey of susceptibilities of *Streptococcus pnemoniae, Haemophilus influenzae,* and *Moraxella catarrhalis* isolates to the 26 antimicrobial agents: a prospective U. S. Study. Antimicrob Agents Chemother 1999; 43:2612–2623.
42b. Benbachir M, Benredjeb S, Boye CS, Dosso M, Belabbes H, Kamoun A, Kaire O, Elmdaghri E. Two-year surveillance of antibiotic resistance in *Streptococcus pneumoniae* in four African cities. Antimicrob Agents Chemother 2001; 45(2):627–629.
43. Woodford N. Epidemiology of the genetic elements responsible for acquired glycopeptide resistance in enterococci. Microb Drug Resist 2001; 7:229–236.
44. Noble WC, Virani Z, Cree RG. Co-transfer of vancomycin and other resistance genes from *Enterococcus faecalis* NCTC 12201 to *Staphylococcus aureus*. FEMS Immunol Med Microbiol 1992; 72:195–198.
45. Hoban DJ, Doern GV, Fluit AC, Roussel-Delvallez M, Jones RN. Worldwide prevalence of antimicrobial resistance in *Streptococcus pneumoniae*, *Haemophilus influenzae* and *Moraxella catarrhalis* in the SENTRY Antimicrobial Surveillance Program, 1997–1999. Clin Infect Dis 2001; 32:S81–S93.
46. Hsueh PR, Teng LJ, Lee LN, Yang PC, Ho SW, Luh KT. Extremely high incidence of macrolide and trimethoprim-sulfamethoxazole resistance among clinical isolates of *Streptococcus pneumoniae* in Taiwan. J Clin Microbiol 1999; 37:897–901.
47. Song JH, Lee NY, Ichiyama S, et al. Spread of drug-resistant *Streptococcus pneumoniae*

in Asian countries: Asian Network for Surveillance of Resistant Pathogens (ANSORP) Study. Clin Infect Dis 1999; 28:1206–1211.
48. Tomasz A, Albino A, Zanati E. Multiple antibiotic resistance in a bacterium with suppressed autolytic system. Nature 1970; 227:138–140.
49. Moreillon P, Markiewicz Z, Nachman S, Tomasz A. Two bactericidal targets for penicillin in pneumococci: autolysis-dependent and autolysis-independent killing mechanisms. Antimicrob Agents Chemother 1990; 34:33–39.
50. Holtje JV, Tuomanen E. The murein hydrolases of *Escherichia coli*: properties, functions and impact on the course of infection in vivo. J Gen Microbiol 1991; 137:441–454.
51. Evers S, Courvalin P. Regulation of VanB-type vancomycin resistance gene expression by the $VanS_B$ two-component regulatory system in *Enterococcus faecalis* V583. J Bacteriol 1996; 179:1302–1309.
52. Liu HH, Tomasz A. Penicillin tolerance in multiply drug-resistant natural isolates of *Streptococcus pneumoniae*. J Infect Dis 1985; 152:365–372.
53. Tauber MG, Zwahlen A. Animal models of meningitis. Meth Enzymol 1994; 235:92–106.
54. Anton N, Blazquez R, Gomez-Garces JL, Alos JI. Study of vancomycin tolerance in 120 strains of *Streptococcus pneumoniae* isolated in 1999 in Madrid, Spain. J Antimicrob Chemother 2001; 47:902–903.
55. Lesher GY, Froelich ED, Gruet MD, et al. 1,8 Naphthyridine derivatives: a new class of chemotherapeutic agents. J Med Pharmacol Chem 1962; 5:1063–1068.
56. Gootz TD, Brighty KE. Chemistry and mechanism of action of the quinolone antibacterials. In: Andriole VT (ed.). The Quinolones. London, England: Academic, 1998, pp. 29–80.
57. Neu HC. Major advances in antibacterial quinolone therapy. Adv Pharmacol 1994; 29:227–262.
57a. Mathai D, Lewis MT, Kugler K, Pfaller MA, Jones RN. (SENTRY). Antibacterial activity of 41 antimicrobials tested against over 2773 bacterial isolates from hospitalized patients with pneumonia: I-results from SENTRY Antimicrobial Surveillance Program (North America, 1998) Diag Microbiol Infect Dis 2001; 39:105–116.
57b. Lee HJ, Park JY, Jang SH, Kim JH, Kim EC, Choi KW. High incidence of resistance to multiple antimicrobials in clinical isolates of *Streptococcus pneumoniae* from a University Hospital in Korea. Clin Infect Dis 1995; 20:826–835.
57c. Felmingham D, Brown DFJ, Soussy CJ. The European Resistance Survey Study Group. European glycopeptide susceptibility survey of gram-positive bacteria, for 1995. Diag Microbiol Infect Dis 1998; 31:563–571.
57d. Chang SC, Hsieh WC, Liu CY. (The Antibiotic Resistance Study Group of Republic of China). High prevalence of antibiotic resistance of common pathogenic bacteria in Taiwan. Diag Microbiol Infect Dis 2000; 36:107–112.
58. Ball P. The quinolones: history and overview. In: Andriole VT (ed.). The Quinolones. London, England: Academic, 1998, pp. 1–28.
59. Sahm DF, Jones ME, Hickey ML, Diankun DR, Mani SV, Thornsberry C. Resistance surveillance of *Streptococcus pneumoniae*, *Haemophilus influenzae* and *Moraxella catarrhalis* isolated in Asia and Europe, 1997–1998. J Antimicrob Chemother 2000; 45:457–466.
59a. Felmingham D. Respiratory pathogens: assessing resistance patterns in Europe and the potential role of grepafloxacin as treatment of patients with infections caused by these organisms. J Antimicrob Chemother 2000; 45 (Topic T2):1–8.
60. Jones ME, Staples AM, Critchley IA, et al. Benchmarking the in vitro activity of moxifloxacin against recent isolates of *Streptococcus pneumoniae*, *Moraxella catarrhalis* and *Haemophilus influenzae*—a European multi-centre study. Diagn Microbiol Infect Dis 2000; 37:203–211.
61. Kato H, Nishimura Y, Imamura R, Niki H, Hiraga S, Suzuki H. New topoisomerase essential for chromosome segregation in *E. coli*. Cell 1990; 63:393–404.
62. Marians KJ. Replication fork progression. In: Neidhardt FC (ed.). *E. coli* and *Salmonella* Cellular and Molecular Biology. Vol. 1. Washington, DC: American Society for Microbiology, 1996, pp. 74–763.

63. Gellert M, Muzuuchi K, O'Dea MH, Itoh T, Tomizawa J. Nalidixic acid resistance: a second genetic character involved in DNA gyrase activity. Proc Natl Acad Sci 1977; 74:4772–4776.
64. Sugino A, Peebles CL, Kruezer KN, Cozzarelli NR. Mechanism of action of nalidixic acid: purification of *Escherichia coli nal*A gene product and its relationship to DNA gyrase and a novel nicking-closing enzyme. Proc Natl Acad Sci 1977; 74:4767–4771.
65. Hooper DC, Wolfson JS. Mechanisms of quinolone action and bacterial killing. In: Hooper DC, Wolfson JS (eds.). Quinolone Antimicrobial Agents. Washington, DC: American Society for Microbiology, 1993, pp. 53–75.
66. Oram M, Fisher LM. 4-Quinolone resistance mutations in the DNA gyrase of *Escherichia coli* clinical isolates identified by using the polymerase chain reaction. Antimicrob Agents Chemother 1991; 35:387–389.
67. Maxwell A. The molecular basis of quinolone action. J Antimicrob Chemother 1992; 30:409–414.
68. Hallett P, Maxwell A. Novel quinolone resistance mutations of the *Escherichia coli* DNA gyrase A protein: enzymatic analysis of mutant proteins. Antimicrob Agents Chemother 1991; 35:335–340.
69. Peng H, Marians KJ. *E. coli* topoisomerase IV, purification, characterization, subunit structure and subunit interactions. J Biol Chem 1993; 268:24,481–24,490.
70. Kato JI, Suzuki H, Ikeda H. Purification and characterization of DNA topoisomerase IV in *Escherichia coli*. J Biol Chem 1992; 267:25,676–25,684.
71. Khodursky AB, Zechdiedrich EL, Cozzarelli NR. Topoisomerase IV is a target of quinolones in *Escherichia coli*. Proc Natl Acad Sci 1995; 92:11,801–11,805.
72. Hoshino K, Kitamura A, Morrissey I, Sato K, Kato JI, Ikeda H. Comparison of inhibition of *Escherichia coli* topoisomerase IV by quinolone with DNA gyrase inhibition. Antimicrob Agents Chemother 1994; 38:2623–2627.
73. Drlica K, Malik M. Fluoroquinolones: action and resistance. Curr Top Med Chem 2003; 3:1349–1364.
74. Ferrero L, Cameron B, Crouzet J. Analysis of *gyr*A and *grl*A mutations in stepwise-selected ciprofloxacin-resistant mutants of *Staphylococcus aureus*. Antimicrob Agents Chemother 1995; 39:1554–1558.
75. Ferrero L, Cameron B, Manse B, et al. Cloning and primary structure of *Staphylococcus aureus* DNA topoisomerase IV: a primary target of fluoroquinolones. Mol Microbiol 1994; 13:641–653.
76. Pan X, Ambler J, Mehtar S, Fisher LM. Involvement of topoisomerase IV and DNA gyrase as ciprofloxacin targets in *Streptococcus pneumoniae*. Antimicrob Agents Chemother 1996; 40:2321–2326.
77. Gootz TD, Zaniewski L, Haskell S, et al. Activity of the new fluoroquinolone trovafloxacin (CP-99,219) against DNA gyrase and topopisomerase IV mutants of *Streptococcus pneumoniae*. Antimicrob Agents Chemother 1996; 40:2691–2697.
78. Pan X, Fisher ML. Targeting of DNA gyrase in *Streptococcus pneumoniae* by sparfloxacin: selective targeting of gyrase or topoisomerase IV by quinolones. Antimicrob Agents Chemother 1997; 41:471–474.
79. Gootz TD, Brighty KE. Fluoroquinolone antibacterials: SAR, mechanism of action, resistance and clinical aspects. Med Res Rev 1996; 16:433–486.
80. Alou L, Ramirez M, Garcia-Rey C, Prieto J, de Lencastre H. *Streptococcus pneumoniae* isolates with reduced susceptibility to ciprofloxacin in Spain: clonal diversity and appearance of ciprofloxacin-resistant epidemic clones. Antimicrob Agents Chemother 2001; 45:2955–2957.
81. Friedman SM, Lu T, Drlica K. A mutation in the DNA gyrase A gene of *Escherichia coli* that expands the quinolone-resistance-determining region. Antimicrob Agents Chemother 2001; 45:2378–2380.
82. Heddle J, Maxwell A. Quinolone-binding pocket of DNA gyrase. Antimicrob Agents Chemother 2002; 46:1805–1815.
83. Ho PL, Que TL, Tsang DN, Ng TK, Chow KH, Seto WH. Emergence of fluoroquinolone

resistance among multiple resistant strains of *Streptococcus pneumoniae* in Hong Kong. Antimicrob Agents Chemother 1999; 43:1310–1313.
84. Bryan LE, Bedard J, Wong S, Chamberland S. Quinolone antimicrobial agents; mechanisms of action and resistance development. Clin Invest Med 1989; 12:14–19.
85. Wolfson JS, Hooper DC. Bacterial resistance to quinolones: mechanisms and clinical importance. Rev Infect Dis 1989; 11:S960–S968.
86. Kaatz GW, Seo SM, Ruble CA. Mechanisms of fluoroquinolone resistance in *Staphylococcus aureus*. J Infect Dis 1991; 163:1080–1086.
87. Kaatz GW, Seo SM. Inducible Nor-A mediated multi-drug resistance in *Staphylococcus aureus*. Antimicrob Agents Chemother 1995; 39:2650–2655.
88. Courvalin P. Plasmid-mediated 4 quinolone resistance: a real or apparent absence. Antimicrob Agents Chemother 1990; 34:681–684.
88a. Blondeau JM, Zhao X, Hansen G, Drlica K. Mutant prevention concentration of fluoroquinolones for clinical isolates of *Streptococcus pnemoniae*. Antimicrob Agents Chemother 2001; 45:433–438.
89. Blondeau JM, Hansen G, Zhao X, Drlica K. Comparison of gatifloxacin (GA), gemifloxacin (GM), levofloxacin (L) and moxifloxacin (M) by the mutation prevention concentration (MPC) using 160 clinical isolates of *Streptococcus pneumoniae* (SP). Paper presented at: 40th Interscience Conference on Antimicrobial Agents and Chemotherapy; Chicago, IL; September 20–22, 2001.
89a. Hansen JM, Drlica K, Hansen GT, Zhao X. Mutant prevention concentration of gemifloxacin for clinical isolates of *Streptococcus pnemoniae*. Antimicrob Agents Chemother 2003; 47(1):440–441.
89b. Blondeau JM, Hansen G. The mutant prevention concentration (MPC) for ciprofloxacin (Cpx) and levofloxacin (Lfx) against non-urinary isolates of *Pseudomonas aeruginosa* (PA) and the relationship to achievable serum drug concentration following IV dosing., 43rd Interscience Conference on Antimicrobial Agents and Chemotherapy, Chicago, IL, September 14–17, 2003. American Society of Microbiology, Washington, DC. Abstract #C2–99.
90. Davidson RJ, Cavalcanti R, Brunton JL, et al. Resistance to levofloxacin and failure of treatment of pneumococcal pneumonia. N Engl J Med 2002; 346:747–750.
90a. Blondeau JM, Hansen G, Zhao X, Drlica K, Borsos S. Effect of inoculum size on the determination of the mutation prevention concentration (MPC) for fluoroquinolones (FQ) against *Streptococcus pneumoniae* (SP). 22nd International Congress of Chemotherapy, Amsterdam, June 30–July 3, 2001. American Society of Microbiology, Washington, DC. Abstract P27.044.
91. Blondeau JM, Hansen G, Metzler KL, Borsos S, Chau J. Optimal killing of *Streptococcus pneumoniae* by gemifloxacin, levofloxacin and moxifloxacin. R Soc Med Press 2002; 76:15–26.
91a. Blondeau JM, Drlica K, Hansen G, Zhao X. The relationship between the mutant prevention concentration (MPC) of fluoroquinolones (FQ) against *Streptococcus pneumoniae* (Sp) and the 24-hour dose response curves., 7th International Symposium of New Quinolones, Edinburgh, Scotland, June 10–12, 2001. Abstract #71.
92. Gillespie SH, Voelker LL, Dickens A. Evolutionary barriers to quinolone resistance in *Streptococcus pneumoniae*. Microb Drug Resist 2002; 8:79–84.
93. Dubreuil L. Concentrations preventing resistance mutations against fluoroquinolones. Presse Med 2002; 31:1807–1809.
94. Kishii R, Takei M, Fukuda H, Hayashi K, Hosaka M. Contribution of the 8-methoxy group to the activity of gatifloxacin against type II topoisomerase of *Streptococcus pneumoniae*. Antimicrob Agents Chemother 2003; 47:77–81.
95. Moreillon P, Wenger A, Caldelari I. Resistance aux antibiotiques chez les pneumocoques [Pneumococcal antibiotic resistance]. Rev Med Suisse Romande 2000; 120:651–659.
96. Blondeau JM, Drlica K, Hansen GT, Zhao X. The relationship between mutant prevention concentration (MPC) and killing by moxifloxacin (M) and levofloxacin (L) of *Streptococcus pnemoniae* (sp). 22nd International Congress of Chemotherapy, Amsterdam, The Netherlands, June 30–July 3, 2001. Abstract p27.110.

4

Management of Glycopeptide-Resistant *Staphylococcus aureus* Infections

A. Peter R. Wilson

1. INTRODUCTION

Before the introduction of penicillin, invasive *Staphylococcus aureus* infections were associated with mortality rates over 90% *(1)*. Although penicillin was initially effective, resistance because of β-lactamase appeared quickly and spread. Within 10 yr, strains were resistant to erythromycin, tetracycline, and chloramphenicol. Methicillin resistance associated with modified penicillin-binding proteins (PBPs) appeared within 2 yr of the introduction of methicillin *(2)*, and over the subsequent decades, strains resistant to an increasing number of antibiotics have spread worldwide. In hospitals, *S. aureus* resistant to multiple antibiotics commonly exceeds the susceptible strains. The emergence of glycopeptide-intermediate *S. aureus* (GISA) and vancomycin-resistant *S. aureus* (VRSA) raised the possibility of infections untreatable by standard antibiotic combinations. New agents are under investigation, but few fulfill the role.

1.1. *Infections Caused by* Staphylococcus aureus

Staphylococcus aureus is the predominant cause of skin and soft tissue infection, which may be localized (furuncles, impetigo, wound infections) or associated with a widespread rash (scalded skin syndrome, toxic shock syndrome). *Staphylococcus aureus* is the most common cause of surgical wound infection. Bacteremia is usually preceded by a localized infection in soft tissue, lung, bone, or intravenous catheter or associated with intravenous drug abuse. The presence of a cardiac murmur suggests endocarditis, which is associated with a mortality of 40–60%, increasing in the presence of an annular or myocardial abscess.

Methicillin-resistant *S. aureus* (MRSA) is now widespread and particularly common in tertiary referral centers *(3)*; it is usually resistant to a wide range of antibiotics. The organism is spread easily in the hospital on the hands of staff and by contamination of their working environment. Colonization is much more common than infection. The common epidemic strains in the United Kingdom are EMRSA-15, EMRSA-16, and EMRSA-3. Prevalence of methicillin resistance is over 30% of *S. aureus* in Italy, France, and Spain *(4)*.

From: *Management of Multiple Drug-Resistant Infections*
Edited by: S. H. Gillespie © Humana Press Inc., Totowa, NJ

MRSA is more likely to cause invasive infection than methicillin-susceptible *S. aureus (5)*. Debilitated, surgical, or immune-suppressed patients are particularly at risk. Recent surgery, pressure sores, intravenous catheterization, or critical illness predispose to bacteremia *(3)*. Patients are more likely to die following bacteremia because of MRSA than methicillin-sensitive *S. aureus* (MSSA). In 84 episodes caused by MRSA, the mortality rate was 58%, compared with 32% in 100 episodes caused by MSSA. The association was independent of other factors, although MRSA carriers were more likely to have had a long hospital stay before infection, previous antibiotic therapy, surgery, urinary catheterization, or blood transfusion *(6)*.

Despite major investment in the containment of MRSA in hospitals by source isolation of patients, use of topical eradication, and closure of beds or units, these organisms have become widespread *(3)*.

1.2. *Current Treatment of* Staphylococcus aureus *Infection*

In the small proportion of cases for which *S. aureus* is susceptible to penicillin, benzyl penicillin is highly effective. However, flucloxacillin or oxacillin is required to treat most MSSA infections. Combination with an aminoglycoside ensures rapid bactericidal activity, but clinical trials have failed to demonstrate an advantage to gentamicin use in the treatment of endocarditis *(7)*. The American Heart Association recommends that gentamicin be used for 3–5 d only except for prosthetic valve endocarditis *(8)*.

Patients allergic to penicillin or those infected with MRSA are treated with vancomycin or teicoplanin. Gentamicin may not improve the outcome of treatment with vancomycin, but at least a 3- to 5-d course is still recommended in endocarditis *(7)*. Vancomycin alone may be associated with slow response of bacteremia. Rifampicin can be added instead of gentamicin.

With the rise in prevalence of MRSA, use of vancomycin and teicoplanin has increased enormously; in many areas, glycopeptides have replaced oxacillin or flucloxacillin as first-line antistaphylococcal agents. As a result, there has been a large increase in hospital spending on antibiotics, and the pressure for emergence of glycopeptide resistance has been considerable. Glycopeptides are the only antibiotics available for treatment in most cases, and delay in adequate treatment is a contributory factor to the increased risk of death. Patients having surgery who are at risk of MRSA colonization may be given glycopeptides instead of the standard prophylaxis.

However, there are few direct comparisons of the glycopeptides for the treatment of MRSA. A randomized trial in soft tissue and respiratory infections reported cure or improvement in 17 of 20 given teicoplanin (400 mg iv qd) compared with 15 of 20 given vancomycin (500 mg iv qds) *(9)*. Although vancomycin is less expensive than teicoplanin, it has to be given by infusion, is nephrotoxic when used with gentamicin, and usually requires serum monitoring. The long serum half-life of teicoplanin requires a loading regimen of three doses at 12-h intervals to achieve therapeutic serum concentrations.

2. GLYCOPEPTIDE-RESISTANT *STAPHYLOCOCCUS AUREUS*

Vancomycin was consistently active against *S. aureus*, including MRSA, until 1996. The first isolate of GISA was from a Japanese patient with a postoperative wound infection *(10)*. GISA probably developed from MRSA with heterogeneous resistance to glycopeptides. These strains are much more common than GISA and contain subpopulations with minimum inhibitory concentrations (MICs) of 8 mg/L. Like GISA, heterogeneous-resistant *S. aureus* are associated with treatment failures. They are not detected by routine sensitivity methods, and various plate methods, as well as the Etest® (AB Biodisk, Solna, Sweden), have been suggested *(11)*.

A survey in Japan of 1149 isolates of MRSA from 203 hospitals reported no case of the original GISA strain (Mu50), but strains heterogeneously resistant to vancomycin comprised 20% of isolates in one hospital and 9% in other teaching hospitals compared with 1% of general hospitals *(12)*. A proportion of the hetero-resistant strains also had an MIC of 8 mg/L or more. Strains with variable susceptibility were present in 20% of isolates in one hospital and in 9% in other teaching hospitals. A later study examined 6625 isolates of MRSA from 278 hospitals, but found no Mu3 or Mu50 isolates *(13)*. Vancomycin-intermediate *S. aureus* (VISA) has been reported from the United States and United Kingdom, although some reports may be because of the screening method used *(14)*. Screening for these organisms should be considered in any patients with persistent MRSA bacteremia despite glycopeptide treatment.

High-level resistance to glycopeptides is very rare, but unlikely to remain so. VRSA has been produced in the laboratory following transfer of vancomycin resistance genes from *Enterococcus faecium* to *S. aureus* in the laboratory *(15)*. There has been one report of VRSA from a dialysis catheter and a foot ulcer of a patient in the United States *(16)*. The MIC of vancomycin was more than128 mg/L, and for teicoplanin, it was 32 mg/L. Vancomycin-resistant *E. faecalis* was also isolated from the patient. A second case in the United States was also associated with a foot ulcer. The organism showed both *mec*A and *van*A genes, and the MIC of vancomycin was 32 mg/L *(17)*.

2.1. *Definitions*

According to the National Committee for Clinical Laboratory Standards (NCCLS) *(18)*, VRSA requires 32 mg/L or more of vancomycin for inhibition. In Japan, the term may be used for organisms with an MIC of 8 mg/L *(19)*.

VISA (GISA) requires 8–16 mg/L of vancomycin for inhibition *(18)*. These organisms show similar reduced susceptibility to teicoplanin.

The term heteroresistant VRSA (hetero-VRSA) is applied to *S. aureus* containing subpopulations of resistant cells derived from a population inhibited by 1–4 mg/L of vancomycin *(19)*. Organisms grown on agar containing vancomycin 4–6 mg/L are selected and further tested; they show an MIC of vancomycin two- to eightfold higher than the original strain. Incubation of these strains in increasing concentrations of vancomycin can select homogeneously resistant organisms that show increased cell wall thickness on electron microscopy *(20)*.

2.2. *Mechanism of Resistance*

High-level vancomycin resistance has been demonstrated in the laboratory as the result of acquisition of the *van*A gene from *E. faecalis (15)*. Presumably, this also accounts for the few clinical reports *(16,17)*. In enterococci, *van*A establishes high-level resistance to vancomycin and teicoplanin by the production of peptidoglycan precursors ending in the depsipeptide D-alanyl-D-lactate instead of the dipeptide

Table 1
Antibiotic Susceptibilities of Glycopeptide-Intermediate Susceptibility *S. aureus*

Antibiotic	*n*	MIC (50 mg/L)	Range	Reference
Vancomycin	35	8	1–8	*22, 34, 35, 38, 46*
Teicoplanin	26	4	0.5–32	*35, 38, 46*
Amoxicillin	19	32	1–>32	*46*
Ampicillin-sulbactam	3	—	8–64	*35*
Gentamicin	6	64	0.25–128	*35, 45*
Rifampicin	3	—	1024–2048	*35*
Trovafloxacin	3	—	0.5–2	*35*
Clinafloxacin	3	—	0.5–1	*35*
Levofloxacin	22	16	0.25–32	*35, 46*
Tetracycline	3	—	0.5–128	*35*
Cotrimoxazole	3	—	0.06–4	*35*
Erythromycin	19	>32	0.12–>32	*46*
Arbekacin	3	—	0.125–2	*45*
Oritavancin (LY333328)	10	2	1–8	*26, 35, 38*
Quinupristin-dalfopristin (RP59500)	10	0.25	0.25–0.5	*34, 35, 38*
Linezolid	10	1	0.5–2	*34, 35, 38*
Tigecycline (GAR-936)	19	0.25	0.06–1	*46*
Daptomycin	22	4	0.5–16	*34, 46*
Everninomycin (SCH27899)	4	—	0.25–1	*38*

D-Ala-D-Ala present in susceptible organisms *(21)*. Complexes can no longer form between glycopeptides and peptidoglycan precursors.

In contrast, GISA produces a thicker cell wall with pentapeptide D-Ala-D-Ala termini that can bind vancomycin *(22)*. Vancomycin is retained at the periphery of the cell wall, growth is slow, and peptidoglycan crosslinking is reduced. An excess of PBP2 is associated with the increase in vancomycin MIC *(23)*. Other changes in peptidoglycan structure and regulation of cell wall synthesis probably contribute, but *van*A, *van*B, and *van*C are absent.

3. TREATMENT

GISA infections usually emerge after prolonged use of vancomycin, often in patients on dialysis or with immune suppression. Treatment has been reported in only a small number of cases (Table 1) and should be determined based on susceptibility testing. Mortality in GISA infections is high, although usually it is attributable to other underlying causes. Infections caused by heteroresistant staphylococci may fail to respond to vancomycin even if the MIC is 1–4 mg/L *(24)*. Nevertheless, combinations of older agents can be effective, and there are new agents in trials at present.

3.1. Vancomycin

Dimerization of vancomycin derivatives has shown that some result in activity against vancomycin-resistant bacteria *(25)*. However, standard vancomycin monotherapy is generally ineffective in GISA infections. In vitro models suggest that very high doses of vancomycin (1.5 g every 12 h) are bactericidal *(26)*. However, in clinical use these doses would carry a greater risk of toxicity. If vancomycin is used to treat staphylococcal lower respiratory tract infection, there is a clear correlation between the area under the 24-h inhibitory curve ($AUIC_{24}$), clinical and microbiological success *(27)*. The $AUIC_{24}$ required for successful outcome was high (>400) and raises the likelihood of clinical failure. In many intensive care units (ICUs), even a modest rise in MIC from 0.5 to 2 mg/L is associated with failure.

3.2. *Combination Regimens*

All GISA remain sensitive to cotrimoxazole, and some are sensitive to chloramphenicol, gentamicin, rifampicin, or tetracycline *(11)*. Combination treatments have been successfully used in combination with surgical drainage (Table 1). Vancomycin may be effective when combined with an aminoglycoside or rifampicin. The latter is known to lower mortality when used with vancomycin for susceptible MRSA infections *(28)*. A combination of rifampicin and cotrimoxazole was effective in treating peritonitis caused by GISA after removal of a continuous ambulatory peritoneal dialysis (CAPD) catheter *(29)*. Another patient was treated for GISA bacteremia with vancomycin, gentamicin, and rifampicin. However, both patients died subsequently. Ampicillin-sulbactam was used with arbekacin in the first GISA infection reported *(30)*. Arbekacin is an aminoglycoside resistant to most modifying enzymes and is bactericidal at 0.5–2 times the MIC. Ampicillin and sulbactam have also been shown to be effective in experimental endocarditis caused by GISA *(31)*.

By acting on different targets in cell wall synthesis, combinations of glycopeptides and β-lactams show additive or synergistic activity against MRSA in vitro *(22)*. In the presence of β-lactams, PBP2a is essential in crosslinking by transpeptidation of the terminal D-Ala, but can only crosslink monomeric disaccharide pentapeptides, not oligomeric muropeptides *(22)*. Competition for the former may account for the synergism between vancomycin and β-lactams.

Some strains of VRSA produced in the laboratory are more sensitive to β-lactams than MRSA *(32)*. Synergy between vancomycin and oxacillin was demonstrated for three strains of GISA, but not against vancomycin-sensitive MRSA. The interaction was more marked in strains with higher vancomycin MICs *(22)* and when high levels of β-lactams were present *(33)*. In a rabbit model of aortic valve endocarditis, vancomycin was not effective against three strains of GISA, and there was no significant reduction in bacterial counts in the vegetation over controls. However, in combination with nafcillin, a four-log reduction in bacterial count was achieved.

3.3. *Monotherapy*

Both linezolid and quinupristin-dalfopristin are licensed and can be used to treat GISA infections.

3.3.1. *Linezolid*

Linezolid, an oxazolidinone, acts by binding to the 50S subunit of the ribosome and prevents formation of the initiation complex. In vitro resistance is uncommon and requires prolonged exposure to low concentrations. Spontaneous mutation to resistance is rare. Linezolid is active against Gram-positive bacteria, including MRSA, irrespective of vancomycin susceptibility (MIC 0.5–2 mg/L) *(34,35)* (Table 1). In a random-

Table 2
Treatment of 10 GISA Infections

Case	Age	Infection	Antibiotics	Duration (d)	Outcome
1	4 mo	Wound infection after heart surgery	Sulbactam/ampicillin, arbekacin	23 d	Cured with debridement
2	59 yr	CAPD peritonitis, diabetes, carcinoma	Multiple drugs (aminoglycosides, rifampicin, cotrimoxazole)	49	Cured, but died 4 mo later
3	66 yr	Bacteremia, diabetes, renal failure, peritoneal dialysis	Vancomycin, gentamicin, rifampicin	28	Infection cleared, but patient died with candidemia at 34 d
4	2 yr	Bacteremia/central-line infection, leukemia	Quinupristin/dalfopristin	10	Cured with drainage
5	79 yr	Bacteremia, chronic obstructive pulmonary disease, chronic hemodialysis	Vancomycin, ceftriaxone, tobramycin	0.5	Died
6	Unknown	Bacteremia	Not known	14	Died
7	63 yr	Catheter-related bacteremia/endocarditis, chronic hemodialysis	Vancomycin, rifampicin, tobramycin	10	Died
8	56 yr	Vertebral osteomyelitis, chronic hemodialysis	Vancomycin, nafcillin, gentamicin	Not stated	Cured, but later died
9	27 yr	Hepatic abscess, biliary stent	Linezolid, cotrimoxazole, doxycycline	6 wk	Cured with drainage
10	45 yr	Pelvic abscess, colon cancer	Vancomycin, ciprofloxacin, metronidazole	15	Died

Source: From refs. *11* and *18*.

ized trial, linezolid (600 mg bid; $n = 240$) and vancomycin (1 g bid; $n = 220$) produced similar rates of cure of infections predominantly caused by MRSA (73.2 vs 73.1%) *(36)*. However, GISA bacteria were not included. Linezolid has been used successfully in one reported case of GISA infection (Table 2), but MRSA resistant to linezolid have already been reported *(37)*.

3.3.2. Quinupristin/Dalfopristin

The streptogramins dalfopristin and quinupristin are available in a synergistic combination in Synercid (Aventis). They act by binding to the 50S subunit of the 70S ribosome so that protein accumulates at the peptidyl transferase site, causing cell death. Resistance develops by changes in the target ribosome, altered permeability, and permeases. The quinupristin/dalfopristin combination was active against GISA in laboratory studies (0.25–0.5 mg/L) (Table 1) *(38)* and has been effective in experimental endocarditis caused by GISA *(39)*. There is one reported clinical case with a successful outcome (Table 2). However, some heteroresistant *S. aureus* have been found resistant (MIC 8 mg/L) *(40)*. Emergence of resistance during treatment has been reported *(41)*. The antibiotic has been associated with numerous side effects, and efficacy has to be weighed against tolerance *(42)*.

3.3.3. *Clinafloxacin, Trovafloxacin, and Sitafloxacin*

GISA has been shown susceptible to clinafloxacin (MIC 0.5–1 mg/L) and trovafloxacin (MIC 0.5–2 mg/L) *(35)* (Table 2). Clinafloxacin is less susceptible to quinolone resistance in staphylococci and more potent than trovafloxacin against MRSA *(43)*. Neither antibiotic is available for clinical use. Sitafloxacin has similar activity against GISA (MIC 0.5–1 mg/L) and is licensed, but reports of clinical experience have not been published *(44)*.

3.4. *Future Alternative Treatments*

A number of agents active against glycopeptide-resistant staphylococci are in various stages of laboratory and clinical trials, but are not yet routinely available. Some, such as everninomycin *(38)* have already been withdrawn following adverse events.

3.4.1. *Daptomycin*

Daptomycin is a cyclic polypeptide of the class *peptolides*, which act by interfering with amino acid transport by the cell membrane and the cytoplasmic membrane potential *(34)*. It is only active against Gram-positive bacteria. In *S. aureus*, daptomycin inhibits incorporation of alanine into peptidoglycan *(45)*. The antibiotic is highly protein bound, and some studies showed treatment of endocarditis at low doses (2–6 mg/kg body weight daily) to fail. Early clinical trials were stopped following adverse reactions, but changes in dosage regimens have allowed resumption of clinical trials *(46)*.

A concentration of 4 mg/L is sufficient to inhibit 50% of GISA (Table 2). In one study, the MIC of daptomycin was 0.5–1 mg/L, but in the presence of albumin, the MIC rose from 0.5 mg/L to 16 mg/L *(47)*. A glass chamber model allowing variation in volumes of culture medium and antibiotics has been used to simulate human serum concentrations of daptomycin, vancomycin, and arbekacin *(45)*. A two-log kill was achieved for daptomycin (3–6 mg/kg body weight daily), but with regrowth at 48 h. There was synergism between daptomycin and arbekacin. Using an in vitro model of vegetation, there was a five- to six-log reduction in number of GISA in 8 h at 6 mg/kg body weight daily, although 10 mg/kg body weight daily was needed to ensure no regrowth at 24 h *(47)*. There have been no reports of treatment of clinical GISA infections.

3.4.2. *Oritavancin (LY333328)*

Oritavancin (LY333328) is a glycopeptide that has potent activity against MRSA and other Gram-positive bacteria. Although susceptibility of GISA is less than MRSA, the difference was less marked than with other glycopeptides (Table 2). There is no clinical experience. In one study, the MIC of three strains of GISA was 1–2 mg/L in Mueller-Hinton broth, but rose to 4–16 mg/L in albumin. An in vitro infection model using variable concentrations of antibiotics in Mueller-Hinton broth was used to simulate serum concentrations expected at doses of 3 mg/kg body weight and 4 mg/kg body weight every 24 h and compared with vancomycin at simulated doses of 1–1.5 g *(26)*. At the lower concentration of oritavancin, regrowth of GISA occurred by 24 h in the presence of albumin. Resistant subpopulations became more prevalent with longer exposure times. Only one strain showed regrowth in the presence of a higher concentration (5 mg/kg body weight).

3.4.3. *Tigecycline (GAR-936)*

Tigecycline (GAR-936) is a glycylcycline derivative of tetracycline and is a broad-spectrum agent that acts by protein inhibition against organisms resistant to other agents. Glycopeptide resistance does not affect activity against staphylococci, and it is 16–32 times more active than teicoplanin, vancomycin, or daptomycin against GISA *(46)*. Daptomycin only reaches similar activity when the medium is supplemented with calcium (75 mg/L). Tigecycline was effective against GISA in an animal model (intraperitoneal murine infection). The median effective dose of tigecycline was 1.9 mg/kg body weight, compared with 6.1 mg/kg body weight daptomycin and 31 mg/kg body weight vancomycin *(46)*. It has not been used in treatment.

3.4.4. *Other Agents*

The cephalosporin RWJ-54428 has been reported as active against four isolates of GISA with an MIC of 2 mg/L *(48)*. Although cephalosporins are generally ineffective against MRSA, this antibiotic has increased affinity against PBP2' and therefore might have a clinical use.

Dalbavancin (BI 397), a semisynthetic derivative of the glycopeptide A-40926, has activity against all Gram-positive organisms tested and has started phase II trials in bacteremia and skin and soft tissue infection *(49)*. Activity against GISA was not reported *(50)*.

Lysostaphin is an endopeptidase produced by *S. simulans*. By hydrolyzing the pentaglycine bridge in the cell wall of *S. aureus*, crosslinks in peptidoglycan are broken, and the cell lyses. Lystostaphin can stimulate formation of inactivating antibodies. The agent has been used against GISA infections in animals *(51)*, but some GISA are resistant, including clinical strains.

4. PREVENTION

As with all staphylococcal infections, the most effective policy to tackle the problem of GISA infection is by prevention of cross-infection. Several guidelines for infection control have been published *(52,53)*. Education programs on hygiene and hand washing are effective, although the benefit is temporary without repeated reinforcement. The pattern in hospitals with good infection control is the emergence of different clones under pressure of exposure to vancomycin or teicoplanin *(27)*. A single-clone outbreak is more likely if cross-infection is frequent. Intended to reduce costs, excessively restrictive antibiotic policies may select for further resistance by overuse of a particular broad-spectrum agent. Nevertheless, strict antibiotic control of cephalosporins is beneficial.

Vancomycin and teicoplanin use must be limited to appropriate indications, diagnostic techniques used to reduce blind therapy, infected prosthetic materials removed rather than treated, and microbiologist or infectious disease physician advice sought in the treatment of staphylococcal disease. Restriction of use of glycopeptides will limit the emergence of GISA, but is increasingly difficult to enforce. Some advocate the planned change of first-line antibiotics every 6 mo to reduce the selective pressure, but results of studies are contradictory *(27)*.

S. aureus is transmitted on hands *(54)* and to a lesser extent by the airborne route. Standard precautions are sufficient to prevent spread *(55)*. Hand washing or disinfection before and after patient contact and source isolation of the patient are essential. Spread of MRSA is likely to occur from unidentified carriers. Universal precautions (e.g., HICPAC) have been introduced in many hospitals and should be started if GISA or VRSA is confirmed *(56)*. These measures are likely to reduce spread of both MRSA and GISA.

5. CONCLUSION

The emergence of *S. aureus* resistant to vancomycin and teicoplanin has long been predicted and is now finally having an effect on clinical practice. The resistant strains are derived from MRSA and appear as likely to cause serious infection as the parent organism. The main defense continues to be emphasis on the control of transmission, particularly in the hospital setting, and judicious use of antibiotics. Once the organism has appeared and spread, treatment may be possible with standard agents determined by the susceptibility profile. Linezolid and quinupristin/dalfopristin are already available for use when there are no effective standard agents. However, both are expensive, and resistance has already emerged. A number of new antibiotics are in development, and some of those may become clinically useful. Clearly, *S. aureus* will continue to evolve means of resisting any new agent as it appears.

REFERENCES

1. Smith IM, Vickers AB. Natural history of 338 treated and untreated patients with staphylococcal septicaemia. Lancet 1960; 1:1318–1321.
2. Jevons MP. "Celbenin" resistant staphylococci. BMJ 1961; 1:124–125.
3. Revised guidelines for the control of methicillin-resistant *Staphylococcus aureus* infection in hospitals. British Society for Antimicrobial Chemotherapy, Hospital Infection Society and the Infection Control Nurses Association. J Hosp Infect 1998; 39:253–290.
4. Voss A, Milatovic D, Wallrauch-Schwarz C, Rosdahl VT, Braveny I. Methicillin-resistant *Staphylococcus aureus* in Europe. Eur J Clin Microbiol Infect Dis 1994; 13:50–55.
5. Pujol M, Pena C, Pallares R, et al. Nosocomial *Staphylococcus aureus* bacteremia among nasal carriers of methicillin-resistant and methicillin-susceptible strains. Am J Med 1996; 100:509–516.
6. Romero-Vivas J, Rubio M, Fernandez C, Picazo JJ. Mortality associated with nosocomial bacteremia due to methicillin-resistant *Staphylococcus aureus*. Clin Infect Dis 1995; 21:1417–1423.
7. Bayer AS. Infective endocarditis. Clin Infect Dis 1993; 17:313–320, quiz 321–322.
8. Wilson WR, Karchmer AW, Dajani AS, et al. Antibiotic treatment of adults with infective endocarditis due to streptococci, enterococci, staphylococci, and HACEK microorganisms. American Heart Association. JAMA 1995; 274:1706–1713.
9. Liu CY, Lee WS, Fung CP, et al. Comparative study of teicoplanin versus vancomycin for the treatment of methicillin-resistant *Staphylococcus aureus* bacteremia. Clin Drug Invest 1996; 12:80–87.

10. Hiramatsu K. Vancomycin-resistant *Staphylococcus aureus*: a new model of antibiotic resistance. Lancet Infect Dis 2001; 1:147–155.
11. Linares J. The VISA/GISA problem: therapeutic implications. Clin Microbiol Infect 2001; 7(suppl. 4):8–15.
12. Hiramatsu K, Aritaka N, Hanaki H, et al. Dissemination in Japanese hospitals of strains of *Staphylococcus aureus* heterogeneously resistant to vancomycin. Lancet 1997; 350:1670–1673.
13. Ike Y, Arakawa Y, Ma X, et al. Nationwide survey shows that methicillin-resistant *Staphylococcus aureus* strains heterogeneously and intermediately resistant to vancomycin are not disseminated throughout Japanese hospitals. J Clin Microbiol 2001; 39:4445–4451.
14. Howe RA, Bowker KE, Walsh TR, Feest TG, MacGowan AP. Vancomycin-resistant *Staphylococcus aureus*. Lancet 1998; 351:602.
15. Noble WC, Virani Z, Cree RG. Co-transfer of vancomycin and other resistance genes from *Enterococcus faecalis* NCTC 12201 to *Staphylococcus aureus*. FEMS Microbiol Lett 1992; 72:195–198.
16. *Staphylococcus aureus* resistant to vancomycin—United States. MMWR Morb Mortal Wkly Rep 2002; 51:565–567.
17. Miller D, Uredaneta V, Weltman A. Vancomycin-resistant *Staphylococcus aureus*—Pennsylvania 2002. MMWR Morb Mortal Wkly Rep 2002; 51:902.
18. National Committee for Laboratory Standards. Methods for dilution antimicrobial susceptibility tests for bacteria that grow aerobically. In: Approved Standard M7-A5. 5th ed. Wayne, PA: National Committee for Clinical Laboratory Standards, 2000.
19. Fridkin SK. Vancomycin-intermediate and -resistant *Staphylococcus aureus*: what the infectious disease specialist needs to know. Clin Infect Dis 2001; 32:108–115.
20. Bobin-Dubreux S, Reverdy ME, Nervi C, et al. Clinical isolate of vancomycin-heterointermediate *Staphylococcus aureus* susceptible to methicillin and in vitro selection of a vancomycin-resistant derivative. Antimicrob Agents Chemother 2001; 45:349–352.
21. Arthur M, Reynolds PE, Depardieu F, et al. Mechanisms of glycopeptide resistance in enterococci. J Infect 1996; 32:11–16.
22. Climo MW, Patron RL, Archer GL. Combinations of vancomycin and β-lactams are synergistic against staphylococci with reduced susceptibilities to vancomycin. Antimicrob Agents Chemother 1999; 43:1747–1753.
23. Moreira B, Boyle-Vavra S, deJonge BL, Daum RS. Increased production of penicillin-binding protein 2, increased detection of other penicillin-binding proteins, and decreased coagulase activity associated with glycopeptide resistance in *Staphylococcus aureus*. Antimicrob Agents Chemother 1997; 41:1788–1793.
24. Ariza J, Pujol M, Cabo J, et al. Vancomycin in surgical infections due to methicillin-resistant *Staphylococcus aureus* with heterogeneous resistance to vancomycin. Lancet 1999; 353:1587–1588.
25. Nicolaou KC, Hughes R, Cho SY, Winssinger N, Labischinski H, Endermann R. Synthesis and biological evaluation of vancomycin dimers with potent activity against vancomycin-resistant bacteria: target-accelerated combinatorial synthesis. Chemistry 2001; 7:3824–3843.
26. Aeschlimann JR, Allen GP, Hershberger E, Rybak MJ. Activities of LY333328 and vancomycin administered alone or in combination with gentamicin against three strains of vancomycin-intermediate *Staphylococcus aureus* in an in vitro pharmacodynamic infection model. Antimicrob Agents Chemother 2000; 44:2991–2998.
27. Schentag JJ. Antimicrobial management strategies for Gram-positive bacterial resistance in the intensive care unit. Crit Care Med 2001; 29(4 suppl.):N100–N107.
28. Burnie J, Matthews R, Jiman-Fatami A, Gottardello P, Hodgetts S, D'Arcy S. Analysis of 42 cases of septicemia caused by an epidemic strain of methicillin-resistant *Staphylococcus aureus*: evidence of resistance to vancomycin. Clin Infect Dis 2000; 31:684–689.

29. Smith TL, Pearson ML, Wilcox KR, et al. Emergence of vancomycin resistance in *Staphylococcus aureus*. Glycopeptide-Intermediate *Staphylococcus aureus* Working Group. N Engl J Med 1999; 340:493–501.
30. Hiramatsu K, Hanaki H, Ino T, Yabuta K, Oguri T, Tenover FC. Methicillin-resistant *Staphylococcus aureus* clinical strain with reduced vancomycin susceptibility. J Antimicrob Chemother 1997; 40:135–136.
31. Backo M, Gaenger E, Burkart A, Chai YL, Bayer AS. Treatment of experimental staphylococcal endocarditis due to a strain with reduced susceptibility in vitro to vancomycin: efficacy of ampicillin-sulbactam. Antimicrob Agents Chemother 1999; 43:2565–2568.
32. Sieradzki K, Tomasz A. Inhibition of cell wall turnover and autolysis by vancomycin in a highly vancomycin-resistant mutant of *Staphylococcus aureus*. J Bacteriol 1997; 179:2557–2566.
33. Howe RA, Wootton M, Bennett PM, MacGowan AP, Walsh TR. Interactions between methicillin and vancomycin in methicillin-resistant *Staphylococcus aureus* strains displaying different phenotypes of vancomycin susceptibility. J Clin Microbiol 1999; 37:3068–3071.
34. Rybak MJ, Hershberger E, Moldovan T, Grucz RG. In vitro activities of daptomycin, vancomycin, linezolid, and quinupristin-dalfopristin against etaphylococci and enterococci, including vancomycin-intermediate and -resistant strains. Antimicrob Agents Chemother 2000; 44:1062–1066.
35. Hershberger E, Aeschlimann JR, Moldovan T, Rybak MJ. Evaluation of bactericidal activities of LY333328, vancomycin, teicoplanin, ampicillin-sulbactam, trovafloxacin, and RP59500 alone or in combination with rifampin or gentamicin against different strains of vancomycin-intermediate *Staphylococcus aureus* by time-kill curve methods. Antimicrob Agents Chemother 1999; 43:717–721.
36. Stevens DL, Herr D, Lampiris H, Hunt JL, Batts DH, Hafkin B. Linezolid versus vancomycin for the treatment of methicillin-resistant *Staphylococcus aureus* infections. Clin Infect Dis 2002; 34:1481–1490.
37. Tsiodras S, Gold HS, Sakoulas G, et al. Linezolid resistance in a clinical isolate of *Staphylococcus aureus*. Lancet 2001; 358:207–208.
38. Tenover FC, Lancaster MV, Hill BC, et al. Characterization of staphylococci with reduced susceptibilities to vancomycin and other glycopeptides. J Clin Microbiol 1998; 36:1020–1027.
39. Vouillamoz J, Tomasz A, Sieradzki K, et al. Efficacy of Synercid (SYN) and/or cefpirome (CP) in the treatment (Rx) of experimental endocarditis (EE) due to glycopeptide intermediate *Staphylococcus aureus* (GISA). In: 40th Interscience Conference on Antimicrobial Agents and Chemotherapy; Toronto, Ontario, Canada: American Society for Microbiology, 2000, p. 56.
40. Werner G, Cuny C, Schmitz FJ, Witte W. Methicillin-resistant, quinupristin-dalfopristin-resistant *Staphylococcus aureus* with reduced sensitivity to glycopeptides. J Clin Microbiol 2001; 39:3586–3590.
41. Dowzicky M, Talbot GH, Feger C, Prokocimer P, Etienne J, Leclercq R. Characterization of isolates associated with emerging resistance to quinupristin/dalfopristin (Synercid) during a worldwide clinical program. Diagn Microbiol Infect Dis 2000; 37:57–62.
42. Lamb HM, Figgitt DP, Faulds D. Quinupristin/dalfopristin: a review of its use in the management of serious Gram-positive infections. Drugs 1999; 58:1061–1097.
43. Roychoudhury S, Catrenich CE, McIntosh EJ, et al. Quinolone resistance in staphylococci: activities of new nonfluorinated quinolones against molecular targets in whole cells and clinical isolates. Antimicrob Agents Chemother 2001; 45:1115–1120.
44. Tanaka M, Wada N, Kurosaka SM, Chiba M, Sato K, Hiramatsu K. In-vitro activity of DU-6859a against methicillin-resistant *Staphylococcus aureus* isolates with reduced susceptibilities to vancomycin. J Antimicrob Chemother 1998; 42:552–553.

45. Akins RL, Rybak MJ. In vitro activities of daptomycin, arbekacin, vancomycin, and gentamicin alone and/or in combination against glycopeptide intermediate-resistant *Staphylococcus aureus* in an infection model. Antimicrob Agents Chemother 2000; 44:1925–1929.
46. Petersen PJ, Bradford PA, Weiss WJ, Murphy TM, Sum PE, Projan SJ. In vitro and in vivo activities of tigecycline (GAR-936), daptomycin, and comparative antimicrobial agents against glycopeptide-intermediate *Staphylococcus aureus* and other resistant Gram-positive pathogens. Antimicrob Agents Chemother 2002; 46:2595–2601.
47. Akins RL, Rybak MJ. Bactericidal activities of two daptomycin regimens against clinical strains of glycopeptide intermediate-resistant *Staphylococcus aureus*, vancomycin-resistant *Enterococcus faecium*, and methicillin-resistant *Staphylococcus aureus* isolates in an in vitro pharmacodynamic model with simulated endocardial vegetations. Antimicrob Agents Chemother 2001; 45:454–459.
48. Swenson JM, Tenover FC. In vitro activity of a new cephalosporin, RWJ-54428, against streptococci, enterococci and staphylococci, including glycopeptide-intermediate *Staphylococcus aureus*. J Antimicrob Chemother 2002; 49:845–850.
49. Steiert M, Schmitz FJ. Dalbavancin (Biosearch Italia/Versicor). Curr Opin Investig Drugs 2002; 3:229–233.
50. Candiani G, Abbondi M, Borgonovi M, Romano G, Parenti F. In-vitro and in-vivo antibacterial activity of BI 397, a new semi-synthetic glycopeptide antibiotic. J Antimicrob Chemother 1999; 44:179–192.
51. Patron RL, Climo MW, Goldstein BP, Archer GL. Lysostaphin treatment of experimental aortic valve endocarditis caused by a *Staphylococcus aureus* isolate with reduced susceptibility to vancomycin. Antimicrob Agents Chemother 1999; 43:1754–1755.
52. From the Centers for Disease Control and Prevention. Interim guidelines for prevention and control of staphylococcal infection associated with reduced susceptibility to vancomycin. JAMA 1997; 278:461–462.
53. Wenzel RP, Edmond MB. Vancomycin-resistant *Staphylococcus aureus*: infection control considerations. Clin Infect Dis 1998; 27:245–249, quiz 250–251.
54. Pittet D, Hugonnet S, Harbarth S, et al. Effectiveness of a hospital-wide programme to improve compliance with hand hygiene. Infection Control Programme. Lancet 2000; 356:1307–1312.
55. Hageman JC, Pegues DA, Jepson C, et al. Vancomycin-intermediate *Staphylococcus aureus* in a home health-care patient. Emerg Infect Dis 2001; 7:1023–1025.
56. Interim guidelines for prevention and control of *Staphylococcal infection* associated with reduced susceptibility to vancomycin. MMWR Morb Mortal Wkly Rep 1997; 46:626–628, 635.

5

Infections Caused by Glycopeptide-Resistant Gram-Positive Bacteria Excluding Staphylococci

Armine Sefton

1. INTRODUCTION

Vancomycin and teicoplanin are the two glycopeptides in clinical use throughout the world. Vancomycin has been in clinical use since 1958, but teicoplanin only since the late 1980s. Glycopeptide resistance in Gram-positive bacteria can be either intrinsic or acquired. Although intrinsic vancomycin resistance in certain organisms predates acquired resistance in enterococci, it is the acquired resistance in enterococci that has increased so dramatically since first reported in the late 1980s by Uttley et al. *(1)*. For instance, a 3-yr analysis of nosocomial bloodstream infections in 49 U.S. hospitals between 1997 and 1999 found that 11% of bacteremias were caused by enterococci; of these enterococci, 3% of *E. faecalis* and 50% of *E. faecium* were vancomycin resistant *(2)*.

In 1989, transfer of the acquired vancomycin resistance (VanR) genes from enterococci to streptococci, *Lactococcus lactis*, and *Listeria* spp was achieved in the laboratory *(3)*. More recently, in vivo spread of vancomycin resistance to other Gram-positive bacteria, such as streptococci and corynebacteria, has happened as well. This is of particular concern as these organisms remained susceptible to glycopeptides for 40 yr.

2. MECHANISM AND EPIDEMIOLOGY

2.1. *Intrinsically Vancomycin-Resistant Gram-Positive Bacteria*

Intrinsically vancomycin resistance occurs in certain *Enterococcus* spp as well as in four other genera of Gram-positive bacteria. The intrinsically vancomycin-resistant enterococci (IVRE) are found in three species: *E. gallinarum, E. casseliflavus,* and *E. flavescens (4)*. However, some authors consider that *E. flavescens* is not a distinct species *(5,6)*. On the other hand, whole-cell protein analysis suggests *E. casseliflavus* and *E. flavescens* constitute a single genospecies *(7)*. Vancomycin resistance in these organisms is conferred by possession of the *van*C gene, which cannot be transferred or acquired *(8)*.

From: *Management of Multiple Drug-Resistant Infections*
Edited by: S. H. Gillespie © Humana Press Inc., Totowa, NJ

The differentiation of IVRE from acquired vancomycin-resistant enterococci (AVRE) and vancomycin-sensitive enterococci can sometimes be difficult. Motility has traditionally been used to distinguish IVRE from *E. faecium*. In addition, many laboratories rely on commercial identification systems for enterococcal identification, but these systems may produce erroneous results *(9,10)*. Distinction by resistance phenotype can also be problematic because of overlap between the minimum inhibitory concentration (MIC) range for IVRE (2 to 32 mg/L) and VanB-mediated resistance in *E. faecium* and *E. faecalis* (4 to >256 mg/L) *(11)*.

2.2. Intrinsically Vancomycin-Resistant Enterococci

IVRE have been isolated both from fecal and nonfecal clinical specimens. Nonhuman sources of IVRE also exist, such as dogs and poultry *(12,13)*. IVRE have been potentially pathogenic to humans, and clinically significant isolates have been reported from blood *(4,8)*, urine *(4,8,14)*, pus and cerebrospinal fluid (CSF) *(4)*, ascitic fluid *(15)*, and wounds *(4,6,14)*.

2.3. Intrinsically Vancomycin-Resistant Nonenterococcal Genera

The four genera of intrinsically vancomycin-resistant nonenterococcal Gram-positive bacteria are *Leuconostoc, Pediococcus, Lactobacillus*, and *Erysipelothrix (16)*. They all have peptidoglycan precursors terminating in D-Ala-D-Lac in a similar fashion to AVRE *(17)* rather than the D-Ala-D-Ser termination found in IVRE *(18)*. *Lactobacillus* spp are part of the normal human gut and vaginal flora *(19)*. *Erysipelothrix* spp are widely disseminated in nature and have been isolated from soil, water, and fish *(20)*, and *Leuconostoc* and *Pediococcus* spp reside in vegetation *(21)*. All of these organisms act as opportunistic pathogens, but have not been known to cause outbreaks.

2.4. Acquired Vancomycin Resistance in Enterococci

Normally, in peptidioglycan synthesis in enterococci, two molecules of D-alanine are joined by a ligase enzyme to form D-Ala-D-Ala, which is then added to the UDP-*N*-acetlymuramyl-tripeptide to form UDP-*N*-acetylmuramyl-pentapeptide. This is incorporated into the growing peptidoglycan strand by a process known as transglycosylation, and it allows the formation of cross-bridges in the peptidoglycan (transpeptidation) to occur. Glycopeptides such as vancomycin act by binding to the D-Ala-D-Ala terminus of the pentapeptide side chain on *N*-acetylmuramic acid. This causes the transglycolase enzyme responsible for transfer of the peptidoglycan precursor to the growing glycan polymer to be inhibited by steric hindrance. Transpeptidase activity may also be inhibited.

Different AVRE have been characterized on both phenotypic and genotypic bases *(22,23)*. VanA enterococci are resistant to high levels of vancomycin and teicoplanin. VanA resistance is caused by a cluster of genes located on a transposon, T1546, which often resides on a plasmid. Expression of these genes results in the synthesis of abnormal peptidoglycan precursors ending in D-Ala-D-Lac rather than D-Ala-D-Ala. Both vancomycin and teicoplanin bind to D-Ala-D-Lac with much lower affinity than to the normal dipeptide product. Resistance is induced by the presence of either drug *(24)*.

VanB glycopeptide resistance in enterococci is mediated by an abnormal ligase, VanB, which is structurally related to VanA ligase. VanB expression (as with VanA) leads to synthesis of abnormal peptidoglycan precursors terminating in D-Ala-D-Lac instead of D-Ala-D-Ala, resulting in loss of binding affinity for vancomycin compared to the normal dipeptide product. VanB enterococci are resistant to a range of vancomycin concentrations, from 4 to more than 1024 mg/L. However, typically they retain susceptibility to teicoplanin, which has not induced resistance *(25)*. VanB resistance is usually chromosomally mediated.

VanA and VanB clusters have been found primarily in *E. faecalis* and *E. faecium.* They are less commonly found in other enterococcal species. VanD is an uncommon phenotype of acquired glycopeptide resistance that has been described in several isolates of *E. faecium* that were resistant to modest levels of vancomycin (MIC 64–128 mg/L) and teicoplanin (MIC 4 mg/L), and VanE has been found in a strain of *E. faecalis* that was resistant to a low concentration of vancomycin (MIC 16 mg/L) but susceptible to teicoplanin *(26,27)*. Rarely, vancomycin-dependent enterococci occur. These are derived from VanA and VanB vancomycin-resistant enterococci (VRE) that develop mutations that prevent them from growing in the absence of glycopeptides *(28)*.

2.5. Acquired Glycopeptide Resistance in Gram-Positive Organisms Other Than Enterococci

Leclercq et al. *(3)* transferred VanA gene of high-level vancomycin resistance from *E. faecium* to *L. monocytogenes* in vitro; a year later, Brisson-Noel et al. *(29)* transferred it to *Bacillus* spp. Biavasco et al. *(30)* transferred vancomycin resistance to *L. monocytogenes* in vitro, as well as to four other species of *Listeria* spp. Fortunately, so far no clinical infections caused by vancomycin-resistant *Listeria* spp have been reported, and in vivo transfer of vancomycin resistance to *Corynebacteria* spp has not been detected. However, sporadic in vivo transfer of the VanA gene from *E. faecium* to *Arcanobacterium haemolyticum* and *Cellulomonas turbata* was reported during an outbreak in an intensive care unit (ICU) in London *(31,32)*. In addition, in 1997 a central-line infection caused by a highly vancomycin-resistant *Bacillus circulans* (MIC to vancomycin >128 mg/L and genetically related to VanA of *E. faecium*) was described in Italy by Fontana and coworkers *(33)*. Fortunately, VanA, coding high-vancomycin resistance together with resistance to aminoglycosides and penicillin, has only been transferred to organisms that generally do not behave as major pathogens and cause infections only sporadically.

2.6. Streptococci

The first in vitro transfer of VanA-type resistance from *E. faecium* to streptococci (*S. sanguis, S. pyogenes, S. lactis/Lactococcus lactis*) was reported in 1989 by Leclercq et al. *(3)*, who detected high-level vancomycin resistance in *S. sanguis* and *S. pyogenes* (MICs to vancomycin were 128 and 512 mg/L, respectively), and low-level resistance in *S. lactis* (MIC 4–8 mg/L). For several years, no further reports of either in vitro transfer or clinical cases of vancomycin resistance in streptococci occurred. Then, in December 1993, Rolston *(34)* reported four bacteremias caused by what were described as "viridans" streptococci in a hematology unit in Houston; the MICs of vancomycin were 8–32 mg/L.

In 1997, two reports of clinical infections caused by vancomycin resistance in streptococci occurred simultaneously, one from France *(35)* and one from Slovakia *(36)*, which were caused by low-level (MIC 16–32 mg/L) vancomycin-resistant *S. bovis* and *S. mitis*, respectively. It was thought that these were most likely caused by VanB or VanB-related genes transferring from enterococci. Strains isolated from both cases were susceptible to teicoplanin, and both occurred in immunocompromised individuals, the *S. bovis* in a child from Africa living in France and who was positive for human immunodeficiency virus (HIV) and the *S. mitis* from a leukemic patient receiving long-term prophylaxis with oral ofloxacin who had also received several courses of intravenous vancomycin *(36)*.

In 1998, Mevius et al. described vancomycin-resistant *Streptococcus gallolyticus* obtained from fecal samples of veal calves screened for glycopeptide resistance *(37)*. Resistant strains were found with both the VanA and VanB genotypes. This was of particular concern as until then resistance of the VanA genotype had not been reported in streptococci, and until 1995, *S. gallolyticus* was classified as a subspecies of *S. bovis*.

3. CLINICAL SIGNIFICANCE AND THERAPY

3.1. *Clinical Significance and Therapeutic Implications for Treatment of Intrinsically Vancomycin-Resistant Nonenterococcal Gram-Positive Bacteria*

There is relatively little data on susceptibility profiles for intrinsically vancomycin-resistant nonenterococcal gram-positive bacteria. However, the data available suggest that they are normally susceptible to a range of antimicrobials, including the β-lactam antibiotics. For example, Swenson et al. *(38)* determined the sensitivities of 85 strains of *Leuconostoc, Lactobacillus*, and *Pediococcus*. They found that although all of the isolates were resistant to vancomycin and teicoplanin (MIC 64 mg/L), only three were resistant to penicillin and all were susceptible to chloramphenicol and imipenem. However, it has been suggested that, in the treatment of serious infections caused by *Lactobacillus* spp, the therapeutic response may be improved by the addition of an aminoglycoside to the β-lactam *(39)*. In contrast, although *Erysipelothrix* spp are highly susceptible to β-lactam agents, the quinolones and clindamycin, they show widespread resistance to aminoglycosides *(40)*.

3.2. *Treatment of Infections Caused by Nonenterococcal Organisms With Acquired Vancomycin Resistance*

Most of the reported infections caused by acquired vancomycin-resistant Gram-positive bacteria other than enterococci have, unsurprisingly, been clinically significant, but it is likely that there are more people who are colonized but not infected by these organisms. Clinical infections have almost entirely occurred in patients who are immunocompromised in some way. The most commonly reported compromising conditions are leukemia, a central vascular catheter *in situ*, and residence in the ICU environment. The most frequently reported risk factor for acquisition of vancomycin-resistant Gram-positive bacteria other than enterococci appears to be prior therapy with broad-spectrum antimicrobials, especially glycopeptides, or quinolones or other drugs that are broad-spectrum drugs also active against anaerobes.

Antimicrobial susceptibility profiles of the streptococci, corynebacterialike organisms, and *Bacillus* spp that were vancomycin-resistant are different and not necessarily multiresistant. For instance, a highly vancomycin-resistant *B. circulans* isolated from a baby with meningitis *(33,41)* was susceptible to six other antibiotics, including amoxicillin/clavulanate, cephalosporins, aminoglycosides, quinolones, rifampicin, cotrimoxazole, but not teicoplanin. Most of the reported organisms, excluding the streptococci and enterococci, that were resistant to vancomycin were also resistant to teicoplanin. In contrast, a vancomycin-resistant *S. mitis* that caused bacteremia in a leukemic patient previously treated with vancomycin *(36)* was susceptible to tetracycline, chloramphenicol, and teicoplanin.

Vancomycin resistance in streptococci *(35,36)* is usually genetically related to the VanB gene of enterococci, and isolates remain susceptible to teicoplanin. However, the possibility of vancomycin resistance, especially if high-level transferring in vivo to vancomycin-susceptible organisms such as *Streptococcus pneumoniae* and β-hemolytic streptococci occurs, should motivate the use of preventive measures to avoid the spread of vancomycin resistance to these organisms, which cause significant mortality and morbidity in humans. Vancomycin-tolerant *S. pneumoniae* has now been reported; this is discussed in more detail in Chapter 3.

3.3. Treatment of Infections Caused by Vancomycin-Resistant Enterococci

VanC enterococci (*E. gallinarum* and *E. casseliflavus*) are relatively uncommon pathogens. In contrast to AVRE, they are typically susceptible to penicillins and other drugs and consequently are less difficult to treat *(22)*. Serious infections with AVRE usually occur in patients with host defenses that are compromised either by disease or therapy or a combination of the two. Sometimes, depending on their antimicrobial susceptibility profiles, infections caused by VRE can be treated with widely available, cheap, and well-established agents like chloramphenicol, doxycycline, or high-dose ampicillin/amoxicillin if the infection is caused by a vancomycin-resistant *E. faecalis*. Nitrofurantoin is also a possibility if the patient is suffering from a lower urinary tract infection. Although the combination of trimethoprim and sulfamethoxazole may appear active against enterococci in vitro, treatment is likely to fail as organisms are able to use exogenous folate *(42)*.

The established treatment of serious enterococcal infections, particularly endocarditis, is combined use of a cell-wall-active agent such as a β-lactam (typically ampicillin or penicillin) or vancomycin and an aminoglycoside to produce a synergistic bactericidal effect *(43)*. High-level resistance to either agent abolishes this synergy. Unfortunately, many isolates of AVRE show high-level resistance to the aminoglycosides. Thus, in all cases of infections caused by vancomycin-resistant Gram-positive bacteria, including enterococci, it is necessary to perform susceptibility testing against a range of agents.

It is a general rule of infectious diseases that foci of infection amenable to drainage should be drained, and infected foreign bodies, such as central venous catheters, should be removed. This is particularly critical when dealing with VRE and may be at least as important as the choice of antimicrobial therapy *(44)*. This is because VRE are frequently multiresistant, and until relatively recently, there were often no licensed drugs available to treat infections caused by some of them.

3.3.1. New Antibiotics

Two new antimicrobial agents (quinupristin/dalfopristin and linezolid) have been licensed for treating vancomycin-resistant infections *(45)*. Quinupristin/dalfopristin

(Synercid) is a streptogramin, which impairs bacterial protein synthesis at both early peptide chain elongation and late peptide chain extrusion steps. It has bacteriostatic activity against vancomycin-resistant *E. faecium*, but is not active against *E. faecalis*. Microbiologically, it is similar to pristinamycin, which is an oral agent only and is relatively poorly absorbed but has been used in France for many years *(46)*. Myalgia/arthralgia appears to the most frequent treatment-limiting adverse effect of Synercid *(45)*.

Linezolid is an oxazolidinone that acts by inhibiting bacterial protein synthesis. Linezolid inhibits formation of the 70S initiation complex by binding to the 50S ribosomal subunit near to the interface with the 30S subunit. This mechanism is unique, and no cross-resistance between oxazolidinones and other protein synthesis inhibitors has been reported *(47)*.

In contrast to Synercid, linezolid has bacteriostatic activity against both vancomycin-resistant *E. faecium* and *E. faecalis*. Linezolid can be given either intravenously or orally and is rapidly and completely absorbed after oral dosing. It is cleared by both renal and nonrenal routes. Studies in patients with renal failure suggest that a decrease in dose may not be necessary. Metabolites do accumulate in renal failure, but their clinical significance is not yet known. Both linezolid and its metabolites are removed during dialysis, so postdialysis dosing is recommended. Adverse effects of linezolid therapy have been predominantly gastrointestinal effects, headache, and taste alteration. In addition, there are reports of it causing thrombocytopenia, but this appears to be largely limited to patients receiving treatment for longer than 14 d. Linezolid resistance has been reported in a small number of *E. faecium* strains; it appears to be secondary to a basepair mutation in the genome encoding for the bacterial 23S ribosome binding site, but currently is very rare.

In addition to Synercid and linezolid, which both have product licenses for clinical use, there are several investigational agents in phase II or III trials for VRE infection *(22,48,49)*. These agents include the glycopeptides oritavancin (previously known as LY333328) *(50)* and daptomycin (an acidic lipopeptide) and the glycylcycline tigecycline (previously known as GAR-936), which is a new tetracycline specifically developed to overcome resistance to earlier tetracyclines *(51)*.

4. PREVENTION OF SPREAD OF GLYCOPEPTIDE-RESISTANT ORGANISMS

It is essential to try to minimize the spread of any infection, but especially of those that are multiresistant and hence difficult to treat. Examples within the hospital setting include infections caused by multiresistant *Acinetobacter* spp and *Klebsiella* spp, methicillin-resistant *Staphylococcus aureus* and VRE. In contrast, patients with infections caused by the intrinsically vancomycin-resistant *Leuconostoc, Pediococcus, Lactobacillus*, and *Erysipelothrix* spp do not normally require isolation as these organisms have not been found to cause outbreaks and are not usually multiresistant. In addition, if an individual is found to be colonized or infected with an IVRE caused by VanC vancomycin (*E. gallinarum* and *E. casseliflavus*), it is probably not necessary to isolate them as in this case resistance is nontransferable *(8,52)*. However, it is a different matter for patients colonized/infected with enterococci with acquired vancomycin resistance. Enterococci are particularly hardy organisms that can resist disinfection and are not destroyed if linen is washed at low temperatures. Preventive measures to minimize their spread should include stringent infection control procedures with isolation of infected patients, especially if they are likely to be excreting large numbers of resistant bacteria and thorough cleaning of ward areas after infected patients have left them. Prudent use of glycopeptides, both in humans and in animals, is also necessary. Further discussion of appropriate infection control methods are found in Chapter 6.

5. CONCLUSIONS

Vancomycin resistance has spread from enterococci to a variety of Gram-positive organisms *(53)*. In addition, vancomycin-resistant mutants of staphylococci (where vancomycin resistance has probably occurred by a different mechanism) have also appeared: In 1997, the first two clinical cases of intermediate VanA *S. aureus* causing systemic infections were reported *(54)* (*see* Chapter 4). Since the mid-1990s, a variety of Gram-positive bacteria, including *A. haemolyticum, C. turbata, L. monocytogenes,* and *Bacillus* spp, have been reported to have acquired VanA or VanB (*S. bovis* and *S. mitis*) resistance genes.

Today, vancomycin resistance has been described in most Gram-positive bacteria with the exception of *S. pneumoniae, S. agalactiae,* and *S. pyogenes* in vivo. However, vancomycin tolerance in *S. pneumoniae* has been reported *(55)*. It would have both major medical and financial implications if, in the future, widespread glycopeptide resistance caused by VanA or VanB were to occur in common community-acquired organisms such as *S. pneumoniae, S. agalactiae*, or *S. pyogenes.*

REFERENCES

1. Uttley AHC, Collins CH, Naidoo J, George RC. Vancomycin resistant enterococci. Lancet 1988; 331:136.
2. Edmond MB, Wallace SE, McClish DK, Pfaller MA, Jones RN, Wenzel RP. Nosocomial bloodstream infections in United States hospitals—a 3-year analysis. Clin Infect Dis 1999; 29:239–244.
3. Leclercq R, Derlot E, Weber M, Courvalin P. Transferable vancomycin and teicoplanin resistance in *E. faecium*. Antimicrob Agents Chemother 1989; 33:10–15.
4. Clark NC, Teixeira L, Facklam R, Tenover FC. Detection and differentiation of *van*C-1, *van*C2 and *van*C-3 glycopeptide resistance genes in enterococci. J Clin Microbiol 1998; 36:2294–2297.
5. Navarro F, Courvalin P. Analysis of genes encoding -Alanine-D-Alanine ligase related enzymes in *Enterococcus casseliflavus* and *Enterococcus flavescens*. Antimicrob Agents Chemother 1994; 38:1788–1793.
6. Leclerq R, Dutka-Malen S, Duval J, Courvalin P. Vancomycin resistance gene *van*C is specific to *Enterococcus gallinarum*. Antimicrob Agents Chemother 1992; 36:2005–2008.
7. Vandamme P, Veracauteren E, Lammer SC, et al. Survey of enterococcal susceptibility patterns in Belgium. J Clin Microbiol 1996; 34:2573–2576.
8. Toye B, Shymanski J, Bobrowska M, Woods W, Ramotar K. Clinical and epidemiologic significance of enterococci intrinsically resistant to vancomycin (possessing the *van*C phenotype). J Clin Microbiol 1997; 35:3166–3170.
9. Cartwright CP, Stock F, Fahle GA, Gill VJ. Comparison of pigment production and motility tests with PCR for reliable identification of intrinsically vancomycin resistant enterococci. J Clin Microbiol 1995; 33:1931–1933.
10. Facklam RR, Collins MD. Identification of *Enterococcus* species isolated from human infections by a conventional test scheme. J Clin Microbiol 1989; 27:731–734.

11. Arthur M, Reynolds PE, Depardieu F, et al. Mechanisms of glycopetide resistance in enterococci. J Infect 1996; 32:11–16.
12. Van Belkum A, Van der Braak N, Thomassen R, Verbrugh H, Encitz H. Vancomycin-resistant enterococci in dogs and cats. Lancet 1996; 348:1038–1039.
13. Van der Braak N, Van Belkum A, Van Kculen M, Vliegenthart J, Verbrugh HA, Encitz HP. Molecular characterisation of vancomycin resistant enterococci from hospitalised patients and poultry products in the Netherlands. J Clin Microbiol 1998; 36:1927–1932.
14. Ruoff KL, De la Maza L, Murtagh M, Spargo JD, Ferraro MJ. Species identities of enterococci isolated from clinical specimens. J Clin Microbiol 1990; 28:435–437.
15. Liassine N, Frei R, Jan I, Auckenthaler R. Characterisation of glycopeptide-resistant enterococci in a Swiss hospital. J Clin Microbiol 1998; 36:1853–1858.
16. Johnson AP, Uttley AH, Woodford N, George RC. Resistance to vancomycin and teicoplanin: an emerging clinical problem. Clin Microbiol Rev 1990; 3:280–291.
17. Billot-Klein D, Gutman L, Sable S, Guittet E, Van Heijenoort J. Modification of the peptidoglycan precursors is a common feature of low-level vancomycin-resistant VanB type enterococcus D366 and of the naturally glycopeptide-resistant species *Lactobacillus casei, Pediococcus pentosaceus, Leuconostoc mesenteroides* and *Enterococcus gallinarum.* J Bacteriol 1994; 176:2398–2405.
18. Reynolds PE, Snalth HA, Maguire AJ, Dutka-Malen S, Courvalin P. Analysis of peptidoglycan precursors in vancomycin-resistant *Enterococcus gallinarum.* Biochem J 1994; 301:5–8.
19. Hillier SL, Moncla BJ. *Peptostreptococcus, Propionobacterium, Eubacterium* and other nonsporeforming anaerobic Gram-positive bacteria. In: Murray PR, Baron EJ, Pfaller MA, Tenover FC, Yolken RH (eds.). Manual of Clinical Microbiology. 6th ed. Washington, DC: ASM, 1995, pp. 587–602.
20. Clarridge JE, Spiegel CA. *Corynebacterium* and miscellaneous irregular Gram-positive rods, *Erysipelothrix* and *Gardnerella.* In: Murray PR, Baron EJ, Pfaller MA, Tenover FC, Yolken RH (eds.). Manual of Clinical Microbiology. 6th ed. Washington, DC: ASM, 1995 pp. 357–378.
21. Ruoff KL. *Leuconostoc, Pediococcus, Stomatococcus* and miscellaneous Gram-positive cocci that grow aerobically. In: Murray PR, Baron EJ, Pfaller MA, Tenover FC, Yolken RH (eds.). Manual of Clinical Microbiology. 6th ed. Washington, DC: ASM, 1995, pp. 315–323.
22. Gold HS. Vancomycin-resistant enterococci: mechanisms and clinical observations. Clin Infect Dis 2001; 33:210–219.
23. Shlaes DM, Etter L, Gutmann L. Synergistic killing of vancomycin-resistant enterococci of classes A, B, and C by combinations of vancomycin, penicillin, and gentamicin. Antimicrob Agents Chemother 1991; 35:776–779.
24. Arthur M, Molinas C, Courvalin P. The VanS-VanR two-component regulatory system controls synthesis of depsipeptide peptidoglycan precursors in *Enterococcus faecium* BM4147. J Bacteriol 1992; 174:2582–2591.
25. Evers S, Courvalin P. Regulation of VanB-type vancomycin resistance gene expression by the VanS(B)-VanR(B) two-component regulatory system in *Enterococcus faecalis* V583. J Bacteriol 1996; 178:1302–1309.
26. Perichon B, Reynolds P, Courvalin P. VanD-type glycopeptide-resistant *Enterococcus faecium* BM4339. Antimicrob Agents Chemother 1997; 41:2016–2018.
27. Fines M, Perichon B, Reynolds P, Sahm DF, Courvalin P. VanE, a new type of acquired glycopeptide resistance in *Enterococcus faecalis* BM4405. Antimicrob Agents Chemother 1999; 43:2161–2164.
28. Van Bambeke F, Chauvel M, Reynolds PE, Fraimow HS, Courvalin P. Vancomycin-dependent *Enterococcus faecalis* clinical isolates and revertant mutants. Antimicrob Agents Chemother 1999; 43:41–47.

29. Brisson-Noel A, Dutka-Malen S, Molinas C, Leclereq R, Courvalin P. Cloning and heterospecific expression of the resistance determinant *van*-A encoding high level resistance to glycopeptides. Antimicrob Agents Chemother 1990; 34:924–927.
30. Biavasco F, Giovanetti E, Miele A. In-vitro co-transfer of Van-A vancomycin resistance between enterococci and *Listeria* of different species. Eur J Clin Microbiol Infect Dis 1996; 15:50–59.
31. Power EG, Abdulla YU, Talsania HG, French G. Van A genes in vancomycin resistant clinical isolates of *Oerskovia turbata* and *Arcanobacterium haemolyticum*. J Antimicrob Chemother 1995; 36:595–600.
32. French G, Abdulla Y, Heathcock R, Poston S, Cameron J. Vancomycin resistance in South London. Lancet 1992; 339:818–819.
33. Fontana R, Ligozzi M, Pedrotti C, Padovani EM, Cornaglia G. Vancomycin resistant *Bacillus circulans* carrying the *van*-A gene responsible for vancomycin resistance in enterococci. Eur J Clin Microbiol Infect Dis 1997; 16:473.
34. Rolston K. The clinical significance of organisms tolerant to vancomycin. Proc Am Soc Microbiol (Atlanta) 1993. Abstract 52.
35. Poyeart-Salmeron C, Pierre C, Quesne G. Emergence of vancomycin resistance in the genus *Streptococcus*: characterization of a Van-B transferable determinant in *Streptococcus bovis*. Antimicrob Agents Chemother 1997; 41:24–29.
36. Krcmery V, Spanik S, Trupl J. First report of vancomycin resistant *Streptococcus mitis* bactaeremia in a patient with acute leukemia after prophylaxis with quinolones and during treatment with vancomycin. J Chemother 1996; 84:325–326.
37. Mevius D, Devriese L, Butaye P, Vandamme P, Verschave M, Valdman K. Isolation of glycopeptide resistant *Streptococcus galolyticus* with Van A and Van B. J Antimicrob Chemother 1998; 42:275–276.
38. Swenson JM, Facklam RR, Thornsberry C. Antimicrobial susceptibility of vancomycin resistant *Leuconostoc, Pediococcus* and *Lactobacillus* species. J Clin Microbiol 1992; 30:2373–2378.
39. Narnnyak SS, Blair ALT, Hughes DF, McElhinney P, Donnelly MR, Corey J. Fatal lung abscess due to *Lactobacillus casei* ss. rhamnosus. Thorax 1992; 47:666–667.
40. Venditti M, Gelfusa V, Tarasi A, et al. Antimicrobial susceptibilities of *Erysipelothrix rhusiopathiae*. Antimicrob Agents Chemother 1990; 34:2038–2040.
41. Krcmery V, Sefton A. Vancomycin resistance in Gram-positive bacteria other than *Enterococcus* spp. Int J Antimicrob Agents 2000; 14:99–105.
42. Goodhart GL. In vivo versus in vitro susceptibility of enterococcus to trimethoprim-sulfamethoxazole: a pitfall. JAMA 1984; 252:2748–2749.
43. Moellering RC Jr. Antimicrobial susceptibility of enterococci: in vitro studies of the action of antibiotics alone and in combination. In: Bisno AL (ed.). Treatment of Endocarditis. New York: Grune and Stratton, 1981, pp. 54–60.
44. Lautenbach E, Schuster MG, Bilker WB, Brennan PJ. The role of chloramphenicol in the treatment of bloodstream infection due to vancomycin-resistant *Enterococcus*. Clin Infect Dis 1998; 27:1259–1265.
45. Linden PK. Treatment options for vancomycin-resistant enterococcal infections. Drugs 2002; 62:425–441.
46. Beauvais P, Filipe G, Berniere J, Carlioc H. Oral prisinamycin for bone and joint infections in children. A report of 50 cases. Arch Fr Pediatr 1981; 38:489–493.
47. Diekema DJ, Jones R. Oxazolidinone antibiotics. Lancet 2001; 358:1975–1982.
48. Rybak MJ. Therapeutic options for Gram-positive infections. J Hosp Infect 2001; 49(suppl. A):S25–S32.
49. Petersen PJ, Bradford PA, Weiss WJ, Murphy TM, Sum PE, Projan SJ. In vitro and in vivo activities of tigeclycline (GAR-936), daptomycin and comparative antimicrobial agents

against glycopetide-intermediate *Staphylococcus aureus* and other resistant Gram-positive pathogens. Antimicrob Agents Chemother 2002; 46:2595–2601.
50. Barrett JF. Oritavancin. Eli Lilly and Company. Curr Opin Investig Drugs 2001; 2:1039–1044.
51. Chopra I. Glycyclines: third-generation tetracycline antibiotics. Curr Opin Pharmacol 2001:1:464–469.
52. Nelson RS. Intrinsically vancomycin resistant Gram positive organisms: clinical relevance and implications for infection control. J Hosp Infect 1999; 42:275–282.
53. Patel R. Enterococcal-type glycopeptide resistance genes in non-enterococcal organisms. FEMS Microbiol Lett 1999; 185:1–7.
54. Hiramatsu K, Hanaki H, Ino T, Yabuta K, Oguri T, Tenover FC. Methicillin resistant *Staphylococcus aureus* clinical strain with reduced vancomycin susceptibility. J Antimicrob Chemother 1997; 40:135–136.
55. Novak R, Henriques B, Charpentier E, Normark S, Tuomanen E. Emergence of vanomycin tolerance in *Streptococcus pneumoniae*. Nature 1999; 399:590–593.

6

Isolation Policies and the Hospital Management of Methicillin-Resistant *Staphylococcus aureus*

A Case of Evidence-Free Medicine?

Sheldon P. Stone

1. INTRODUCTION

The incidence of patient colonization, infection, and death caused by methicillin-resistant *Staphylococcus aureus* (MRSA) continues to rise in UK hospitals *(1,2)*. Whereas the first-line antibiotics to treat infection are quite clear (teicoplanin or vancomycin) *(3,4)* and the role and limited efficacy of topical eradication with mupirocin *(3,5)* is understood, the measures aimed at reducing the spread of this organism through screening of asymptomatic carriers and the use of isolation measures are controversial *(6–11)*. Until recently, the most thorough review of the evidence was provided by the national working party revising the UK national guidelines *(3)*. Most of the evidence came from expert opinion or consensus. Even that evidence considered to come from "well designed experimental studies" was of an observational or quasi-experimental nature.

The 1998 revised guidelines recognized that increasing levels of MRSA meant that the more stringent control measures previously recommended were no longer feasible in many hospitals with endemic MRSA *(3)*. A more flexible "targeted approach" depending on the level of risk posed to individual patient groups was recommended. Even so, the rationale and cost-effectiveness *(12)* of these more "relaxed" guidelines were widely disputed *(12)*. The UK Hospital Infection Society agreed on a consensus statement in February 2000 (unpublished data) proposing further relaxation and suggesting that no more should be done for MRSA than for any other hospital-acquired infection (hand hygiene and surveillance), reserving the most intensive isolation measures for those most at risk from invasive or difficult-to-treat disease. It pointed out that the scientific basis for a coherent approach to control was lacking. So, is the widespread use and recommendation *(3,13–16)* of isolation and screening simply a case of evidence-free medicine?

Since the 2000 consensus statement, there has been a systematic review, with epidemiological and economic modeling, of the evidence for the effectiveness and cost-

From: *Management of Multiple Drug-Resistant Infections*
Edited by: S. H. Gillespie © Humana Press Inc., Totowa, NJ

Table 1
Threats to Validity

Potential confounders considered:

- Antibiotic use
- Length of stay
- Bed occupancy
- Pre-existing trends
- Trends in numbers colonized on admission
- Staffing levels
- Workload
- Seasonal effects
- MRSA strain change

Potential sources of bias:

- Case-mix changes (selection bias)
- Changes in screening practice (detection bias)
- Changes in laboratory methods (detection bias)

Reporting bias: Resulting from selective reporting or publication of experimental or quasi-experimental results. Likely to result from unplanned intervention studies in which choice of outcome not independent of knowledge of data. Usually, reporting bias can be expected to result in the over-representation of positive results (successful interventions) in the literature.

Regression to mean effects: A statistical phenomenon distorting results in comparative studies because of the nonrandom selection of initial observations. The distortion occurs since, on average, an extreme observation will be followed by a less-extreme observation and may affect unplanned studies in which the intervention is prompted by a higher than usual level of MRSA.

Statistical conclusion validity. Inappropriate statistical analysis threatens the validity of statistical conclusions. In the present context, inappropriate analyses usually take the form of assuming that outcomes are independent when this assumption cannot be justified (since MRSA is infectious).

effectiveness of different isolation policies *(17)*. The aim of this chapter is to summarize the methods, findings, limitations, and implications of this review.

At the very outset, the review team realized that most outbreak reports and intervention studies are observational and quasi-experimental, and in such studies *(18)*, there may be plausible alternative explanations for changes in MRSA that have usually been attributed to isolation measures. These threats to the validity of inference include stochastic (chance) effects arising from the nature of the epidemic process *(19)* and the presence of potential confounders (effect modifiers) and bias arising from experimental design (*see* Table 1). Systematic assessment of these was a particular and unique feature of the review, and the findings should inform not only the design of future studies, but also the nature of audit and surveillance activity by infection control teams (ICTs). The team's approach was also informed by the observation *(3)* that a lack of epidemiological modeling makes it difficult to assess the effectiveness and cost-effectiveness of interventions when the successful outcome is an event not occurring.

Table 2
Data Extracted

Details of all populations under investigation (e.g., whole hospital, specialist unit)
Details of patient isolation, screening, and other infection control measures (e.g., eradication of carriage, antibiotic restriction, hand hygiene, feedback, ward closures)
Information on outcomes (e.g., infection, colonization, bacteremia, death)
Details of potential confounders and aspects of study design that might introduce bias (*see* Table 1)

2. SYSTEMATIC REVIEW

The team searched MEDLINE, EMBASE, CINAHL, SIGLE, and Cochrane Library databases, without language restriction, for articles published to the end of 2000 that covered the main subject areas of MRSA, screening, patient isolation, and outbreak control. Studies with economic data or analysis were also included. Nearly 4400 abstracts were appraised, and over 250 full papers were reviewed and selected for data extraction if they mentioned endemic or epidemic MRSA in a hospital setting, had a clear isolation policy, and had a MRSA-related outcome.

The original review protocol accepted studies without imposing quality restrictions, but the sheer volume of papers necessitated changing this so that the minimum requirement was a component of prospective data collection or that, if entirely retrospective, comparisons should be planned and not prompted by any part of the outcome data. No such restrictions were imposed on studies using the most intensive forms of isolation, such as isolation wards (IWs) or nurse cohorting (NC) (i.e., designated nurses for the care of MRSA-affected patients on wards with non-MRSA patients), as these interventions have the greatest implications for resource allocation and service organization. A particular feature of the review was the team's recognition that formally implemented studies were the exception, and that in principle, the efficacy of interventions could be evaluated even in apparently noncomparative studies, given sufficient reporting details and appropriate analysis *(20,21)*.

Data extracted (*see* Table 2) from each accepted study was summarized in table form; the study period was divided into phases, if appropriate, according to major change in isolation or other infection control policy. Authors were contacted in writing if isolation or screening policies, or their timing, were unclear. Formal meta-analysis was considered inappropriate because of heterogeneity in study design and patient populations.

The strength of evidence in each study was evaluated by examining the study design, quality of data, size of effect, and presence of plausible alternative explanations because of confounders and biases and characterized as none, weak, evidence, or stronger evidence. The team was explicit that this characterization of evidence was not a formal scale, and that such assessments necessarily have a subjective element. Formal scoring systems that assess quality were not used as these yield inconsistent results *(22)*, and the team considered that these might have lent a misplaced concreteness to their conclusions.

Table 3
Study Interventions and Settings

	Isolation ward	Nurse cohorting	Other isolation policy
Number of studies	18	9	19
Duration of studies	3 mo–15 yr	3.5 mo–4 yr	1 mo–9 yr
Setting: entire hospital or a group of hospitals	16	3	6
Setting: a hospital unit (e.g., burn, ICU, neonatal)	2	6	12
Screening	18	9	14
Eradication	12	5	8
Hand hygiene program	8	2	6

The reviewers accepted 46 studies; 18 described the use of IW, 9 described the use of NC, and 19 described the use of other isolation policies (cohorting on general wards, single-room isolation, barrier nursing) (Table 3). Half the studies were set in entire hospitals and the remainder in hospital units, except for one, which used survey data from multiple hospitals *(23)*. In nearly all studies, there were multiple simultaneous infection control interventions. There was huge variation in the length of studies and the number of patients involved (Table 3).

3. FINDINGS

3.1. Clinical Studies

There were few *(24–27)* formally planned prospective studies with predefined pre- and postintervention periods. The striking finding was that systematic assessment and adjustment for potential confounders was lacking, and that measures to reduce selection or detection bias were rare (for example, using diagnostic criteria when the main outcome was infection or recording changes in case mix). Regression to the mean effects and confounders (seasonal effects and changes in antibiotic use, length of stay, strain type, case mix, or numbers colonized on admission) were considered plausible alternative explanations of outcome in many studies. The predominance of unplanned retrospective reports for which comparisons were suggested by observed outcomes suggested that many study designs were highly vulnerable to reporting bias (especially apparently successful short outbreak reports). Only one study made any explicit adjustments for confounders in the analysis *(23)*, and statistical methods to analyze outcome were considered inappropriate (because of either insufficient reporting or assumptions that outcomes were independent) in all but two studies *(23,28)*.

In a third of studies, no conclusions could be drawn as to the effect of isolation, and in studies with multiple simultaneous interventions, it was not possible to assess the relative contribution of individual measures. Most others provided evidence consistent with reduction of MRSA by combined measures, including isolation. In half of these, the evidence was considered weak because of poor design, major confounders, or risk of systematic biases. There were two studies that presented evidence consistent with

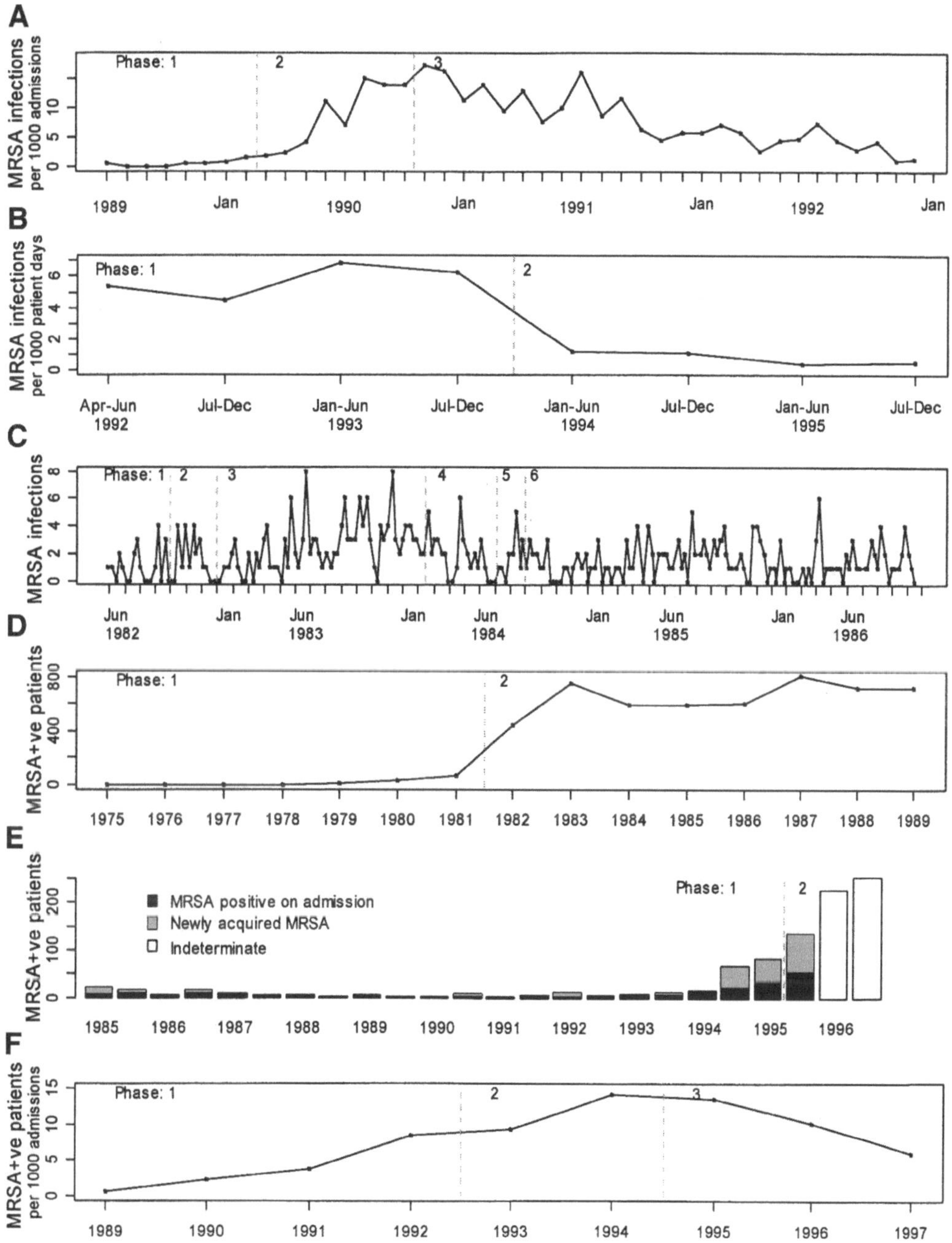

Fig. 1. Outcome of studies presenting the strongest evidence: A, nurse cohorting *(34)*; B, single-room isolation *(35)*; C, isolation ward *(29)*; D, isolation ward *(30)*; E, isolation ward *(31)*; F, single-room isolation *(32,33)*. Table 4 provides explanatory text.

immediate isolation reducing transmission, but there were plausible alternative explanations *(23,28)*. The strongest evidence, however, came from six larger and longer time series, with large changes in MRSA numbers, detailed information on interventions, and relative absence of plausible alternative explanations (Table 4; Fig. 1).

Table 4
Isolation Studies Presenting Strongest Evidence

Ref.	Setting and study population	Design	Main interventions	Patient outcomes	Assessment of evidence
31	Teaching hospital (1000 beds)	Retrospective interrupted time series; two phases 9.5 and 2.5 yr	Continual operation of isolation ward; screening, ward closure, and eradication policies relaxed slightly in phase 2.	221 MRSA acquisitions, 206 colonized on admission, 61 uncertain; number colonized on admission and acquisitions stable and low for 9.5 yr; major increase in both 1 yr prior to control policy changes; increases continued after the changes	Stronger evidence supporting control of MRSA for 9.5 yr by combined measures, followed by eventual control failure related to rise in numbers colonized on admission or to change in strain rather than changed control measures
30	Teaching hospital (1200 beds) initially free of MRSA	Retrospective interrupted time series; two phases: 7 and 8 yr	Isolation ward throughout; additional measures in phase 2 included segregated areas for highly susceptible MRSA-free patients with prescreening of admissions and transfers in; handwashing education; antibiotic restriction	Total MRSA increased rapidly in phase 1 and during the first 2 yr of phase 2; numbers were slightly lower during the next 3 yr, but subsequently increased and appeared to stabilize at a high endemic level	Stronger evidence that combined control measures in both phases failed to prevent MRSA from spreading and becoming endemic
29	Teaching hospital (645 beds)	Retrospective interrupted time series (4.5 yr); six phases: 4, 3, 13.5, 4, 1.5, 26 mo	Initial isolation mainly single rooms plus some cohorting (phases 1–3), changing to mainly isolation ward (phases 4–6); simultaneous changes to screening, eradication, and other measures	Approx 408 MRSA infections; incidence of MRSA infection increased in phase 3, was sustained at a higher level, then decreased in phase 4 from 3 to 4 per wk, and remained at a reduced level (1–2 per wk)	Stronger evidence supporting efficacy of combined measures in reducing incidence, but many potential confounders not recorded

34	Teaching hospital (1500 beds)	Prospective interrupted time series; three phases: 8, 8, and 26 mo; phases and end point not predefined	Phases 1 and 2 had minimal isolation and screening; Phase 3 had single-room isolation and cohorting, contact screening, prompt discharge of MRSA cases; topical eradication with neomcyin nasal cream in phase 1 and with mupirocin in phases 2 and 3	476 infected patients; number of infections increased throughout phases 1 and 2, peaked at start of phase 3, then declined slowly to a very low level	Stronger evidence supporting control of a major outbreak by interventions; no information on many confounders
32, 33	Teaching hospital (1300–1600 beds)	Hybrid retrospective/ prospective interrupted time series; three phases: 4, 2, 3 yr	Phase 1 had no control measures; phase 2 had single-room isolation, screening, mupirocin; Phase 3 was the same as phase 2 plus hand hygiene education and feedback program	1771 MRSA colonizations and infections; 158 bacteremias; incidence of total MRSA and bacteremias increased each year in phase 1, stabilized in phase 2, then fell sharply, especially in phase 3	Stronger evidence supporting control by interventions; some potential confounders, but these provided less-plausible explanations for the changes
35	Pediatric ICU (20 beds)	Hybrid retrospective (phase 1, 21 mo) and prospective (phase 2, 24 mo) interrupted time series	Phase 1 had screening for last 11 mo; phase 2 had single-room isolation, cohorting, screening, feedback, handwashing education, barrier nursing, chlorhexidine soap, and other measures	MRSA infection numbers were 50 in phase 1 and 6 in phase 2; MRSA infection incidence showed sharp reduction after intervention and remained at a low level	Stronger evidence supporting conclusion that interventions reduced MRSA infections; regression to mean and Hawthorne effects supplied less-plausible alternative explanations

Three of these studies presented conflicting evidence of the effectiveness of IWs (with other measures) in reducing MRSA infection hospital wide. One reduced infection *(29)*; one did not *(30)*; and one resulted in control for many years until a change in strain or an increase in the number of patients colonized on admission overwhelmed the institution *(31)*.

One presented evidence that single room isolation with screening, eradication, and an extensive hand-hygiene program reduced MRSA infection and colonization hospital wide *(32,33)*. One provided evidence that nurse cohorting in single rooms with screening and eradication reduced infection hospitalwide *(34)*. One pediatric intensive care unit (ICU) study provided evidence that single-room isolation and patient cohorting in bays with screening, feedback of infection rates, and hand hygiene education reduced infection *(35)*. There was little comprehensive and consistent information on economic costs and virtually no attempt to consider the opportunity costs attributable to preventing MRSA (i.e., the lost opportunities to use resources, such as empty beds in isolation wards, to meet other health care needs).

3.2. Modeling Studies

The modeling study was able to address some of the economic issues. In brief, stochastic and deterministic compartmental models were used to investigate the long-term transmission dynamics of MRSA with both hospital and community populations considered, but all transmission was assumed to occur in the hospital. Models studied the impact of a fixed-capacity isolation ward in a 1000-bed hospital. Hospital size, length of stay, MRSA clearance, and patient discharge and readmission rates were kept fixed, and the number of beds in the isolation ward, screening rate, the transmissibility of the organism, and the date the isolation ward was opened were varied. Local cost data from the Royal Free NHS Trust, Hampstead, were coupled to models to produce economic evaluations. The costs of an unisolated bed day, screening, laboratory tests, and antibiotics were kept fixed, but a range of values was employed for the extra cost of an isolated bed day, additional length of stay attributable to MRSA, and the proportion of MRSA patients infected.

The key finding was that equilibrium endemic prevalences of MRSA in hospitals with fixed-capacity isolation facilities were dependent on the detection rate of MRSA patients, the number of isolation beds available, and the transmissibility of the organism. Improving either the detection rate or the isolation capacity decreased endemic levels provided the other was not the limiting factor. The larger the isolation capacity (Fig. 2) and the sooner the isolation area opened (Fig. 3), the greater the reduction in prevalence, with ultimate eradication often possible only when the isolation ward was opened early, although a large enough unit might reduce endemic levels even when opened after many years (Fig. 4).

Although a paucity of reliable information on key parameter values hampered economic evaluations, substantial savings might be achieved over 10 yr. However, under a wide range of plausible parameter values, substantial savings could be achieved over 10 yr provided the burden of unused isolation ward capacity and staff time was not too great (Fig. 5). The additional length of stay attributable to MRSA was a key influence, so that for shorter lengths of stay, the smaller units were the most cost-effective; with longer stays, the larger units were the most cost-effective. Under many scenarios, long-

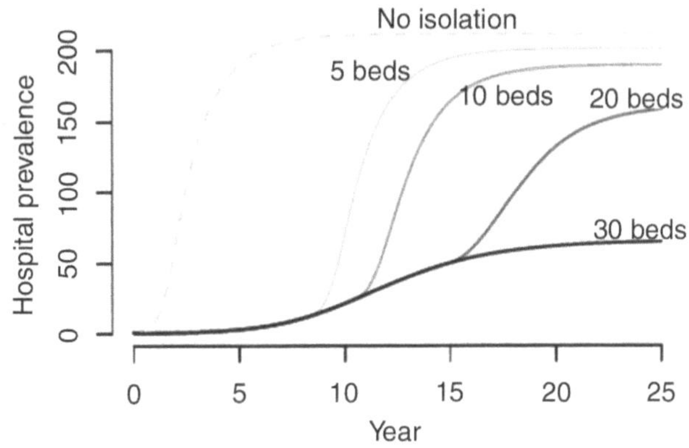

Fig. 2. Effect of changing the size of the isolation ward.

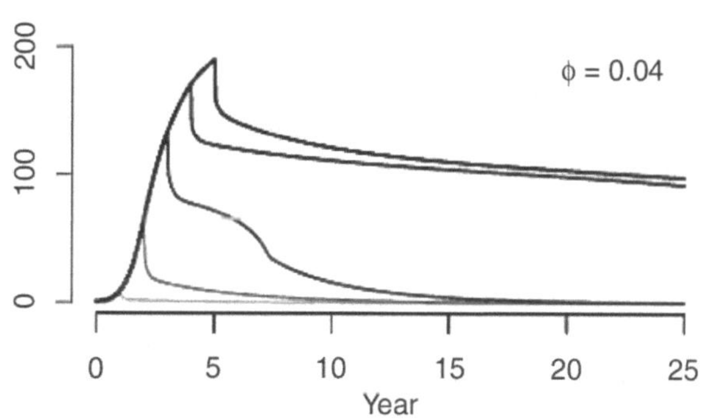

Fig. 3. Isolation ward with 30 beds opening after 0, 1, 2, 3, 4, and 5 yr of endemic MRSA.

term control failure occurred because of saturation of isolation facilities as the number colonized on admission rose. However, even when such control failure occurred, the isolation ward delayed the rate at which prevalence increased and reduced the ultimate endemic level compared to a policy of no isolation (Fig. 2). The team concluded that, taken as a whole, the review emphasized the need to collect adequate data frequently enough to enable the effects of interventions to be interpreted more easily, and that the six studies with the strongest evidence and the results of the modeling provided testable hypotheses for future prospective studies.

4. CONCLUSIONS

So what does the review tell us about the evidence base for isolation? The review, with its highly comprehensive search strategy, and inclusion criteria that examined a wide variety of study designs, avoids the limitations of narrative reviews where study selection may be biased by authors' prejudices. It has some potential limitations. Unpublished studies or conference abstracts were nor not included mainly because their potential benefit would likely be limited in observational studies *(36)*. Although all but two studies presented inappropriate analysis of data, the team chose not to re-analyze the data using more appropriate statistical methods either because data was

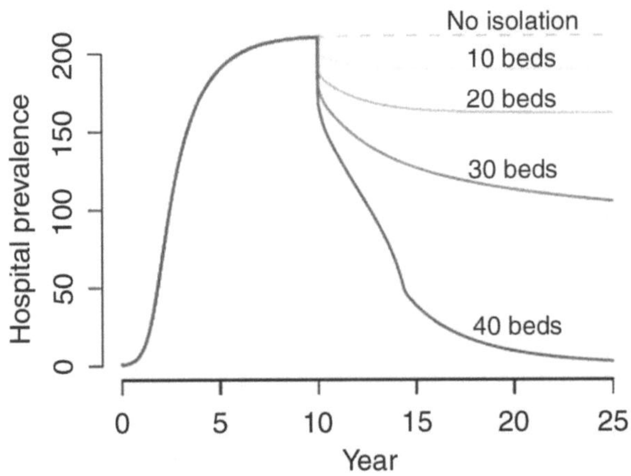

Fig. 4. Effect of isolation ward opened after 15 yr of endemic MRSA.

insufficient or because of the threats to validity that little would be gained. Their qualitative assessment of the evidence has a subjective element in that the plausibility of many of the threats to validity in individual studies is itself dependent on other observational research that is subject to similar limitations. Such assessments necessarily have a subjective element. Opportunity costs were excluded from the economic modeling.

The original intention of the review was to try to model the flexible "targeted approach" of the revised UK guidelines with respect to different patient groups, virulence, epidemicity, and strain type. Although it was possible to do so for virulence and epidemicity, there was insufficient information concerning different patient groups. Although the team recorded meticulous details of the isolation measures and screening strategies (site, frequency, target population) in each study, it was not possible to identify the single most effective isolation or screening measure. The review could not even tell which combination of measures were most effective at reducing transmission, which eradicated MRSA, and which were the most cost-effective in different clinical situations.

What can be concluded from the evidence base is, first, that major methodological weaknesses and inadequate reporting in published research into the effectiveness of isolation measures mean that many plausible alternative explanations for reductions in MRSA associated with interventions cannot be ruled out. No well-designed studies allowed the role of isolation measures alone to be assessed. The full report of the review *(17)* produced guidelines to facilitate the planning and publication of better quality studies and also suggested that an audit system that enables ICTs to collect and use data on potential effect modifiers, alongside current MRSA surveillance systems, needs to be designed, piloted, and evaluated. This might help ICTs plan interventions and interpret their outcomes. Much of the information required (Table 1) is already available in many National Health Service Hospital Trusts, but requires modest investment in resources, including information technology (IT) packages, to make such a system viable.

The second conclusion is that, despite the limitations of existing research, as systematically documented by the review, there was evidence that concerted interventions that include an isolation policy can substantially reduce MRSA transmission, even in

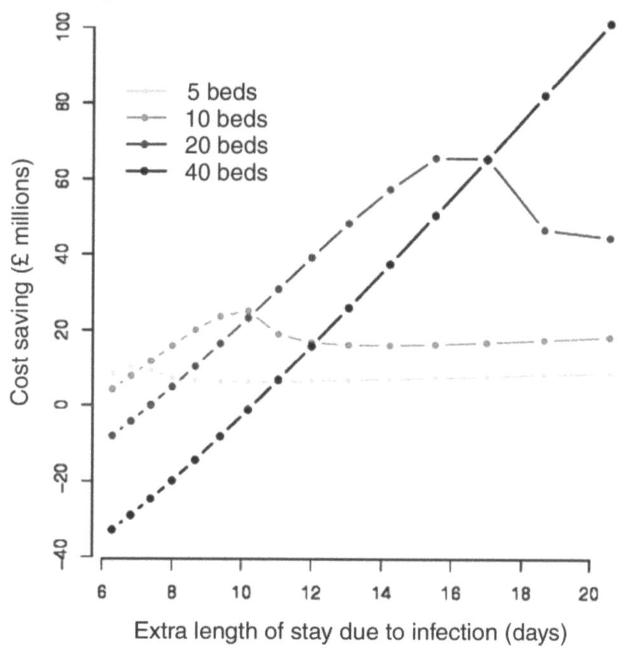

Fig. 5. Total cost savings over 10 years, using IW for endemic MRSA.

settings with a high level of endemic MRSA. Less evidence was found to suggest that current isolation measures recommended in many countries *(3,13–16)* are ineffective, and these should continue to be applied until further research establishes otherwise. What appears as a clear hypothesis from the modeling is that the isolation, screening facilities, and resources need to be in scale with the problem.

4.1. Future Research

Future research should concentrate on prospective planned comparisons, with predefined pre- and postintervention periods and systematic assessment and adjustment for potential confounders as necessary. Randomized controlled trials (RCTs) with cluster randomization by hospital or specialist unit are one possibility. Priority research questions include those involving an examination of the effects of isolation wards that are an adequate size in hospitals with endemic MRSA; of single-room isolation with an extensive hand hygiene program, screening, and eradication; and of nurse cohorting with screening and eradication. Study designs that permit the identification of the effects of both individual interventions and combined interventions should be considered.

There is also much work to be done on providing accurate economic assessments of the costs of MRSA control, including the opportunity costs. Indeed, the key parameter in the economic modeling was the extra length of stay attributable to MRSA, but there is no information in the literature in this regard; research is required to establish this in different patient groups. Methodological research for the analysis of data generated by outbreak investigations is also required. Specifically, a formal assessment of different approaches to analyzing time series count data that typically arise from hospital epidemics would be valuable and would aid interpretation of routine data collection.

The continued rise of MRSA *(1)* and the emergence of GISA (glycopeptide-intermediate *S. aureus*) strains *(37,38)* and GRSA (glycopeptide-resistant *S. aureus*) *(39,40)*, which further reduces therapeutic options *(41)*, make reduction of MRSA and implementation of well-designed interventional studies to inform the choice of control measures even more important. This review, together with modeling, helps to set limitations of current research, proposes better data collection and analysis, and suggests research designs and priorities.

REFERENCES

1. Public Health Laboratory Service. The first year of the Department of Health's mandatory MRSA bacteraemia surveillance scheme in acute NHS Trusts in England: April 2001–March 2002. CDR Wkly 2002; 12:20. Available at: www.org.uk/publications/cdr/2002/mrsa2502.pdf. Accessed on December 20, 2002.
2. Crowcroft NS, Catchpole M. Mortality from methicillin resistant *Staphylococcus aureus* in England and Wales: analysis of death certificates. BMJ 2002; 325:1390–1391.
3. Revised guidelines for the control of methicillin-resistant *Staphylococcus aureus* infection in hospitals. British Society for Antimicrobial Chemotherapy, Hospital Infection Society and the Infection Control Nurses Association. J Hosp Infect 1998; 39:253–290.
4. Michel M, Guttman L. Methicillin resistant *Staphylococcus aureus*: therapeutic realities and possibilities. Lancet 1997; 349:1901–1906.
5. Dacre J, Emmerson AM, Jenner EA. Gentamicin-methicillin-resistant *Staphylococcus aureus*: epidemiology and containment of an outbreak. J Hosp Infect 1986; 7:130–136.
6. Boyce JM. Nosocomial staphylococcal infections. Ann Intern Med 1981; 95:241–242.
7. Stone SP. Managing methicillin-resistant *Staphylococcus aureus* in hospital: the balance of risk. Age Ageing 1997; 26:165–168.
8. Barrett SP, Teare EL, Sage R. Methicillin resistant *Staphylococcus aureus* in three adjacent health districts of south-east England 1986–91. J Hosp Infect 1993; 24:313–325.
9. Bell SM. Recommendations for control of the spread of methicillin resistant *Staphylococcus aureus* infection. Med J Aust 1982; 2:472–474.
10. Cookson BD. Is it time to stop searching for MRSA. BMJ 1997; 31:664–666.
11. Teare EL, Barrett SP. Is it time to stop searching for MRSA? Stop the ritual of tracing colonised people. BMJ 1997; 314:665–666.
12. Rahman M, Sanderson PJ, Bentley AH, et al. Control of MRSA. J Hosp Infect 2000; 44:151–153.
13. Garner JS, Simmons BP. CDC Guideline for Isolation Precautions in Hospitals. Atlanta, GA: US Department of Health and Human Services, Public Health Service, Centers for Disease Control, 1983. HHS publication (CDC) 83-8314; Infect Control 1983; 4:245–325; Am J Infect Control 1984; 12:103–163.
14. Garner JS, Hospital Infection Control Practices Advisory Committee. Guideline for isolation precautions in hospitals. Infect Control Hosp Epidemiol 1996; 17:53–80; Am J Infect Control 1996; 24:24–52.
15. Ministry of Health, Wellington, New Zealand. Guidelines for the control of methicillin-resistant *Staphylococcus aureus* in New Zealand. August 2002. Available at: www.moh.gov.nz/cd/mrsa.
16. Management Policy for Methicillin-Resistant *Staphylococcus aureus*. Guideline No. 35A. Leiden: WIP, 1994.
17. Cooper BS, Stone SP, Kibbler CC, et al. Isolation policies and screening practices in the hospital management of methicillin resistant *Staphylococcus aureus*: a systematic review with epidemiological and economic modelling. Health Technology Assessment Report 2003. In press. Available at: www.hta.nhsweb.nhs.uk.

18. Cook TD, Campbell DT. Quasi-Experimentation: Design and Analysis Issues for Field Settings. Chicago: Rand McNally College Publications, 1979.
19. Cooper BS, Medley GF, Scott GM. Preliminary analysis of the transmission dynamics of nosocomial infections: stochastic and management effects. J Hosp Infect 1999; 43:131–147.
20. Grimes DA, Schulz KF. Descriptive studies: what they can and cannot do. Lancet 2002; 359:145–149.
21. Grimes DA, Schulz KF. Cohort studies: marching towards outcomes. Lancet 2002; 359:341–345.
22. Juni P, Witschi A, Bloch R, Egger M. The hazards of scoring the quality of clinical trials for meta-analysis. JAMA 1999; 282:1054–1060.
23. Esveld MI, de Boer AS, Notenboom AJ, van Pelt W, van Leeuwen WJ. Secondary infection with methacillin resistant *Staphylococcus aureus* in Dutch hospitals (July 1994–June 1996). Ned Tijdschr Geneeskd 1999; 143:205–208.
24. Blumberg LH, Klugman KP. Control of methicillin-resistant *Staphylococcus aureus* bacteraemia in high-risk areas. Eur J Clin Microbiol Infect Dis 1994; 13:82–85.
25. Kac G, Buu-Hoi A, Herisson E, Biancardini P, Debure C. Methicillin-resistant *Staphylococcus aureus*. Nosocomial acquisition and carrier state in a wound care center. Arch Dermatol 2000; 136:735–739.
26. Ribner BS, Landry MN, Gholson GL. Strict versus modified isolation for prevention of nosocomial transmission of methicillin-resistant *Staphylococcus aureus*. Infect Control 1986; 7:317–320.
27. Yoshida J, Kuroki S, Akazawa K, et al. The order of ward rounds influences nosocomial infection. A 2-year study in gastroenterologic surgery patients. J Gastroenterol 1995; 30:718–724.
28. Jernigan JA, Titus MG, Groschel DH, Getchell-White S, Farr BM. Effectiveness of contact isolation during a hospital outbreak of methicillin-resistant *Staphylococcus aureus*. Am J Epidemiol 1996; 143:496–504.
29. Duckworth GJ, Lothian JL, Williams JD. Methicillin-resistant *Staphylococcus aureus*: report of an outbreak in a London teaching hospital. J Hosp Infect 1988; 11:1–15.
30. Faoagali JL, Thong ML, Grant D. Ten years' experience with methicillin-resistant *Staphylococcus aureus* in a large Australian hospital. J Hosp Infect 1992; 20:113–119.
31. Farrington M, Redpath C, Trundle C, Coomber S, Brown NM. Winning the battle but losing the war: methicillin-resistant *Staphylococcus aureus* (MRSA) infection at a teaching hospital. QJM 1998; 91:539–548.
32. Harbarth S, Martin Y, Rohner P, Henry N, Auckenthaler R, Pittet D. Effect of delayed infection control measures on a hospital outbreak of methicillin-resistant *Staphylococcus aureus*. J Hosp Infect 2000; 46:43–49.
33. Pittet D, Hugonnet S, Harbarth S, et al. Effectiveness of a hospital-wide programme to improve compliance with hand hygiene. Infection Control Programme. Lancet 2000; 356:1307–1312.
34. Coello R, Jimenez J, Garcia M, et al. Prospective study of infection, colonization and carriage of methicillin-resistant *Staphylococcus aureus* in an outbreak affecting 990 patients. Eur J Clin Microbiol Infect Dis 1994; 13:74–81.
35. Cosseron-Zerbib M, Roque Afonso AM, Naas T, et al. A control programme for MRSA (methicillin-resistant *Staphylococcus aureus*) containment in a paediatric intensive care unit: evaluation and impact on infections caused by other micro-organisms. J Hosp Infect 1998; 40:225–235.
36. The Cochrane Effective Practice and Organisation of Care (EPOC) Review Group. Cochrane Library Database. 2000.
37. Hiramatsu K, Hanaki H, Ino T. Methicillin resistant *Staphylococcus aureus* clinical strain with reduced vancomycin susceptibility. J Antimicrob Chemother 1997; 40:135–136.

38. *Staphylococcus aureus* with reduced susceptibility to vancoycin—Illinois 1999. MMWR Morb Mortal Wkly Rep 2000; 48:1165–1167.
39. Vancomycin resistant *Staphylococcus aureus*, Pennsylvania, 2002. MMWR Morb Mortal Wkly Rep 2002; 51; 902.
40. Centers for Disease Control and Prevention. *Staphylococcus aureus* resistant to vancomycin—United States, 2002. MMWR Morb Mortal Wkly Rep 2002; 51:565–567.
41. Perry CN, Jarvis B. Linezolid: a review of its use in the management of serious gram positive infections. Drugs 2001; 61:525–551.

II

Gram-Negative Pathogens

7

The Management of Resistant *Acinetobacter* Infections in the Intensive Therapy Unit

Nicola Baker and Peter Hawkey

1. INTRODUCTION

Acinetobacter species are ubiquitous Gram-negative bacteria widespread in nature. In the clinical setting, they have been isolated from the hospital environment and from the skin of health care workers. Although initially considered nonpathogenic, certain species of the genus *Acinetobacter*, particularly *A. baumannii*, are increasingly recognized as important nosocomial pathogens, particularly in intensive care unit (ICU) settings. With the increased use of invasive clinical procedures and expanding number of ICU beds, the prevalence of *Acinetobacter* infections is increasing. Also, there has been a rapid increase in resistance to all the major classes of antibiotics for *Acinetobacter*. Controlling the spread of *Acinetobacter* spp and the management of infections caused by these organisms poses a major challenge for the future.

2. LABORATORY IDENTIFICATION OF *ACINETOBACTER*

The genus *Acinetobacter* comprises a heterogeneous group of Gram-negative coccobacilli that are strictly aerobic, nonmotile, oxidase negative, and catalase positive. They grow readily on routinely used laboratory media, although the use of selective media that suppresses the growth of other microorganisms can aid isolation from clinical samples *(1,2)*.

Over the past three decades, there have been numerous changes to the taxonomy of these bacteria. Until 1986, just one species (*Acinetobacter calcoaceticus*) with two subspecies (var *anitratus* and var *lwoffii*) *(3)* or two species (*Acinetobacter calcoaceticus* and *Acinetobacter lwoffii*) *(4)* were described. In 1986, Bouvet and Grimont *(5)* described a simple classification system containing 12 genomic species based on DNA–DNA hybridization studies. Since this time, a variety of genotypic methods have been used to identify genomic species of acinetobacters, including ribotyping *(6)*, transfer RNA (tRNA) spacer fingerprinting *(7)*, amplified fragment length polymorphism (AFLP) *(8)*, and amplified ribosomal DNA restriction analysis (ARDRA) *(9)*. To date, these methods have resulted in the description of more than 20 genomic species; only a small number of these have species names *(10–14)*. It is not

From: *Management of Multiple Drug-Resistant Infections*
Edited by: S. H. Gillespie © Humana Press Inc., Totowa, NJ

Table 1
Classification of *Acinetobacter* Species

	Genospecies number (DNA group)	
Species name	Bouvet et al. *(5,10)*	Tjernberg and Ursing *(11)*
A. calcoaceticus	1	1
A. baumannii	2	2
UN	3	3
UN	Ungrouped	13TU
A. haemolyticus	4	4
A. junii	5	5
UN	6	6
A. johnsonii	7	7
A. lwoffii	8	8TU
UN	9	8TU
UN	10	10
UN	11	11
A. radioresistens	12	12
UN	13	14TU
UN	14	Not done
UN	15	Not done
UN	16	Ungrouped
UN	17	Not done
UN	Not done	17TU
A. venetianus	Not done	Not done
A. ursingii	Not done	Not done
A. schlindleri	Not done	Not done

Abbr: UN, unnamed species.

within the scope of this chapter to discuss these in detail; however, Table 1 gives an overview of the species identified.

Many of the difficulties in eliciting the clinical significance of individual species stem from this constantly changing and confusing nomenclature combined with the technical difficulties of universally applying molecular methods for identification. Furthermore, studies have repeatedly demonstrated that the differentiation of these organisms using phenotypic characteristics is unreliable *(15–17)*. This is particularly the case for those strains belonging to DNA groups 1 (*A. calcoaceticus*), 2 (*A. baumannii*), 3, and 13TU, which are phenotypically very similar. It has been suggested that these groups should be referred to as the *A. calcoaceticus–A. baumannii* complex *(15)*.

Very few clinical laboratories have the facilities available for accurate discrimination of species into genomic groups, and presumptive identification of genomic species is often made using commercial identification systems such as API 20NE (Bio-Merieux). This system uses a panel of 20 biochemical tests, the results of which are compared to those in a database of organisms. Repeated studies have demonstrated that such systems are unable to identify species of *Acinetobacter (17,18)* reliably, so definitive identification requires the use of DNA-based methods. This fact is often not recognized by many laboratories; as a result, the identification of common species such as *A. baumannii* and association with particular clinical and epidemiological situations may not be truly representative. With the increasing use of genetic techniques, it is likely that the clinical significance of many other species of *Acinetobacter* will be better characterized in the future.

3. EPIDEMIOLOGY OF *ACINETOBACTER* INFECTIONS

Sporadic cases of *Acinetobacter* infections are seen in many hospitals and in a variety of patient settings. However, outbreaks of infection caused by endemic strains are increasingly described, particularly in ICUs.

Acinetobacter spp are some of the most common Gram-negative bacteria found as natural residents of human skin. Studies have shown that they are carried on the skin of up to 40% of healthy individuals, particularly in moist areas such as the axillae, groin, and toe webs *(19)*. Carriage rates in hospitalized patients are significantly higher *(20)*. This has been postulated as caused by reduced hygiene standards among hospitalized patients and the warm, humid atmosphere of hospital beds, which is supported by the observation that colonization is more frequent in summer months *(21)*.

Two studies using DNA-based techniques demonstrated that much of this colonization is caused by species of *Acinetobacter* not commonly associated with clinical infection *(19,20)*. The majority of isolates were *A. lwoffii* (genospecies 8/9), *A. johnsonii*, genospecies 15BJ, or *A. radioresistens*. *A. baumannii*, the species most commonly isolated from nosocomial infections, very rarely colonize healthy individuals or the skin of hospitalized patients.

In contrast, very high rates of *A. baumannii* carriage have been described during outbreaks of infection in ICUs. Frequent colonization of the skin, throat, respiratory, and digestive tracts has been described in ICU patients. In one study of adult patients in a French ICU, 33% developed oropharyngeal or rectal carriage of *A. baumannii* or *Klebsiella pneumoniae* within a median period of 9 d *(22)*. Similarly, 20% of patients screened in a UK ICU became colonized with *Acinetobacter* spp, which was most commonly identified as *A. baumannii (23)*. Studies of patients with burns demonstrated colonization rates with *A. baumannii* of over 50%, mainly because of superficial wound colonization *(24–26)*.

High rates of colonization of the respiratory tract have also been described in outbreaks involving mechanically ventilated patients *(27,28)*. In one study, 45% of tracheostomies were colonized with *Acinetobacter* spp *(29)*.

Although colonization of the digestive tract is not generally considered an important source of *Acinetobacter*, several studies have demonstrated significant rectal carriage of *A. baumannii* in ICU patients *(30,31)*. It has been suggested that this site represents a major source of multidrug-resistant organisms that contribute substantially to the burden of colonization in ICU settings.

A number of case-control studies have identified factors associated with the acquisition of *Acinetobacter* spp by ICU patients. The independent factors predisposing to colonization with *Acinetobacter* spp were increasing severity of underlying illness (as defined by the APACHE II score), longer length of stay in the ICU, prolonged mechanical ventilation, increasing number of intravenous lines, and previous antimicrobial therapy with third-generation cephalosporins, aminoglycosides, or fluoroquinolones *(22,32–37)*.

All of these studies point toward the fact that the acquisition of *Acinetobacter* in the ICU setting is generally an isolated event that occurs after admission, either as a result of cross-transmission from other colonized patients or as a result of spread from a contaminated environment. The relative importance of these different modes of spread is still a matter of much debate and is discussed in detail here.

Recent advances in methods for demonstrating the relatedness of individual strains of *Acinetobacter* have enabled detailed studies that provide more precise information regarding the sources of outbreaks and the modes of transmission within ICUs. In many routine clinical laboratories, techniques such as biotyping and antibiograms are employed to identify possible relatedness of *Acinetobacter* isolates. As has described Section 2, commercial biotyping systems have a low discriminatory capacity, especially for most commonly isolated species. Antibiotic susceptibility patterns, although useful as a screening tool, are unreliable as a method of typing *(38)*. Many unrelated strains may show identical antibiotic susceptibilities, and the pattern of resistance of endemic strains may change over time.

More sophisticated methods of typing have been used over the years, including serotyping, phage typing, bacteriocin typing, plasmid profiles, and cell envelope protein electrophoresis *(39,40)*. Few of these have shown sufficient discrimination between strains or reliability to be useful in clinical settings. However, these methods have largely been superseded by molecular techniques such as ribotyping *(41)*, analysis of restriction length polymorphisms in chromosomal DNA by pulsed field gel electrophoresis (PFGE) *(42,43)*, and polymerase chain reaction (PCR) fingerprinting. PCR fingerprinting methods used for typing clinical strains have included ARDRA *(44)*, random amplified polymorphic DNA (RAPD) analysis *(45,46)*, AFLP fingerprinting *(47,48)*, infrequent-restriction site PCR (IRS-PCR) *(49)*, and repetitive extragenic palindromic sequence-based PCR (REP-PCR) *(50)* as well as other methods.

All of these methods have shown excellent discrimination between clinical isolates, but at present there is no agreed standard method for the typing of strains of *Acinetobacter* spp. One study that compared 73 isolates of *A. calcoaceticus–A.baumannii* complex by ribotyping and PFGE concluded that PFGE was more discriminatory *(43)*, but others have shown comparable results with both techniques *(51)*. Comparable results have also been obtained for a variety of PCR-based methods, including ADRA, RAPD, and AFLP *(52)*. One advantage of ribotyping together with PCR fingerprinting methods is that they have the ability to identify various genomic species of *Acinetobacter*, including the *A. calcoaceticus–A. baumannii* complex, because each genospecies produces a unique banding pattern. PFGE, although highly discriminatory between strains, does not have the ability to identify organisms to the genomic species level.

Although there is much debate over the optimal methods, it is agreed that accurate typing to identify related and nonrelated strains of *Acinetobacter* is an essential component of the management of infections in any ICU, particularly when outbreaks occur or infections are endemic. Accurate typing of strains relies on a combination of techniques that includes simple methods such as antibiotic sensitivities or phenotypic testing together with at least one molecular technique. The exact methods used depend very much on local expertise and availability. However, a better understanding of *Acinetobacter* infections will require the introduction of standardized methods that enable data to be correlated between hospitals and laboratories.

4. CLINICAL SPECTRUM OF *ACINETOBACTER* INFECTIONS

Acinetobacter spp have been isolated from a wide variety of clinical specimens, including blood, respiratory tract secretions, urine, cerebrospinal fluid (CSF), and feces. However, determining the significance of clinical isolates is often not straightforward because *Acinetobacter* spp are prevalent in the natural environment and are commonly found as colonizers of both healthy individuals and hospitalized patients *(20)*, although increased use of identification methods capable of identifying genomic species should overcome this state of affairs. Despite this, *Acinetobacter* spp have been associated with a number of opportunistic infections in critically ill patients, including pneumonia, bacteremia, endocarditis, meningitis, wound and soft tissue infections, and urinary tract infections (UTIs) *(39,53)*. The distribution of infections does not differ significantly from that of other Gram-negative organisms causing infections in the ICU, with the lower respiratory tract and urinary tract the most common sites.

4.1. Respiratory Tract Infection

Nosocomial respiratory tract infections are the most frequently seen *Acinetobacter* infections occurring in the hospital *(1,39,53)*. Numerous large outbreaks of pneumonia have been described in ICUs, most commonly associated with mechanical ventilation. Data from the Centers for Disease Control and Prevention (CDC) National Nosocomial Infection Surveillance (NNIS) suggested that 4% of all nosocomial pneumonias are caused by *Acinetobacter* spp *(54)*, and *Acinetobacter* is the fourth most common isolate associated with nosocomial pneumonia in the ICU setting *(55)*. In the European Prevalence of Infection in Intensive Care (EPIC) study, *Acinetobacter* spp accounted for 10% of all cases of pneumonia *(56)*. A number of risk factors for the development of nosocomial *Acinetobacter* pneumonia have been identified, including mechanical ventilation, tracheostomy, length of stay in the ICU, increasing age, presence of underlying pulmonary disease, and recent surgery *(33,36,40,53)*.

Nosocomial pneumonia caused by *Acinetobacter* spp is frequently severe, and complications such as cavitation, pleural effusion, bronchopleural fistula formation, and secondary bacteremia have been described *(1)*. Overall mortality rates ranging from 30 to 75% have been reported, figures that are much higher than documented nosocomial pneumonias caused by many other bacteria *(53)*. Much of the increased mortality is probably because of the severity of underlying illness in patients who acquire *Acinetobacter* spp. However, a recent study in a Spanish ICU demonstrated an attributable mortality of 53% in patients with *A. baumannii* respiratory tract infections *(57)*. When this group of patients was compared to a matched cohort of patients from whom *Acinetobacter* was not isolated, the estimated risk of death reached 4.0, and the excess length of stay was 13 d.

4.2 Bacteremia

The frequency of *Acinetobacter* bacteremia ranges between studies, depending on the population mix and clinical setting *(24,58–60)*. Data from bacteremias reported to the Public Health Laboratory Service (PHLS) in England and Wales suggest that 1.5% of nosocomial bacteremias in England are caused by *Acinetobacter* spp, and similar figures have been described in US hospitals *(61)*. Most cases of bacteremia are caused by *A. baumannii*, but other species have been less commonly reported *(58,62,63)*. Bacteremias are frequently polymicrobial *(64,65)*.

Almost all reported cases of *Acinetobacter* bacteremia are acquired in the hospital, and of these, the majority are associated with ICU admission *(58,60,64)*. In adults, the most commonly identified predisposing conditions are immunosuppression, malignancy, burns, and trauma, which reflect the opportunistic nature of this infection *(58,65)*. Small case-control studies have documented a number of factors that are associated with the development of bacteremia in adult ICU patients, including prior colonization with *Acinetobacter* spp, the use of broad-spectrum antibiotics (particularly third-generation cephalosporins), mechanical ventilation, and exposure to invasive procedures such as placement of intravascular or urinary catheters, tracheostomy, or recent surgery *(24,59,64,65)*. Two studies have demonstrated that the risk of bacteremia in colonized patients is as high as 18–20% *(60,66)*.

In up to 50% of all reported cases, the source of bacteremia is unknown *(58,60,65)*. The most common of the identified sources are the respiratory tract, surgical wounds, intravenous catheters, burns, and the urinary tract. The exact contribution of each varies according to the patient population studied and the definitions used, although the respiratory tract is invariably the most common identifiable source *(58,65,67)*.

Although considered to be an opportunistic infection, studies have shown that 24–30% of patients develop severe sepsis, and significant numbers have septic shock *(60,64)*. In one study, 30% of patients developed disseminated intravascular coagulation (DIC) *(60)*. The crude mortality associated with *Acinetobacter* bacteremia is high and varies between studies from 27 to 52% *(24,58,60,64,65)*. In general, the prognosis appears to be determined by the patient's underlying condition, and death directly related to *Acinetobacter* bacteremia is uncommon. Mortality is higher among patients with malignancies and burns, but tends to be lowest in trauma patients *(65)*. Risk factors for increased mortality identified in a small case series included infection with *A. baumannii*, presence of septic shock at the onset of bacteremia, mechanical ventilation, the presence of a rapidly fatal underlying disease, pneumonia as a primary focus, and inappropriate antimicrobial treatment *(60,64)*.

4.3. *Meningitis*

Meningitis caused by *Acinetobacter* spp is rare. The majority of cases are nosocomial, occurring after neurosurgical procedures in ICU patients treated with antibiotics. Almost, but not exclusively, all cases are caused by *A. baumannii*. In the largest case series reported, the most common risk factor was the presence of communication between the CSF and the environment, such as a ventriculostomy or a CSF fistula *(68)*. The heavy use of antibiotics in neurosurgical ICUs appears to play a substantial role in the development of infection. In the case series described here, simply reducing antibiotic usage resulted in control of the outbreak.

Meningitis may occur acutely or follow a more subacute course with an insidious onset. Reported mortality rates have varied from 20 to 27% *(39)*. Up to 30% of patients may have a petechial rash, which can lead to confusion over the diagnosis, particularly because *Acinetobacter* may look similar to *Neisseria meningitidis* on a Gram stain of the CSF *(1)*.

4.4. *Urinary Tract Infection*

Acinetobacter spp have been described as a cause of 2–61% of nosocomial UTIs *(40)*. The risk factors for infection are similar to those for bacteremias, and most patients have indwelling urinary catheters. The huge variation in incidence between studies probably reflects the difficulty in diagnosing infection in the presence of bacteriuria in this situation. Bacteremia is a very rare consequence of urinary tract infection.

4.5. *Soft Tissue Involvement*

Colonization of burns, traumatic wounds, and postoperative wounds with *Acinetobacter* spp is not uncommon, particularly in ICU settings. Differentiating between wound colonization and infection can often be difficult. However, cellulitis surrounding intravenous catheter sites and caused by *Acinetobacter* has been described *(69)*. There have been infrequent reports of extensive soft tissue necrosis adjacent to colonized wounds *(60)* and synergistic necrotizing fasciitis in conjunction with *Streptococcus pyogenes (1)*. Acinetobacter colonization of extremity wounds was frequently observed in casualties of the Vietnam War. In many of these cases, colonization of wounds was followed 3–5 d later by bacteremia *(70)*. In several large case series, 4–27% of all *Acinetobacter* bacteremias occurred as a result of infected surgical or burn wounds *(58,60,64)*.

4.6. *Other Infections*

There are infrequent reports in the literature of a number of other infections caused by *Acinetobacter*, including prosthetic and native valve endocarditis, endophthalmitis following trauma, corneal ulceration caused by soft contact lens contamination, osteomyelitis, peritonitis in patients undergoing continuous peritoneal dialysis, septic arthritis, and liver abscesses *(1,39)*. All of these are rare, but the pattern of infections caused by *Acinetobacter* spp appears to be increasing as improved techniques for isolation and identification of organisms are developed and as the opportunities in clinical practice for infection to develop expand.

5. THE PROBLEM OF ANTIBIOTIC RESISTANCE

One problem associated with *Acinetobacter* spp has been their intrinsic resistance to multiple antibiotics and their particular propensity to acquire antibiotic resistance rapidly. In the most recent surveillance reports, a high incidence of resistance among clinical isolates of *Acinetobacter* spp has been reported to a range of antibiotics, including aminoglycosides, third-generation cephalosporins, fluoroquinolones, extended-spectrum penicillins, and monobactams *(71–74)*.

In a study conducted in more than 100 ICUs in five European countries, resistance rates to ciprofloxacin, gentamicin, piperacillin, and ceftazidime frequently exceeded 50% *(71)*. There was wide variation in resistance patterns detected in different countries, which is likely to reflect both species distribution and differences in the use of antibiotics. A study of 595 *Acinetobacter* spp isolates in the United Kingdom demonstrated that 89% of *A. baumannii* were resistant to ceftazidime, and more than 40% showed resistance to ciprofloxacin or gentamicin *(74)*.

The carbapenems retain the most activity, but reports have demonstrated increasing resistance to both imipenem and meropenem *(75,76)*. Outbreaks of infection have been described in which sulbactam or colistin are the only antibiotics to which isolates of *A. baumannii* are susceptible *(77–79)*.

Species of *Acinetobacter* other than *A. baumannii,* such as *A. lwoffii, A. johnsonii,* and *A. junii,* are less commonly associated with nosocomial infections and are generally more susceptible to antibiotics *(39)*. However, there is some evidence that resistance in these species is increasing.

6. MECHANISMS OF ANTIBIOTIC RESISTANCE

The full extent of the mechanisms by which *Acinetobacter* spp develop resistance to different classes of antibiotics is yet to be elucidated. A variety of mechanisms has been described that confer resistance to all the major classes of antibiotics. It is not within the scope of this text to describe these mechanisms in detail, but the following discussion gives an overview of their complexities and extent.

6.1. *β-Lactams*

As with other Gram-negative bacilli, the main mechanism of resistance to β-lactam antibiotics is the production of β-lactamases encoded either by the chromosome or by transferable plasmids. Table 2 shows the properties of some of the β-lactamases that have been described in *Acinetobacter* spp.

Early studies demonstrated the high frequency of β-lactamases in clinical strains of *Acinetobacter* spp. One study in Spain isolated the β-lactamase TEM-1 from 16% of *A. baumannii* isolates and cephalosporinases from 98% of strains *(81)*. In France, 81% of strains of *A. calcoaceticus* produced β-lactamases, the majority of which were of the TEM type *(80)*. As many as 32% of strains possessed multiple β-lactamases conferring resistance to both penicillins and cephalosporins. It has been shown that a high percentage of clinical isolates of *A. baumannii* have increased production of the inducible chromosomal β-lactamase Amp-C, and that this enzyme plays an important role in mediating β-lactam resistance *(84)*.

However, these mechanisms do not fully explain the increasing resistance of *Acinetobacter* strains to either extended-spectrum cephalosporins or carbapenems, which have long been the mainstay of therapy. Reports from Turkey and more recently France have described the presence of a plasmid-encoded, extended-spectrum β-lactamase (ESBL) PER-1 in clinical isolates of *Acinetobacter* spp *(86,87)*. This enzyme confers resistance to all penicillins, monobactams, and cephalosporins, including ceftazidime.

There have been numerous reports of carbapenem hydrolyzing β-lactamases isolated from *Acinetobacter* spp *(88–97)*, and their emergence has been declared a "global sentinel event" *(99)*. Metalloenzymes of the IMP type have been described in isolates from areas as diverse as Cuba *(100)*, Hong Kong *(95)*, Japan *(97)*, Italy *(92)*, and the United Kingdom *(93)*. These enzymes possess strong carbapenemase activity and have been linked to clinical resistance to imipenem and meropenem, as well as broad-spectrum cephalosporins; there are signs they are becoming more common, probably because of the increasing use of carbapenems in the ICU. More frequently reported to now have been the OXA-type β-lactamases, which have very weak carbapenemase activity *(88–91)*. However, they have been isolated from 35% of clinical isolates of *A. baumannii* and are associated with clinical resistance to the carbapenems *(84)*.

Despite their wide prevalence in strains of *Acinetobacter* spp, β-lactamases cannot explain *in toto* the high level of resistance to many β-lactam antibiotics that is seen in

Table 2
Outline of Some β-Lactamases Identified in *Acinetobacter* Species

β-Lactamase	Location of gene	Substrate	Properties	Reference
TEM-1	Plasmid	Penicillins	Common in nearly all Gram-negative bacteria; inhibited by clavulinic acid	*80, 81*
TEM-2	Plasmid	Penicillins	Similar to TEM-1	
CARB-5	Plasmid	Penicillins	Inhibited by clavulinic acid	*82*
ACE-1 ACE-2 ACE-3 ACE-4	Chromosome	Cephalosporins	Confers resistance to cephalosporins; possesses some activity against penicillins; no activity against aztreonam or the broad-spectrum cephalosporins, only ACE-1 hydrolyses cefuroxime	*39, 40*
Amp-C	Chromosomal	Cephalosporins	Inducible β-lactamase. Poorly inhibited by clavulanic acid.	*83, 84*
PER-1	Plasmid	ESBL[a]	Confers resistance to all β-lactam antibiotics, including aztreonam; no activity against carbapenems; inhibited by clavulanic acid	*85–87*
OXA-21 ARI-1 (OXA-23) OXA-24-27	Plasmid	Carbapenems	Class D, nonmetalloenzymes with weak carbapenemase activity	*88–91*
IMP-1 IMP-2 IMP-4 IMP-5 VIM-2	Plasmid and integrons	Carbapenems	Metalloenzymes with potent carbapenemase activity; confers resistance to carbapenems and all β-lactam classes except monobactams	*92–98*

[a]Extended-spectrum β-lactams (e.g., ceflasidime, cefotaxime, cefotriaxome).

clinical isolates. Other mechanisms, including the expression of altered penicillin-binding proteins and reduced permeability of the outer membrane, have also been suggested that may confer a level of intrinsic resistance *(101,102)*. The outer membrane permeability of *Acinetobacter* species to β-lactams has been 1–3% of that of *Escherichia coli*, probably as a result of the production of smaller outer membrane pores or reduced numbers of porins *(102)*. The loss of outer membrane porins has been demonstrated in clinical strains of *A. baumannii* showing resistance to imipenem, suggesting that, as in *Pseudomonas aeruginosa*, this mechanism plays a significant role in the development of carbapenem resistance *(103,104)*. It seems likely that a combination of mechanisms, including β-lactamases, reduced permeability, and perhaps also altered protein targets, combines to create the high-level resistance to β-lactam antibiotics that is seen in clinical strains of *Acinetobacter*.

6.2. Aminoglycosides

The aminoglycosides are widely used for the treatment of infections caused by *Acinetobacter* spp, largely as a result of their synergy when combined with β-lactams. However, resistance to these agents is rapidly increasing. Bacteria become resistant to aminoglycosides by three main mechanisms: alteration of the ribosomal target, reduction of uptake, and enzymatic modification of the drug. The majority of resistance in clinical isolates of *Acinetobacter* spp is caused by the latter.

Three types of aminoglycoside-modifying enzymes exist: acetylating (AAC), phosphorylating (APH), and adenylating (ANT). All three types have been described in *Acinetobacter* spp, the most common of which are AAC(3)-I, ANT(3")-I, AAC(3)-II, AAC(6)-I, ANT(2"), APH(3)-I, and APH(3')-VI *(105,106)*. Different enzymes have a different substrate range and so confer specific patterns of aminoglycoside resistance that enable determination of their presence. For example, the enzyme AAC(3)-I confers resistance to gentamicin alone, whereas AAC(3')-VI confers resistance to kanamycin, amikacin, and isepamicin *(40)*.

However, the situation is complicated by the fact that many strains of *Acinetobacter* possess more than one enzyme, particularly as some are present in the chromosome (contributing to intrinsic resistance) and others are plasmid mediated. Most of the genes encoding these commonly detected aminoglycoside enzymes have now been sequenced, enabling their detection by PCR, which has greatly enhanced understanding of the mechanism of resistance acquisition. Studies have shown that these genes may be present on plasmids or transposons or within integron-type structures, which means they can readily be transmitted between strains and genomospecies.

In a recent study of 24 resistant isolates of *A. baumannii* from 11 countries worldwide, all strains produced at least one aminoglycoside-modifying enzyme, and these enzymes were similar in all strains *(106)*. Transfer of resistance to sensitive strains was observed for 9 isolates.

6.3. Fluoroquinolones

Resistance to ciprofloxacin has developed rapidly among *Acinetobacter* spp. Studies have shown that much of this resistance is because of mutations in codons 82 and 83 of the *gyr*A gene encoding a subunit of DNA gyrase. This mechanism is almost identical to that described in isolates of *E. coli*, and confers a moderate level of resistance to quinolones. Much higher minimum inhibitory concentrations (MICs) to ciprofloxacin are seen in some strains of *Acinetobacter*, which is largely because of additional mutations in the *Par*C gene encoding a subunit of the topoisomerase IV molecule *(40,107)*.

Another possible mechanism by which *Acinetobacter* display reduced sensitivity to quinolones is by decreased accumulation of the drug because of either decreased permeability of the outer membrane or increased efflux from the cell. The contribution of reduced membrane permeability was discussed in Section 6.1. Efflux pump mechanisms have been well described in *P. aeruginosa* that account for their intrinsic resistance to a number of antibiotics and contribute to quinolone resistance *(108,109)*. A report of a novel efflux-type protein from an isolate of *A. baumannii* that mediated resistance to aminoglycosides and reduced susceptibility to fluoroquinolones, among other drugs, suggests that this mechanism may also play a role in *Acinetobacter* spp *(110)*. Further evidence for the role of efflux pumps has been reported in the activity of the efflux pump inhibitor MC107,110 on reducing the MIC of nalidixic acid in its presence *(111)*.

6.4. Other Antibiotics

Resistance to antibiotics other than the β-lactams, aminoglycosides, or quinolones is less well understood and clinically less important. Resistance to the tetracyclines is mediated by two efflux proteins, Tet A and Tet B, which have both been described in clinical isolates of *A. baumannii (112)*. Tet A confers resistance to tetracycline but not minocycline, whereas Tet B confers resistance to both. So far, the resistance mechanisms that result in clinical resistance to the newer tetracycline derivatives, the glycyclines (e.g., tigecycline) have not been identified.

High-level trimethoprim resistance has been described in which the encoding genes are transferred by plasmids and associated with the acquisition of multiple antibiotic resistance. However, the exact mechanisms have not been delineated *(113)*. Resistance to chloramphenicol has been described as a result of a transferable plasmid or chromosomally located gene, CAT-1. This gene encodes an intracellular enzyme that inactivates the antibiotic *(39,81)*.

7. OPTIONS FOR ANTIBIOTIC THERAPY

There have been few clinical trials to determine the most effective antibiotic therapy for *Acinetobacter* infections, which in any case would be greatly influenced by local resistance patterns. Most studies have reported the use of extended-spectrum penicillins, third-generation cephalosporins (e.g., ceftazidime), carbapenems, quinolones, or aminoglycosides. Although some mild-to-moderate infections may be treated with one antibiotic, many require combination antibiotic therapy, usually with a β-lactam antibiotic plus an aminoglycoside.

However, for many strains of *Acinetobacter* spp, these options are now either lost or severely limited. The management of *Acinetobacter* infections should always be based on local resistance patterns and the results of accurate sensitivity testing. In particular, β-lactam antibiotics should be used with caution because of the high prevalence of inducible β-lactamases. The emergence of multiresistant strains of *Acinetobacter* has led to the search for novel antibiotics or antibiotic combinations that retain some activity against these organisms.

Reports of moderate success, in vitro at least, have been described for combination therapy with some of the commonly used antibiotics. Imipenem combined with an aminoglycoside had synergistic activity against multidrug-resistant *A. baumannii* isolates *(114)*, and similar findings were reported for combinations of a quinolone and amikacin for isolates with low quinolone MICs (<2 mg/L) *(115)*. Bactericidal synergy has also been demonstrated when carbenicillin and aminoglycosides are combined, even in the presence of moderate aminoglycoside resistance *(117)*. Variable success has been achieved with combinations of imipenem and ciprofloxacin, but half of all the strains tested showed no evidence of synergy *(117)*. Despite these observations, any increase in activity above that observed for either drug alone is minimal, and the use of these combinations in the face of frank in vitro resistance to either or both antibiotics is unlikely to prove clinically successful.

There has been much interest in recent years in the use of β-lactamase inhibitors as therapy for *Acinetobacter* infections. Although tazobactam and clavulanic acid have been successfully used in combination with β-lactam antibiotics to treat *Acinetobacter* infections, the most useful of these agents is sulbactam. In addition to its inhibition of β-lactamases, sulbactam also possesses intrinsic antimicrobial activity against *Acinetobacter* spp.

Several large studies have shown susceptibility rates exceeding 80% of *Acinetobacter* spp to ampicillin-sulbactam *(118)*. In vitro data suggest that ampicillin-sulbactam is consistently more active against *Acinetobacter* spp than many of the cephalosporins, ciprofloxacin, and gentamicin and retains greater activity than most other β-lactam/β-lactamase inhibitor combinations *(119)*. Imipenem and meropenem generally remain more active *(120)*, although two studies have shown ampicillin-sulbactam to be superior *(119,121)*.

It appears that most of the susceptibility of *Acinetobacter* spp is caused by sulbactam itself. This observation is supported by animal models of *A. baumannii* endocarditis and pneumonia, in which the use of sulbactam alone has shown superior activity to many antibiotics with an efficacy similar to imipenem *(40,122)*. Clinical studies have demonstrated the effectiveness of ampicillin-sulbactam in the treatment of severe multidrug-resistant *Acinetobacter* infections, including bacteremia *(60)*, ventilator-associated pneumonia *(123)*, and meningitis *(124)*. In one study, the use of ampicillin-sulbactam was compared with use of sulbactam alone for the treatment of nonsevere *A. baumannii* infections, with both agents showing success in over 94% of cases *(125)*.

Despite these reports of success, it should be noted that the blood–brain barrier penetration to sulbactam is poor in the absence of inflammation, and this may account for the reports of clinical failure of therapy in cases of meningitis *(118)*.

Although the use of sulbactam either alone or in combination shows promise as a novel therapy for *Acinetobacter* infections, other treatment options are clearly needed. Resistance to colistin has generally remained low (9% in one large UK study), and there have been outbreaks of *A. baumannii* reported in which this remains the only active antibiotic *(74)*. There have been limited reports of clinical success with the use of intravenous colistin for the management of *Acinetobacter* meningitis and other infections *(126,127)*. Intrathecal colistin has also been used to treat a case of ventriculitis caused by a carbapenem-resistant strain of *A. baumannii (128)*. Despite this, animal models of *A. baumannii* pneumonia have shown disappointing results *(129)*, and a poor response rate was shown with the use of this agent alone in a clinical study of patients with multidrug-resistant *A. baumannii* pneumonia *(127)*. Therefore, although colistin may be useful in certain infections because of multidrug-resistant *Acinetobacter* spp, it does not appear to be useful in the management of *Acinetobacter* pneumonias. The use of this drug is also severely limited by its toxic effects, most notably nephrotoxicity, neurotoxicity, and neuromuscular blockade.

A few reports have documented the good in vitro susceptibility of *Acinetobacter* spp to tetracyclines, particularly minocycline *(74,130)*. A single study using a mouse model of *A. baumannii* pneumonia reported synergy between doxycycline and amikacin and suggested that this may be a useful alternative to imipenem therapy *(131)*. However, tetracyclines are merely bacteriostatic, and there is very little clinical data to support their use in the treatment of severe *Acinetobacter* infections. There has been renewed interest in the tetracyclines as a result of the new agent tigecycline, which is a derivative of minocycline. Several studies have shown high levels of in vitro susceptibility of clinical isolates of *Acinetobacter* spp to tigecycline, but it does not appear to have any major advantage over minocycline *(74,132)*.

Although resistance to ciprofloxacin is increasing, there have been promising reports regarding some of the new fluoroquinolones, which have a greater potency against a variety of bacterial species. Two studies showed that all of the newer quinolones, including clinafloxacin, gatifloxacin, gemifloxacin, trovofloxacin, moxifloxacin, and sparfloxacin, exhibit 4- to 16-fold greater activity against *A. baumannii* isolates than ciprofloxacin *(133,134)*. Despite this significantly greater activity compared to ciprofloxacin, resistance to all these quinolones is still observed, with more than 50% of strains showing reduced susceptibility in one study *(133)*. Outbreak strains are significantly more resistant to all these agents than sporadic strains, suggesting that resistance is likely to develop rapidly once these agents are more widely used as alternatives to clinical therapy *(134)*.

In vitro studies suggest that the susceptibility of *Acinetobacter* spp to rifampicin is poor; in fact, the majority of strains show evidence of resistance (MIC > 4 mg/L) *(130)*. Despite this, a study using a mouse model of pneumonia demonstrated excellent efficacy of rifampicin as monotherapy against three strains of multiresistant *A. baumannii* *(135)*. Several studies have shown synergy on combination of rifampicin with colistin, sulbactam, or imipenem, but this is variable between strains *(135–138)*. The use of rifampicin as monotherapy is certainly not recommended because of the rapid development of resistance, but it does appear to have a potential role as adjunctive therapy in multiresistant *Acinetobacter* infections. At present, there is no accepted cutoff level for rifampicin resistance in Gram-negative bacteria other than *Neisseria* spp or *Haemophilus* spp. Exactly how MIC values correlate with clinical effectiveness needs further elucidation before rifampicin combinations are widely used.

Obviously, with increasing reports of infections caused by strains of *A. baumannii* that have very limited sensitivities, there are concerns regarding options for the management of infections in the future. The introduction of the fourth-generation cephalosporins cefepime and cefpirome, which have greater activity against organisms with inducible β-lactamases, provided some hope, but resistance to these agents is already widespread *(73,84)*.

This highlights the importance of searching for novel antibacterial agents. Recent reports have demonstrated the potential role of polycationic peptides as agents active against Gram-negative bacteria, including clinical isolates of *A. baumannii (139,140)*. These molecules are polypeptides isolated from a wide range of animal, plant, and bacterial species. They are thought to act by crossing the outer membrane of Gram-negative bacteria, inserting themselves into the cytoplasmic membrane, and then causing death by a variety of mechanisms. These agents, which include compounds such as buforin II, cecrophin P1, and margainin II, appear to have a rapid in vitro bactericidal effect against multiresistant *A. baumannii (140)*. Significant synergy is also seen with combinations of margainin II, a compound produced by the African clawed frog, and β-lactam antibiotics. Obviously, further studies of these and other similar compounds are required. To date, very little is known about their in vivo activity or toxicity, but their potential value as an alternative therapy is promising.

8. PREVENTION OF INFECTION IN THE ICU

Numerous studies have documented the presence of *Acinetobacter* spp in the hospital environment, particularly within ICUs. Heavy environmental contamination is most frequently seen in the areas immediately surrounding colonized patients *(141)*. However, using molecular typing methods, endemic or outbreak strains of *Acinetobacter* spp have been found in any number of sites, including floors and horizontal work surfaces, door handles, sinks, curtains, and bed rails *(51,142–144)*. Outbreaks of infection have been traced to a variety of environmental sources, including mattresses *(25)*, curtains *(144)*, pillows *(145)*, computer keyboards *(146)*, arterial pressure transducers *(147)*, room humidifiers *(69)*, and contaminated ventilator equipment *(46,148,149)*.

One of the factors that may contribute to environmental contamination is the unusual ability of *Acinetobacter* spp to survive in the environment. Studies have shown that many species of *Acinetobacter*, including *A. baumannii*, can survive for long periods in dry conditions. Buxton et al. demonstrated the survival of *A. baumannii* for 7 d on an air-dried washcloth believed to be the source of an outbreak *(150)*. Other investigators have demonstrated the recovery of outbreak strains of *A. baumannii* after several weeks in dry conditions in the laboratory *(151,152)*. Genomic species of *Acinetobacter* associated with nosocomial infection had significantly greater desiccation tolerance, as were freshly isolated strains *(153)*. This prolonged survival may account at least in part for the extended nature of many outbreaks of *Acinetobacter* described.

A number of reports have highlighted the importance of the hands of health care workers in the persistence of outbreaks of *A. baumannii* infections. Outbreak strains of *A. baumannii* have been isolated from the hands of health care workers *(154)*. In one outbreak, epidemiological data demonstrated the source of infection was computer keyboards, which were repeatedly contaminated by the hands of staff on the unit *(146)*. It seems likely that unrecognized contamination of inanimate objects and the subsequent spread of organisms on the hands of health care workers plays a significant role in the cross-transmission of *Acinetobacter* spp in the ICU setting. Cross-transmission is further aided by the propensity of *Acinetobacter* to survive for such prolonged periods in the environment.

These observations are highlighted by the fact that many outbreaks of *Acinetobacter* in ICUs have been controlled by a number of simple measures, including strict adherence to infection control practices such as handwashing and the wearing of disposable gloves and aprons and regular decontamination of the environment *(28,142,155,156)*. Simple cleaning of bed spaces with water and detergent should generally be adequate, but during an outbreak or when *Acinetobacter* is endemic, additional measures, such as frequent changing of curtains or pillows, may be necessary. In outbreak situations, the use of environmental screening coupled with molecular typing of any *Acinetobacter* spp isolated is essential to detect the need for further control measures. Long-term persistence of strains of *Acinetobacter* spp in the ICU environment has been described, indicating that continued surveillance even during periods without an outbreak may be necessary in those units where outbreaks have occurred in the past *(23)*.

A small number of outbreak reports have demonstrated that contact isolation, such as that employed for the control of methicillin-resistant *Staphylococcus aureus* (MRSA), and adherence to the above infection control measures is insufficient to prevent the spread of *A. baumannii (27,47,52,157)*. This suggests that the airborne mode of spread may play a significant role in transmission. In this situation, patient isolation or closure of the unit may be necessary to control significant outbreaks of infection.

Prophylactic treatment with selective digestive decontamination (SDD) has been suggested as a strategy to reduce the number of colonized patients in an ICU. One study demonstrated a significant reduction in fecal and pharyngeal carriage of multiresistant *A. baumannii* in patients treated with a combination of polymixin E and tobramycin *(158)*. Similar results have also been obtained in studies of decolonization of other Gram-negative organisms *(159)*. Despite these encouraging results, gut carriage is not the sole source of colonization. SDD has no effect on skin carriage and so cannot be used as an isolated control measure. Furthermore, while no resistance to polymixin was demonstrated in the study described here, there are concerns regarding the widespread use of antibiotics for decontamination, which may simply increase resistance in the future. SDD may be useful as an additional control measure in prolonged outbreaks of multiresistant *Acinetobacter* infections, but its efficacy has yet to be proven as a routine control measure.

It has been shown that epidemic strains of *Acinetobacter* are significantly more resistant to antibiotics than sporadic strains *(151,160,161)*. In addition, as already described, the use of broad-spectrum antibiotics is a significant risk factor for *A. baumannii* acquisition. These findings suggest that a major factor contributing to the development of prolonged outbreaks of *Acinetobacter* is the selection pressure of antibiotics, which encourages colonization of patients with multidrug-resistant bacteria. Reduction in *Acinetobacter* acquisition and infections may be achieved by controlling the use of broad-spectrum antibiotics, particularly β-lactams. This can be achieved using strict antibiotic policies together with a multidisciplinary approach involving microbiologists and infectious diseases specialists in the management of infections in ICUs. A small number of outbreaks have been successfully controlled using antibiotic restriction either alone or with other measures *(37,38,155)*.

The reason why *Acinetobacter* infections are so common in the ICU setting is likely to be multifactorial, involving an interaction of environmental contamination, inadequate adherence to infection control measures, and the selection pressure of broad-spectrum antibiotics. It therefore follows that effective control of these infections will also rely on a multifaceted approach that addresses all these factors.

9. CONCLUSIONS

Acinetobacter species, particularly *A. baumannii*, contribute significantly to nosocomial infections in ICUs. Using sensitive typing techniques, the acquisition of endemic strains and numerous outbreaks of infection have been described that place a huge burden on health care resources. The success of these bacteria in the hospital setting appears to be related to their ability to survive for long periods in the environment and to acquire resistance to multiple antibiotics. Many strains of *A. baumannii* have been identified that are resistant to multiple classes of antibiotics, including third- and fourth-generation cephalosporins, aminoglycosides, fluoroquinolones, and carbapenems. As a result, options for the management of infections caused by *Acinetobacter* spp are severely limited, and treatment often relies on the use of novel or toxic antibiotic regimens.

Preventing further spread of multiresistant *Acinetobacter* obviously depends on the rapid introduction of effective control strategies. It appears that multiple approaches are necessary to prevent their emergence and spread in ICU settings; these approaches include strict adherence to infection control practices, frequent environmental surveillance and decontamination, rapid detection and isolation of colonized patients, and control of antibiotic usage. In the meantime, the race is on to develop new antimicrobial agents or combinations that retain activity against these bacteria.

REFERENCES

1. Allen DM, Hartman BJ. *Acinetobacter* species. In: Mandell GL, Bennett JE, Dolin R (eds.). Mandell, Douglas, and Bennetts Principles and Practice of Infectious Diseases. 5th ed. London: Churchill-Livingstone, 2000, pp. 2339–2344.
2. Jawad A, Hawkey PM, Heritage J, Snelling AM. Description of Leeds *Acinetobacter* Medium, a new selective and differential medium for isolation of clinically important *Acinetobacter* spp, and comparison with Herellea agar and Holton's agar. J Clin Microbiol 1994; 32:2353–2358.
3. Juni E. Genus III *Acinetobacter* Brisou and Prevot 1954. In: Kreig NR, Holt JG (eds.). Bergeys Manual of Systematic Bacteriology. Vol. 1. Baltimore, MD: Williams and Wilkins, 1984, pp. 303–307.
4. Skerman VBD, McGowan V, Sneath PA. Approved lists of bacterial names. Int J Syst Bacteriol 1980; 30:225–420.
5. Bouvet PJM, Grimont PAD. Taxonomy of the genus *Acinetobacter* with the recognition of *Acinetobacter baumannii* sp nov, *Acinetobacter haemolyticus* sp nov, *Acinetobacter johnsonnii* sp nov, and *Acinetobacter junii* sp nov, and emended descriptions of *Acinetobacter calcoaceticus* and *Acinetobacter lwoffii*. Int J Syst Bacteriol 1986; 36: 228–240.
6. Gerner-Smidt P. Ribotyping of the *Acinetobacter calcoaceticus–Acinetobacter baumannii* complex. J Clin Microbiol 1992; 30:2680–2685.
7. Jansen P, Coopman R, Huys G, et al. Evaluation of the DNA fingerprinting method AFLP as a new tool in bacterial taxonomy. Microbiology 1996; 142:1881–1893.
8. Ehrenstein B, Bernard AT, Dijkshoorn L, et al. *Acinetobacter* species identification using tRNA spacer fingerprinting. J Clin Microbiol 1996; 34:2414–2420.
9. Vaneechoutte M, Dijkshoorn L, Tjernberg I, et al. Identification of *Acinetobacter* genomic species by amplified ribosomal DNA restriction analysis. J Clin Microbiol 1995; 33:11–15.
10. Bouvet PJM, Jean-Jean S. Delineation of new proteolytic genomic species in the genus *Acinetobacter*. Res Microbiol 1989; 140:291–299.
11. Tjernberg I, Ursing J. Clinical strains of *Acinetobacter* classified by DNA–DNA hybridisation. APMIS 1989; 97:595–605.
12. Nishimura Y, Ino T, Lizuka H. *Acinetobacter radioresistens* sp nov isolated from cotton and soil. Int J Syst Bacteriol 1988; 38:209–211.
13. Jansen P, Maqueli K, Coopman R, et al. Discrimination of *Acinetobacter* genomic species by AFLP fingerprinting. Int J Syst Bacteriol 1997; 49:1179–1187.
14. Nemec A, De Baere T, Tjernberg I, et al. *Acinetobacter ursingii* sp nov and *Acinetobacter schlindleri* sp nov, isolated from human clinical specimens. Int J Syst Evolut Microbiol 2001; 51:1891–1899.
15. Gerner-Scmidt P, Tjernberg I, Ursing J. Reliability of phenotypic tests for identification of *Acinetobacter* species. J Clin Microbiol 1991; 29:277–282.
16. Bernard AT, Dijkshoorn L, Van der Toom J, et al. Phenotypic characterisation of strains of 13 DNA–DNA hybridisation groups by means of the Biolog system. J Med Microbiol 1995; 42:113–119.

17. Bernards AT, van der Toom J, van Boven CPA, et al. Evaluation of the ability of a commercial system to identify *Acinetobacter* genomic species. Eur J Clin Microbiol Infect Dis 1996; 15:303–308.
18. Jawad A, Snelling AM, Heritage J, Hawkey PM. Exceptional desiccation tolerance of *Acinetobacter radioresistens*. J Hosp Infect 1998; 39:235–240.
19. Berlau J, Aucken H, Malnick H, Pitt T. Distribution of *Acinetobacter* species on skin of healthy humans. Eur J Clin Microbiol Infect Dis 1999; 3:179–183.
20. Seifert H, Dijkshoorn L, Gerner-Smidt P, et al. Distribution of *Acinetobacter* species on human skin: comparison of phenotypic and genotypic identification methods. J Clin Microbiol 1997; 35:2819–2825.
21. Kloos WE, Musselwhite MS. Distribution and persistence of *Staphylococcus, Micrococcus* species and other aerobic bacteria on human skin. Appl Microbiol 1975; 30:381–385.
22. Garrouste-Orgeas M, Marie O, Rouveau M, et al. Secondary carriage with multi-resistant *Acinetobacter baumannii* and *Klebsiella pneumoniae* in an adult intensive care unit population: relationship with nosocomial infections and mortality. J Hosp Infect 1996; 34:279–289.
23. Webster CA, Crowe M, Humphreys H, Towner KJ. Surveillance of an adult intensive care unit for long-term persistence of a multi-resistant strain of *Acinetobacter baumannii*. Eur J Clin Microbiol Infect Dis 1998; 17:171–176.
24. Wisplinghoff H, Perbix W, Seifert H. Risk factors for nosocomial bloodstream infections due to *Acinetobacter baumannii*: a case-control study of adult burn patients. Clin Infect Dis 1999; 28:59–66.
25. Sheretz RJ, Sullivan ML. An outbreak of infections with *Acinetobacter calcoaceticus* in burn patients: contamination of patients' mattresses. J Infect Dis 1985; 151:252–258.
26. Fjita K, Lilly HA, Ayliffe GAJ. Spread of resistant Gram negative bacilli in a burns unit. J Hosp Infect 1982; 3:29–37.
27. Allen D, Green HT. Hospital outbreak of multiresistant *Acinetobacter anitratus*: an airborne mode of spread. J Hosp Infect 1987; 9:110–119.
28. Mah MW, Memish ZA, Cunningham G, Bannatyne RM. Outbreak of *Acinetobacter baumannii* in an intensive care unit associated with tracheostomy. Am J Infect Control 2001; 29:282–288.
29. Rosenthal SL. Source of *Pseudomonas* and *Acinetobacter* species found in human culture material. Am J Clin Pathol 1974; 62:807–811.
30. Timsit J-F, Garant V, Musset B, et al. The digestive tract is a major site for *Acinetobacter baumannii* colonisation in intensive care unit patients. J Infect Dis 1993; 168:1336–1337.
31. Corbella X, Pujol M, Ayati J, et al. Relevance of digestive tract colonisation in the epidemiology of nosocomial infections due to multiresistant *Acinetobacter baumannii*. Clin Infect Dis 1996; 23:239–234.
32. Wong TH, Tan BH, Ling ML, Sang C. Multi-resistant *Acinetobacter baumannii* on a burns unit—clinical risk factors and prognosis. Burns 2002; 28:349–357.
33. Lortholary O, Fagan JY, Hoi AC, et al. Nosocomial acquisition of multi-resistant *Acinetobacter baumannii*: risk factors and prognosis. Clin Infect Dis 1995; 20:790–796.
34. Mulin B, Alan D, Viel JF, et al. Risk factors for nosocomial colonisation with multi-resistant *Acinetobacter baumannii*. Eur J Clin Microbiol Infect Dis 1995; 14:569–576.
35. Scerpella EG, Wanger AR, Amitige L, et al. Nosocomial outbreak caused by a multiresistant clone of *Acinetobacter baumannii*: results of the case-control and molecular epidemiologic investigations. Infect Control Hosp Epidemiol 1995; 16:92–97.
36. Peacock JE, Sorrell L, Sottie FD, et al. Nosocomial respiratory tract colonisation and infection with aminoglycoside resistant *Acinetobacter calcoaceticus* var. *anitratus*: epidemiologic characteristics and clinical significance. Infect Control Hosp Epidemiol 1988; 9:302–308.
37. Villers D, Espaze E, Costel-Burel M, et al. Nosocomial *Acinetobacter baumannii* infections: microbiological and clinical epidemiology. Ann Intern Med 1998; 129:182–189.

38. Seifert H, Schulze A, Baginski R, Pulverer G. Comparison of four different typing methods for epidemiologic typing of *Acinetobacter baumannii.* J Clin Microbiol 1994; 32:1816–1819.
39. Bergogne-Berezin E, Towner KJ. *Acinetobacter* spp as nosocomial pathogens: microbiological, clinical and epidemiological features. Clin Microbiol Rev 1996; 9:148–165.
40. Towner KJ (ed.). Clinical importance and antibiotic resistance of *Acinetobacter* spp. Proceedings of a symposium held on 4–5 November 1996 at Eilat, Israel. J Med Microbiol 1997; 46:721–746.
41. Biendo M, Laurans G, Lefebvre JF, et al. Epidemiologic study of an *Acinetobacter baumannii* outbreak by using a combination of antibiotyping and ribotyping. J Clin Microbiol 1999; 37:2170–2175.
42. Gouby A, Carles Nurit MJ, Bouziges N, et al. Use of pulsed-field gel electrophoresis for investigation of hospital outbreaks of *Acinetobacter baumannii.* J Clin Microbiol 1992; 30:1588–1591.
43. Seifert H, Gerner-Schmidt P. Comparison of ribotyping and pulsed-field gel electrophoresis for molecular typing of *Acinetobacter* isolates. J Clin Microbiol 1995; 33:1402–1407.
44. Bernards AT, de Beaufort AJ, Dijkshoorn L, van Boven CPA. Outbreak of septicaemia in neonates caused by *Acinetobacter junii* investigated by amplified ribosomal DNA restriction analysis (ARDRA) and four typing methods. J Hosp Infect 1997; 35:129–140.
45. Levidiotou S, Galanakis E, Vrioni G, et al. A multi-resistant *Acinetobacter baumannii* outbreak in a general intensive care unit. In Vivo 2002; 16:117–122.
46. Mathai E, Kaufmann ME, Richard VS, et al. Typing of *Acinetobacter baumannii* isolated from hospital acquired respiratory infections in a tertiary care centre in southern India. J Hosp Infect 2001; 47:159–162.
47. Kooleman JGM, Parevliet GA, Dijkshoorn L, et al. Nosocomial outbreak of multi-resistant *Acinetobacter baumannii* on a surgical ward: epidemiology and risk factors for acquisition. J Hosp Infect 1997; 37:113–123.
48. Janssen P, Dijkshoorn L. High resolution DNA fingerprinting of *Acinetobacter* outbreak strains. FEMS Microbiol Lett 1996; 42:191–194.
49. Wu T-L, Su L-H, Leu H-S, et al. Molecular epidemiology of nosocomial infection associated with multi-resistant *Acinetobacter baumannii* by infrequent restriction-site PCR. J Hosp Infect 2002; 51:27–32.
50. Snelling A, Gerner-Smidt P, Hawkey PM, et al. Validation of whole-cell repetitive extragenic palindromic sequence-based PCR (REP-PCR) for typing strains belonging to the *Acinetobacter calcoaceticus–Acinetobacter baumannii* complex and application of the method to the investigation of a hospital outbreak. J Clin Microbiol 1996; 47:1179–1187.
51. van Dessel H, Kamp-Hopmans TEM, Fluit AC, et al. Outbreak of a susceptible strain of *Acinetobacter* species 13 (sensu Tjernberg and ursing) in an adult neurosurgical intensive care unit. J Hosp Infect 2002; 51:89–95.
52. Kooleman JGM, Stoof J, Biesmans DJ, et al. Comparison of amplified ribosomal DNA restriction analysis, random amplified polymorphic DNA analysis and amplified fragment length polymorphism fingerprinting for identification of *Acinetobacter* genomic species and typing of *Acinetobacter baumannii.* J Clin Microbiol 1998; 36:2522–2529.
53. Bergogne-Berezin E. The increasing role of *Acinetobacter* species as nosocomial pathogens. Curr Infect Dis Rep 2001; 3:440–444.
54. Schaberg DS, Culver D, Gaynes R. Major trends in the microbial aetiology of nosocomial infections. Am J Med. 1991; 91:725–755.
55. Jarvis WR, Martone WJ. Predominant pathogens in hospital infections. J Antimicrob Chemother 1992; 29(suppl. A):19–24.
56. Vincent J-L, Bihari DT, Suter PM, et al. The prevalence of nosocomial infection in intensive care units in Europe. Results of the European Prevalence of Infection in Intensive Care (EPIC) study. JAMA 1995; 274:639–644.

57. Garcia-Garmendia JL, Artiz-Lyba C, Garnacho-Montero J, et al. Mortality and the increase in length of stay attributable to the acquisition of *Acinetobacter* in critically ill patients. Crit Care Med 1999; 27:1794–1799.
58. Wisplinghoff H, Edmond MB, Pfaller MA, et al. Nosocomial bloodstream infections caused by *Acinetobacter* species in United States hospitals: clinical features, molecular epidemiology and antimicrobial susceptibility. Clin Infect Dis 2000; 31:690–697.
59. Garcia-Garmendia J-L, Ortiz-Leyba C, Garnacho-Montero J, et al. Risk factors for *Acinetobacter baumannii* nosocomial bacteraemia in critically ill patients: a cohort study. Clin Infect Dis 2001; 33:939–946.
60. Cineros JM, Reyes MJ, Pachon J, et al. Bacteraemia due to *Acinetobacter baumannii*: epidemiology, clinical findings and prognostic features. Clin Infect Dis 1996; 22:1026–1032.
61. Nosocomial Infection National Surveillance Service (NINSS). Surveillance of Hospital-Acquired Bacteraemia in English Hospitals, 1997–2000. PHLS, 2002.
62. Linde H-J, Hahn J, Holler E, et al. Septicaemia due to *Acinetobacter junii.* J Clin Microbiol 2002; 40:2696–2697.
63. Ku SC, Hsueh PR, Yang PC, Luh KT. Clinical and microbiological characteristics of bacteraemia caused by *Acinetobacter lwoffii.* Eur J Clin Microbiol Infect Dis 2000; 19:501–505.
64. Seifert H, Strate A, Pulverer G. Nosocomial bacteraemia due to *Acinetobacter baumannii*: clinical features, epidemiology and predictors of mortality. Medicine (Baltimore) 1995; 74:340–349.
65. Tilley PAG, Roberts FJ. Bacteraemia with *Acinetobacter* species. Risk factors and prognosis in different clinical settings. Clin Infect Dis 1994; 18:896–900.
66. Seifert H, Baginski R, Schulze A, Pulverer G. The distribution of *Acinetobacter* species in clinical culture materials. Int J Med Microbiol Virol Parasitol Infect Dis 1993; 279:544–552.
67. Ng TK, Ling JM, Cheng AF, Norrby SR. A retrospective study of clinical characteristics of *Acinetobacter* bacteraemia. Scand J Infect Dis. 1996; 101(suppl.):26–32.
68. Siegman-Igra Y, Bar-Yosef S, Gorea A, Avram J. Nosocomial *Acinetobacter* meningitis secondary to invasive procedures: report of 25 cases and review. Clin Infect Dis 1993; 17:843–849.
69. Gervich DH, Grout CS. An outbreak of nosocomial *Acinetobacter* infections from humidifiers. Am J Infect Control 1985; 13:210–215.
70. Tong MJ. Septic complications of war wounds. JAMA 1972; 219:1044–1047.
71. Hanberger H, Garcia-Rodriguez J-A, Gobernado M, et al. Antibiotic susceptibility among aerobic Gram-negative bacilli in intensive care units in five European countries. JAMA 1999; 281:67–71.
72. Sader HS, Jones RN, Gales AC, et al. Antimicrobial susceptibility for pathogens isolated from patients in Latin American medical centres with a diagnosis of pneumonia: analysis of results from the SENTRY antimicrobial surveillance program (1997). SENTRY Latin American Study Group. Diagn Microbiol Infect Dis 1998; 32:289–301.
73. Pfaller MA, Jones RN, Biedenbach DJ. Antimicrobial resistance trends in medical centers using carbapenems: report of 1999 and 2000 results from the MYSTIC program (USA). Diagn Microbiol Infect Dis 2001; 41:177–182.
74. Henwood CJ, Gatwood T, Wraner M, et al. Antibiotic resistance among clinical isolates of *Acinetobacter* in the UK, and in vitro evaluation of tigecycline (GAR-936). J Antimicrob Chemother 2002; 49:479–487.
75. Afzal-Shah M, Livermore DM. Worldwide emergence of carbapenems-resistant *Acinetobacter* spp. J Antimicrob Chemother 1998; 41:576–577.
76. Da Silva GJ, Leitao GJ, Peixe L. Emergence of carbapenem-hydrolysing enzymes in *Acinetobacter baumannii* clinical isolates. J Clin Microbiol 1999; 37:2109–2110.
77. Corbella X, Montero A, Pujol M, et al. Emergence and rapid spread of carbapenems resistance during a large and sustained hospital outbreak of multi-resistant *Acinetobacter baumannii.* J Clin Microbiol 2000; 38:4086–4095.

78. Go ES, Urban C, Burns J, et al. Clinical and molecular epidemiology of *Acinetobacter* infections sensitive only to polymixin B and sulbactam. Lancet 1994; 344:1329–1332.
79. Fierobe L, Lucet JC, Decre D, et al. An outbreak of imipenem-resistant *Acinetobacter baumannii* in critically ill surgical patients. Infect Control Hosp Epidemiol 2001; 22:35–40.
80. Joly-Gouillou ML, Bergogne-Berezin E, Phillippou A. Distribution of β-lactamases and phenotype analysis in clinical strains of *Acinetobacter calcoaceitcus*. J Antimicrob Chemother 1988; 22:597–604.
81. Vila J, Marcos A, Marco F, et al. In vitro antimicrobial production of β-lactamases, aminoglycoside modifying enzymes and chloramphenicol acetyltransferase by and susceptibility of clinical isolates of *Acinetobacter baumannii*. Antimicrob Agents Chemother 1993; 37:138–141.
82. Paul G, Joly-Gouillou ML, Bergogne-Berezin E, et al. Novel carbenicillin-hydrolysing β-lactamase (CARB-5) from *Acinetobacter calcoaceticus* var. *anitratus*. FEMS Microbiol Lett 1989; 59:45–50.
83. Bou G, Martinez-Beltran J. Cloning, nucleotide sequencing and analysis of the gene encoding an Amp-C β-lactamase in *Acinetobacter baumannii*. Antimicrob Agents Chemother 2000; 44:428–432.
84. Danes C, Navia MM, Ruiz J, et al. Distribution of β-lactamases in *Acinetobacter baumannii* clinical isolates and the effect of Syn2190 (AmpC inhibitor) on the MICs of different β-lactam antibiotics. J Antimicrob Chemother 2002; 50:261–264.
85. Vahaboglu H, Coskunkan F, Tansel O, et al. Clinical importance of extended-spectrum β-lactamase (PER-1-type)-producing *Acinetobacter* spp and *Pseudomonas aeruginosa* strains. J Med Microbiol 2001; 50:642–645.
86. Vahaboglu H, Ozturk R, Aygun F, et al. Widespread detection of PER-1-type extended spectrum β-lactamases among nosocomial *Acinetobacter* and *Pseudomonas aeruginosa* isolates in Turkey: a national multicenter study. Antimicrob Agents Chemother 1997; 41: 2265–2269.
87. Poirel L, Karim A, Mercat A, et al. Extended-spectrum β-lactamase producing strain of *Acinetobacter baumannii* isolated from a patient in France. J Antimicrob Chemother 1999; 43:157–158.
88. Paton R, Miles RS, Hood J, Amyes SGB. ARI-1: β-lactamase mediated imipenem resistance in *Acinetobacter baumannii*. Int J Antimicrob Agents 1993; 2:81–88.
89. Vila J, Navia M, Ruiz J, Casals C. Cloning and nucleotide sequence analysis of a gene encoding an OXA-derived β-lactamase in *Acinetobacter baumannii*. Antimicrob Agents Chemother 1997; 41:2757–2759.
90. Bou G, Oliver A, Martinez-Beltran J. OXA-24, a novel Class D β-lactamase with carbapenemase activity in an *Acinetobacter baumannii* clinical strain. Antimicrob Agents Chemother 2000; 44:1556–1561.
91. Afzal-Shah M, Woodford N, Livermore DM. Characterisation of OXA-25, OXA-26 and OXA-27, molecular class D β-lactamases associated with carbapenems resistance in clinical isolates of *Acinetobacter baumannii*. Antimicrob Agents Chemother 2001; 45:583–588.
92. Cornaghia G, Riccio ML, Mazzariol A, et al. Appearance of IMP-1 metallo β-lactamase in Europe. Lancet 1999; 353:899–900.
93. Tysall L, Stockdale MW, Chadwick PR, et al. IMP-1 carbapenemase detected in an *Acinetobacter* clinical isolate from the UK. J Antimicrob Chemother 2002; 49:215–224.
94. Riccio ML, Franceschini N, Boscli B, et al. Characterisation of the metallo β-lactamase determinant of *Acinetobacter baumannii* AC-54/97 reveals the existence of bla_{IMP} allelic variants caused by the gene cassettes of different phylogeny. Antimicrob Agents Chemother 2000; 44:1229–1235.
95. Chu Y-W, Afzal-Shah M, Houang ETS, et al. IMP-4, a novel metallo β-lactamase from nosocomial *Acinetobacter* spp collected in Hong Kong between 1994 and 1998. Antimicrob Agents Chemother 2001; 45:710–714.

96. Yum JH, Yi K, Lee H, et al. Molecular characterisation of metallo β-lactamase producing *Acinetobacter baumannii* and *Acinetobacter* genospecies 3 from Korea: identification of two new integrons carrying the bla_{VIM} gene cassettes. J Antimicrob Chemother 2002; 49:837–840.
97. Takahshi A, Yomoda S, Kobayashi I, et al. Detection of carbapenemase-producing *Acinetobacter baumannii* in a hospital. J Clin Microbiol 2000; 38:526–529.
98. Da Silva GJ, Correia M, Vital C, et al. Molecular characterization of bla(IMP-5), a new integron-borne metallo-β-lactamase gene from an *Acinetobacter baumannii* nosocomial isolate in Portugal. FEMS Microbiol Lett 2002; 215:33–39.
99. Richet HM, Mohammed J, McDonald LC, Jarvis WR. Building communication networks: international network for the study and prevention of emerging antimicrobial resistance. Emerg Infect Dis 2001; 7:319–322.
100. Perez AN, Baet IG, Robledo EH, et al. Metallo β-lactamases in *Acinetobacter calcoaceticus*. Med Sci Res 1996; 24:315–317.
101. Obara M, Nakae T. Mechanisms of resistance to β-lactam antibiotics in *Acinetobacter calcoaceticus*. J Antimicrob Chemother 1991; 28:791–800.
102. Sato K, Nakae T. Outer membrane permeability of *Acinetobacter calcoaceticus* and its implications in antibiotic resistance. J Antimicrob Chemother 1991; 36:585–586.
103. Bou G, Cervero G, Dominguez MA, et al. Characterisation of a nosocomial outbreak caused by a multiresistant *Acinetobacter baumannii* strain with a carbapenem-hydrolysing enzyme: high level carbapenems resistance is not due solely to the presence of β-lactamases. J Clin Microbiol 2000; 38:3299–3305.
104. Clark RB. Imipenem resistance among *Acinetobacter baumannii*: association with reduced expression of a 33–36 kDa outer membrane protein. J Antimicrob Chemother 1996; 38:245–251.
105. Lambert T, Rudant E, Bouvet P, Courvalin P. Molecular basis of aminoglycoside resistance in *Acinetobacter* spp. J Med Microbiol 1997; 46:731–735.
106. Seward RJ, Lambert T, Towner KJ. Molecular epidemiology of aminoglycoside resistance in *Acinetobacter* spp. J Med Microbiol 1998; 47:455–462.
107. Seward RJ, Towner KJ. Molecular epidemiology of quinolone resistance in *Acinetobacter* spp. Clin Microbiol Infect 1998; 4:248–254.
108. Poole K, Srikumar R. Multidrug efflux in *Pseudomonas aeruginosa*: components, mechanisms and clinical resistance. Curr Top Med Chem 2001; 1:59–71.
109. Nakajima A, Sugimoto Y, Yoneyama H, Nakae T. High level fluoroquinolones resistance in *Pseudomonas aeruginosa* due to the interplay of the mexAB-OprM efflux pump and the DNA gyrase mutation. Microbiol Immunol 2002; 46:391–395.
110. Magnet S, Courvalin P, Lambert T. Resistance-nodulation-cell division-type efflux pump involved in aminoglycoside resistance on *Acinetobacter baumannii* strain BM4454. Antimicrob Agents Chemother 2001; 45:3375–3380.
111. Ribera A, Ruiz J, Jimenez de Anta T, Vila J. Effect of an efflux pump inhibitor on the MIC of nalidixic acid for *Acinetobacter baumannii* and *Stenotrophomonas maltophilia* clinical studies. J Antimicrob Chemother 2002; 49:697–702.
112. Guardabassi L, Dijkshoorn L, Collard JM, Olsen JE, Dalsgaard A. Distribution and in vitro transfer of tetracycline resistance determinants in clinical and aquatic *Acinetobacter* strains. J Med Microbiol 2000; 49:929–936.
113. Goldstein FW, Labigne-Rousel A, Gerbaud G, et al. Transferrable plasmid mediated antibiotic resistance in *Acinetobacter*. Plasmid 1983; 10:138–147.
114. Marques MB, Brookings ES, Moser SA, et al. Comparative in vitro antimicrobial susceptibilities of nosocomial isolates of *Acinetobacter baumannii* and synergistic activities of nine antimicrobial combinations. Antimicrob Agents Chemother 1997; 41:881–885.
115. Bajaksouzian S, Visalli MA, Jacobs MR, Appelbaum PC. Activities of levofloxacin, ofloxacin, and ciprofloxacin alone and in combination with amikacin, against acineto-

bacters as determined by checkerboard and time-kill studies. Antimicrob Agents Chemother 1997; 41:1073–1076.
116. Ramphal R, Kluge RM. *Acinetobacter calcoaceticus* variety *anitratus*: an increasing nosocomial problem. Am J Med Sci 1979; 277:57–66.
117. Ermertcan S, Hosgor M, Tunger O, Cosor G. Investigation of synergism of meropenem and ciprofloxacin against *Pseudomonas aeruginosa* and *Acinetobacter* strains isolated from intensive care unit infections. Scand J Infect Dis 2001; 33:818–821.
118. Levin AS. Multiresistant *Acinetobacter* infections: a role for sulbactam combinations in overcoming an emerging worldwide problem. Clin Microbiol Infect 2002; 8:144–153.
119. Doubyas J, Tzouvelekis LS, Tsakris A. In vitro activity of ampicillin/sulbactam against multiresistant *Acinetobacter calcoaceticus* var *anitratus* clinical isolates. J Antimicrob Chemother 1994; 34:298–300.
120. Murray PR, Jones RN, Allen SD, et al. Multilaboratory evaluation of the in vitro activity of 13 β-lactam antibiotics against 1474 clinical isolates of aerobic and anaerobic bacteria. Diagn Microbiol Infect Dis 1993; 16:191–203.
121. Urban C, Go E, Mariano N, et al. Effect of sublactam on infections caused by imipenem-resistant *Acinetobacter calcoaceticus* biotype *anitratus*. J Infect Dis 1993; 167:448–451.
122. Rodriguez-Hernandez M-J, Cuberos L, Pichardo C, et al. Sulbactam efficacy in experimental models caused by susceptible and intermediate *Acinetobacter baumannii* strains. J Antimicrob Chemother 2001; 47:479–482.
123. Wood GC, Hane SC, Cruce MA, et al. Comparison of ampicillin-sulbactam and imipenem-cilastatin for the treatment of *Acinetobacter* ventilator associated pneumonia. Clin Infect Dis 2002; 34:1425–1430.
124. Jimenez-Mejias ME, Pachon J, Becerril B, et al. Treatment of multidrug-resistant *Acinetobacter baumannii* meningitis with ampicillin/sulbactam. Clin Infect Dis 1997; 24:932–935.
125. Corbella X, Ariza J, Ardanuy C, et al. Efficacy of sulbactam alone and in combination with ampicillin in nosocomial infections caused by multiresistant *Acinetobacter baumannii*. J Antimicrob Chemother 1998; 42:793–802.
126. Jimenez-Mejias ME, Becerril B, Marquez-Rivas FJ, et al. Successful treatment of multidrug-resistant *Acinetobacter baumannii* meningitis with intravenous colistin silfomethate sodium. Eur J Clin Microbiol Infect Dis 2000; 19:970–971.
127. Levin LS, Barone AA, Penco J, et al. Intravenous colistin as therapy for nosocomial infections caused by multidrug-resistant *Pseudomonas aeruginosa* and *Acinetobacter baumannii*. Clin Infect Dis 1999; 28:1008–1011.
128. Fernandez-Viladrich P, Corbella X, Corral L, et al. Successful treatment of ventriculitis due to carbapenem-resistant *Acinetobacter baumannii* with intraventricular colistin sulfomethate sodium. Clin Infect Dis 1999; 28:916–917.
129. Montero A, Ariza J, Corbella X, et al. Efficacy of colistin versus β-lactams, aminoglycosides and rifampin as monotherapy in a mouse model of pneumonia caused by multiresistant *Acinetobacter baumannii*. Antimicrob Agents Chemother 2002; 46: 1946–1952.
130. Appelmann MD, Belzberg H, Citron DM, et al. In vitro activities of non-traditional antimicrobials against multiresistant *Acinetobacter baumannii* strains isolated in an intensive care unit outbreak. Antimicrob Agents Chemother 2000; 44:1035–1040.
131. Rodriguez-Hernandez M-J, Pachon J, Pichardo C, et al. Imipenem, doxycycline and amikacin in monotherapy and in combination in *Acinetobacter baumannii* experimental pneumonia. J Antimicrob Chemother 2000; 45:493–501.
132. Betriu C, Rodriguez-Avial I, Sanchez BA, et al. In vitro activities of tigecycline (GAR-936) against recently isolated clinical bacteria in Spain. Antimicrob Agents Chemother 2002; 46:892–895.

133. Vila J, Ribera A, Marco F, et al. Activity of clinafloxacin compared with six other quinolones against *Acinetobacter baumannii* clinical isolates. J Antimicrob Chemother 2002; 49:471–477.
134. Heinemann B, Wisplinghoff H, Edmond M, Seifert H. Comparative activities of ciprofloxacin, clinafloxacin, gatifloxacin, gemifloxacin, levofloxacin, moxifloxacin and trovofloacin against epidemiologically defined *Acinetobacter baumannii* strains. Antimicrob Agents Chemother 2000; 44:2211–2213.
135. Wolff M, Joly-Guillou M-L, Farinotti R, Carbon C. In vivo efficacies of combinations of β-lactams, β-lactamase inhibitors, and rifampin against *Acinetobacter baumannii* in a mouse pneumonia model. Antimicrob Agents Chemother 1999; 43:1406–1411.
136. Giamarellos-Bourboulis EJ, Xirouchaki E, Giamarrellou H. Interactions of colistin and rifampin on multidrug-resistant *Acinetobacter baumannii.* Diagn Microbial Infect Dis 2001; 40:117–120.
137. Hogg GM, Barr JG, Webb CH. In vitro activity of the combination of colistin and rifampicin against multidrug-resistant strains of *Acinetobacter baumannii.* J Antimicrob Chemother 1998; 41:494–495.
138. Tascini C, Menichetti F, Bozza S, et al. Evaluation of the activities of two-drug combinations of rifampicin, polymixin B and ampicillin/sulbactam against *Acinetobacter baumannii.* J Antimicrob Chemother 1998; 42:270–271.
139. Hancock REW, Chapple DS. Peptide antibiotics. Antimicrob Agents Chemother 1999; 43:1317–1323.
140. Giacometti A, Cirioni O, Del Prete MS, et al. Comparative activities of polycationic peptides and clinically used antimicrobial agents against multidrug resistant nosocomial isolates of *Acinetobacter baumannii.* J Antimicrob Chemother 2000; 46:807–810.
141. Levin AS, Gobara S, Caio MF, et al. Environmental contamination by multidrug resistant *Acinetobacter baumannii* in an intensive care unit. Infect Control Hosp Epidemiol 2001; 22:717–720.
142. Roberts SA, Findlay R, Long SDR. Investigation of an outbreak of multidrug resistant *Acinetobacter baumannii* in an intensive care unit. J Hosp Infect 2001; 48:228–232.
143. Debast SB, Meis JF, Melchers WT, Hoogkamp-Korstange JA, Voss A. Use of interrepeat PCR fingerprinting to investigate an *Acinetobacter baumannii* outbreak in an intensive care unit. Scand J Infect Dis 1996; 28:577–581.
144. Das I, Lambert P, Hill D, et al. Carbapenem-resistant *Acinetobacter* and role of curtains in an outbreak in intensive care. J Hosp Infect 2002; 50:110–114.
145. Weernink A, Severin WPJ, Tjernberg I, Dijkshoorn L. Pillows, an unexpected source of *Acinetobacter.* J Hosp Infect 1995; 29:189–199.
146. Neely AN, Maley MP, Warden GD. Computer keyboards as reservoirs for *Acinetobacter baumannii* in a burn hospital. Clin Infect Dis 1999; 29:1358–1360.
147. Beck-Sague C, Jarvis W, Brook J, et al. Epidemic bacteraemia due to *Acinetobacter baumannii* in five intensive care units. Am J Epidemiol 1990; 132:723–733.
148. Cefai C, Richards J, Gould FK, McPeake A. An outbreak of *Acinetobacter* respiratory tract infection resulting from incomplete disinfection of ventilatory equipment. J Hosp Infect 1990; 15:177–182.
149. Hartstein AI, Rashad AL, Liebler JM, et al. Multiple intensive care unit outbreak of *Acinetobacter calcoaceticus* subspecies *anitratus* respiratory infection and colonisation associated with contaminated reusable ventilator circuits and resuscitation bags. Am J Med 1988; 85:624–631.
150. Buxton AE, Anderson RL, Werdegar D, Atlas E. Nosocomial respiratory tract infection and colonisation with *Acinetobacter calcoaceticus*—epidemiologic characteristics. Am J Med 1978; 65:507–513.
151. Jawad A, Seifert H, Snelling AM, Heritage J, Hawkey PM. Survival of *Acinetobacter*

baumannii on dry surfaces: comparison of outbreak and sporadic isolates. J Clin Microbiol 1998; 36:1938–1941.
152. Wendt C, Dietze B, Dietza E, Ruden H. Survival of *Acinetobacter baumannii* on dry surfaces. J Clin Microbiol 1997; 35:1394–1397.
153. Jawad A, Heritage J, Snelling AM, Gascoyne-Binzi DM, Hawkey PM. Influence and relative humidity and suspending menstrua on survival of *Acinetobacter* spp on dry surfaces. J Clin Microbiol 1996; 34:2881–2887.
154. Podnos YD, Cinat ME, Wilson S, et al. Eradication of multi-drug resistant *Acinetobacter* from an intensive care unit. Surg Infect 2001; 2:297–301.
155. Horrevorts A, Bergman K, Kollee L, et al. Clinical and epidemiological investigations of *Acinetobacter* genospecies 3 in a neonatal intensive care unit. J Clin Microbiol 1995; 33:1567–1572.
156. Simor AE, Lee M, Vearncombe M, et al. An outbreak due to multiresistant *Acinetobacter baumannii* in a burn unit: risk factors for acquisition and management. Infect Control Hosp Epidemiol 2002; 23:261–267.
157. Bernards AT, Frenay HM, Lim BT, et al. Methicillin resistant *Staphylococcus aureus* and *Acinetobacter baumannii*: an unexpected difference in epidemiologic behaviour. Am J Infect Control 1998; 26:544–551.
158. Augusti C, Pujol M, Argerich MJ, et al. Short-term effect of application of selective decontamination of the digestive tract on different body site reservoir ICU patients colonised by multi-resistant *Acinetobacter baumannii.* J Antimicrob Chemother 2002; 49:205–208.
159. Taylor ME, Oppenheim BA. Selective decontamination of the gastrointestinal tract as an infection control measure. J Hosp Infect 1991; 17:271–278.
160. Dijkshoorn L, Aucken H, Gerner-Smidt P, et al. Comparison of outbreak and nonoutbreak *Acinetobacter baumannii* strains by genotypic and phenotypic methods. J Clin Microbiol 1996; 34:1519–1525.
161. Kooleman JG, van der Bijl MW, Stoof J, Vandenbroucke-Grauls CM, Savelkoul PH. Antibiotic resistance is a major risk factor for epidemic behaviour of *Acinetobacter baumannii.* Infect Control Hosp Epidemiol 2001; 22:284–288.

8

Drug-Resistant *Helicobacter pylori*

Peter J. Jenks

1. INTRODUCTION

Helicobacter pylori is a Gram-negative, microaerobic, spiral bacterium that colonizes the stomachs of approximately half the world's population *(1)*. Infection with *H. pylori* is associated with chronic gastritis and peptic ulceration, and the bacterium is also considered a risk factor for the development of gastric adenocarcinoma and mucosa-associated lymphoid tissue (MALT) lymphoma *(2–4)*. The recognition of an etiologic link between *H. pylori* and severe gastroduodenal disease has revolutionized the management of these conditions and means that this gastric pathogen is a major public health concern.

Eradication of *H. pylori* from the gastric and duodenal mucosa of infected patients is the most important goal in the management of peptic ulcer disease and other *H. pylori*–associated conditions *(5)*. The survival capabilities of *H. pylori* within the stomach make this difficult, and although the bacterium appears susceptible to many antibiotics in vitro, few are effective in clinical practice. There is evidence that many antibiotics fail to achieve therapeutic concentration at the site of infection, and the organism's slow rate of growth and metabolism, as well as the presence of so-called sanctuary sites *(6)*, contribute to its relative in vivo resistance.

Effective treatment requires multidrug regimens consisting of two antibiotics (usually selected from clarithromycin, metronidazole, amoxicillin, and tetracycline) combined with acid suppressants or bismuth compounds *(7)*. Although several controlled clinical trials have shown that current first-line regimens are effective in most patients, a significant proportion fail therapies in clinical trials, and success rates are frequently as low as 70% in everyday clinical practice *(8)*. Factors that adversely affect the outcome of standard treatments for *H. pylori* infection include advanced age, smoking, high pretreatment intragastric bacterial load, bacterial genotype, and host genetic polymorphisms of the cytochrome P450 isoenzymes specifically involved in the metabolism of proton pump inhibitors (*see* ref. *9* for review). Side effects associated with multi-drug regimens are relatively common, and patient education and compliance-enhancing programs are particularly important for successful eradication of infection *(10)*.

However, as is the case for many other infectious diseases, resistance to the antibiotic component of the regimen is the major cause of treatment failure. Widespread

From: *Management of Multiple Drug-Resistant Infections*
Edited by: S. H. Gillespie © Humana Press Inc., Totowa, NJ

antimicrobial use has resulted in a worldwide increase in the prevalence of antibiotic resistance in *H. pylori (11,12)*, and it is becoming an increasingly important problem in the clinical management of *H. pylori* infection. The threat that resistance poses to current eradication regimens makes it essential to safeguard the already-limited number of treatment options as alternative agents have yet to be developed.

2. EPIDEMIOLOGY OF RESISTANCE

Resistance in *H. pylori* parallels the level of general antibiotic use in a particular region *(13–15)*. Resistance to the 5-nitromidazoles is common, affecting 10 to 50% of clinical strains isolated in developed countries and virtually all strains from developing countries *(13)*. Metronidazole is commonly used to treat anaerobic and parasitic infections, and metronidazole resistance in *H. pylori* is associated with prior use of this antibiotic in certain patient groups *(16–20)*. Although there has been some debate as to the clinical impact of metronidazole resistance, meta-analyses have established beyond doubt that resistance to the 5-nitroimidazole component of the regimen is an important predictor of treatment failure, reducing the chance of success by approx 20% *(21–23)*.

The prevalence of clarithromycin resistance ranges from 0 to 20% and reflects the use of macrolides, particularly to treat respiratory tract infections *(13)*. In the majority of cases, clarithromycin-resistant strains emerge after spontaneous mutation of the 23S ribosomal RNA (rRNA) gene after exposure to the drug *(24–27)*. When clarithromycin-based triple therapy is given to a patient harboring a resistant strain, eradication rates fall by more than 50% *(21–23)*.

Until recently, it was generally accepted that tetracycline resistance was rare in *H. pylori*, with rates less than 2% *(28,29)*. However, in certain areas where there has been an increase in tetracycline use, resistant isolates are emerging at a rate of 5 to 7% of isolates *(30–34)*. The first reported amoxicillin-resistant strains were isolated from dyspeptic patients in Italy and the United States *(35)*, and although resistance was lost in vitro, it was associated with a marked reduction in treatment efficacy *(36)*. Subsequent reports described the isolation of both stable and unstable amoxicillin-resistant isolates *(37,38)*. Although high resistance rates have been reported in certain countries *(33)*, this may reflect variations in susceptibility testing; the overall prevalence of amoxicillin resistance remains low.

In general, increased use and exposure to antibiotics has resulted in a significant rise in both the prevalence of resistance and in strains exhibiting resistance to multiple antibiotics *(11,12,28,32,39)*.

3. MECHANISMS OF RESISTANCE

Although bacterial resistance genes are frequently carried on extrachromosomal elements such as plasmids or transposons, all resistance mechanisms so far described in *H. pylori* have been chromosomally mediated. In addition, although many strains of *H. pylori* are competent for natural transformation *(40)* and there is evidence for frequent recombination *(41)*, the transfer of genetic material appears to play a relatively minor role in the acquisition of resistance, with the majority arising because of *de novo* mutation. An initial analysis of membrane-associated efflux systems suggested that active efflux does not play a role in the intrinsic resistance of *H. pylori* to a number of antibiotics, including metronidazole and the macrolides *(42)*.

3.1. Nitroimidazole Resistance

Once they have entered the cell by diffusion, the antimicrobial toxicity of the 5-nitromidazoles is dependent on reduction of its nitro moiety to the nitro anion radical and other compounds, including nitroso and hydroxylamine derivatives *(43)*. These reduction products are damaging to macromolecules and have been shown to cause DNA degradation and strand breakage *(43,44)*.

Early biochemical studies demonstrated that the pyruvate oxidoreductase enzyme of *H. pylori* was able to reduce metronidazole via flavodoxin *(45,46)*. However, insertional inactivation of pyruvate oxidoreductase is lethal, implying that the bacterium is unable to use compensatory metabolic pathways *(47)*. This suggests that the ability to downregulate synthesis of pyruvate oxidoreductase in response to metronidazole could contribute resistance, but is unlikely to result in complete protection from this antibiotic.

In 1998, Goodwin and coworkers reported that oxygen-insensitive nicotinamide adenine dinucleotide phosphate (NADPH) nitroreductase activity was associated with susceptibility to metronidazole in *H. pylori (48)*. It was proposed that this enzyme reduces the nitro group of metronidazole through sequential two-electron reductions to active metabolites, and that resistance arose from mutational inactivation of the underlying gene, *rdx*A *(48)*. Several groups have since shown that resistance is associated with many different alterations of the *rdx*A gene, including missense and frameshift mutations and deletions and insertion of transposable elements *(48–54)*.

Although the majority of metronidazole resistance arises by *de novo* mutation of the *rdx*A gene *(48)*, interspecies transfer of a mutant *rdx*A allele has been demonstrated *(55)*. It has been demonstrated that inactivation of other reductase-encoding genes, including *frx*A (which encodes NADPH flavin oxidoreductase [FrxA]) and *fdx*B (which encodes ferredoxinlike protein), is also associated with resistance to metronidazole *(56–60)*. However, the fact that the majority of strains tested on a worldwide basis contain inactivating mutations within *rdx*A suggests a pivotal role for this gene in determining susceptibility to metronidazole in *H. pylori*, and that these other mechanisms are relatively unimportant or are involved in the transition to high-level resistance once inactivation of the *rdx*A gene has occurred *(59,60)*. The report by one group that resistance may arise after inactivation of *frx*A alone might challenge current thinking on this subject *(57,58)*, but more work on these isolates has cast doubt on the validity of this finding *(61)*.

It is possible that other mechanisms of metronidazole resistance remain to be discovered in *H. pylori*, and these most likely involve additional nitroreductases or other enzymes that maintain an intracellular redox potential sufficiently low to activate metronidazole-reducing pathways *(45–47,62–65)*. Mutations affecting DNA repair systems *(66,67)* and activity of the antioxidant defense enzyme alkyl hydroperoxide reductase *(68,69)* also appear to contribute to the resistant phenotype. Interstrain differences in the activity of nitroreductases and ability to neutralize toxic metronidazole metabolites and repair DNA damage are likely to account for the wide variations in the baseline susceptibility of individual *H. pylori* strains to metronidazole.

Based on their in vitro activity, the nitrofuran group of compounds, which includes nitrofurantoin and furazolidone, appears a particularly promising source of alternative agents for metronidazole in *H. pylori* eradication regimens *(70–72)*. Despite this, nitrofurantoin-containing therapy failed to eradicate *H. pylori* infection from mice *(73)* and performed inadequately in clinical practice, particularly in the presence of metronidazole resistance *(74)*. In contrast, a number of recent clinical trials have demonstrated that furazolidone-containing short-term triple therapies are effective in the treatment of *H. pylori* infection *(70,71,75,76)*. Like the 5-nitroimidazoles, the biological activity of these nitroaromatic compounds is largely derived from reductive metabolism of the nitro moiety of the parent compound; in *H. pylori* this is predominantly performed by FrxA and to a lesser extent pyruvate oxidoreductase *(77)*.

Although nitrofuran resistance has been described *(78,79)*, it is difficult to assess the significance of these reports because the breakpoint for resistance in an organism like *H. pylori* is difficult to define. Inactivation of *rdx*A, *frx*A, and *fdx*B genes does not alter the susceptibility of *H. pylori* to the nitrofurans *(73,77,79)*, and further analysis of these "resistant" strains has failed to identify a definitive resistance mechanism.

3.2. Macrolide Resistance

Macrolide activity is mediated by ribosomal binding, which leads to an interruption in protein elongation. The major cause of macrolide resistance in *H. pylori* is lack of binding to the 23S subunit of the bacterial ribosome because of point mutations in the peptidyltransferase-encoding region of domain V of 23S rRNA *(80–82)*. The mutation is usually an A-to-G transition mutation at position 2142 or 2143, but in a few cases, it may be an A-to-C transversion mutation at position 2142 *(81)*. Two additional mutations, A2115G and G2141A, also have been described in the same strain *(83)*, but neither has been reported subsequently. *H. pylori* contains two copies of 23S rRNA gene; for most strains of *H. pylori*, mutation occurs in both 23S rRNA copies *(82)*.

The A2142G mutations are usually associated with higher resistance levels (minimum inhibitory concentration [MIC] $\geq$ 64 µg/mL) than those of the A2143G type (MIC $\leq$ 32 µg/mL) *(84,85)*. Changes in nucleotide sequence are thought to induce a change in free energy and conformation within the ribosome that is least for the A2142G and A2143G substitutions. These A-to-G mutants have a competitive growth advantage, and other mutations are probably less common or not found at all because they have a greater effect on fitness or are lethal *(86)*.

3.3. β-Lactam Resistance

Amoxicillin acts by disrupting synthesis of the bacterial cell wall, and resistance in other bacterial species occurs because of β-lactamase production or structural alterations in one of the penicillin-binding proteins (PBPs) or other proteins involved in cell wall synthesis. Examination of the genome sequences of *H. pylori* failed to reveal any β-lactamase homologues *(87,88)*, and although a *H. pylori*–specific β-lactamase has since been described *(89)*, the resistant phenotype is not dependent on expression of this enzyme *(36–38,90,91)*.

A number of PBPs have been described in *H. pylori (90,92–94)*, and amoxicillin binds almost exclusively to the 72-kDa PBP 1A *(93)*. Further evidence that this PBP might be involved in resistance was provided when reduced labeling of PBP 1 by biotinylated amoxicillin was demonstrated in an amoxicillin-resistant strain generated in vitro *(91)*. Molecular studies have since confirmed that stable amoxicillin resistance results from point mutations within the PBP 1A gene *(91,95,96)*. Nonstable amoxicillin resistance is probably the result of decreased expression of PBP 4 *(90)*.

3.4. Tetracycline Resistance

Tetracycline inhibits protein synthesis by binding to the 30S ribosomal subunit and blocking the fixation of the aminoacyl-transfer RNA to the acceptor site on the messenger RNA–ribosome complex. In other bacteria, resistance is commonly because of an energy-dependent efflux across the cell membrane or proteins that confer ribosomal protection by reducing ribosomal affinity for tetracycline or by competing for ribosomal binding. Other mechanisms include enzymatic inactivation of tetracycline and mutations in the 16S rRNA genes that affect the binding of tetracycline. The few tetracycline-resistant *H. pylori* strains that have been studied contain the $AGA_{926–928}{\rightarrow}TTC$ mutation within the 16S rRNA gene that affects h31 of the primary binding site and is likely to alter the affinity of the ribosome for the antibiotic *(97)*.

3.5. Fluoroquinolone Resistance

Fluoroquinolones are not commonly used in *H. pylori* eradication regimens because they are associated with low eradication rates and the emergence of secondary resistance *(98)*. Fluoroquinolone resistance in *H. pylori*, which is rising with increased general use *(29,30)*, is associated with mutations in *gyr*A, which encodes the A subunit of DNA gyrase *(99)*.

3.6. Rifamycin Resistance

Rifabutin-containing regimens have been effective in clinical practice *(100)*, although they should probably be restricted for use against multiresistant strains. Resistance is rare and results from mutation within the β-subunit of the DNA-dependent RNA polymerase encoded by the *rpo*B gene *(101–103)*.

4. METHODS OF SUSCEPTIBILITY TESTING

Laboratory antimicrobial susceptibility testing of strains from individual patients is designed to predict responses to therapy and influence the clinician's choice of antibiotics. Comparison of prevalence of resistant strains is frequently made to monitor the spread of resistant bacteria, both nationally and internationally, and detect changes from the normal pattern of susceptibility.

Agar dilution is generally regarded as the gold standard method of susceptibility testing for *H. pylori (104,105)* and is highly reproducible, but laborious and time consuming *(106,107)*. The epsilometer (Etest®; AB Biodisk, Solna, Sweden) is frequently used because, although it is expensive, it is easier to perform and has good reproducibility *(107,108)*. Although disk diffusion is generally not recommended for bacterial species that need long incubation periods because of the pattern of antibiotic release from the disk, this method is cheap and easy to perform and has been reliable in *H. pylori* when test methods are well controlled *(107,109–111)*. Both the Etest and disk testing have the advantage that they allow visualization of resistant subpopulations within the zone of inhibition.

Until recently, methods of susceptibility testing of *H. pylori* suffered from a lack of consistency of base medium, inoculum, and incubation, all of which influence the outcome of testing *(112,113)*; conflicting results were frequently found when different techniques were compared *(107,109,110,113–116)*. Although a certain lack of consistency might be expected for a slow-growing organism that requires specific growth conditions, there is also evidence that susceptibility testing could be performed with high accuracy and relate to treatment efficacy *(114,117,118)*. When performed appropriately, there is good correlation with all methods for the testing of clarithromycin, tetracycline, and amoxicillin, and disk testing would appear an adequate choice for these agents.

Testing for metronidazole susceptibility is more difficult because the distribution of MICs is continuous, resistant subpopulations are frequently present, and results are more easily affected by test conditions. Although the Etest is usually recommended, even this method may overestimate resistance *(107,119,120)*, and more than one testing method may be appropriate, particularly for strains close to the breakpoint.

In an attempt to improve agreement in reporting and encourage centers to reassess the importance of routine susceptibility testing, there has been a recent trend toward standardization of testing *(104,121,122)*. These methods are relatively straightforward and should mean that culture and susceptibility testing of *H. pylori* can now be performed in most hospital laboratories. Refinement of protocols and participation in quality control schemes will improve reproducibility of testing and will allow national and international surveillance of antibiotic resistance, both to monitor the prevalence of resistant strains and to guide empirical treatment based on local resistance patterns.

4.1. Interpretation of Results

Currently, the interpretation of susceptibility data is confusing because in vitro susceptibility does not necessarily correlate with in vivo efficacy, and a clear consensus regarding what defines resistance is needed before accurate prediction of individual responses to therapy is possible. Although the presence of resistance to clarithromycin is highly predictive of treatment failure, the relationship between susceptibility determined in vitro and clinical outcome for other antibiotics is less clear. In particular, methods for assessing resistance to metronidazole and amoxicillin are frequently not predictive of clinical outcome. This is largely because current breakpoints have been adopted from similar, but not identical, organisms; whether these levels correlate with those required to eradicate infection from the gastric mucosa have not been defined by clinical trials. This is particularly true in the case of metronidazole, for which in vivo susceptibility is likely influenced by variations in gastric pit microenvironmental conditions (such as oxygen tension and redox potential), which are known to influence the activity of metronidazole-reducing enzymes *(123)*.

Residual nitroreductase activity may in part explain why strains that appear resistant on in vitro susceptibility testing can be eradicated by nitroimidazole-containing regimens, although the antimicrobial activity of the other components of these regimens and duration of therapy are probably the most important determinants of treatment outcome in this situation *(123)*. Testing standardization and reproducible susceptibility testing are important preliminary steps toward the establishment of interpretative criteria based on trials in which the in vitro susceptibility of a large population of isolates is correlated with the pharmacokinetic profile of the drug and, most importantly, the clinical efficacy of a regimen.

5. MOLECULAR METHODS OF SUSCEPTIBILITY TESTING

A rapid and useful alternative to conventional susceptibility testing is to use molecular methods to detect resistance markers in bacteria or directly in gastric biopsy specimens, and several genotype-based methods have been developed to identify the limited number of point mutations that cause macrolide resistance in *H. pylori*. These mutations were initially detected using polymerase chain reaction (PCR) and sequencing *(81,82)* or PCR and restriction fragment length polymorphism analysis *(80,81,85, 124,125)*.

Rapid detection can now be achieved using mutant-specific oligonucleotide probe–based assays such as a PCR–oligonucleotide ligation assay *(84)*, PCR–line probe assay *(26,126)* and DNA enzyme-linked immunoassay (DEIA) *(127)*. The introduction of LightCycler technology has led to the development of real-time PCR-based methods to detect mutations associated with resistance *(128,129)*. Both real-time PCR and DEIA have been modified for use directly on gastric biopsy samples, permitting resistance testing without the need for culture *(25,130)*.

Other methods used to detect clarithromycin-resistant mutants include 3'-mismatch primers *(131)*, preferential homoduplex formation *(24)*, and an rRNA-based whole-cell *in situ* hybridization using a set of fluorescently labeled oligonucleotide probes *(132)*. This last approach allows the simultaneous detection of *H. pylori* with a 16S rRNA probe and resistant mutant with a 23S rRNA probe *(132)*.

Because resistance to metronidazole is associated with multiple changes within *rdx*A and possibly other reductase-encoding genes, it has not been possible to develop simple genotype-based assays capable of detecting nitroimidazole resistance. Despite this, preliminary results indicate that testing for the absence of the RdxA protein would identify the majority of metronidazole-resistant clinical isolates and may be useful for predicting which strains will respond poorly to metronidazole-containing eradication regimens *(133,134)*. One major advantage of using this approach is that it would identify all resistant strains that carry mutations affecting expression of the *rdx*A gene, including those that have not yet been identified by nucleotide sequence analysis.

Further advances in the understanding of the underlying mechanisms of metronidazole resistance in *H. pylori* will have important implications for the development of assays capable of detecting metronidazole resistance in *H. pylori*. Likewise, further examination of the mutations associated with tetracycline and amoxicillin resistance may make it possible to develop molecular screening tests for resistance to these antimicrobial agents.

Although the availability of tests for other antibiotics would strengthen the case for more routine use of molecular tests, it is currently unclear how readily these tests will be accommodated into the routine diagnostic microbiology laboratory, particularly given the rigorous quality indicators to satisfy accreditation requirements *(135)*. Nonetheless, molecular-based assays for resistance detection offer an attractive alternative to obtain susceptibilities to antibiotics with greater accuracy and speed, as well as the possibility of a same-day result *(135)*.

6. RESISTANCE TO SUSCEPTIBILITY TESTING

Although basing therapy on pretreatment laboratory susceptibility data may significantly improve the eradication rate *(136)*, cost implications and the convenience of non-culture-based diagnostic tests mean that laboratory susceptibility testing is rarely performed before empirical therapy commences. Indeed, international consensus statements advocate the empirical management of *H. pylori* infection in primary care

(7,137), and in many centers, such testing is only deemed practical and cost-effective for patients who have repeatedly failed treatment. Consequently, selection of the most appropriate first-line eradication therapy is critical for preventing primary failure and the subsequent emergence of resistant strains as a result of suboptimal therapy *(138)*. Although it is recommended that this choice is based on local susceptibility patterns, which vary geographically and within specific treatment groups, remarkably few countries have regional surveillance programs. A recent survey in the United Kingdom revealed that only 7 of 49 Public Health Laboratory Service (PHLS) laboratories undertook routine culture and susceptibility testing of *H. pylori (122)*, confirming that few laboratories are equipped or experienced to provide such a service. As discussed in the section on methods of susceptibility testing, this is likely to reflect the methodological problems of testing an organism that is slow growing and requires specific growth conditions and reflect the difficulty of interpreting susceptibility data that do not necessarily correlate with in vivo efficacy. However, the increase in resistance emphasizes the need for community surveillance of *H. pylori* that would allow timely adaptation of treatment regimens to changes in resistance patterns.

Although the success rates of current first-line treatments are far from ideal, ultimate eradication rates of 95 and 99% can be achieved after appropriately chosen second and third courses of therapy without recourse to susceptibility testing *(139)*. Consequently, many clinicians argue that sensitivity testing is unlikely to improve the results of logically chosen, but empirical, treatments without a prohibitive increase in costs. The use of repeated "blind" courses of antibiotics seems particularly difficult to justify at a time when bacterial drug resistance is recognized as a global problem and strategies to combat its spread advocate antibiotic use based on microbiological results *(140–143)*.

In *H. pylori* infection, antibiotic therapy based on the results of culture and susceptibility testing has been shown to give a significant improvement in eradication rate *(136)*. Furthermore, the antimicrobial components of *H. pylori* eradication regimens cause marked ecological disturbances in the oral, gastric, and intestinal microflora that lead to decreased colonization resistance and overgrowth of potentially pathogenic and drug-resistant organisms *(144,145)*. In addition, there is overwhelming evidence that resistance in *H. pylori* emerges as a result of suboptimal therapy and hence is driven by inappropriate and, often, repeated treatment *(19,138,146)*. Routine pretreatment susceptibility testing would therefore not only provide a far more rational approach to the use of antibiotics, but would be predicted to reduce the emergence of resistant strains associated with treatment failure and extend the useful life of these agents for the treatment not only of *H. pylori* infections, but also other infections as well *(146)*.

Although at present susceptibility testing is not a prerequisite for successful eradication of *H. pylori* from individual patients, this will change as more and more people are treated for *H. pylori* infection and the proportion of patients colonized with resistant strains continues to rise. This change in the epidemiology of *H. pylori* infection will eventually mean that the savings that can be made by avoiding patient follow-up and repeat treatment costs will outweigh the expense of acquiring specimens by endoscopy *(147)*. In certain regions, it may soon become cost-effective to obtain pretreatment antibiotic susceptibility testing, especially if minimally invasive and less-expensive procedures to obtain specimens reliably for culture become widely available *(148–*

150). Reproducible laboratory methods for ascertaining resistance and the establishment of clinically relevant interpretative guidelines will be increasingly important in allowing a more rational approach to the use of currently available drug regimens.

7. CONCLUSIONS

A worldwide increase in the prevalence of antibiotic resistance in *H. pylori* combined with the expense of currently used antimicrobial regimens means that there is a need to evaluate alternative antibiotics for combination therapy of *H. pylori* infections. An indication of the scale of the problem is given by the fact that a number of "old" antibiotics, as well as various bioactive compounds from natural sources *(151–153)*, have been assessed for bactericidal activity against *H. pylori*. Although a number of alternatives to antibiotic-based therapies are currently being assessed, including mucoprotective agents, antiadhesive oligosaccharides, cationic peptides, and probiotics, there is little evidence to suggest that any of these compounds have outstanding therapeutic potential.

Continuing investigation of the molecular pathogenesis of *H. pylori* and particularly analysis of two complete genome sequences *(87,88)* will continue to identify potential targets for antimicrobial development. Similarly, genome-based techniques will allow the identification of candidates with potential for vaccine development. However, although such approaches may ultimately lead to new prophylactic and therapeutic options, these agents remain some distance from clinical practice. In the meantime, it would appear prudent to take appropriate steps to optimize the use, and hence prolong the effectiveness, of currently available regimens. The widespread adoption of pretreatment susceptibility testing would represent an important step forward in this process.

ACKNOWLEDGMENTS

Peter J. Jenks is supported by an Advanced Fellowship for Medical, Dental, and Veterinary Graduates from the Wellcome Trust, United Kingdom (061599).

REFERENCES

1. Warren JR. Unidentified curved bacilli on gastric epithelium in chronic active gastritis. Lancet 1983; 1:1273.
2. Blaser MJ. *Helicobacter pylori*: microbiology of a "slow" bacterial infection. Trends Microbiol 1993; 1:255–260.
3. Parsonnet J, Friedman GD, Vandersteed DP, et al. *Helicobacter pylori* infection and the risk of gastric cancer. N Engl J Med 1991; 325:1127–1129.
4. Parsonnet J, Hansen S, Rodriguez L, et al. *Helicobacter pylori* infection and gastric lymphoma. N Engl J Med 1994; 330:1267–1271.
5. Hunt RH, Smaill FM, Fallone CA, Sherman PM, Veldhuyzen van Zanten SJ, Thomson AB. Implications of antibiotic resistance in the management of *Helicobacter pylori* infection: Canadian Helicobacter Study Group. Can J Gastroenterol 2000; 14:862–868.
6. Atherton JC, Cockayne A, Balsitis M, Kirk GE, Hawkey CJ, Spiller RC. Detection of the intragastric sites at which *Helicobacter pylori* evades treatment with amoxycillin and cimetidine. Gut 1995; 36:670–674.
7. Malfertheiner P, Megraud F, O'Morain C, et al. Current concepts in the management of *Helicobacter pylori* infection—the Maastricht 2-2000 consensus report. Aliment Pharmacol Ther 2002; 16:167–180.

8. Qasim A, O'Morain CA. Treatment of *Helicobacter pylori* infection and factors influencing eradication. Aliment Pharmacol Ther 2002; 16(suppl. 1):24–30.
9. Jenks PJ. Causes of failure of eradication of *Helicobacter pylori*. BMJ 2002; 325:3–4.
10. Lee M, Kemp JA, Canning A, Enag C, Tataronis G, Farraye FA. A randomized controlled trial of an enhanced patient compliance program for *Helicobacter pylori* therapy. Arch Intern Med 1999; 159:2312–2316.
11. van der Wouden EJ, van Zwet AA, Vosmaer GD, Oom JA, de Jong A, Kleibeuker JH. Rapid increase in the prevalence of metronidazole-resistant *Helicobacter pylori* in the Netherlands. Emerg Infect Dis 1997; 3:385–389.
12. Lopez-Brea M, Domingo D, Sanchez I, Alarcon T. Evolution of resistance to metronidazole and clarithromycin in *Helicobacter pylori* clinical isolates from Spain. J Antimicrob Chemother 1997; 40:279–281.
13. Mégraud F. Epidemiology and mechanism of antibiotic resistance in *Helicobacter pylori*. Gastroenterology 1998; 115:1278–1282.
14. Palmer DL. Epidemiology of antibiotic resistance. J Med 1980; 11:255–262.
15. Mégraud F. Antibiotic resistance in *Helicobacter pylori* infection. Br Med Bull 1998; 54:207–216.
16. Banatvala N, Davies GR, Abdi Y, et al. High prevalence of *Helicobacter pylori* metronidazole resistance in migrants to east London: relationship with previous nitroimidazole exposure and gastrointestinal disease. Gut 1994; 35:1562–1566.
17. Becx MC, Janssen AJ, Clasener HA, de Koning RW. Metronidazole-resistant *Helicobacter pylori*. Lancet 1990; 335:539–540.
18. Glupczynski Y, Burette A, Koster ED, et al. Metronidazole resistance in *Helicobacter pylori*. Lancet 1990; 335:976–977.
19. Jenks PJ, Labigne A, Ferrero RL. Exposure to metronidazole in vivo readily induces resistance in *Helicobacter pylori* and reduces the efficacy of eradication therapy in mice. Antimicrob Agents Chemother 1999; 43:777–781.
20. Rautelin H, Seppala K, Renkonen OV, Vainio U, Kosunen TU. Role of metronidazole in therapy of *Helicobacter pylori* infections. Antimicrob Agents Chemother 1992; 36:163–166.
21. van der Wouden EJ, Thijs JC, van Zwet AA, Sluiter WJ, Kleibeuker JH. The influence of in vitro nitroimidazole resistance on the efficacy of nitroimidazole containing anti-*Helicobacter pylori* regimens: a meta-analysis. Am J Gastroenterol 1999; 94:1751–1759.
22. Houben MH, Van De Beek D, Hensen EF, Craen AJ, Rauws EA, Tytgat GN. A systematic review of *Helicobacter pylori* eradication therapy—the impact of antimicrobial resistance on eradication rates. Aliment Pharmacol Ther 1999; 13:1047–1055.
23. Dore MP, Leandro G, Realdi G, Sepulveda AR, Graham DY. Effect of pretreatment antibiotic resistance to metronidazole and clarithromycin on outcome of *Helicobacter pylori* therapy: a meta-analytical approach. Dig Dis Sci 2000; 45:68–76.
24. Maeda S, Yoshida H, Matsunaga H, et al. Detection of clarithromycin-resistant *Helicobacter pylori* strains by a preferential homoduplex formation assay. J Clin Microbiol 2000; 38:210–214.
25. Marais A, Monteiro L, Occhialini A, Pina M, Lamouliatte H, Mégraud F. Direct detection of *Helicobacter pylori* resistance to macrolides by a polymerase chain reaction/DNA enzyme immunoassay in gastric biopsy specimens. Gut 1999; 44:463–467.
26. van Doorn LJ, Debets-Ossenkopp YJ, Marais A, et al. Rapid detection, by PCR and reverse hybridization, of mutations in the *Helicobacter pylori* 23S rRNA gene, associated with macrolide resistance. Antimicrob Agents Chemother 1999; 43:1779–1782.
27. Matsuoka M, Yoshida Y, Hayakawa K, Fukuchi S, Sugona K. Simultaneous colonisation of *Helicobacter pylori* with and without mutations in the 23S rRNA gene in patients with no history of clarithromycin exposure. Gut 1999; 45:503–507.
28. Midolo PD, Korman MG, Turnidge JD, Lambert JR. *Helicobacter pylori* resistance to tetracycline. Lancet 1996; 347:1194–1195.

29. Debets-Ossenkopp YJ, Herscheid AJ, Pot RG, Kuipers EJ, Kusters JG, Vandenbroucke-Grauls CM. Prevalence of *Helicobacter pylori* resistance to metronidazole, clarithromycin, amoxycillin, tetracycline and trovafloxacin in The Netherlands. J Antimicrob Chemother 1999; 43:511–515.
30. Boyanova L, Stancheva I, Spassova Z, Katzarov N, Mitov I, Koumanova R. Primary and combined resistance to four antimicrobial agents in *Helicobacter pylori* in Sofia, Bulgaria. J Med Microbiol 2000; 49:415–418.
31. Kim JJ, Reddy R, Lee M, et al. Analysis of metronidazole, clarithromycin and tetracycline resistance of *Helicobacter pylori* isolates from Korea. J Antimicrob Chemother 2001; 47:459–461.
32. Kwon DH, Kim JJ, Lee M, et al. Isolation and characterization of tetracycline-resistant clinical isolates of *Helicobacter pylori*. Antimicrob Agents Chemother 2000; 44:3203–3205.
33. Realdi G, Dore MP, Piana A, et al. Pretreatment antibiotic resistance in *Helicobacter pylori* infection: results of three randomized controlled studies. Helicobacter 1999; 4: 106–112.
34. Wu H, Shi XD, Wang HT, Liu JX. Resistance of *Helicobacter pylori* to metronidazole, tetracycline and amoxycillin. J Antimicrob Chemother 2000; 46:121–123.
35. Dore MP, Piana A, Carta M, et al. Amoxycillin resistance is one reason for failure of amoxycillin-omeprazole treatment of *Helicobacter pylori* infection. Aliment Pharmacol Ther 1998; 12:635–639.
36. Dore MP, Osato MS, Realdi G, Mura I, Graham DY, Sepulveda AR. Amoxycillin tolerance in *Helicobacter pylori*. J Antimicrob Chemother 1999; 43:47–54.
37. van Zwet AA, Vandenbrouke-Grauls CM, Thijs JC, van der Wouden EJ, Gerrits MM, Kusters JG. Stable amoxycillin resistance in *Helicobacter pylori*. Lancet 1998; 352:1595.
38. Han SR, Bhakdi S, Maeurer MJ, Schneider T, Gehring S. Stable and unstable amoxicillin resistance in *Helicobacter pylori*: should antibiotic resistance testing be performed prior to eradication therapy? J Clin Microbiol 1999; 37:2740–2741.
39. Heep M, Kist M, Strobel S, Beck D, Lehn N. Secondary resistance among 554 isolates of *Helicobacter pylori* after failure of therapy. Eur J Clin Microbiol Infect Dis 2000; 19: 538–541.
40. Nedenskov-Sorensen P, Bukholm G, Bovre K. Natural competence for genetic transformation in *Campylobacter pylori*. J Infect Dis 1990; 161:365–366.
41. Achtman M, Azuma T, Berg DE, et al. Recombination and clonal groupings within *Helicobacter pylori* from different geographical regions. Mol Microbiol 1999; 32:459–470.
42. Bina JE, Alm RA, Uria-Nickelsen M, Thomas SR, Trust TJ, Hancock RE. *Helicobacter pylori* uptake and efflux: basis for intrinsic susceptibility to antibiotics in vitro. Antimicrob Agents Chemother 2000; 44:248–254.
43. Edwards DI. Nitroimidazole drugs—action and resistance mechanisms. I. Mechanisms of action. J Antimicrob Chemother 1993; 31:9–20.
44. Sisson G, Jeong JY, Goodwin A, et al. Metronidazole activation is mutagenic and causes DNA fragmentation in *Helicobacter pylori* and in *Escherichia coli* containing a cloned *H. pylori rdx*A+ (nitroreductase) gene. J Bacteriol 2000; 182:5091–5096.
45. Hughes NJ, Chalk PA, Clayton CL, Kelly DJ. Identification of carboxylation enzymes and characterization of a novel four-subunit pyruvate:flavodoxin oxidoreductase from *Helicobacter pylori*. J Bacteriol 1995; 177:3953–3959.
46. Kaihovaara P, Höök-Nikanne J, Uusi-Oukari M, Kosunen TU, Salaspuro M. Flavodoxin-dependent pyruvate oxidation, acetate production and metronidazole reduction by *Helicobacter pylori*. J Antimicrob Chemother 1998; 41:171–177.
47. Hughes NJ, Clayton CL, Chalk PA, Kelly DJ. *Helicobacter pylori por*CDAB and *oor*DABC genes encode distinct pyruvate:flavodoxin and 2-oxoglutarate:acceptor oxidoreductases which mediate electron transport to NADP. J Bacteriol 1998; 180:1119–1128.

48. Goodwin A, Kersulyte D, Sisson G, Veldhuyzen van Zanten SJ, Berg DE, Hoffman PS. Metronidazole resistance in *Helicobacter pylori* is due to null mutations in a gene (*rdx*A) that encodes an oxygen-insensitive NADPH nitroreductase. Mol Microbiol 1998; 28:383–393.
49. Tankovic J, Lamarque D, Delchier JC, Soussy CJ, Labigne A, Jenks PJ. Frequent association between alteration of the *rdx*A gene and metronidazole resistance in French and North African isolates of *Helicobacter pylori*. Antimicrob Agents Chemother 2000; 44:608–613.
50. Debets-Ossenkopp YJ, Pot RG, van Westerloo DJ, et al. Insertion of mini-IS605 and deletion of adjacent sequences in the nitroreductase (*rdx*A) gene cause metronidazole resistance in *Helicobacter pylori* NCTC11637. Antimicrob Agents Chemother 1999; 43: 2657–2662.
51. Jenks PJ, Ferrero RL, Labigne A. The role of the *rdx*A gene in the evolution of metronidazole resistance in *Helicobacter pylori*. J Antimicrob Chemother 1999; 43:753–758.
52. Kwon DH, Pena JA, Osato MS, Fox JG, Graham DY, Verslovic J. Frameshift mutations in *rdx*A and metronidazole resistance in North American *Helicobacter pylori* isolates. J Antimicrob Chemother 2000; 46:793–796.
53. Solcà NM, Bernasconi MV, Piffaretti JC. Mechanism of metronidazole resistance in *Helicobacter pylori*: comparison of the *rdx*A gene sequences in 30 strains. Antimicrob Agents Chemother 2000; 44:2207–2210.
54. Wang G, Wilson TJ, Jiang Q, Taylor DE. Spontaneous mutations that confer antibiotic resistance in *Helicobacter pylori*. Antimicrob Agents Chemother 2001; 45:727–733.
55. Pot RG, Kusters JG, Smeets LC, VanTongeren W, Vandenbroucke-Grauls CM, Bart A. Interspecies transfer of antibiotic resistance between *Helicobacter pylori* and *Helicobacter acinonychis*. Antimicrob Agents Chemother 2001; 45:2975–2976.
56. Bilardi C, Marais A, Cantet F, Birac C, Mégraud F. Characterization of the *rdx*A and *frx*A genes in metronidazole resistant *Helicobacter pylori* strains. Gut 2000; 47(suppl. 1):A2.
57. Kwon DH, El-Zaatari FA, Kato M, et al. Analysis of *rdx*A and involvement of additional genes encoding NAD(P)H flavin oxidoreductase (FrxA) and ferredoxin-like protein (FdxB) in metronidazole resistance of *Helicobacter pylori*. Antimicrob Agents Chemother 2000; 44:2133–2142.
58. Kwon DH, Kato M, El-Zaatari FA, Osato MS, Graham DY. Frame-shift mutations in NAD(P)H flavin oxidoreductase encoding gene (*frx*A) from metronidazole resistant *Helicobacter pylori* ATCC43504 and its involvement in metronidazole resistance. FEMS Microbiol Lett 2000; 188:197–202.
59. Jeong JY, Mukhopadhyay AK, Dailidiene D, et al. Sequential inactivation of *rdx*A (HP0954) and *frx*A (HP0642) nitroreductase genes causes moderate and high-level metronidazole resistance in *Helicobacter pylori*. J Bacteriol 2000; 182:5082–5090.
60. Jeong JY, Berg DE. Mouse-colonizing *Helicobacter pylori* SS1 is unusually susceptible to metronidazole due to two complementary reductase activities. Antimicrob Agents Chemother 2000; 44:3127–3132.
61. Jeong JY, Mukhopadhyay AK, Akada JK, Dailidiene D, Hoffman PS, Berg DE. Roles of FrxA and RdxA nitroreductases of *Helicobacter pylori* in susceptibility and resistance to metronidazole. J Bacteriol 2001; 183:5155–5162.
62. Hoffman PS, Goodwin A, Johnsen J, Magee K, Veldhuyzen van Zanten SJ. Metabolic activities of metronidazole-sensitive and -resistant strains of *Helicobacter pylori*: repression of pyruvate oxidoreductase and expression of isocitrate lyase activity correlate with resistance. J Bacteriol 1996; 178:4822–4829.
63. Mendz GL, Trend MA. Intracellular redox status and antibiotic resistance in enterogastric microaerophilic bacteria: evidence for the "scavenging of oxygen" hypothesis. Redox Rep 2001; 6:179–181.
64. Jorgensen MA, Trend MA, Hazell SL, Mendz GL. Potential involvement of several nitroreductases in metronidazole resistance in *Helicobacter pylori*. Arch Biochem Biophys 2001; 392:180–191.

65. Mendz GL, Mégraud F. Is the molecular basis of metronidazole resistance in microaerophilic organisms understood? Trends Microbiol 2002; 10:370–375.
66. Chang KC, Ho SW, Yang JC, Wang JT. Isolation of a genetic locus associated with metronidazole resistance in *Helicobacter pylori*. Biochem Biophys Res Commun 1997; 236:785–788.
67. Thompson SA, Blaser MJ. Isolation of the *Helicobacter pylori recA* gene and involvement of the *recA* region in resistance to low pH. Infect Immun 1995; 63:2185–2193.
68. Trend MA, Jorgensen MA, Hazell SL, Mendz GL. Oxidases and reductases are involved in metronidazole sensitivity in *Helicobacter pylori*. Int J Biochem Cell Biol 2001; 33: 143–153.
69. McAtee CP, Hoffman PS, Berg DE. Identification of differentially regulated proteins in metronidazole resistant *Helicobacter pylori* by proteome techniques. Proteomics 2001; 1:516–521.
70. Segura AM, Gutierrez O, Otero W, Angel A, Genta RM, Graham DY. Furazolidone, amoxycillin, bismuth triple therapy for *Helicobacter pylori* infection. Aliment Pharmacol Ther 1997; 11:529–532.
71. Xiao SD, Liu WZ, Hu PJ, Xia DH, Tytgat GN. High cure rate of *Helicobacter pylori* infection using tripotassium bismuthate, furazolidone and clarithromycin triple therapy for 1 week. Aliment Pharmacol Ther 1999; 13:311–315.
72. Coudron PE, Stratton CW. In-vitro evaluation of nitrofurantoin as an alternative agent for metronidazole in combination antimicrobial therapy against *Helicobacter pylori*. J Antimicrob Chemother 1998; 42:657–660.
73. Jenks PJ, Ferrero RL, Tankovic J, Thiberge JM, Labigne A. Evaluation of nitrofurantoin combination therapy of metronidazole-sensitive and -resistant *Helicobacter pylori* infections in mice. Antimicrob Agents Chemother 2000; 44:2623–2629.
74. Graham DY, Saeed MA, Hoffman J, El-Zimaity HM, Kwon DH, Osato MS. Nitrofurantoin quadruple therapy for *Helicobacter pylori* infection: effect of metronidazole resistance. Aliment Pharmacol Ther 2001; 15:513–518.
75. Dani R, Queiroz DM, Dias MG, et al. Omeprazole, clarithromycin and furazolidone for the eradication of *Helicobacter pylori* in patients with duodenal ulcer. Aliment Pharmacol Ther 1999; 13:1647–1652.
76. Liu WZ, Xiao SD, Shi Y, et al. Furazolidone-containing short-term therapies are effective in the treatment of *Helicobacter pylori* infection. Aliment Pharmacol Ther 1999; 13: 317–322.
77. Sisson G, Goodwin A, Raudonikiene A, et al. Enzymes associated with reductive activation and action of nitazoxanide, nitrofurans, and metronidazole in *Helicobacter pylori*. Antimicrob Agents Chemother 2002; 46:2116–2123.
78. Mendonca S, Ecclissato C, Sartori MS, et al. Prevalence of *Helicobacter pylori* resistance to metronidazole, clarithromycin, amoxicillin, tetracycline, and furazolidone in Brazil. Helicobacter 2000; 5:79–83.
79. Kwon DH, Lee M, Kim JJ, et al. Furazolidone- and nitrofurantoin-resistant *Helicobacter pylori*: prevalence and role of genes involved in metronidazole resistance. Antimicrob Agents Chemother 2001; 45:306–308.
80. Versalovic J, Shortridge D, Kibler K, et al. Mutations in 23S rRNA are associated with clarithromycin resistance in *Helicobacter pylori*. Antimicrob Agents Chemother 1996; 40:477–480.
81. Occhialini A, Urdaci M, Doucet-Populaire F, Bébéar MC, Lamouliatte H, Mégraud F. Macrolide resistance in *Helicobacter pylori*: rapid detection of point mutations and assays of macrolide binding to ribosomes. Antimicrob Agents Chemother 1997; 41:2724–2728.
82. Taylor DE, Ge Z, Purych D, Lo T, Hiratsuka K. Cloning and sequence analysis of two copies of a 23S rRNA gene from *Helicobacter pylori* and association of clarithromycin resistance with 23S rRNA mutations. Antimicrob Agents Chemother 1997; 41:2621–2628.

83. Hultén K, Gibreel A, Skold O, Engstrand L. Macrolide resistance in *Helicobacter pylori*—mechanism and stability in strains from clarithromycin-treated patients. Antimicrob Agents Chemother 1997; 41:2550–2553.
84. Stone GG, Shortridge D, Versalovic J, et al. A PCR-oligonucleotide ligation assay to determine the prevalence of 23S rRNA gene mutations in clarithromycin-resistant *Helicobacter pylori*. Antimicrob Agents Chemother 1997; 41:712–714.
85. Versalovic J, Osato MS, Spakovsky K, Dore MP, Reddy R. Point mutations in the 23S rRNA gene of *Helicobacter pylori* associated with different levels of clarithromycin resistance. J Antimicrob Chemother 1997; 40:283–286.
86. Wang G, Rahma MS, Taylor DE. Multiplex sequence analysis demonstrated the competitive growth advantage of the A-to-G mutants of clarithromycin-resistant *Helicobacter pylori*. Antimicrob Agents Chemother 1999; 43:683–685.
87. Alm RA, Ling LS, Moir DT, et al. Genomic-sequence comparison of two unrelated isolates of the human gastric pathogen *Helicobacter pylori*. Nature 1999; 397:176–180.
88. Tomb JF, White O, Kervalage AR, et al. The complete genome sequence of the gastric pathogen *Helicobacter pylori*. Nature 1997; 388:539–547.
89. Mittl PR, Luthy L, Hunziker P, Grutter MG. The cysteine-rich protein A from *Helicobacter pylori* is a β-lactamase. J Biol Chem 2000; 275:17,693–17,699.
90. Dore MP, Graham DY, Sepulveda AR. Different penicillin-binding profiles in amoxicillin-resistant *Helicobacter pylori*. Helicobacter 1999; 4:154–161.
91. DeLoney CR, Schiller NL. Characterization of an in vitro-selected amoxicillin-resistant strain of *Helicobacter pylori*. Antimicrob Agents Chemother 2000; 44:3368–3373.
92. DeLoney CR, Schiller NL. Competition of various β-lactam antibiotics for the major penicillin-binding proteins of *Helicobacter pylori*: antibacterial activity and effects on bacterial morphology. Antimicrob Agents Chemother 1999; 44:2702–2709.
93. Harris AG, Hazell SL, Netting AG. Use of digoxigenin-labelled ampicillin in the identification of penicillin-binding proteins in *Helicobacter pylori*. J Antimicrob Chemother 2000; 45:591–598.
94. Krishnamurthy P, Parlow MH, Schneider J, et al. Identification of a novel penicillin-binding protein from *Helicobacter pylori*. J Bacteriol 1999; 181:5107–5110.
95. Paul R, Postius S, Melchers K, Shafer KP. Mutations of the *Helicobacter pylori* genes *rdx*A and *pbp*1 cause resistance against metronidazole and amoxicillin. Antimicrob Agents Chemother 2001; 45:962–965.
96. Gerrits MM, Schuijffel D, van Zwet AA, Kuipers EJ, Vandenbroucke-Grauls CM, Kusters JG. Alterations in penicillin-binding protein 1A confer resistance to β-lactam antibiotics in *Helicobacter pylori*. Antimicrob Agents Chemother 2002; 46:2229–2233.
97. Trieber CA, Taylor DE. Mutations in the 16S rRNA genes of *Helicobacter pylori* mediate resistance to tetracycline. J Bacteriol 2002; 184:2131–2140.
98. Stone JW, Wise R, Donovan IA, Gearty J. Failure of ciprofloxacin to eradicate *Campylobacter pylori* from the stomach. J Antimicrob Chemother 1988; 22:92–93.
99. Moore RA, Beckthold B, Wong S, Kureishi A, Bryan LE. Nucleotide sequence of the *gyr*A gene and characterization of ciprofloxacin-resistant mutants of *Helicobacter pylori*. Antimicrob Agents Chemother 1995; 39:107–111.
100. Perri F, Festa V, Clemente R, Quitadamo M, Andriulli A. Rifabutin-based "rescue therapy" for *Helicobacter pylori* infected patients after failure of standard regimens. Aliment Pharmacol Ther 2000; 14:311–316.
101. Heep M, Odenbreit S, Beck D, et al. Mutations at four distinct regions of the *rpo*B gene can reduce the susceptibility of *Helicobacter pylori* to rifamycins. Antimicrob Agents Chemother 2000; 44:1713–1715.
102. Heep M, Beck D, Bayerdorffer E, Lehn N. Rifampin and rifabutin resistance mechanism in *Helicobacter pylori*. Antimicrob Agents Chemother 1999; 43:1497–1499.

103. Heep M, Rieger U, Beck D, Lehn N. Mutations in the beginning of the *rpo*B gene can induce resistance to rifamycins in both *Helicobacter pylori* and *Mycobacterium tuberculosis*. Antimicrob Agents Chemother 2000; 44:1075–1077.
104. National Committee for Clinical Laboratory Standards. Performance Standards for Antimicrobial Susceptibility Testing. Sixth Informational Supplement M100 S9, 19,1. Villanova, PA: National Committee for Clinical Laboratory Standards, 1999.
105. Glupczynski Y, Andersen LP, Lopez-Brea M, Mégraud F. Towards standardization of antimicrobial susceptibility testing of *Helicobacter pylori*: preliminary results by a European Multicentre Study Group. Gut 1998; 43(suppl. 2):A47.
106. Knapp CC, Ludwig MD, Washington JA. In vitro activity of metronidazole against *Helicobacter pylori* as determined by agar dilution and agar diffusion. Antimicrob Agents Chemother 1991; 35:1230–1231.
107. Chaves S, Gadanho M, Tenreiro R, Cabrita J. Assessment of metronidazole susceptibility in *Helicobacter pylori*: statistical validation and error rate analysis of breakpoints determined by disk diffusion test. J Clin Microbiol 1999; 37:1628–1631.
108. Cederbrant G, Kahlmeter G, Ljungh A. The E test for antimicrobial susceptibility testing of *Helicobacter pylori*. J Antimicrob Chemother 1993; 31:65–71.
109. Hirschl MA, Hirschl MM, Rotter ML. Comparison of three methods for determination of the susceptibility of *Helicobacter pylori* to metronidazole. J Antimicrob Chemother 1993; 32:45–49.
110. DeCross AJ, Marshall BJ, McCallum RW, Hoffman SR, Barrett LJ, Guerrant RL. Metronidazole susceptibility testing for *Helicobacter pylori*: comparison of disk, broth, and agar dilution methods and their clinical relevance. J Clin Microbiol 1993; 31:1971–1974.
111. Xia HX, Keane CT, Beattie S, O'Morain CA. Standardization of disk diffusion test and its clinical significance for susceptibility testing of metronidazole against *Helicobacter pylori*. Antimicrob Agents Chemother 1994; 38:2357–2361.
112. Henriksen TH, Brorson O, Schoyen R, Thoreson T, Lia A. A simple method for determining resistance of *Helicobacter pylori*. J Clin Microbiol 1997; 35:1424–1426.
113. Hartzen SH, Andersen LP, Bremmelgaard A, et al. Antimicrobial susceptibility testing of 230 *Helicobacter pylori* strains: importance of medium, inoculum, and incubation time. Antimicrob Agents Chemother 1997; 41:2634–2639.
114. van der Wouden EJ, de Jong A, Thijs JC, Kleibeuker JH, van Zwet AA. Subpopulations of *Helicobacter pylori* are responsible for discrepancies in the outcome of nitroimidazole susceptibility testing. Antimicrob Agents Chemother 1999; 43:1484–1486.
115. Piccolomini R, Di Bonaventura G, Catamo G, Carbone F, Neri M. Comparative evaluation of the E test, agar dilution, and broth microdilution for testing susceptibilities of *Helicobacter pylori* strains to 20 antimicrobial agents. J Clin Microbiol 1997; 35:1842–1846.
116. Midolo PD, Bell JM, Lambert JR, Turnidge JD, Grayson ML. Antimicrobial resistance testing of *Helicobacter pylori*: a comparison of Etest and disk diffusion methods. Pathology 1997; 29:411–414.
117. Thijs JC, Van Zwet AA, Thijs WJ, Van der Wouden EJ, Kooy A. One-week triple therapy with omeprazole, amoxycillin and tinidazole for *Helicobacter pylori* infection: the significance of imidazole resistance. Aliment Pharmacol Ther 1997; 11:305–309.
118. van der Wouden EJ, Thijs JC, Van Zwet AA, Kooy A, Klebeuker JH. The influence of metronidazole resistance on the efficacy of ranitidine bismuth citrate triple therapy regimens for *Helicobacter pylori* infection. Aliment Pharmacol Ther 1999; 13:297–302.
119. Hachem CY, Clarridge JE, Reddy R, et al. Antimicrobial susceptibility testing of *Helicobacter pylori*. Diagn Microbiol Infect Dis 1996; 24:37–41.
120. Mégraud F, Lehn N, Lind T, et al. Antimicrobial susceptibility testing of *Helicobacter pylori* in a large multicenter trial: the MACH2 study. Antimicrob Agents Chemother 1999; 43:2747–2752.

121. King A. Recommendations for susceptibility tests on fastidious organisms and those requiring special handling. J Antimicrob Chemother 2001; 48(suppl. S1):77–80.
122. McNulty C, Owen R, Tompkins D, et al. *Helicobacter pylori* susceptibility testing by disc diffusion. J Antimicrob Chemother 2002; 49:601–609.
123. Van der Wouden EJ, Thijs JC, Van Zwet AA, Kleibeuker KH. Nitroimidazole resistance in *Helicobacter pylori.* Aliment Pharmacol Ther 2000; 14:7–14.
124. Ménard A, Santos A, Mégraud F, Oleastro M. PCR-restriction fragment length polymorphism can also detect point mutation A2142C in the 23S rRNA gene, associated with *Helicobacter pylori* resistance to clarithromycin. Antimicrob Agents Chemother 2002; 46:1156–1157.
125. Szczabara F, Dhaenens L, Vincent P, Husson MO. Evaluation of rapid molecular methods for detection of clarithromycin resistance in *Helicobacter pylori.* Eur J Clin Microbiol Infect Dis 1997; 16:162–164.
126. van Doorn LJ, Glupczynski Y, Kusters JG, et al. Accurate prediction of macrolide resistance in *Helicobacter pylori* by a PCR line probe assay for detection of mutations in the 23S rRNA gene: multicenter validation study. Antimicrob Agents Chemother 2001; 445: 1500–1504.
127. Pina M, Occhialini A, Monteiro L, Doermann HP, Mégraud F. Detection of point mutations associated with resistance of *Helicobacter pylori* to clarithromycin using by hybridization in liquid phase. J Clin Microbiol 1998; 36:3285–3290.
128. Matsumura M, Hikiba Y, Ogura K, et al. Rapid detection of mutations in the 23S rRNA gene of *Helicobacter pylori* that confers resistance to clarithromycin treatment to the bacterium. J Clin Microbiol 2001; 39:691–695.
129. Gibson JR, Saunders NA, Burke B, Owen RJ. Novel method for rapid determination of clarithromycin sensitivity in *Helicobacter pylori.* J Clin Microbiol 1999; 37:3746–3748.
130. Chisholm SA, Owen RJ, Teare EL, Saverymuttu S. PCR-based diagnosis of *Helicobacter pylori* infection and real-time determination of clarithromycin resistance directly from gastric biopsy specimens. J Clin Microbiol 2001; 39:1217–1220.
131. Alarcon T, Domingo D, Prieto N, Lopez-Brea M. PCR using 3'-mismatched primers to detect A2142C mutation in 23S rRNA conferring resistance to clarithromycin in *Helicobacter pylori* clinical isolates. J Clin Microbiol 2000; 38:923–925.
132. Trebesius K, Panthel K, Strobel S, et al. Rapid and specific detection of *Helicobacter pylori* macrolide resistance in gastric tissue by fluorescent in situ hybridisation. Gut 2000; 46:608–614.
133. Latham SR, Owen RJ, Elviss NC, Labigne A, Jenks PJ. Differentiation of metronidazole-sensitive and -resistant *Helicobacter pylori* by immunoblotting with antisera to the RdxA protein. J Clin Microbiol 2001; 39:3052–3055.
134. Latham SR, Labigne A, Jenks PJ. Production of the RdxA protein in metronidazole-susceptible and -resistant isolates of *Helicobacter pylori* cultured from treated mice. J Antimicrob Chemother 2002; 49:675–678.
135. Owen RJ. Molecular testing for antibiotic resistance in *Helicobacter pylori.* Gut 2001; 50:285–289.
136. Toracchio S, Cellini L, Di Campli E, et al. Role of antimicrobial susceptibility testing on efficacy of triple therapy in *Helicobacter pylori* eradication. Aliment Pharmacol Ther 2000; 14:1639–1643.
137. NIH Consensus Conference. *Helicobacter pylori* in peptic ulcer disease. JAMA 1994; 272:65–69.
138. Huang JQ, Hunt RH. Treatment after failure: the problem of "non-responders." Gut 1999; 45(suppl. 1):I40–I44.
139. Gisbert JP, Pajares JM. Review article: *Helicobacter pylori* "rescue" regimen when proton pump inhibitor-based triple therapies fail. Aliment Pharmacol Ther 2002; 16:1047–1058.

140. Wise R, Hart C, Cars O, et al. Antimicrobial resistance. BMJ 1998; 317:609–610.
141. Harrison PF, Lederberg J (eds.). Antimicrobial resistance: issues and options. Washington, DC: National Academy Press, 1998.
142. House of Lords Select Committee on Science and Technology. Seventh Report. Resistance to Antibiotics and Other Antimicrobial Agents. London: Stationery Office, 1998.
143. Department of Health Standing Medical Advisory Committee Subgroup on Antimicrobial Resistance. UK Antimicrobial Resistance Strategy and Action Plan. London: Department of Health, 2000.
144. Stark CA, Adamsson I, Edlund C, et al. Effects of omeprazole and amoxycillin on the human oral and gastrointestinal microflora in patients with *Helicobacter pylori* infection. J Antimicrob Chemother 1996; 38:927–939.
145. Adamsson I, Nord CE, Lundquist P, Sjostedt S, Edlund C. Comparative effects of omeprazole, amoxycillin plus metronidazole versus omeprazole, clarithromycin plus metronidazole on the oral, gastric and intestinal microflora in *Helicobacter pylori*–infected patients. J Antimicrob Chemother 1999; 44:629–640.
146. Hazell SL. Will *Helicobacter pylori* be the next organism for which we will have exhausted our treatment options. Eur J Clin Microbiol Infect Dis 1999; 18:83–86.
147. Breuer T, Graham DY. Costs of diagnosis and treatment of *Helicobacter pylori* infection: when does choosing the treatment regimen based on susceptibility testing become cost effective? Am J Gastroenterol 1999; 94:725–729.
148. Ferguson DA, Jiang C, Chi DS, Laffan JJ, Li C, Thomas E. Evaluation of two string tests for obtaining gastric juice for culture, nested-PCR detection, and combined single- and double-stranded conformational polymorphism discrimination of *Helicobacter pylori*. Dig Dis Sci 1999; 44:2056–2062.
149. Graham DY. Antibiotic resistance in *Helicobacter pylori*: implications for therapy. Gastroenterology 1998; 115:1272–1277.
150. Qureshi WA, Graham DY. Antibiotic-resistant *H. pylori* infection and its treatment. Curr Pharm Des 2000; 6:1537–1544.
151. Jonkers D, van den Broek E, van Dooren I, et al. Antibacterial effect of garlic and omeprazole on *Helicobacter pylori*. J Antimicrob Chemother 1999; 43:837–839.
152. O'Gara EA, Hill DJ, Maslin DJ. Activities of garlic oil, garlic powder, and their diallyl constituents against *Helicobacter pylori*. Appl Environ Microbiol 2000; 66:2269–2273.
153. Huwez FU, Thirlwell D, Cockayne A, Ala'Aldeen DA. Mastic gum kills *Helicobacter pylori*. N Engl J Med 1998:1946.

9
The Management of Antibiotic-Resistant *Neisseria gonorrhoeae*

Catherine A. Ison and Jonathan Ross

1. INTRODUCTION

Gonorrhea is a common cause of bacterial sexually transmitted infection (STI), and in many countries (such as the United Kingdom), it is second only to chlamydial infection *(1)*. In many industrialized countries, the epidemiology of gonorrhea has changed in the last 15–20 yr. After the advent of acquired immunodeficiency syndrome (AIDS) in 1984, there was a rapid decline in the number of cases of STIs, including gonorrhea, reaching a trough in 1990–1991. This decline was followed initially by small increases in the number of cases, which has been sustained with significant increases in STIs in the last 5 yr *(1)*.

Neisseria gonorrhoeae, the causative agent of gonorrhea, is an obligate human pathogen that exhibits phase and antigenic variation and can cause repeated episodes of infection in the same host, appearing as a new infection on each occasion. This diversity exhibited by *N. gonorrhoeae* is believed to result from its ability for horizontal gene exchange and for recombination, which in vivo probably occurs during mixed infections. *Neisseria gonorrhoeae* is inherently susceptible to most antimicrobial agents, but as successive therapeutic agents have been introduced, resistance has either been acquired by the acquisition of plasmids from other organisms, such as *Haemophilus*, or resistant mutants have emerged under selective pressure of continual usage. The ability of this pathogen both to evade the immune response and to develop resistance to most therapeutic agents presents a challenge for the management of gonococcal infections.

2. RECOMMENDED THERAPIES

Patients with gonorrhea are usually treated empirically—after a provisional diagnosis is made based on microscopy—when named as the contact of an infected patient or if syndromic management guidelines are being followed. In the initial absence of antimicrobial sensitivity data, up-to-date information on the epidemiological patterns of antibiotic resistance is essential in making a rational choice of therapy. By convention, the antimicrobial chosen as first-line therapy should be effective against at least 95% of local isolates *(2,3)*.

From: *Management of Multiple Drug-Resistant Infections*
Edited by: S. H. Gillespie © Humana Press Inc., Totowa, NJ

Table 1
Guidelines for First-Line Treatment of Gonorrhea

	First-line therapy	Therapy if resistance suspected
UK national guidelines *(6)*	Ciprofloxacin 500 mg, single dose Ofloxacin 400 mg, single dose	Ceftriaxone 250 mg Cefotaxime 500 mg im, single dose
	Ampicillin 2 g or 3 g plus probenecid 1 g, single dose (only where regional prevalence of penicillin resistance is less than 5%)	Spectinomycin 2 g im, single dose
WHO guidelines *(5)*	Ciprofloxacin 500 mg, single dose	Dependent on antimicrobial sensitivities
	Azithromycin 2 g, single dose Ceftriaxone 125 mg im, single dose Cefixime 400 mg, single dose Spectinomycin 2 g im, single dose Kanamycin 2 g im, single dose (only in regions where in vitro resistance is low) Trimethoprim (80 mg) plus sulfamethoxazole (400 mg); 10 tablets as a single dose daily for 3 d (only in regions where in vitro resistance is low)	
CDC guidelines *(4)*	Cefixime 400 mg, single dose	Dependent on antimicrobial sensitivities
	Ceftriaxone 125 mg im, single dose	Also consider spectinomycin 2 g im, single dose
	Ciprofloxacin 500 mg, single dose Ofloxacin 400 mg, single dose Levofloxacin 250 mg, single dose	

The third-generation cephalosporins and quinolones generally have good activity against *N. gonorrhoeae* and form the backbone of most recommended regimens (Table 1) *(4–6)*, but the high levels of quinolone resistance in some regions of the world are now limiting the usefulness of these agents. In both the United Kingdom and the United States, treatment guidelines have been updated, and although noting the increase in strains of gonorrhea that have reduced susceptibility and resistance to quinolones, they continue to recommend ciprofloxacin and ofloxacin as options for first-line therapy. These guidelines are currently under review, however, because of recent increases in ciprofloxacin resistance.

The different national and international guidelines make a number of specific recommendations about choosing appropriate therapy (Table 1). The UK guidelines suggest that all imported infections (i.e., those acquired abroad) should be considered penicillin and tetracycline resistant and possibly quinolone resistant, with second-line therapy therefore appropriate *(6)*. The US guidelines suggest avoiding quinolones as first-line therapy when the infection has been acquired in Hawaii or California, Asia, or the Pacific *(4)*.

2.1. Factors Affecting the Choice of Therapy

A variety of demographic and epidemiological factors have been associated with antimicrobial resistance to *N. gonorrhoeae* and may help the clinician choose appropriate treatment. Such information, however, is imprecise and cannot always be relied on to predict resistance in individual patients *(7)*. The factors that may influence the choice of therapy include membership in high-risk groups, local epidemiology, patient choice, concurrent treatment for *Chlamydia trachomatis*, sexual history, cost and antibiotic availability, safety of clinic staff, site of infection, cultural factors, and miscellaneous factors.

2.1.1. High-Risk Groups

A history of foreign travel by the patient or the patient's partner to areas with high levels of endemic resistance to usual first-line antibiotics may alter the choice of therapy. Gay men are more likely to be infected with *mtr* strains of *N. gonorrhoeae*, which may reduce sensitivity to penicillin and tetracyclines *(8)*.

2.1.2. Local Epidemiology

The availability of high-quality local epidemiological data about antimicrobial resistance to guide empirical therapy may influence drug choice at a population level, and availability of sensitivity testing will also affect the choice of antibiotic for an individual, particularly when treatment failure occurs.

2.1.3. Patient Choice

Oral, rather than parenteral, therapy is usually preferred by the patient. Directly observed single-dose therapy avoids the risk of poor adherence.

2.1.4. Concurrent Treatment for Chlamydia trachomatis

Genital coinfection with *C. trachomatis* is found in 20–40% of patients with gonorrhea. Concurrent treatment for chlamydia is therefore often given in addition to antibiotics for the gonorrhea, usually with a tetracycline or macrolide *(2)*. This may provide effective therapy for some, but by no means all, penicillin- and quinolone-resistant strains of *Neisseria gonorrhoeae*.

2.1.5. Sexual History

If a patient fails to respond to treatment, it usually implies reinfection or resistance. A history of unprotected intercourse with a potentially infected partner makes reinfection more likely, and the absence of such a history raises the possibility of resistance and the need to use a different antibiotic.

2.1.6. Cost and Antibiotic Availability

The availability of antibiotics varies in different areas of the world; even when available, high cost may limit their use.

2.1.7. Safety of Clinic Staff

The use of parenteral therapy raises the risk of needle-stick injuries. Such concerns are of particular importance where human immunodeficiency virus (HIV) infection is highly prevalent and highlights the need for sterile equipment and appropriate training for those giving injections. Where there is a risk of disposable syringes being reused, parenteral therapy may need to be avoided *(9)*.

2.1.8. Site of Infection

Spectinomycin is a less-effective agent for the treatment of pharyngeal infections *(10)* and therefore may not be an appropriate choice for gay men.

2.1.9. Cultural Factors

In some cultures, there is a perception that oral medication is less efficacious than an injection. This may need to be reflected in the choice of regimen *(9)*.

2.1.10. Miscellaneous

Choice of treatment may also be altered by drug allergy and pregnancy and for children. Quinolones particularly should be avoided in pregnancy and young children because of concerns (based on animal studies) about damage to cartilage in developing joints, although current Centers for Disease Control and Prevention (CDC) guidelines recommend that they can be used in children weighing over 45 kg because cartilage damage has never been described in humans *(4)*.

3. MECHANISMS OF RESISTANCE

3.1. Penicillin

Penicillin is a β-lactam antibiotic that kills bacteria by binding to the transpeptidases and endopeptidases, also known as penicillin-binding proteins (PBPs), involved in the crosslinking of the peptide chains of peptidoglycan, the backbone of the bacterial cell wall. Integrity of the cell wall is essential for bacterial viability; hence, inhibition of cell wall synthesis is bactericidal. *Neisseria gonorrhoeae* have four PBPs, of which two (PBP 1 and 2) are essential for cell viability *(11)* and are potential targets for antimicrobial agents. When penicillin was first used for therapy for gonorrhea, gonococcal isolates were very susceptible (minimum inhibitory concentrations [MICs] 0.004–0.01 mg/L), but decreased susceptibility, which was chromosomally mediated, emerged very quickly; in the 1970s, isolates therapeutically resistant to penicillin were reported (MIC $\geq$ 2 mg/L) *(12)*. High levels of resistance were not encountered until strains of *N. gonorrhoeae* were reported in 1976 that had acquired plasmids encoding for the production of penicillinase *(13,14)*.

3.1.1. Chromosomal Resistance to Penicillin

Chromosomally mediated resistant *N. gonorrhoeae* (CMRNG) are now known to have mutations in a series of genes (*pen*A, *mtr*, *pen*B, *pon*A1, and *pen*C) *(11)* that are acquired in a stepwise manner and result in increasing levels of resistance to penicillin and tetracycline. The gene *pen*A encodes for PBP 2, and resistant isolates with an altered gene exhibit decreased rates of acetylation to penicillin *(15)*. This has resulted from the acquisition of divergent sequences from commensal *Neisseria*, leading to multiple amino acid changes, of which the most frequent is an insertion at Asp345a *(16)*, and these isolates exhibit low levels of decreased susceptibility to penicillin.

Further increases in resistance are dependent on the *mtr* locus, which confers nonspecific resistance to a number of antibiotics and hydrophobic agents through overexpression of the MtrC-MtrD-MtrE efflux pump *(17,18)*. However, *mtr* alone does not increase resistance, but requires the *pen*B locus *(19)*, which has been correlated with mutations in the *por* gene *(20)* for expression. Acquisition of these three loci will result in decreased susceptibility, but two other loci, *pon*A1 *(21)* and *pen*C *(11)*, have been shown necessary for full resistance to be expressed.

The gene *pon*A1 encodes for PBP 1, and unlike the alterations in PBP 2, the sequence is conserved; the resistant forms of PBP 1 have a single base change, resulting in an amino acid change at position 421 from leucine to proline *(11)*. As yet, the identity of *pen*C is unknown. The overall effect of these loci results in a change in permeability of the cell wall to penicillin such that the antibiotic cannot get through or is actively transported out of the wall. CMRNG continue to be a therapeutic problem in many parts of the world and contribute to the decline in usefulness of this agent.

3.1.2. Plasmid-Mediated Resistance to Penicillin

Penicillinase-producing *N. gonorrhoeae* (PPNG) carry low molecular weight plasmids that encode for the TEM-1 β-lactamase produced in the periplasmic space of the gonococcus and breaks the β-lactam ring of penicillin, rendering the antibiotic inactive. PPNG were initially found to carry plasmids of either 3.2 MDa or 4.4 MDa, which had originated in Africa and Asia, respectively, and for many years were known respectively as the African and Asian plasmids *(13,14,22)*. These plasmids are thought to have been acquired from *Haemophilus*, but are now species restricted in that they can only be transferred between gonococci. However, they are not self-mobilizable and require the presence of a 24.5-MDa conjugative plasmid in the donor strain for transfer to occur, a plasmid already present in some isolates of *N. gonorrhoeae (23)*. Subsequently, PPNG carrying plasmids of differing molecular weights have been reported and named by their geographical site of isolation; all these plasmids have been shown to be related, but carry deletions of various sizes in nonfunctional parts of the plasmid *(24)*.

PPNG have spread worldwide. In some countries, the prevalence has now declined, and many of the infections seen are imported from parts of the world where the prevalence remains high, such as the western Pacific region *(25)*.

3.2. Cephalosporins

Cephalosporins are β-lactam antibiotics modified to resist the action of penicillinase. There are several generations, each with increasing levels of β-lactamase resistance. Ceftriaxone, a third-generation cephalosporin not affected by the β-lactamase produced by PPNG, is recommended treatment for gonorrhea. This is a highly active antimicrobial agent, although it is given intramuscularly by injection; cefixime, an oral cephalosporin, is sometimes used as an alternative.

Therapeutic failure to these cephalosporins has not been documented, so the original recommended dose of 250 mg in some protocols has been reduced to 125 mg *(4,26)*. However, this is a concern as decreased susceptibility has been detected by laboratory methods *(27)*. Cross-resistance has been demonstrated between penicillin and the earlier cephalosporins, such as cefuroxime. The chromosomal mutations responsible for penicillin resistance also confer reduced susceptibility to the cephalosporins *(28)*. The combination of decreasing susceptibility and lowering of the dosage seems an obvious approach for selecting resistant strains, particularly in parts of the world where ceftriaxone is readily available and may be an off-patent, less-potent form of the drug.

3.3. *Spectinomycin*

Spectinomycin is an aminocyclitol compound that inhibits protein synthesis. Resistance to spectinomycin is single step and results in high levels of resistance (MICs > 64 mg/L); the cause is reported to be mutations in 16S rRNA *(29)*. Resistance has been sporadic *(30–33)* and has not widely spread, suggesting that this agent may be suitable as an alternative therapy when other drugs are no longer useful. Spectinomycin has not been widely used and has been difficult to obtain as pharmaceutical companies have stopped production.

3.4. *Quinolones*

Ciprofloxacin is a 4-quinolone with DNA gyrase (GyrA) and topoisomerase IV (ParC) bacterial targets in *N. gonorrhoeae*. These enzymes are responsible for the supercoiling of bacterial DNA and essential for growth and division; hence, inhibition by quinolones is bactericidal *(34)*. *Neisseria gonorrhoeae* were exquisitely sensitive to ciprofloxacin when it was first introduced, but in vitro studies showed that resistant strains could be selected for on sequential increments of ciprofloxacin with resulting mutations in multiple sites, first of the *gyr*A gene and in strains exhibiting higher levels of resistance also in the *par*C gene *(35)*.

Unfortunately, clinical isolates with ever-increasing levels of resistance to ciprofloxacin have appeared, almost certainly because of overuse and misuse of the quinolones in parts of the world where resistance is most prevalent, such as the western Pacific region. The quinolone-resistant *N. gonorrhoeae* (QRNG) exhibit cross-resistance to other quinolones; this results from multiple mutations, resulting in amino acid substitutions in *gyr*A and *par*C *(36–38)*. Porin changes and efflux mechanisms may also contribute to enhance the levels of resistance. Newer quinolones have been produced, such as moxifloxacin, but their primary target site is ParC, which is of secondary importance in gonococci and hence is unlikely to be a useful alternative *(39)*. Resistance to ciprofloxacin in *N. gonorrhoeae* is currently limited to chromosomal mutations. However, a recent report of plasmid-meditated resistance in a clinical isolate of *Klebsiella pneumoniae*, which was transferable to other *Enterobacteriaceae*, is particularly worrying *(40)*.

3.5. *Azithromycin*

Azithromycin is a macrolide that, like erythromycin, inhibits protein synthesis by binding to the 50S ribosome and inhibiting the elongation of the peptide chains. Azithromycin is not generally used as the drug of choice for gonorrhea; it more commonly is used for chlamydial infection. However, increasing resistance in gonococci to other antimicrobial agents has led to its recommendation as alternative therapy for resistant infections. Ideally, it should be used at a 2-g dose to prevent or delay the emergence of resistance, but many patients find this dosage difficult to tolerate; therefore, the 1-g dose is chosen although it has given an unacceptable level of clinical failure *(41)*. Resistance to macrolides in other bacteria includes efflux mechanisms and alteration of the target by the production of enzymes or mutations that reduce affinity for the ribosomal target.

In *N. gonorrhoeae*, resistance to azithromycin has only recently emerged. Mutations in the *mtr* operon, in the promotor regions of *mtr*R and *mtr*C genes *(42–44)*, have been detected in gonococcal isolates showing reduced susceptibility (MICs 0.25–0.5 mg/L). Another macrolide pump, encoded by the *mef* genes, has now been found in clinical isolates of gonococci and may be implicated in resistance *(45)*. Modification of the ribosomal target by methylases *(46)* and mutations in the 23S rRNA have also been described in gonococci *(47)*.

3.6. Tetracycline

Tetracycline inhibits bacterial growth by affecting protein synthesis. It is not generally recommended for first-line therapy for gonorrhea, but it is inexpensive and widely available. It is used in parts of the world where more effective alternatives either are not available or are too expensive. Tetracycline resistance either can be low level and chromosomally mediated (MIC 2–8 mg/L), resulting from multiple chromosomal mutations *(48)*, or can be high level (MIC ≥ 16 mg/L) and plasmid mediated *(49)*. High-level resistance was first reported in 1985 and is the result of the acquisition of the TetM determinant inserted into the conjugative plasmid of gonococci. Tetracycline-resistant *N. gonorrhoeae* (TRNG) have spread widely, probably because of their ability to mobilize between both gonococci and other genera found in the lower genital tract *(50)* and to the widespread use of this antibiotic.

3.7. Aminoglycosides

The aminoglycosides kanamycin and gentamicin affect bacterial growth by inhibiting protein synthesis. Kanamycin is mentioned in some guidelines as an alternative therapy, and use of gentamicin has been reported. However, efficacy data and definitions of resistance in vitro are not clear *(51,52)*.

3.8. Cotrimoxazole

Cotrimoxazole is a combination of sulfamethoxazole and trimethoprim, which are administered orally in a multidose regimen; it has been used occasionally for the treatment of gonorrhea. Both agents inhibit the synthesis of tetrahydrofolate acid. Sulfamethoxazole is an analogue of para aminobenzoic acid and competitively inhibits the formation of dihydropteric acid; trimethoprim binds to dihydrofolate reductase and inhibits the formation of tetrahydrofolate acid. In the absence of tetrahydrofolate acid, which serves as a carrier of methyl groups, the production of purines and thymidine are affected; hence, DNA synthesis is affected. There are reports of increasing resistance in areas such as Tanzania *(53)*, where cotrimoxazole is used, but true levels may be unknown because of the technical difficulties in determining susceptibility in vitro.

4. DETECTION OF RESISTANCE

Patients who fail therapy may harbor an isolate that is exhibiting resistance or may be reinfected. Susceptibility testing in vitro can be very useful for confirming the presence of a resistant isolate in a particular patient; in many laboratories, each gonococcal isolate is tested to a range of antimicrobial agents currently used for therapy. The aim of susceptibility testing is to predict the outcome of therapy, to detect the emergence of resistance, and to monitor drifts in susceptibility. For gonococcal infections, identification of PPNG using the chromogenic cephalosporin nitrocefin to detect β-lactamase is often done first *(54)*. The reagent is initially yellow and turns quickly pink/red when the β-lactam ring is broken. Alternative methods, such as the starch iodine test, are occasionally used when resources are not available to purchase nitrocefin *(55)*.

4.1. Disk Diffusion

The method of choice for routine testing of other types of resistance is probably disk diffusion, by which antibiotic-containing disks are placed on a lawn of bacteria; the zones of inhibition are measured and compared to control strains. For gonococci, this method can be difficult because *N. gonorrhoeae* is a fastidious organism that requires an enriched medium for growth, which may contain nutrients that influence the activity of some antibiotics. Strains requiring nutrition may grow at reduced rates, making comparison with control strains difficult. There are methods recommended by the World Health Organization (WHO) *(56)*, National Committee for Clinical Laboratory Standards (NCCLS) *(57)*, and the British Society of Antimicrobial Chemotherapy (BSAC) *(58)*, among others.

Although these methods vary primarily in the medium used and the content of the disks, each can be successful if carefully performed with an appropriate panel of control strains for interpretation. The results obtained can be correlated with clinical outcome. Susceptible strains have less than a 5% likelihood of treatment failure; resistant strains may be associated with more than a 15% chance of treatment failure; and intermediate resistance or decreased susceptibility have a 5–15% possibility of treatment failure *(59)*. The E-test, a paper strip containing varying concentrations of antibiotic that is placed onto a lawn of bacteria, can also be used. A zone of inhibition is obtained that gives an indication of the MIC. These tests are commercially available and expensive, but can be useful for laboratories that isolate few gonococci.

4.2. Agar Dilution Techniques

An alternative to disk diffusion is the use of the breakpoint agar dilution technique, which categorizes strains as susceptible or resistant *(60)*. This is particularly useful for screening for high-level resistance, for which single concentrations may be used (e.g., growth on agar containing 0.5 mg/L ciprofloxacin indicates an MIC ≥ 1 mg/L). The use of the agar dilution method to determine the full MIC of isolates to an antibiotic is not appropriate for routine or daily use for gonococci.

There are three methodologies in regular use in different parts of the world; these differ primarily in the agar base used: GC agar base (NCCLS, North America) *(57)*, Isosensitest (Australia) *(61)*, and Diagnostic Sensitivity Agar (Europe) *(62)*. The different bases can affect the breakpoint that indicates resistance; the most important is for penicillin, which can be either 2 mg/L or higher (GC agar base) or 1 mg/L or higher (Isosensitest and DST agar). Other antimicrobial agents are largely unaffected. Determination of the MIC is most appropriate for use in surveillance programs and is undertaken at reference or specialized laboratories.

4.3. Molecular Techniques

Conventional susceptibility testing requires a viable organism, which can only be obtained by culturing the specimen from the patient. However, with increasing use of nucleic acid amplification tests (NAATs) for the detection of *N. gonorrhoeae*, less susceptibility data will be available; hence, the data will be less representative. In essence, molecular detection of resistance in *N. gonorrhoeae* should be possible because most of the genes involved are recognized.

The detection of plasmid-mediated resistance is the simplest, and amplification methods have been described for both penicillin *(63)* and tetracycline *(64,65)*. The chromosomal mutations responsible for penicillin resistance are also documented and should be detectable using probes or microarrays. Resistance to ciprofloxacin is the result of mutations at multiple sites on both the *gyr*A and *par*C genes; although methods for detecting mutations have been described *(66,67)*, it has been difficult to identify common changes that would predict therapeutic resistance. The approach that holds the most promise is the use of DNA microarrays, and preliminary results indicate that it should be explored more extensively *(68)*.

5. TREATMENT OF RESISTANT INFECTIONS

5.1. Relationship of Level of Resistance (MIC) to Treatment Failure

The relationship between in vitro sensitivity (minimum inhibitory concentration [MIC]) and clinical response is closely correlated for most antibiotics used to treat gonorrhea, but treatment failure in "sensitive" isolates and clinical success in "resistant" isolates can occur. The interpretation of quinolone in vitro sensitivity tests may be particularly difficult. Some studies have found close agreement between reported sensitivity and clinical response *(69)*, but wide discrepancies were seen in others *(70)*.

The interpretation and comparison of studies that have assessed in vitro antibiotic sensitivity is limited by a lack of consistency in the methodologies used in different laboratories in different countries. Thus, the sensitivity of an isolate may also vary according to minor differences in laboratory procedure or reagents.

5.2. Relationship Between Drug Dosage and Treatment Failure

In the early days of penicillin use, low-level resistance could be overcome by increasing the dose of the antibiotic. The pharmacokinetics of the drug and toxicity associated with higher drug levels limit the usefulness of this approach, and clinical failure can still occur even with "adequate" drug levels *(71)*. It does, however, remain essential to use an adequate treatment dose of antibiotic to prevent the development of resistance in those who are initially sensitive to individual agents.

5.3. Test of Cure to Ensure Resolution

Guidelines vary regarding advisement whether a repeat test should be performed after treatment (test of cure) to ensure resolution of infection. Because sensitivity testing cannot always predict clinical response and microbiological clearance does not always accompany clinical resolution, a test of cure is worth performing if the patient will return for a follow-up examination. Either treatment failure or reinfection may result in a positive test of cure, although the sexual history may help differentiate the two; in either case, retreatment is required, usually with an alternative antibiotic, unless a clear history of re-exposure to a known sensitive isolate is given.

5.4. Appropriate Advice for the Patient

Following the initial diagnosis appropriate explanation about the infection, preferably with clear written information, should be given to the patient. The patient should be advised to avoid sex until his or her partner has been seen, the antibiotic therapy is finished, and the test of cure is negative. Arrangements should be made for the partner to be seen, screened, and offered empirical antibiotics. In women, it is appropriate to provide information on the risk of pelvic inflammatory disease (approx 8–10%) and associated infertility, ectopic pregnancy, and chronic pelvic pain.

6. SURVEILLANCE OF ANTIMICROBIAL RESISTANCE

A range of antimicrobial agents have been used as first-line therapies for gonorrhea, but resistance continues to emerge and spread, so there is a real concern that gonorrhea will become increasingly difficult to treat *(72)*. Surveillance programs, therefore, are essential to inform the choice of an appropriate antimicrobial agent by providing reliable data on the susceptibility profiles of the gonococcal population. There are established surveillance programs in the United States *(73)*, Canada *(74)*, Australia *(75)*, and the Netherlands *(76)*; these have shown that long-term surveillance is possible and can provide valuable temporal data. A global surveillance program, the Gonococcal Antimicrobial Surveillance Program (GASP), was initiated in 1990 by the World Health Organization *(77)*, but is currently most active in the Americas, the Caribbean, and the western Pacific region *(72)*.

An important consideration of any surveillance program is that data should be comparable between laboratories; this is dependent on the development of training and quality assurance programs. As resistant gonorrhea increases unabated, there have been additional programs established, such as in West Africa *(78)* and England and Wales *(79,80)*. The challenge remains to produce comparable data worldwide using a number of procedures that have a common methodology but small and significant differences. It seems probable that this will be achieved best using a robust panel of control strains to establish breakpoints for resistance that enable gonococcal isolates to be categorized as susceptible or resistant.

7. CONCLUSION

Surveillance programs have shown that penicillin is no longer a suitable first-line treatment for gonorrhea unless good data are available to indicate that the local gonococcal population is susceptible. In the western Pacific region, widespread resistance was found, with levels of total penicillin resistance (PPNG and CMRNG) for 80% of total isolates tested in China and 89.3% in the Philippines in the year 2000. Resistance to quinolones was also found in many parts of this region, with levels increasing from 1999 to 2000 *(25)*. Surveillance programs have also noted that resistance to quinolones can differ between regions of the same national program *(80)*, giving valuable information to inform local choice of therapy.

Neisseria gonorrhoeae continues to spread and cause increasing numbers of infections in many parts of the world. It remains a challenge to manage gonococcal infections effectively as antibiotic resistance increases and is of worldwide importance. A real concern is the lack of new antimicrobial agents specifically for the treatment of gonorrhea, so it is imperative that surveillance programs are sustained to prolong the useful life of current therapies.

REFERENCES

1. PHLS, DHSS&PS and the Scottish ISD(D)5 Collaborative Group. Sexually Transmitted Infections in the UK: New Episodes Seen at Genitourinary Medicine Clinics, 1991–2001. London: Public Health Laboratory Service, 2002.
2. Fitzgerald M, Bedford C. National standards for the management of gonorrhoea. Int J STD AIDS 1996; 7:298–300.
3. Handsfield HH, McCutchan JA, Corey L, Ronald AR. Evaluation of new anti-infective drugs for the treatment of uncomplicated gonorrhea in adults and adolescents. Infectious Diseases Society of America and the Food and Drug Administration. Clin Infect Dis 1992; 15(suppl. 1):S123–S130.
4. Centers for Disease Control. CDC Sexually Transmitted Diseases Guidelines 2002—Gonococcal Infections. 2002. Available at: http://www.cdc.gov/std/treatment/4-2002TG.htm#Gonococcal. Accessed September 9, 2003.
5. World Health Organization. WHO Guidelines for the Management of Gonococcal Infections. 2001. Available at: http://www.who.int/STIManagemntguidelines/who_hiv_aids_2001.01/003.htm#3.1. Accessed September 9, 2003.
6. Bignell C. 2001 National Guideline for the Management of Gonorrhoea in Adults. Clinical Effectiveness Group of MSSVD/AGUM. 2001. Available at: http://www.mssvd.org.uk/PDF/CEG2001/gc%200601.PDF. Accessed September 9, 2003.
7. Goodfellow A, Standley T, Ross JD. Predicting penicillin resistance in patients with gonorrhoea. Sex Transm Infect 1999; 75:190.
8. Morse SA, Lysko PG, McFarland L, et al. Gonococcal strains from homosexual men have outer membranes with reduced permeability to hydrophobic molecules. Infect Immun 1982; 37:432–438.
9. Tapsall J. Antimicrobial Resistance to *Neisseria gonorrhoeae*. Geneva, Switzerland: World Health Organization, 2001. WHO/CDS/CSR/DRS/2001.3.
10. Kraus SJ. Incidence and therapy of gonococcal pharyngitis. Sex Transm Dis 1979; 6: 143–147.
11. Ropp PA, Hu M, Olesky M, Nicholas RA. Mutations in *pon*A, the gene encoding penicillin-binding protein 1, and a novel locus, *pen*C, are required for high-level chromosomally mediated penicillin resistance. Antimicrob Agents Chemother 2002; 46:769–777.
12. Faruki H, Kohmescher RN, McKinney WP, Sparling PF. A community-based outbreak of infection with penicillin-resistant *Neisseria gonorrhoeae* not producing penicillinase (chromosomally mediated resistance). N Engl J Med 1985; 313:607–611.
13. Ashford WA, Golash RG, Hemming VG. Penicillinase-producing *Neisseria gonorrhoeae*. Lancet 1976; 2:657–658.
14. Percival A, Rowlands J, Corkhill JE, et al. Penicillinase-producing gonococci in Liverpool. Lancet 1976; 2:1379–1382.
15. Spratt BG. Hybrid penicillin-binding proteins in penicillin-resistant strains of *Neisseria gonorrhoeae*. Nature 1988; 332:173–176.
16. Brannigan, JA, Tirodimos IA, Zhang QY, Dowson CG, Spratt BG. Insertion of an extra aminoacid is the main cause of the low affinity of penicillin-binding protein 2 in penicillin resistant strains of *Neisseria gonorrhoeae*. Mol Microbiol 1990; 4:913–919.
17. Hagman KE, Pan W, Spratt BG, Balthazar JT, Judd RC, Shafer WM. Resistance of *Neisseria gonorrhoeae* to antimicrobial hydrophobic agents is modulated by the *mtr*RCDE efflux system. Microbiology 1995; 141:611–622.
18. Delahay RM, Robertson BD, Balthazar JT, Shafer WM, Ison CA. Involvement of the gonococcal MtrE protein in the resistance of *Neisseria gonorrhoeae* to toxic hydrophobic agents. Microbiology 1997; 143:2127–2133.
19. Sparling PF, Sarubbi FA Jr, Blackman E. Inheritance of low-level resistance to penicillin, tetracycline and chloramphenicol in *Neisseria gonorrhoeae*. J Bacteriol 1975; 124:740–749.

20. Gill MJ, Simjee S, Al-Hattawi K, Robertson BD, Easmon CSF, Ison CA. Gonococcal resistance to β-lactams and tetracycline involves mutation in loop 3 of the porin encoded at the *pen*B locus. Antimicrob Agents Chemother 1998; 42:2799–2803.
21. Ropp PA, Nicholas RA. Cloning and characterization of the *pon*A gene encoding penicillin-binding protein 1 from *Neisseria gonorrhoeae* and *Neisseria meningitidis*. J Bacteriol 1997; 179:2783–2787.
22. Roberts M, Elwell LP, Falkow S. Molecular characterization of two β-lactamase-specifying plasmids isolated from *Neisseria gonorrhoeae*. J Bacteriol 1977; 131:557–563.
23. Roberts MC. Plasmids of *Neisseria gonorrhoeae* and other *Neisseria* species. Clin Microbiol Rev 1989; 2(suppl.):S18–S23.
24. Pagotto F, Aman AT, Ng LK, Teung KH, Brett M, Dillon JA. Sequence analysis of the family of penicillinase-producing plasmids of *Neisseria gonorrhoeae*. Plasmid 2000; 43:24–34.
25. WHO Western Pacific Region Gonococcal Antimicrobial Surveillance Programme. Surveillance of antibiotic resistance in *Neisseria gonorrhoeae* in the WHO Pacific Region, 2000. Commun Dis Intell 2001; 25:274–277.
26. Bignell CJ. European guideline for the management of gonorrhoea. Int J STD AIDS 2001; 12(suppl. 3):27–29.
27. Schwebke JR, Whittington W, Rice RJ, Handsfield HH, Hale J, Holmes KK. Trends in susceptibility of *Neisseria gonorrhoeae* to ceftriaxone from 1985 through 1991. Antimicrob Agents Chemother 1995; 39:917–920.
28. Ison CA, Bindayna KM, Woodford N, Gill MJ, Easmon CSF. Penicillin and cephalosporin resistance in gonococci. Genitourin Med 1990; 66:351–356.
29. Galimand M, Gerbaud G, Courvalin P. Spectinomycin resistance in *Neisseria* spp due to mutations in 16S rRNA. Antimicrob Agents Chemother 2000; 44:1365–1366.
30. Boslego JW, Tramont EC, Takafuji ET, et al. Effect of spectinomycin use on the prevalence of spectinomycin resistant and of penicillinase-producing *Neisseria gonorrhoeae*. N Engl J Med 1987; 317:272–278.
31. Spectinomycin-resistant penicillinase producing *Neisseria gonorrhoeae*—California. MMWR Morb Mortal Wkly Rep 1981; 30:221–222.
32. Zenilman JM, Nims LJ, Menegus MA, Nolte F, Knapp JS. Spectinomycin-resistant gonococcal infections in the United States, 1985–86. J Infect Dis 1987; 156:1002–1004.
33. Easmon CSF, Ison CA, Bellinger CM, Harris JRW. Emergence of resistance after spectinomycin treatment for gonorrhoea due to β–lactamase-producing strain of *Neisseria gonorrhoeae*. BMJ 1982; 284:1604–1605.
34. Drlica K, Zhao X. DNA gyrase, topisomerase IV, and the 4-quinolones. Microbiol Mol Biol Rev 1997; 61:377–392.
35. Belland RJ, Morrison SG, Ison C, Huang WM. *Neisseria gonorrhoeae* acquires mutations in analogous regions of *gyr*A and *par*C in fluoroquinolone-resistant isolates. Mol Microbiol 1994; 14:371–380.
36. Trees DL, Sandul AL, Whittington WL, Knapp JS. Identification of novel mutation patterns in the *par*C gene of ciprofloxacin-resistant isolates of *Neisseria gonorrhoeae*. Antimicrob Agents Chemother 1998; 42:2103–2105.
37. Trees DL, Sandul AL, Neal SW, Higa H, Knapp JS. Molecular epidemiology of *Neisseria gonorrhoeae* exhibiting decreased susceptibility and resistance to ciprofloxacin in Hawaii, 1991–1999. Sex Transm Dis 2001; 28:309–314.
38. Knapp JS, Fox KK, Trees DL, Whittington WL. Fluoroquinolone resistance in *Neisseria gonorrhoeae*. Emerg Infect Dis 1997; 3:33–38.
39. Shultz TR, Tapsall JW, White PA. Correlation of in vitro susceptibilities to newer quinolones of naturally-occurring quinolone-resistant *Neisseria gonorrhoeae* strains with changes in GyrA and ParC. Antimicrob Agents Chemother 2001; 45:734–738.

40. Martinez-Martinez L, Pascual A, Jacoby GA. Quinolone resistance from a transferable plasmid. Lancet 1998; 351:797–799.
41. Young H, Moyes A, McMillan A. Azithromycin and erythromycin resistant *Neisseria gonorrhoeae* following treatment with azithromycin. Int J STD AIDS 1997; 8:299–302.
42. Zaratonnelli L, Borthagaray G, Lee E-H, Shafer WM. Decreased azithromycin susceptibility of *Neisseria gonorrhoeae* due to *mtr*R mutations. Antimicrob Agents Chemother 1999; 43:2468–2472.
43. Xia M, Whittington WL, Shafer WM, Holmes KK. Gonorrhoea among men who have sex with men: an outbreak caused by a single genotype of erythromycin-resistant *Neisseria gonorrhoeae* with a single-base pair deletion in the *mtr*R promotor region. J Infect Dis 2000; 181:2080–2082.
44. Shafer WM, Veal WL, Lee EH, Zarantonelli L, Balthazar JT, Roquette C. Genetic organization and regulation of antimicrobial efflux system possessed by *Neisseria gonorrhoeae* and *Neisseria meningitidis*. J Mol Microbiol Biotechnol 2001; 3:219–224.
45. Luna VA, Cousin S Jr, Whittington WL, Roberts MC. Identification of the conjugative *mef* genes in clinical *Acinetobacter junii* and *Neisseria gonorrhoeae* isolates. Antimicrob Agents Chemother 2000; 44:2503–2506.
46. Roberts MC, Chung WO, Roe D, et al. Erythromycin-resistant *Neisseria gonorrhoeae* and oral commensal *Neisseria* spp. carry known rRNA methylase genes. Antimicrob Agents Chemother 1999; 43:1367–1372.
47. Ng L-K, Martin I, Liu G, Bryden L. Mutation in 23S rRNA associated with macrolide resistance in *Neisseria gonorrhoeae*. Antimicrob Agents Chemother 2002; 46:3020–3025.
48. Johnson SR, Morse SA. Antibiotic resistance in *Neisseria gonorrhoeae*, genetics and mechanisms of resistance. Sex Transm Dis 1988; 15:217–224.
49. Morse SA, Johnson SR, Biddle JW, Roberts MC. High-level tetracycline resistance in *Neisseria gonorrhoeae* is result of acquisition of streptococcal *tet*M determinant. Antimicrob Agents Chemother 1986; 30:664–670.
50. Knapp JS, Johnson SR, Zenilman JM, Roberts MC, Morse SA. High-level tetracycline resistance resulting from TetM in strains of *Neisseria* spp, *Kingella denitrificans*, and *Eikenella corrodens*. Antimicrob Agents Chemother 1988; 32:765–767.
51. Daly CC, Hoffman I, Hobbs M, et al. Development of an antimicrobial susceptibility surveillance system for *Neisseria gonorrhoeae* in Malawi. J Clin Microbiol 1997; 35:2985–2988.
52. Lkhamsuren E, Shultz TR, Limnios EA, Tapsall JW. The antibiotic susceptibility of *Neisseria gonorrhoeae* isolated in Ulaanbaatar, Mongolia. Sex Transm Infect 2001; 77:218–219.
53. West B, Changalucha J, Grooskurth H, et al. Antimicrobial susceptibility, auxotype and plasmid content of *Neisseria gonorrhoeae* in northern Tanzania: emergence of high-level plasmid mediated tetracycline resistance. Genitourin Med 1995; 71:9–12.
54. O'Callaghan CH, Morris A, Kirby SM, Shingler AH. Novel method for detection of β-lactamases by using chromogenic cephalosporin substrate. Antimicrob Agents Chemother 1972; 1:283–288.
55. Livermore DM, Brown DFJ. Detection of β-lactamase-mediated resistance. J Antimicrob Chemother 2001; 48(suppl. S1):59–64.
56. World Health Organization. Bench-Level Manual for Sexually Transmitted Diseases. Geneva, Switzerland: World Health Organization. WHO/VDT/89. 1989, p. 443.
57. National Committee for Clinical Laboratory Standards. Approved Standard: Performance Standards for Antimicrobial Disk Susceptibility Tests. 5th ed. Villanova, PA: National Committee for Clinical Laboratory Standards. 2003 Document M2-A8.
58. King A. Recommendations for susceptibility tests on fastidious organisms and those requiring special handling. J Antimicrob Chemother 2001; 48(suppl.):77–80.
59. Ison CA, Martin DM. Gonorrhoea. In: Morse SA, Ballard R (eds.). Atlas of Sexually Transmitted Diseases. London: Harcourt Health Sciences, 2002, pp. 109–125.

60. Ison CA, Branley NS, Kirtland K, Easmon CSF. Surveillance of antibiotic resistance in clinical isolates of *Neisseria gonorrhoeae*. BMJ 1991; 303:1307.
61. Members of the Australian Gonococcal Surveillance Programme. Penicillin sensitivity of gonococci in Australia: development of Australian gonococcal surveillance programme. Br J Vener Dis 1984; 60:226–230.
62. Ison CA, Martin IMC, London Gonococcal Working Group. Susceptibility of gonococci isolated in London to therapeutic antibiotics: establishment of a London surveillance programme. Sex Transm Infect 1999; 75:107–111.
63. Palmer HM, Leeming JP, Turner A. A multiplex polymerase chain reaction to differentiate β-lactamase plasmids of *Neisseria gonorrhoeae*. J Antimicrob Chemother 2000; 45:777–782.
64. Xia M, Pang Y, Roberts MC. Detection of two groups of 25.2 MDa Tet M plasmids by polymerase chain reaction of the downstream region. Mol Cell Probes 1995; 9:327–332.
65. Ison CA, Tekki N, Gill MJ. Detection of the *tet*M determinant in *Neisseria gonorrhoeae*. Sex Transm Dis 1993; 20:329–333.
66. Deguchi T, Yasuda M, Nakano M, et al. Rapid screening of point mutations of the *Neisseria gonorrhoeae gyr*A gene associated with decreased susceptibilities to quinolones. J Clin Microbiol 1996; 34:2255–2258.
67. Deguchi T, Yasuda M, Nakano M, et al. Rapid screening of point mutations of *Neisseria gonorrhoeae par*C associated with resistance to the quinolones. J Clin Microbiol 1997; 35:948–950.
68. Ng L-K, Sawatzky P, Martin IE, Booth S. Characterisation of ciprofloxacin resistance in *Neisseria gonorrhoeae* isolates in Canada. Sex Transm Dis 2002; 29:780–788.
69. Rahman M, Alam A, Nessa K, et al. Treatment failure with the use of ciprofloxacin for gonorrhea correlates with the prevalence of fluoroquinolone-resistant *Neisseria gonorrhoeae* strains in Bangladesh. Clin Infect Dis 2001; 32:884–889.
70. Ng PP, Chan RK, Ling AE. Gonorrhoea treatment failure and ciprofloxacin resistance. Int J STD AIDS 1998; 9:323–325.
71. O'Mahony C, Timmins D. Treatment failure using double dose ciprofloxacin in a case of highly resistant gonorrhoea. Genitourin Med 1992; 68:274–275.
72. Ison CA, Dillon JR, Tapsall J. The epidemiology of global antibiotic resistance among *Neisseria gonorrhoeae* and *Haemophilus ducreyi*. Lancet 1998; 351(suppl.):8–11.
73. Schwarcz SK, Zenilman JM, Schnell D, et al. National surveillance of antimicrobial resistance in *Neisseria gonorrhoeae*. JAMA 1990; 264:1413–1417.
74. Dillon JR. National microbiological surveillance of the susceptibility of gonococcal isolates to antimicrobial agents. Can J Infect Dis 1992; 3:202–206.
75. Australian Gonococcal Surveillance Program. Penicillin sensitivity of gonococci in Australia: development of Australian gonococcal surveillance program. Genitourin Med 1988; 61:147–151.
76. Van de Laar MJW, van Duynhoven YTPH, Dessens M, van Santen M, van Klingeren B. Surveillance of antibiotic resistance in *Neisseria gonorrhoeae* in the Netherlands, 1997–95. Genitourin Med 1997; 73:510–517.
77. World Health Organization. Global Surveillance Network for Gonococcal Antimicrobial Susceptibility. Geneva, Switzerland: World Health Organization. WHO/VDT/90–452.
78. Mayaud P, West B, Lloyd-Evans N, Seck K. GASP-WAR: West African network to tackle gonorrhoea. Lancet 2002; 359:173.
79. GRASP Steering Group. The Gonococcal Resistance to Antimicrobials Surveillance Programme (GRASP) Year 2000 Report. London: Public Health Laboratory Service, 2001.
80. GRASP Steering Group. The Gonococcal Resistance to Antimicrobials Surveillance Programme (GRASP) Year 2001 Report. London: Public Health Laboratory Service, 2002.

10

Management of Urinary Tract Infections Caused by Multiresistant Organisms

Jeremy M. T. Hamilton-Miller

1. INTRODUCTION

During the 1970s and 1980s, there was much interest in the treatment of urinary tract infections (UTIs). The engine that drove the clinical trials was that many novel antibiotics (e.g., β-lactams and early fluoroquinolones) were being produced, resulting in many phase II and III clinical trials because UTIs, especially complicated infections, proved a good test bed for therapeutic efficacy of these compounds. There were also many protocols designed to develop shortened courses of treatment, typified by a prolonged (but ultimately unsuccessful) dalliance with "single-dose therapy" *(1)*, and investigations into the possible usefulness of antibody-coated bacteria as a marker of upper tract involvement. In recent years, there have been fewer trials because the fewer new compounds becoming available have been mainly for lower respiratory tract infection (e.g., new macrolides and fluoroquinolones) or specifically aimed at multiresistant Gram-positive cocci (e.g., linezolid and quinupristin/dalfopristin), which do not commonly give rise to UTIs. Thus, recent research in this field has mainly consisted of meta-analyses and surveys of resistance and bacterial virulence factors.

1.1. Definitions

It is unfortunate that the two key elements in the topic under discussion in this chapter, namely, *urinary tract infection* and *multiresistant*, have been defined in different ways, leading to the confusing situation of one expert uncertain as to exactly what another means. Under these circumstances, the nonexpert may be completely baffled.

It is important to remember that a UTI is strictly defined in terms of the concentration of pathogenic microorganisms in a specimen (i.e., the laboratory findings are decisive). For many years, the presence of an infection was defined following the criteria laid down by Kass *(2)*: $\geq 10^5$ or more colony forming units per milliliter (CFU/mL) of a midstream urine (MSU) or "clean catch" specimen (two consecutive separate specimens in the case of an asymptomatic patient) or 10^4 CFU/mL in a catheter specimen. This definition was largely adhered to by the British Society of Antimicrobial Chemotherapy *(3)*. However, more recently, definitions have become increasingly complex, and thus more difficult to understand and, most important, to apply in practice.

From: *Management of Multiple Drug-Resistant Infections*
Edited by: S. H. Gillespie © Humana Press Inc., Totowa, NJ

Table 1
Antibiotic Resistance in *Escherichia coli* From Outpatients With Urinary Tract Infections

	Percentage of strains sensitive to antibiotic					
Country and survey year	Ampicillin/ amoxicillin	Coamoxiclav	Trimethoprim cotrimoxazole	Fluoro- quinolone	First-generation cephalosporin	Reference
Israel, 1995	48		69			*68*
Italy, 1996	45	85	70			*69*
United Kingdom, 1997	52	96	76	99	77	*70*
Finland, 1998	70		76	96	93	*70*
Germany/ Austria/ Switzerland	58	86	<70	90	95	*70*
France, 1997	59	63	78	98		*70*
Spain, 1998	70	84	57	70	61	*70*
Latin America, 1997	40	60	43	85	75	*71*
Canada	61	81	85	99	90	*72*
United States, 1996	66		82	>99	72	*73*
United States, 1999			83	98	72	*74*

A joint Infectious Diseases Society of America/Food and Drug Administration (IDSA/FDA) guideline published in 1992 *(4)* produced a scheme that is briefly summarized as follows: $\geq 10^3$ CFU/mL for acute uncomplicated infections in females; $\geq 10^4$ CFU/mL for acute uncomplicated pyelonephritis and in males; $\geq 10^5$ CFU/mL in complicated or recurrent infections and in asymptomatic patients (those who study these guidelines in the original should be aware of the misprints in its crucial Table 1).

Kunin *(5)* disagreed with certain of these recommendations and suggested seven "modified diagnostic criteria." Johnson et al. *(6)* later gave the following definition:

> UTI was defined by the presence in urine of one or more significant organisms, including Gram-negative bacilli, at $\geq 10^2$ cfu/mL (regardless of the presence of other organisms), as well as enterococci or streptococci at $\geq 10^3$ CFU/mL and staphylococci at $\geq 10^4$ CFU/mL, so long as a significant Gram-negative bacillus was not also present and the specimen contained no more than two different Gram-positive organisms.

The main practical problem lies with the largely unquestioning acceptance of the criteria proposed by Stamm et al. *(7)*, namely, that the presence of coliforms in concentrations of 10^2 CFU/mL or higher is a significant finding. Apart from the fact that the original supposed validation of this figure is mathematically questionable (for example, according to the Poisson distribution, a urine specimen containing 10^2 CFU/mL could show "no growth" using the methods described), in many laboratories such low concentrations cannot be detected; for example, automated systems using Multipoint techniques inoculate less than 1 μL of urine.

For resolution of the problems of definition outlined above, one must turn to regulatory criteria. Drugs are licensed for clinical use in certain specific indications at recommended doses; the decision to grant a license depends on performance in clinical trials. Scrutiny of 20 such trials carried out for regulatory purposes in the treatment of UTIs carried out since 1987 (selected at random from my files) involving β-lactams and fluoroquinolones showed that all used a criterion of 10^5 CFU/mL or above. This is the evidence base on which the efficacy of these antibiotics should be judged. As Kunin *(5)* stated: "It is reasonable to assume that anti-infective drugs that eradicate infection in patients who have bacterial counts of $\geq 10^5$ would be equally effective in patients who have lower counts, *but this hypothesis needs to be confirmed*" (italics added).

As yet, this has not been done. Low-count bacteriuria, if indeed such an entity exists, may be a different disease from that generally recognized as UTI; as such, it may respond differently to antibiotics. Indeed, Fihn et al. *(8)* have suggested that it may be more difficult to treat than a typical UTI. This needs to be tested, but further consideration clearly lies outside the scope of this chapter.

The definition of multiresistant offers fewer problems, although it is unfortunately also not clear-cut. Dictionary definitions of *multi* and *multiple* use words such as "several" and "many," which do not give a numerical lower limit. For the purposes of this chapter, a multiresistant organism is assumed to be one that has acquired resistance to more than one antibiotic customarily regarded as active against that species or one such as *Enterococcus* spp, *Pseudomonas aeruginosa*, or *Acinetobacter* spp, which are intrinsically resistant to many of the commonly used antimicrobial agents.

1.2. Antibiotic Resistance in Urinary Pathogens

Ampicillin (or amoxicillin) and trimethoprim (with or without sulfonamide) used to be first-choice antibiotics for the treatment of urinary infections. Over the period of more than 30 yr for which these antibiotics have been available, the susceptibility base has been eroded, mainly because of the transfer of plasmids; now, neither can be regarded as first-line treatment (*see* Table 1). Resistance is now emerging to drugs regarded as second line, such as coamoxiclav and oral cephalosporins, and in some countries (e.g., Spain), the fluoroquinolones also are already becoming less effective. Thus, it is prudent now to regard all urinary pathogens as potentially multiresistant.

2. Antibiotic Treatment of Different Types of UTI

2.1. Urethral Syndrome

Urethral syndrome is a condition found in approx 50% of patients who present to their family doctor with any or all of urinary frequency, dysuria, and urgency, yet no significant bacteriuria can be found. This perplexes and frustrates patient and physician alike as the etiology is multifactorial and obscure *(9)*; thus, the treatment is unsatisfactory. Fortunately, the condition is almost always self-limiting, and patients should be reassured about this.

Microorganisms seem to play a minor role; an early suggestion that lactobacilli were responsible was based on faulty evidence and conclusions *(10)*. If *Ureaplasma urealyticum* or *Mycoplasma hominis* is found, long-term, low-dose macrolides or tetracyclines have been suggested *(11)*. Stamm et al. *(12)* reported doxycycline superior to placebo.

Diagnosis of a microbial cause of the urethral syndrome requires detailed laboratory investigations, notably the examination of segmented urine specimens; presence of larger numbers of organisms in the first voided sample (voided bladder 1, VB_1) than in the MSU from a symptomatic patient might be suggestive. It should be noted that because of the difficulties, especially under family practice conditions, of distinguishing the urethral syndrome from classical "cystitis," many patients for whom this condition recurs will have had repeated courses of antibiotics and thus are likely to harbor multiresistant organisms.

2.2. Infections Confined to the Bladder

2.2.1. Symptomatic

A symptomatic infection confined to the bladder is commonly referred to by patients and physicians as *cystitis*. Although this a useful term because it enables both parties to understand what the other means, it is not strictly correct as there is no inflammation of the bladder wall. As noted in the Section 2.1, symptoms do not distinguish between the urethral syndrome and true bladder infection; thus, culture of an MSU is necessary. Screening for the presence of nitrite and pyuria using an appropriate dipstick is particularly useful both in the laboratory and in the family doctor's office. In the latter venue, positive results of both tests from an MSU are highly suggestive of a significant bacteriuria and call for the empirical prescription of an antibiotic.

In the United Kingdom, ampicillin or trimethoprim have been the most widely used compounds for such "best guess" use; in the United States, cotrimoxazole has been preferred. However, the gradual buildup over the years of resistance to these compounds has necessitated a change in prescribing practice. Thus, in many locations, urinary pathogens, even those causing an isolated episode in uncomplicated circumstances (e.g., in a 25-yr-old female with no previous history) must be regarded as potentially multiresistant. An oral cephalosporin (e.g., cefaclor), coamoxiclav, or nitrofurantoin (in the delayed-release formulation) would be an appropriate choice. Naturally, in regions where resistance levels are known to be lower (i.e., $\leq 10\%$), trimethoprim may be used empirically.

In the United States, the recommendation of the IDSA *(13)* was to use cotrimoxazole unless the proportion of resistance is more than 10–20%; this figure was later refined, on cost-efficiency grounds, to more than 20% *(14)*. Otherwise, a fluoroquinolone should be used. Three days of treatment is generally regarded as sufficient; it should be noted that, following this regimen, inhibitory concentrations of antibiotic will remain in the urine even on the fifth day because of the long half-life of trimethoprim and the great intrinsic activity of the fluoroquinolones. Norfloxacin, on scientific grounds, is the fluoroquinolone of choice for the treatment of urinary infections, although ciprofloxacin seems to be very widely used.

If infections are recurrent, culture of an MSU is mandatory to obtain information about resistance patterns. These patients will have received multiple courses of antibiotics in the recent past, and the infecting organisms are much more likely to show resistance. Considerable guidance can be obtained from past records and should show whether the recurrences tend to be reinfections or relapses. Again, an oral first-generation cephalosporin, coamoxiclav, nitrofurantoin, or a fluoroquinolone would be a suitable choice. Management of recurrent infections is discussed in Section 2.5.

In infants and young children, the American Academy of Pediatrics *(15)* suggests parenteral treatment (a first- or third-generation cephalosporin, an aminoglycoside, ampicillin, or ticarcillin) for 24–48 h, followed by a switch to oral amoxicillin, cotrimoxazole, or a cephalosporin. The recommendation is that the course should be continued for 7–14 d. Two recent meta-analyses *(16,17)* showed that cure rates after "short course" (from one dose to 4 d) treatment were significantly lower than following a "standard course" (5 to 14 d).

In the elderly, urinary infections are generally regarded as complicated *(18,19)*. Treatment for 7–14 d for symptomatic infections is recommended.

It is surprising that little effort has been made to discover which treatment results in the most rapid relief of symptoms because this is what is the greatest concern to the patient. Symptoms have usually disappeared after 3 d, which is one good reason for limiting the length of treatment to this period because patients are unlikely to continue treatment when symptoms have abated. There appear to be only three studies in which this question was addressed *(20–22)*; these showed, respectively, that enoxacin was better than cefuroxime axetil, coamoxiclav was better than cotrimoxazole, and pefloxacin was better than norfloxacin.

2.2.2. *Asymptomatic*

In pregnancy, most urinary infections are asymptomatic; the reason for this phenomenon is unknown. Pregnancy *per se* does not seem to be a factor predisposing to infection, but as there are possible deleterious consequences to both mother and fetus, it is important to detect infections and treat them. Unlike the situation for symptomatic infections, for which choice of antibiotic must be empirical, initiation of treatment in pregnancy can await the receipt of results of sensitivity testing. A 7-d course of ampicillin is the preferred choice, with an oral cephalosporin, nitrofurantoin, or a sulfonamide as alternatives if the infecting strain is resistant *(23)*. A meta-analysis *(24)* showed that treatment of asymptomatic bacteriuria during pregnancy reduced the incidence of pyelonephritis, of preterm delivery, and of low birth weight babies.

There is controversy as to whether it is necessary to treat asymptomatic infections in patients who are not pregnant. At one extreme, "covert" bacteriuria is regarded as beneficial, protecting the bladder from invasion by a more virulent strain *(25)*; at the other extreme, it is seen as a stepping-stone toward symptomatic bacteriuria. It was our policy at the Urinary Infection Clinic at the Royal Free Hospital (referred to hereafter as the RFH clinic) to treat asymptomatic infections that had been correctly diagnosed (i.e., if two separate MSUs yielded $\geq 10^5$ CFU/mL) in patients with a history of recurrent infections. It was also found that many patients reported feeling very much better following such treatment, underlining the difficulty of defining *asymptomatic* because individuals are known to have widely varying discomfort thresholds. Asymptomatic infections can be treated in exactly the same way as symptomatic ones, but with the advantage that selection of antibiotic can be according to the result of sensitivity testing rather than an empirical decision.

In the elderly, infections commonly are asymptomatic, and most authorities suggest that treatment is useless as there will almost inevitably be recurrences. Despite this advice, treatment is often given (*see* ref. *26* and references cited therein). However, it should be remembered that presentation of UTI in the elderly may be atypical (e.g., as confusion, reduced ability to cope, or incontinence) *(27)*, and that these effects can be reversed by treatment, with benefit to both the patient and the caregivers. It is surprising that there are no trials of antibiotic prophylaxis in the elderly to solve the important problem of whether lasting benefit can accrue by keeping the urine uninfected; at the RFH clinic prophylaxis was effective in ambulatory patients up to the age of 90 yr.

The whole question of the cause of symptoms in UTI is unexplained despite much research, so gauging their importance is more difficult. There seems to be no correlation between any virulence factor and the severity of symptoms produced. The simplistic and widely accepted explanation that symptoms are caused by an acidic urine is certainly untrue *(28)*: relief gained by drinking solutions of sodium or potassium citrate is untested by clinical trial and, if it occurs, may well be the result of water loading *(29)*.

2.3. *Pyelonephritis*

Infections of the upper urinary tract may not always be accompanied by symptoms regarded as typical (e.g., fever, rigors, loin pain, sweating, vomiting, accompanied by significant bacteriuria and pyuria). As many as 50% of cases of apparent cystitis may be associated with upper tract involvement.

Many patients with pyelonephritis present to the emergency department extremely ill, and once the diagnosis has been made, antibiotic treatment must clearly be started on an empirical basis. This must assume that a resistant pathogen is present. For many years, a combination of ampicillin and gentamicin was recommended, although as late as 1991, this had not been evaluated in a published study *(30)*. By that time, resistance to ampicillin was becoming so common that this regimen in most cases amounted to monotherapy.

Bergeron *(31)* remarked, in view of failure rates of 25–60% reported in various antibiotic trials, "A close look at the available data is disturbing." He suggested that, because the infecting bacteria are protected in the renal medulla, bactericidal levels at the site of infection are necessary, and he preferred fluoroquinolones and aminoglycosides to β-lactams. Sandberg et al. *(32)*, using circumstantial evidence, attributed the high recurrence rate observed following treatment with β-lactams (both penicillins and cephalosporins) to a failure to eradicate the infecting organism from the vaginal flora, leading to an increased chance of relapse.

There is agreement, without much evidence, that treatment should last at least 10 d and maybe up to 20 d *(33)*, although there have been suggestions that this period can be shortened to 5 d *(34,35)*. A recent clinical trial showed that a 7-d course of ciprofloxacin *(36)* resulted in a 90% cure rate when assessed at 22–48 d.

Only the first few days of a course of treatment have to be parenteral; patients feel better very quickly, and many can be discharged after 2 or 3 d to continue treatment orally with an appropriate antibiotic (e.g., ciprofloxacin, cotrimoxazole, or cefixime), depending on the sensitivity of the infecting organisms, which by that time will have been established. This management strategy, "switch therapy," is cost-effective as well as convenient for the patient *(37)*.

Notwithstanding this discussion, it is clear that not all patients with pyelonephritis require intravenous therapy; patients not seriously ill (no severe sepsis, obstruction, or renal foci) respond equally well to treatment by mouth *(38)*. Millar et al. *(39)*, in a trial of β-lactam antibiotics for pyelonephritis during pregnancy, showed that outpatient

Table 2
Etiology of Complicated Urinary Tract Infections (n = 838 patients)

Causal organism	Incidence (%)
Escherichia coli	48.9%
Klebsiella spp	17.2
Pseudomonas aeruginosa	6.2
Proteus mirabilis	6
Enterobacter spp	4.1
Citrobacter spp	3.5
Staphylococci	2.9
Enterococci	2.8
Morganella morganii	2.2
Serratia spp	2.2
Other Gram negatives[a]	3.1
Group B streptococci	1.6

Source: From refs. *75–78*.
[a]Other than those named here.

treatment with intravenous ceftriaxone followed by cephalexin was as effective as inpatient treatment with intravenous cefazolin followed by cephalexin; they concluded that not only did the former management offer substantial cost-saving, but also it prevented separation of women from their families.

It is important to monitor the progress of treatment by examining an MSU taken 1 to 2 d after treatment initiation; the presence of even low numbers of bacteria in such a specimen, which will contain high concentrations of antibiotic, suggests that the infection is likely to persist when treatment has stopped *(35)*.

2.4. Complicated Infections

Definitions of a complicated infection vary somewhat, but one widely accepted is that it is a UTI in the presence of a catheter or if there are anatomical or other abnormalities of the tract. The abnormalities may include residual urine (>100 mL when the patient has finished voiding); obstruction (e.g., by a tumor, stone, or hypertrophic prostate); reflux; reduced renal function; or kidney transplant. Complicated UTI is more common in elderly females, and UTI in males is by definition complicated *(4)*.

Causal organisms are often other than *Escherichia coli* (Table 2) because predisposing factors allow species not specifically equipped to colonize and infect the urinary tract (e.g., *Staphylococcus epidermidis* and enterococci) to gain a foothold and multiply. As recurrence is a feature in such patients, they will have received many courses of antibiotics in the past, and their infecting organisms are thus likely to be multiresistant. Further, many cases of complicated UTI will have been nosocomially acquired and thus be caused by organisms that have survived in the hospital environment by virtue of acquiring resistance.

A wide variety of antibiotics has been used in the treatment of complicated UTI, often in the context of phase III studies of novel agents (*see* Section 1.). Provided the infecting organism is sensitive, no particular agent has proved better than another (*see*, e.g., data for several trials involving ciprofloxacin, ofloxacin, ceftazidime, ceftriaxone, and imipenem/cilastatin and numerous comparators in refs. *40–44)*.

Thus, in day-to-day practice, the antibiotic most commonly used will be, according to the formulary of the particular hospital, a fluoroquinolone (e.g., ciprofloxacin), a third-generation cephalosporin (e.g., cefotaxime or ceftriaxone), or an aminoglycoside (e.g., gentamicin). Clearly, the choice of treatment in each specific instance must be guided absolutely by results of sensitivity testing, so vancomycin might be necessary for an enterococcus, or a fourth-generation cephalosporin such as cefepime would be used if an *Enterobacter* sp is responsible.

As expected, cure rates are dependent on the type of underlying abnormality, and if meaningful results are to be obtained from comparative clinical trials, it is essential that appropriately matched and well-described groups are tested. Late follow-up MSUs (i.e., 4 wk after the end of treatment) are essential as a test of cure as recurrence will be often observed; this is because the factors that make for a complicated scenario are also predisposing factors, underlying again that the defense mechanisms of the urinary tract against infection are predominantly mechanical.

Although clearly one of the objectives in managing complicated UTI is the ultimate reversal of any predisposing factors, with the exception of removing a catheter, this is difficult to achieve in practice. During 18 yr of experience in the RFH clinic more than 1000 patients were seen, about 30% of whom had a predisposing factor; many were referred for possible surgical intervention to correct abnormalities, but with very few exceptions, this was only possible in the case of stone removal.

Intuitively, it would be expected that a longer course of treatment would be required for complicated than for simple UTI, and recommendations are for a duration of 7–14 d. However, the evidence base for this is very slight, and it may well be that shorter courses would be equally effective.

2.5. *Management of Recurrence*

Recurring UTIs are either relapses (the original infecting organism reappears) or reinfections (a new organism causes an infection). It can be argued that relapses suggest a failure to eradicate the original organism, in which case more intensive treatment (a higher dose for a longer period) may be effective. On the other hand, a reinfection may imply some deficit in the patient's defense mechanisms. Notwithstanding such possible differences, many recurrences can be prevented using appropriate antimicrobial prophylaxis, whether or not a patient appears to have predisposing factors.

This management strategy is based on maintaining an antibacterial barrier in the bladder urine or eliminating potentially uropathogenic organisms (i.e., coliforms) from the gut flora for periods of up to 1 yr. The most widely used agents for this purpose have been antifolates *(45)* and nitrofurantoin *(46)*; however, with the increasing rates of resistance to trimethoprim, this agent is rapidly losing its value. Nitrofurantoin has remained effective, with breakthroughs because of intrinsically resistant species (e.g., *Proteus* spp or *Pseudomonas aeruginosa*) very unusual. Alternatives are a first-generation cephalosporin or fluoroquinolone. Methenamine salts, which generate formaldehyde in the bladder provided the urine is kept sufficiently acidic, are less effective.

Table 3
Schedule of Specimens Required for Diagnosis of Bacterial Prostatitis

Specimen	Description
Urine, voided bladder 1 (VB_1)	First 10 mL (urethral washout)
Urine, VB_2	Midstream specimen
Expressed prostatic excretion	Fluid produced after prostatic massage
Urine, VB_3	First 10 mL after prostatic massage

It is essential not to start such long-term, low-dose prophylaxis until the urine has been rendered sterile by a conventional course of treatment. Follow-up at intervals by culture of MSU and rectal swab is recommended. Breakthrough infections should be treated in accordance with results of sensitivity tests, and prophylaxis should be restarted as soon as the infection has been cured. Over 70% of patients benefit from this type of regimen, and most of these recurrences cease when patients stop taking prophylaxis after 12 mo.

Self-administered antibiotics are advocated by some *(47,48)*, but at the RFH clinic we preferred the highly effective and inexpensive strategy of long-term prophylaxis because this can be instituted and monitored by the patient's family doctor without the need to attend the hospital *(46,49)*.

There is often terminological confusion between (low-dose) prophylactic use of antibiotics described here and the suppressive use. There are two important differences: In prophylaxis, a low dose is used (typically, one-quarter of the therapeutic dose daily); starting with a sterile urine, the aim is to maintain the status quo. Suppression describes the taking of antibiotics in full dose continuously in the face of an otherwise uncontrollable infection, such as may occur in the presence of a stone, with the object of keeping the bacterial population under control as much as possible. It is clearly very important to monitor at regular intervals the infecting organism for resistance to the suppressive antibiotic used.

2.6. *Prostatitis*

The proper management of prostatitis has been bedeviled over the years by inadequate diagnosis. Thus, much of the literature is confusing and actually misleading.

It is essential to appreciate that there are four different types of prostatitis, only two of which have a microbiological etiology *(50)*. Discussion of the other two types, nonbacterial prostatitis and prostatodynia, is beyond the scope of this chapter.

Diagnosis of infective prostatitis requires close collaboration among physician, microbiologist, and patient because the production and analysis of segmented urine specimens must be carried out (Table 3). After culture of the four specimens on appropriate media, bacterial prostatitis can be confirmed if the bacterial density in expressed prostatic excretion (EPS) and VB_3 exceeds that in VB_1, most convincingly if by a factor of 10. A UTI often accompanies bacterial prostatitis, which can confuse the issue, because VB_2 (the MSU) will then contain a high concentration of bacteria.

Table 4
Etiological Agents in Prostatitis

Escherichia coli	80%
Pseudomonas aeruginosa, Serratia spp, *Klebsiella* spp, *Proteus* spp	10–15%
Enterococci	5–10%
Staphylococci	Occasionally
Other causes: Gonococci, *Mycobacterium tuberculosis, Salmonella* spp, clostridia, parasites, yeasts, fungi have been reported	
Suggested but unproven: chlamydia, mycoplasmas	

Adapted from ref. *79*.

Under these circumstances, a short course of treatment should be administered with an antibiotic that does not penetrate the prostate (*see* discussion in this section below), such as ampicillin or nitrofurantoin, and that is active against the organisms in VB_2; the test is repeated after 2 or 3 d. It is not uncommon to find a mixed infection, most commonly with Gram-negative rods and enterococci, some or all of which may be multiresistant. There are numerous other uncommon, and in some cases suggested but as yet unproven, microbial causes (Table 4). It is unfortunate that often a diagnosis of prostatitis is made by urologists without the appropriate microbiological evidence *(51)*.

Treatment of acute prostatitis is relatively simple because there is an inflammatory response that allows antibiotics to penetrate the normally impervious prostate. Meares *(50)* recommended ampicillin (to cover enterococci) plus gentamicin, followed by a switch to appropriate, culture-specific, oral therapy, with a total course of 30 d. This length of treatment ensures eradication of the infecting organisms and reduces the chance of establishing a chronic infection.

On the other hand, treatment of chronic bacterial prostatitis has disappointing results. This is to some extent a consequence of the nature of the infecting organisms, but mainly because of the difficulties in obtaining adequate antibiotic concentrations at the site of infection in the absence of the brisk inflammatory response found in the acute form. A further complication is the common occurrence of prostatic stones *(52)*, which may harbor bacteria in their interstices and thus act as a nidus for reinfection.

A considerable amount of pharmacokinetic work has been done to study antibiotic access to the prostate *(53)*, much using the dog model, but this can be misleading because in normal dogs the prostatic secretions are acidic ($pH \leq 6.4$); in men with chronic bacterial prostatitis, secretions were found *(54)* to be alkaline (about pH 8.4). However, it is clear that many antibiotics, such as penicillins, cephalosporins, and aminoglycosides, usually used for treatment of infections caused by Gram-negative bacteria penetrate very poorly and thus fail to eradicate the infection. However, as such antibiotics will often cure, at least temporarily, the concomitant UTI, this may be reported by some as success. This is an example of the misleading information available on this topic.

Before the introduction of the fluoroquinolones, only trimethoprim was effective in chronic prostatitis; the cure rate was only about 30–40%, with courses of cotrimoxazole lasting 4–16 wk *(50)*. Fluoroquinolones are now the drugs of choice and are given in full dosage for at least 1 mo and sometimes longer; cure rates of 60–90% have been reported *(55)*. In some cases, the infection cannot be controlled, and suppressive treatment (discussed in Section 2.5.) is indicated. Surgical intervention may be necessary as a last resort.

2.7. Catheter-Associated Infections

The interpretation of microbiological results from catheter specimen urines (CSUs) is one of the most difficult laboratory problems presenting to the medical microbiologist. The first confounding factor is the assumption that the specimen has been correctly taken (i.e., from the sampling port as fresh-flowing urine rather than from the bag). Next, a catheter will become colonized, usually with several microbial species, after a few days, and thus the CSU will give mixed growth. Third, biofilm forms on the catheter surface *(56)*, which contains a sessile mixed culture embedded in glycocalyx. Thus, the flora of the CSU (the planktonic moiety) does not necessarily represent the entire resident flora of the catheter. The fact that many patients with catheters are incidentally receiving antibiotics excreted in the urine also blurs the picture.

The general rule is for watchful waiting and close liaison with the clinician; in particular, the presence and sensitivity patterns of such resistant species as *Pseudomonas aeruginosa* and *Candida* should be noted. If a symptomatic episode with positive blood culture occurs, this information can be very helpful in deciding on immediate empirical antibiotic treatment, which would usually be with an aminoglycoside, third-generation cephalosporin, or fluoroquinolone, depending on local practice.

Persistent colonization of the catheter with *Candida* spp in at-risk patients should be handled by bladder washout with either amphotericin B solution or oral fluconazole.

Much experience has occurred in specialist centers, particularly those with a catheter care team, and much can be learned from this *(57)*, chiefly in terms of prevention.

3. ALTERNATIVES TO ANTIBIOTICS

First-line antibiotics (*see* Section 1.2.) are now of limited usefulness, and second-line agents are now the empirical drugs of choice. There are ominous signs that, in some locations, resistance is now also making serious inroads into the latter, for the time being leaving only fluoroquinolones and nitrofurantoin as viable oral agents in some cases. This situation has encouraged the exploration of ways that the use of antibiotics can be minimized by preventive interventions.

SolcoUrovac is a vaccine comprised of heat-killed bacteria representative of those commonly causing UTIs. It has been used intravaginally and intramuscularly in phase II trials to prevent recurrent infections. Results so far are encouraging *(58,59)*. Another vaccine, UroVaxom or Uro-Munal, consisting of proteins extracted from *E. coli* administered orally, has been reported to be effective in preventing symptomatic infections in female adults and children *(60,61)*.

The use of probiotics (*Lactobacillus rhamnosus* GR-1 and *L. fermentum* RC-14), applied topically to the vagina, has been suggested *(62)*, and some success in preventing recurrent infections was claimed in pilot studies. The strategy here is to prevent colonization of the vagina by uropathogenic coliforms, thereby removing this reservoir of potentially infecting organisms. It should be noted that probiotic strains commonly used for other purposes (e.g., *Lactobacillus* strain GG) are not necessarily suitable for the prevention of UTI *(62,63)*.

Cranberry juice has been popularized as prophylaxis for recurrent UTI based on the ability of the proanthocyanidin component to inhibit adherence of P-fimbriate *E. coli* to uroepithelial cells. Although modest beneficial effects of consuming adequate amounts of cranberry juice have been demonstrated in specific patient groups *(63,64)*, doubt has been expressed concerning the mechanisms *(65,66)*.

4. CONCLUSIONS

As Kunin *(67)* pointed out, most of the scientific groundwork used today for the rational diagnosis and treatment of UTI was laid 40 yr ago. There may be answers now to why some patients are more susceptible than others and why some bacterial strains have greater uropathogenicity than others, but there is no response to the gradual whittling away of useful antibiotics. In terms of practical patient management, this is the most fundamental problem now facing the medical community and related disciplines, and it is one that we fail to address at our peril.

REFERENCES

1. Bailey RR. Single Dose Therapy of Urinary Tract Infections. Sydney, Australia: ADIS Health Science Press, 1983.
2. Kass EH. Asymptomatic infections of the urinary tract. Trans Am Assoc Phys 1956; 69: 56–63.
3. Report. The clinical evaluation of antibacterial drugs. J Antimicrob Chemother 1989; 23(suppl. B):1–39.
4. Rubin RH, Shapiro ED, Andriole VT, Davis RJ, Stamm WE. Evaluation of new anti-infective drugs for the treatment of urinary tract infection. Clin Infect Dis 1992; 15(suppl. 1):S216–S227.
5. Kunin CM. Guidelines for the evaluation of new anti-infective drugs for the treatment of urinary tract infection: additional considerations. Clin Infect Dis 1992; 15:1041–1044.
6. Johnson JR, Tiu FS, Stamm WE. Direct antimicrobial susceptibility testing for acute urinary tract infections in women. J Clin Microbiol 1995; 33:2316–2323.
7. Stamm WE, Counts GW, Running KR, Fihn S, Turck M, Holmes KK. Diagnosis of coliform infections in acutely dysuric women. N Engl J Med 1982; 307:463–468.
8. Fihn S, Johnson C, Stamm WE. *Escherichia coli* urethritis in women with symptoms of acute urinary tract infection. J Infect Dis 1988; 157:196–199.
9. Hamilton-Miller JMT. The urethral syndrome and its management. J Antimicrob Chemother 1994; 33(suppl. A):63–73.
10. Hamilton-Miller JMT, Brumfitt W, Smith GW. Are fastidious organisms an important cause of dysuria and frequency? The case against. In: Asscher AW, Brumfitt W (eds.). Microbial Diseases in Nephrology. Chichester, UK: Wiley, 1986, pp. 19–30.
11. Cardozo L. Postmenopausal cystitis. BMJ 1996; 313:129.
12. Stamm WE, Running K, McKevitt M, Counts GW, Turck M, Holmes KK. Treatment of the acute urethral syndrome. N Engl J Med 1981; 304:956–958.
13. Warren JW, Abrutyn E, Hebel JR, Johnson JR, Schaeffer A. Guidelines for antimicrobial treatment of uncomplicated acute bacterial cystitis and acute pyelonephritis in women. Clin Infect Dis 1999; 29:745–759.
14. Le TP, Miller LG. Empirical therapy for uncomplicated urinary tract infections in an era of increasing antimicrobial resistance: a decision and cost analysis. Clin Infect Dis 2001; 33: 615–621.
15. American Academy of Pediatrics. Practice parameter: the diagnosis, treatment, and evaluation of the initial urinary tract infection in febrile infants and young children. Pediatrics 1999; 103:843–852.

16. Tran D, Muchant DG, Asronoff SC. Short-course versus conventional length antimicrobial therapy for uncomplicated lower urinary tract infections in children: a meta-analysis of 1279 patients. J Pediatr 2001; 139:93–99.
17. Keren R, Chan E. A meta-analysis of randomized, controlled trials comparing short- and long-course antibiotic therapy for urinary tract infections in children. Pediatrics 2002; 109:e70. Available at: http://www.pediatrics.org/cgi/content/full/109ts/e70.
18. Nicolle LE. A practical guide to the management of complicated urinary tract infection. Drugs 1997; 53:583–592. Accessed September 12, 2002.
19. Nicolle LE. A practical guide to antimicrobial management of complicated urinary tract infection. Drugs Aging 2001; 18:243–254.
20. Brumfitt W, Hamilton-Miller JMT, Walker S. Enoxacin relieves symptoms of recurrent urinary infections more rapidly than cefuroxime axetil. Antimicrob Agents Chemother 1993; 37:1558–1559.
21. Fancourt GJ, Matts SGF, Mitchell CJ. Augmentin (amoxycillin–clavulanic acid) compared with co-trimoxazole in urinary tract infections. BMJ 1984; 289:82–83.
22. Guibert J, Mazeman E, Colau LC, Delavault, P. Cystite aigue chez la femme de plus de 50 ans: efficacite de la pefloxacine en dose unique et de la norfloxacine prescrite pendant 10 jours. Press Med 1993:22:288–292.
23. Ovalle A, Levancini M. Urinary tract infections in pregnancy. Curr Opin Urol 2001; 11: 55–59.
24. Smaill F. Antibiotics for asymptomatic bacteriuria in pregnancy. Cochrane Data Syst Rev 2000; 2:CD000490.
25. Asscher AW, Chick S, Radford N, et al. Natural history of asymptomatic bacteriuria in non-pregnant women. In: Brumfitt W, Asscher AW (eds.). Urinary Tract Infection. London: Oxford University Press, 1973, pp. 51–61.
26. Walker S, McGeer A, Simor AE, Armstrong-Evans M, Loeb M. Why are antibiotics prescribed for asymptomatic bacteriuria in institutionalized elderly people? Can Med Assoc J 2000; 163:273–277.
27. Choudhury SL, Brocklehurst JC. Urinary infections in the elderly. In: Brumfitt W, Hamilton-Miller JMT, Bailey RR (eds.). Urinary Tract Infections. London: Chapman and Hall, 1998, pp. 229–243.
28. Brumfitt W, Hamilton-Miller JMT, Cooper J, Raeburn A. Relationship of urinary pH to symptoms of "cystitis." Postgrad Med J 1990; 66:727–729.
29. Gargan RA, Hamilton-Miller JMT, Brumfitt W. Effect of alkalinisation and increased fluid intake on bacterial phagocytosis and killing in urine. Eur J Clin Microbiol Infect Dis 1993; 12:534–539.
30. Johnson JR, Lyons MF, Pearce W, et al. Therapy for women hospitalized with acute pyelonephritis: a randomized trial of ampicillin versus trimethoprim-sulfamethoxazole for 14 days. J Infect Dis 1991; 163:325–330.
31. Bergeron MG. Treatment of pyelonephritis in adults. Med Clin North Am 1995; 79:619–649.
32. Sandberg T, Alestig K, Eilard T, et al. Aminoglycosides do not improve the efficacy of cephalosporins for treatment of acute pyelonephritis in women. Scand J Infect Dis 1997; 29:175–179.
33. Myrier A, Guibert J. Diagnosis and drug treatment of acute pyelonephritis. Drugs 1992; 44:356–367.
34. Bailey RR, Peddie BA. Treatment of acute urinary tract infection in women. Ann Intern Med 1987; 107:430.
35. Kincaid-Smith P. Acute pyelonephritis. In: Brumfitt W, Hamilton-Miller JMT, Bailey RR (eds.). Urinary Tract Infections. London: Chapman and Hall 1998, pp. 281–292.
36. Talan DA, Stamm WE, Hooton TM, et al. Comparison of ciprofloxacin (7 days) and trimethoprim-sulfamethoxazole (14 days) for acute uncomplicated pyelonephritis in women. JAMA 2000; 283:1583–1590.

37. Hamilton-Miller JMT. Switch therapy: the theory and practice of early change from parenteral to non-parenteral antibiotic administration. Clin Microbiol Infect 1996; 2:12–19.
38. Mombelli G, Pezzoli R, Pinoja-Lutz G, Monotti R, Marone C, Franciolli M. Oral versus intravenous ciprofloxacin in the initial empirical management of severe pyelonephritis or complicated urinary tract infections. Arch Intern Med 1999; 159:53–58.
39. Millar LK, Wing DA, Paul RH, Grimes DA. Outpatient treatment of pyelonephritis on pregnancy: a randomized controlled trial. Obstet Gynecol 1995; 86:560–564.
40. Wilson APR, Gruneberg RN. Ciprofloxacin: 10 Years of Clinical Experience. Oxford, UK: Maxim Medical, 1997.
41. Monk JP, Campoli-Richards DM. Ofloxacin: a review of its antibacterial activity, pharmacokinetic properties and therapeutic use. Drugs 1987; 33:346–391.
42. Rains CP, Bryson HM, Peters DH. Ceftazidime: an update of its antibacterial activity, pharmacokinetic properties and therapeutic efficacy. Drugs 1995; 49:577–617.
43. Davis R, Bryson HM. Ceftriaxone: a pharmacoeconomic evaluation of its use in the treatment of serious infections. PharmacoEconomics 1994; 6:249–269.
44. Clissold SP, Todd PA, Campoli-Richards DM. Imipenem/cilastatin: a review of its antibacterial activity, pharmacokinetic properties and therapeutic efficacy. Drugs 1987; 33:183–241.
45. Nicolle LE, Ronald AR. Recurrent urinary tract infection and its prevention. In: Brumfitt W, Hamilton-Miller JMT, Bailey RR (eds.). Urinary Tract Infections. London: Chapman and Hall, 1998, pp. 293–301.
46. Brumfitt W, Hamilton-Miller JMT. Efficacy and safety profile of long-term nitrofurantoin in urinary infections: 18 years' experience. J Antimicrob Chemother 1998; 42:363–371.
47. Schaeffer AJ, Stuppy BA. Efficacy and safety of self-start therapy in women with recurrent urinary tract infections. J Urol 1999; 161:207–211.
48. Gupta K, Hooton TM, Roberts PL, Stamm WE. Patient-initiated treatment of uncomplicated recurrent urinary tract infections in young women. Ann Intern Med 2001; 135:9–16.
49. Brumfitt W, Hamilton-Miller JMT. Prophylactic antibiotics for recurrent urinary tract infections. J Antimicrob Chemother 1990; 25:505–512.
50. Meares EM. Prostatitis: diagnosis, aetiology and management. In: Brumfitt W, Hamilton-Miller JMT, Bailey RR (eds.). Urinary Tract Infections. London: Chapman and Hall, 1998, pp. 217–228.
51. Collins MMcN, Fowler FJ, Elliott DB, Albertsen PC, Barry MJ. Diagnosing and treating chronic prostatitis: do urologists use the four-glass test? Urology 2000; 55:403–407.
52. Peeling WB, Griffiths GJ. Imaging of the prostate by ultrasound. J Urol 1984; 132:217–224.
53. Sharer WC, Fair WR. The pharmacokinetics of antibiotic diffusion in chronic bacterial prostatitis. Prostate 1982; 3:139–148.
54. Fair WR, Crane DB, Schiller N, Heston WDW. Reappraisal of treatment in chronic bacterial prostatitis. J Urol 1979; 121:437–441.
55. Lipsky BA. Prostatitis and urinary infection in men: what's new, what's true? Am J Med 1999; 106:327–334.
56. Donlan RM. Biofilm formation: a clinically relevant microbiological process. Clin Infect Dis 2001; 33:1387–1392.
57. Pearman JW. Catheter care. In: Brumfitt W, Hamilton-Miller JMT, Bailey RR (eds.). Urinary Tract Infections. London: Chapman and Hall, 1998, pp. 303–316.
58. Uehling DT, Hopkins WJ, Beierle LM, Kryger JV, Heisey DM. Vaginal mucosal immunization for recurrent urinary tract infection: extended phase II clinical trial. J Infect Dis 2001; 183(suppl. 1):S81–S83.
59. Nayir A, Emre S, Sirin A, Bulut A. The effects of vaccination with inactivated uropathogenic bacteria in recurrent urinary tract infections of children. Vaccine 1995; 13:987–990.

60. Schulman CC, Corbusier A, Michiels H, Taezner HJ. Oral immunotherapy of recurrent urinary tract infections: a double-blind placebo-controlled multicenter study. J Urol 1993; 150:917–921.
61. Lettgen B. Prevention of recurrent urinary tract infections in female children. Curr Ther Res 1996; 57:464–475.
62. Reid G, Bruce AW. Selection of *Lactobacillus* strains for urogenital probiotic applications. J Infect Dis 2001; 183(suppl. 1):S77–S80.
63. Kontiokari T, Sundqvist K, Nuutinen M, Pokka T, Koskela M, Uhari M. Randomised trial of cranberry-ligonberry juice and *Lactobacillus* GG drink for the prevention of urinary tract infections in women. BMJ 2001; 322:1571–1573.
64. Avorn J, Monane M, Gurwitz JH, Glynn RJ, Choodnovskiy I, Lipsitz LA. Reduction of bacteriuria and pyuria after ingestion of cranberry juice. JAMA 1994; 271:751–754.
65. Hamilton-Miller JMT. Reduction of bacteriuria and pyuria using cranberry juice. JAMA 1994; 272:588.
66. Dearing MD, Appel HM, Schultz JC. Why do cranberries reduce incidence of urinary tract infections? J Ethnopharmacol 2002; 80:211.
67. Kunin CM. Perspectives of a long-time observer. J Infect Dis 2001; 183(suppl. 1):S9–S11.
68. Weber G, Riesenberg K, Schlaeffer F, Peled N, Borer A, Yagupsky P. Changing trends in frequency and antimicrobial resistance of urinary pathogens in outpatient clinics and a hospital in Southern Israel, 1991–1995. Eur J Clin Microbiol Infect Dis 1997; 16:834–838.
69. Fanos V, Khoory BJ. Antimicrobial survey of urinary tract isolates from a pediatric department. J Chemother 1999; 11:255–259.
70. Felmingham D, Arakawa S. Resistance among urinary pathogens: experience outside the USA. Clin Drug Invest 2001; 21(suppl. 1):7–11.
71. Sader HS, Jones RN, Winokur PL, et al. Antimicrobial susceptibility of bacteria causing urinary tract infections in Latin American hospitals: results from the SENTRY Antimicrobial Surveillance Program (1997). Clin Microbiol Infect 1999; 5:478–487.
72. Blondeau JM, Vaughan D. A review of antimicrobial resistance in Canada. Can J Microbiol 2000; 46:867–877.
73. Gupta K, Scholes D, Stamm WE. Increasing prevalence of antimicrobial resistance among uropathogens causing acute complicated cystitis in women. JAMA 1999; 281:736–738.
74. Karlowski JA, Jones ME, Thornsberry C, Critchley I, Kelly LJ, Sahm DF. Prevalence of antimicrobial resistance among urinary tract pathogens isolated from female outpatients across the US in 1999. Int J Antimicrob Agents 2001; 18:121–127.
75. Cox CE, Holloway WJ, Geckler RW. A multicenter comparative study of meropenem and imipenem/cilastatin in the treatment of complicated urinary tract infections in hospitalized patients. Clin Infect Dis 1995; 21:86–92.
76. Klimberg IW, Cox CE, Fowler CL, King W, Kim SS, Callery-D'Amico S. A controlled trial of levofloxacin and lomefloxacin in the treatment of complicated urinary tract infection. Urology 1998; 51:610–615.
77. Pittman W, Moon JO, Hamrick LC, Cox CE, Clark J, Childs S, Pizzuti D, Fredericks J, St Clair P. Randomized double-blind trial of high- and low-dose fleroxacin versus norfloxacin for complicated urinary tract infection. Am J Med 1993; 94(suppl. 3A):101S–104S.
78. Gottlieb PL. Comparison of enoxacin versus trimethoprim-sulfamethoxazole in the treatment of patients with complicated urinary tract infection. Clin Ther 1995; 17:493–502.
79. Roberts RO, Lieber MM, Bostwick DG, Jacobsen SJ. A review of clinical and pathological prostatitis syndromes. Urology 1997; 49:809–821.

11

Management of Multiple Drug-Resistant *Salmonella* Infections

Christopher M. Parry

1. INTRODUCTION

Salmonellae are found widely in nature both as commensals in the gastrointestinal tracts of domesticated and wild mammals, reptiles, birds, and insects and as pathogens in animals and humans. *Salmonella typhi* is restricted to humans and causes typhoid fever, which in the preantibiotic era was associated with considerable morbidity and mortality. Other *Salmonella* serotypes are an important cause of food poisoning and occasional systemic infections. The increasing levels of antimicrobial resistance in *Salmonella* combined with their ability to cause serious disease means this group of bacteria is of considerable public health importance.

2. BACKGROUND

Salmonellae are Gram-negative bacilli and are members of the family Enterobacteriacae. The majority of salmonellae are classified as a single species, *Salmonella enterica*, with six subspecies and more than 2000 serotypes based the O (somatic) and H (flagellar) antigens. *Salmonella enterica* subspecies *enterica* serotype *typhi* (abbreviated *Salmonella typhi*), *S. paratyphi*, and *S. sendai* are highly adapted to humans, with no other known host. Other serotypes are adapted to specific hosts, such as *S. dublin* in cattle and *S. enterica* subspecies *arizonae* in reptiles, and only cause occasional infection in humans; some have a wider host range, including animals and humans, such as *S. typhimurium* and *S. enteritidis*.

Salmonella typhi, *S. paratyphi A*, and *S. paratyphi B* are responsible for the syndrome of typhoid or enteric fever *(1,2)*. Such infections occur in areas that lack adequate sanitation and clean water. Although once common in Europe and the United States, cases are now restricted to the resource-poor countries of Asia, Africa, South and Central America, and the Caribbean and Pacific islands. Cases in the industrialized countries are mostly restricted to travelers returning from endemic regions *(3,4)*. Worldwide, there are estimated to be more than 16 million cases of typhoid fever each year, with up to 600,000 deaths. Transmission is person to person by the fecal-oral route, principally via contaminated water or food. Convalescent and long-term carriers are the principle sources of transmission, and there are no environmental or zoonotic reservoirs.

From: *Management of Multiple Drug-Resistant Infections*
Edited by: S. H. Gillespie © Humana Press Inc., Totowa, NJ

In industrialized countries, the nontyphi *Salmonella* serotypes are invariably associated with consumption of inadequately cooked foods of animal origin, such as meat, poultry eggs, and dairy products, contaminated with *Salmonella (1,5)*. Manufactured foods, such as ice cream, powdered milk products and infant formula, and ready-to-eat snacks, have been the source of widespread outbreaks *(1)*. Although most illness is foodborne, occasional waterborne outbreaks have been described, and institutional and hospital outbreaks may occur *(6,7)*. Infections linked to exotic pets, particularly reptiles, are recognized in some areas.

In the United States, there are estimated to be 1 to 3 million cases of *Salmonella* infection that result in 400–600 deaths each year *(5)*. The most common nontyphi serotypes are *S. typhimurium*, *S. enteritidis*, *S. virchow*, and *S. hadar*. In resource-poor countries, particularly sub-Saharan Africa, infections caused by these nontyphi serotypes are associated with a much higher incidence of invasive disease with a high mortality *(8,9)*. Children under the age of 5 yr and adults with human immunodeficiency virus (HIV) infection are particularly affected. The routes of transmission are less clear in these areas.

Typhoid fever commonly affects children and young adults aged 3 to 25 yr and typically presents after a week or more with a high fever, abdominal symptoms, a headache, and a dry cough *(1,2)*. Complications occur in 10 to 15% of patients, and gastrointestinal bleeding, intestinal perforation, and encephalopathy are the most important. After the resolution of symptoms, relapse, reinfection, and chronic fecal or urinary carriage may occur. The average mortality rate with treatment is less than 1%.

The nontyphoidal salmonellae commonly cause acute diarrhea that is indistinguishable from gastroenteritis caused by other gastrointestinal pathogens *(1,5)*. The illness is self-limiting, lasting less than a week; the main complication is dehydration, and the mortality is less than 0.5%. Low-level convalescent fecal carriage is common for a month or more, particularly in children, but chronic carriage is rare *(10)*. Bacteremia may complicate gastroenteritis in about 5–10% of individuals. The prognosis is good unless there is underlying immunosuppression or the patient is very young or elderly *(11,12)*. Primary bacteremia, without gastrointestinal symptoms, occurs in people with severe underlying disease, immunosuppression, or acquired immunodeficiency syndrome (AIDS) and is associated with significant mortality *(11,13)*. Bacteremia is more common with specific serotypes, such as *S. choleraesuis*, *S. virchow*, and *S. dublin*. Focal infections at extraintestinal sites complicate approx 5 to 10% of bacteremias. Septic arthritis, osteomyelitis, endovascular infections, endocarditis, meningitis, pneumonia, pleurisy, appendicitis, choleycystitis, peritonitis, urinary tract infections, and abscesses in various locations are all described *(1,14)*.

Decreased gastric acidity, changes in the normal gastrointestinal flora because of prior antibiotics, and gastrointestinal surgery predispose to *Salmonella* infections *(1,2,5)*. Very young children, the elderly, and immunocompromised patients are the most likely to develop severe or fatal disease. Invasive nontyphoidal salmonellosis is associated with impaired host immunity such as occurs in lymphoproliferative disease, organ transplants, systemic lupus erythematosis, cancer, liver disease, diabetes mellitus, corticosteroid therapy, interleukin-12 (IL-12) deficiency, and HIV infection *(1,5,9)*. Infections such as bartonellosis, malaria, schistosomiasis, histoplasmosis, and sickle cell disease characterized by phagocytic overload are also predisposing factors.

3. ANTIMICROBIAL RESISTANCE

Chloramphenicol resistance in *S. typhi* emerged as a major problem in 1972, with outbreaks in Mexico, India, Vietnam, Thailand, Korea, and Peru *(1,2)*. These *S. typhi* were also resistant to sulfonamides, tetracycline, and streptomycin, but amoxicillin and trimethoprim-sulfamethoxazole remained effective alternative drugs. At the end of the 1980s and early 1990s, *S. typhi* developed resistance simultaneously to chloramphenicol, trimethoprim, sulfamethoxazole and ampicillin and caused outbreaks in China, India, Pakistan, Bangladesh, Vietnam, the Middle East, and Africa *(1,2)*. Multidrug resistant (MDR) *S. typhi* and *S. paratyphi A* are still common in many areas of Asia and some countries in Africa, although they have declined in some areas *(15–17)*. The resistance genes are typically encoded on 100–120 megadaltons, IncHI plasmids and include *bla* (TEM-1; ampicillin), *cat*I (chloramphenicol), *dhfr*1b or *dhfrvVII* (trimethoprim), *sul*II (sulfonamide), and *str*AB (streptomycin) *(18–20)*.

Among the nontyphoidal *Salmonella* serotypes, antimicrobial resistance was recognized in the mid-1960s *(1,21)*. Antimicrobial drug resistance and multiple resistance (to four or more drugs) became common in *S. typhimurium* phage types DT29, DT204, DT193, and DT204c and in other serotypes, such as *S. newport (21,22)*. Plasmid-mediated resistance developed to a wide range of antimicrobials, including ampicillin, chloramphenicol, gentamicin, kanamycin, streptomycin, sulfonamides, tetracyclines, and trimethoprim. Currently, although *S. typhimurium* DT104 with chromosomal resistance to ampicillin, chloramphenicol, streptomycin, sulfonamide, and tetracyclines (R-type ACSSuT), and sometimes with additional trimethoprim and ciprofloxacin resistance, is an important concern *(23)*, new serotypes, such as *S. typhimurium* DT204b, continue to appear *(24)*. Similar resistance in nontyphi serotypes is also a problem in developing countries and has a more critical impact because the alternative antimicrobials are often unavailable or unaffordable *(8,25)*.

3.1. *Multidrug-Resistant* Salmonella typhimurium *DT104*

MDR *S. typhimurium* DT104, R-type ACSSuT, was first isolated in the United Kingdom from exotic birds in the early 1980s and appeared in humans in 1989 *(23)*. This serotype has now become common in cattle, poultry, pigs, and sheep in the United Kingdom, and human infection has been associated with the consumption of chicken, beef, pork sausages, and meat paste and to a lesser extent with contact with food animals *(26)*. Infections in food animals and humans have been recognized in several European countries, the United States, Canada, Israel, Turkey, and Japan *(23,27–30)*. In the United States, *S. typhimurium* with the R-ACSSuT resistance pattern increased from 0.6% in 1979–1980 to 34% in 1996, and the majority of these isolates were DT104 *(27)*.

The complete spectrum of resistance R-type ACSSuT is chromosomally encoded *(29,31–33)*. The overall gene complex, known as Salmonella genomic island 1 (SGI1), consists of a sequence of approx 14 kilobases (kb), which contain two integrons, one encodes resistance for ampicillin (CARB-2; PSE-1) and the other resistance for streptomycin, with the intervening plasmid-derived sequences coding for resistance to chloramphenicol and tetracyclines. Isolates of DT104 contain the same gene cassettes irrespective of origin (food animal or human) or country of origin *(33)*. SGI1 has been found in *S. typhimurium* DT12 and DT120, although these appear to be instances for which DT104 has changed its phage type *(34)*, and in other serotypes such as *S. paratyphi B* and *S. agona (31,35)*. More recently, isolates with plasmid-mediated resistance to trimethoprim and chromosomal low-level fluoroquinolone resistance have been isolated *(23,36)*. By 2000 in England and Wales, 10% of DT104 isolates were resistant to trimethoprim, 9% had low-level resistance to ciprofloxacin, and 1% were resistant to the full R-type ACSSuTTmCp$_L$ *(23)*.

3.2. Resistance to the Fluoroquinolones

Fluoroquinolones, such as ciprofloxacin and ofloxacin, have potent in vitro activity against salmonellae and rapid bactericidal activity against MDR strains. Epidemics of MDR *S. typhi* and *S. paratyphi* in developing countries have been managed successfully with fluoroquinolone therapy, and these drugs have become widely used for treating endemic disease in areas where MDR strains are common *(2,37)*. The fluoroquinolones have also proved useful for the treatment of multiresistant nontyphi *Salmonella* infections *(1,5)*.

The quinolones act by inhibiting the action of DNA gyrase, resulting in the disruption of DNA replication, followed by cell death. Mutants conferring resistance to quinolones can be grouped into two types, both of which involve chromosomal genes. Mutants either produce an alteration in the DNA gyrase or alternatively mediate changes at the cell surface, decreasing the uptake of a range of antimicrobial drugs or affecting energy-dependent efflux systems *(38)*. Single-point mutations in *gyr*A that confer resistance to quinolone drugs occur in the conserved region of the N-terminal domain of the A subunit close to the catalytic Tyr122 site, termed the quinolone-resistance-determining region (QRDR). Typical mutations result in the replacement of serine at position 83 by phenylalanine, leucine, tyrosine, or tryptophan and aspartate at position 87 by glycine, tyrosine, or asparagine *(38–47)*. Mutations may also occur in the *gyr*B and *par*C genes or in the *mar*A or *sox*R genes, affecting drug efflux *(38,43)*.

Single-point mutations in the *gyr*A gene confer resistance to the quinolone nalidixic acid and low-level resistance to fluoroquinolones. The minimum inhibitory concentration (MIC) to ciprofloxacin is typically 0.125–1.0 mg/L compared to the wild-type MIC, which is 0.03 mg/L or less *(4,46)*. Although reported as susceptible by disk testing using recommended breakpoints to fluoroquinolones, these organisms have MICs to fluoroquinolones 10-fold higher than fully susceptible strains, and infections with these strains do not respond reliably to treatment *(48)*. It is probable that these fluoroquinolone breakpoints for salmonellae will change in the near future, although in practice the presence of nalidixic acid resistance is a good marker of low-level fluoroquinolone resistance *(2,48,49)*.

Isolates of *S. typhi, S. paratyphi*, and other serotypes with low-level fluoroquinolone resistance have become a major problem in Asia *(16,50–52)*. Such isolates are also isolated from travelers returning from these endemic areas *(3,4,53)*. In England and Wales in 2000, 36% of *S. typhi* isolates and 22% of *S. paratyphi A* had low-level resistance to ciprofloxacin *(4)*. Most patients infected with these strains had recently returned from countries of the Indian subcontinent, and 52% of the *S. typhi* strains were also MDR.

Among the nontyphi serotypes, in England and Wales in 1999 low-level ciprofloxacin resistance was found in 8% of *S. typhimurium*, 8% of *S. enteritidis*, 39%

of *S. virchow*, and 70% of *S. hadar* isolates *(21)*. Resistant isolates have been associated with foreign travel *(21,53)*. In animal isolates, the level of resistance was considerably higher, with up to 78% in turkeys and 38% in chickens *(38)*. A survey in the United States in 1994–1995 of 4008 isolates of *Salmonella* revealed 21 (0.5%) resistant to nalidixic acid and 1 (0.02%) resistant to ciprofloxacin *(54)*. In France in 1995 and 1996, human and animal (cattle, pigs, or poultry) isolates of *S. typhimurium* showed an increase of nalidixic acid resistance from 8.5% in 1995 to 18.6% in 1996 *(55)*. In Denmark, low-level resistance in *S. enteritidis* increased from 0.8% in 1995 to 8.5% in 2000 *(56)*. Low-level resistance was found in an average of 14.3% of nontyphi serotypes in a recent survey in the Asia-Pacific region, ranging from 3.9% in Australia to 27.4% in Taiwan *(57)*.

There are a few reports of human infections with salmonellae fully resistant to fluoroquinolones *(41,44,58–61)*. If characterized, isolates usually have two or more point mutations in *gyr*A with variable additional mutations in *gyr*B or *par*C or mutations leading to the overexpression of *sox*R or *mar*A, resulting in altered levels of AcrB or OmpF *(38,44,58,61)*. The appearance of full resistance in *S. choleraesuis* is particularly disturbing as this serotype has a propensity to cause invasive disease *(41)*.

3.3. Resistance to Extended-Spectrum Cephalosporins

From 1988, nontyphi *Salmonella* isolates with resistance to extended-spectrum β-lactamases (ESBLs) have been increasingly reported. Isolates have been reported from countries in North and West Africa, South America, the Middle East, Turkey, Greece, countries of eastern Europe and Russia, India, East Asia, and the United States.

Resistance generally results from the production of Ambler class A or C ESBLs (Table 1). Class A enzymes confer resistance to oxyimino-β-lactams such as cefotaxime, ceftazidime, and aztreonam, but are not active against cephamycins and can be inactivated by clavulanic acid and similar inhibitors *(62–88)*. Class C enzymes, AmpC β-lactamases, are cephalosporinases capable of hydrolyzing all β-lactams to some extent. Overexpression confers resistance to all the β-lactam drugs, including the cephamycins, but not cefipime, cefpirome, and the carbapenems, and they are not inhibited by clavulanic acid *(72,74,75,77,89–95)*. The description of *S. typhimurium* containing SHV-9 (an ESBL) and CMY-7 (an AmpC β-lactamase), is a worrying development *(75)*.

A recent study reported that 1.6% of 431 *Salmonella* isolates evaluated from Europe, the Americas, and the western Pacific region expressed an ESBL phenotype *(96)*. The incidence of human *Salmonella* strains with extended-spectrum cephalosporin resistance in the United States increased from 0.1% in 1996 to 0.5% in 1998 *(97)*. In a multiprovince study in Canada, more than 1000 independent isolates of *S. typhimurium* were examined for the presence of ESBLs, and only 1 isolate was positive, with an SHV-2a enzyme *(71)*. In the United Kingdom, 0.08% of 18,178 isolates were resistant to extended-spectrum cephalosporins in 1998, with most acquired during foreign travel *(98)*. In small studies from India, 3–8% of nontyphoidal salmonellae blood culture isolates had an ESBL *(72)*, and in one study in Turkey, 19 of 75 isolates contained an ESBL *(99)*.

Although there have been anecdotal reports from the Indian subcontinent of extended-spectrum cephalosporin resistance in *S. typhi*, thus far there have been few

Table 1
Ambler Class A and C Extended-Spectrum β-Lactamases and Cephalosporinases in *Salmonella*

β-Lactamase	Country	Serotype	Reference
Class A			
TEM-3	France, Tunisia	*Typhimurium, kedougou, enteritidis*	*62, 63*
TEM-27	Spain	*Othmarschen*	*64*
TEM-52	Turkey	*Typhimurium*	*65*
SHV-2	Tunisia, France, Argentina, Canada, Poland, India	*Typhimurium, wein*	*66–72*
SHV-5	Argentina, India, Romania	*Seftenberg, typhimurium*	*68, 73, 74*
SHV-9	Australia	*Typhimurium*	*75*
SHV-12	Italy, Senegal	*Enteritidis*, 35:c:1,2	*76, 77*
CTX-M-2	Algeria, Argentina	*Mbandaka, typhimurium, agona, infantis, enteritidis, oranienberg*	*68, 78–80*
CTX-M-3	Poland, Taiwan	*Typhimurium, enteritidis, anatum*	*70, 82*
CTX-M-4	Russia, Greece, Hungary	*Typhimurium*	*81, 83*
CTX-M-5	Greece, Latvia	*Typhimurium*	*84, 85*
CTX-M-6	Greece	*Typhimurium*	*84*
CTX-M-9	Spain	*Virchow*	*86*
CTX-M-15	India	Various	*72*
PER-1	Turkey	*Typhimurium*	*87*
PER-2	Argentina	*Typhimurium*	*88*
OXA-9	Argentina	Various	*80*
Class C			
CMY-2	United States, Algeria, Italy, Romania	*Typhimurium, seftenberg, heidelberg*	*74, 77, 89–92*
CMY-4	Tunisia	*Wein*	*93*
CMY-6	India	Various	*72*
CMY-7	Australia, India	*Typhimurium*	*72, 75*
DHA-1	France, Romania, Saudi Arabia	*Enteritidis, typhimurium*	*74, 94, 95*

clear reports. Isolates of *S. paratyphi A* from Pakistan and *S. typhi* from Bangladesh have demonstrated high-level resistance to ceftriaxone, but were not characterized further *(100,101)*.

3.4. Emergence and Dissemination of Resistance Determinants

Antibiotic-resistant *Salmonella* disease may result from infection with a resistant strain or the development of resistance during the course of treatment. The emergence of resistance during treatment has been described because of either the transfer of an antibiotic resistance plasmid from other enterobacteriacae to salmonellae in the gastrointestinal tract *(62,81,102,103)* or in the context of subtherapeutic antibiotic concentrations at the site of infection or inadequate abscess drainage *(48)*. Initial infection with a resistant isolate is probably more common and may occur because of the clonal dissemination of an MDR *Salmonella* strain through a population or the transfer of the resistance plasmid through multiple *Salmonella* strains *(104,105)*.

A variety of plasmid restriction patterns and chromosmal pulse field types have been described in MDR *S. typhi* and nontyphi salmonellae *(25,28,90,106,107)*. In particular areas, however, particular clones predominate and produce less-diverse pulse field types among MDR strains than those fully susceptible *(107)*. For the fluoroquinolones, resistance is mediated by point mutations. Spontaneous point mutations will always occur in a large population of *Salmonella*, and occasional mutants resistant to nalidixic acid were evident in salmonellae prior to the widespread use of fluoroquinolones *(108)*. Once the strain has developed resistance, either by mutation or by the acquisition of resistance genes, selection by antimicrobials will lead to the preferential transmission of those strains with dissemination within the community.

Genes that mediate resistance to the β-lactams, aminoglycosides, trimethoprim, and chloramphenicol have spread into the many serotypes of *Salmonella* carried on mobile genetic elements such as plasmids, transposons, and integrons. R-Factor plasmids, carrying antimicrobial resistance genes, are commonly found in the normal Gram-negative flora of the gastrointestinal tract and may be transferred to potential pathogens such as *Salmonella (109)*. The pattern of resistance carried on these plasmids appear to have evolved by the sequential addition of integrons or transposons carrying different arrays of antibiotic resistance genes *(18,79,80,110–112)*.

Dissemination of resistance strains will be favored where transmission is easy, such as in areas with poor clean water supplies and adequate sanitation and in hospitals if infection control practices are poor. The emergence and dissemination of resistant strains is also facilitated by the pressure of widespread, and often indiscriminate, antimicrobial use. Transmission within the community is particularly encouraged if inadequate treatment leads to increased convalescent fecal carriage and, as a result, increased onward transmission as secondary cases. In multiresistant strains, any of the antibiotics to which the strain is resistant will inevitably select for the full complement of resistance determinants. Therefore, dissemination of an MDR replicon may not depend on the use of a specific antibiotic, but rather may be a result of more general antimicrobial use.

In developed countries, antimicrobial drug resistance in nontyphoidal *Salmonella* has been considered the consequence of the widespread use of antimicrobial agents therapeutically, prophylactically, or for growth promotion (feed additives) in food-producing animals. Antimicrobials such as ceftiofur, an extended-spectrum injectable cephalosporin, and the fluoroquinolones enrofloxacin, danofloxacin, marbofloxacin, and sarafloxacine have all been approved for therapeutic veterinary use *(21,38,56,113)*.

Epidemiological evidence for the link between resistance in animals and humans is shown by the close identity between molecular types of animal- and human-derived strains *(28,38,90)*. In developing countries, overuse of antimicrobials in humans and poor living conditions that favor the rapid dissemination of strains are the principle driving forces encouraging the development of resistance.

4. TREATMENT

4.1. Typhoid

In endemic areas, many typhoid fever cases are managed outside the hospital with antibiotics and bed rest. For those requiring hospital admission, good nursing care, careful fluid and electrolyte balance, adequate nutrition, and prompt recognition and

Table 2
Antibiotic Regimens in Typhoid Fever and Invasive Nontyphoidal Salmonellosis

Antibiotic	Dose	Divided daily doses	Route	Duration: nonsevere typhoid fever[a]	Duration: severe or complicated typhoid fever[a,b,c]
Chloramphenicol[d]	50–100 mg/kg body weight per day; reduce dose to 30 mg/kg body weight per day when fever ceases	4	Oral (intramuscular/ intravenous)	14–21 d	14–21 d
Amoxicillin	75–100 mg/kg body weight per day	3	Oral/intramuscular/ intravenous	14 d	14 d
Cotrimoxazole (trimethoprim-sulfamethoxazole)[e]	8 mg trimethoprim + 40 mg sulfamethoxazole/kg body weight per day	2–3	Oral/intramuscular/ intravenous	14 d	14 d
Ciprofloxacin[f]	15–25 mg/kg body weight per day	2	Oral/intravenous	5–7 d	10–14 d
Ofloxacin[f]	10–20 mg/kg body weight per day	2	Oral/intravenous	5–7 d	10–14 d
Pefloxacin[f]	800 mg	2	Oral/intravenous	5–7 d	10–14 d
Ceftriaxone	50–80 mg/kg body weight per day	1–2	Intramuscular/ intravenous	7–10	10–14 d
Cefotaxime	100–150 mg/kg body weight per day	3–4	Intramuscular/ intravenous	7–10 d	10–14 d
Cefixime[g]	20–30 mg/kg body weight per day	2	Oral	7–10 d	
Azithromycin[g]	8–10 mg/kg body weight per day	1	Oral	7 d	

[a]Refer to text for duration of treatment in nontyphoidal salmonellosis.

[b]In intestinal perforation, antibiotic treatment should also cover other aerobic and anaerobic gastrointestinal bacteria contaminating the peritoneum.

[c]In severe typhoid (characterized by delerium, obtundation, coma, or shock), dexamethasone should be given in an initial dose of 3 mg/kg body weight by slow intravenous infusion over 30 min, followed by 1 mg/kg body weight dexamethasone given at the same rate every 6 h for 8 additional doses.

[d]May cause bone marrow depression.

[e]May cause allergic reactions and nephrotoxicity. Not suitable for children younger than 2 yr or pregnant women.

[f]Isolates with low-level fluoroquinolone resistance (nalidixic acid resistance) may not respond.

[g]Not recommended for invasive nontyphoidal salmonellosis or severe typhoid.

treatment of complications are as important as effective antibiotics. Chloramphenicol, amoxicillin, or trimethoprim-sulfamethoxazole are still used for the treatment of typhoid fever in areas of the world where the bacteria are fully sensitive to these drugs and the fluoroquinolones are not available or affordable *(2)* (Table 2). These drugs are inexpensive, rarely associated with side effects, and usually produce relief of symptoms within 5 to 7 d. Unfortunately, 2 to 3 wk of treatment is required, and although cure rates are about 95%, relapse rates vary between 1 and 7%; 2 to 10% of patients are convalescent excretors *(1,2)*.

Resistance to chloramphenicol, ampicillin, and cotrimoxazole is invariably high level and leads to treatment failure. Fluoroquinolones have proved to be safe and effective drugs for such strains. In randomized controlled trials in fluoroquinolone-susceptible *S. typhi*, they have been rapidly effective even with courses less than 7 d *(2,37,114,115)*. Fever and symptoms usually resolve in less than 4 d. The cure rates exceed 96%, with relapse and persistent carriage rates of less than 2% *(2)*.

Fluoroquinolones are not usually recommended for pediatric use because of worries, based on evidence from experimental animals, about possible joint or tendon damage. However, there is now a large body of evidence concerning the compassionate use of a prolonged course of fluoroquinolones in children with cystic fibrosis and a short course in children with dysentery and enteric fever; this evidence suggests that they are safe to use *(116–119)*. In some countries, they are still not approved for use in children. In areas endemic for MDR typhoid, where low-level fluoroquinolone-resistant strains are uncommon, the fluoroquinolones are the current treatment of choice for adults with typhoid and for children older than 2 yr with typhoid. Short-course regimens are particularly useful in epidemic containment *(37)*.

The main problem with the use of fluoroquinolones has been the emergence of low-level resistance. For *S. typhi* with low-level fluoroquinolone resistance, short-course (<7 d) fluoroquinolone treatment results in high failure rates *(46,48,120)*. Unfortunately, these strains are often also MDR, so the choice of drugs is limited. If alternative antimicrobials are unavailable, high doses of fluoroquinolone for 7 to 10 d may be successful in about 90% of patients, but fever clearance times are long (7 d or more), and convalescent fecal carriage can be as high as 20% *(2)*.

The third-generation cephalosporins (parenteral ceftriaxone, cefotaxime, or cefoperazone and oral cefixime) are also effective drugs for typhoid *(115,121–123)*. In randomized controlled trials with the third-generation cephalosporins, principally ceftriaxone and cefixime, fever clearance times averaged 1 wk, with treatment failure rates of 5 to 10%, relapse rates of 3 to 6%, and fecal carriage rates less than 3% *(2)*. Azithromycin has also emerged as a new typhoid treatment. Using a treatment course of 5 to 7 d, the cure rate has been 95%, with relapse and convalescent fecal carriage rates less than 3% *(114,120,123)*. Fever and symptoms usually resolve within 4 to 7 d. The third-generation cephalosporins and azithromycin are both effective for MDR strains with low-level fluoroquinolone resistance. Aztreonam and imipenem are potential third-line drugs.

In severe typhoid, fluoroquinolones or third-generation cephalosporins should be given for a minimum of 10 d *(121,124)*. Patients with typhoid perforation require resuscitation with fluids, blood, and oxygen as appropriate, followed by surgery *(125)*. Early intervention is crucial as delay increases mortality. Patients require additional parenteral antibiotics to cover enteric bacteria contaminating the peritoneal cavity. Mortality rates vary between 10 and 32%. Intestinal hemorrhage is usually not severe and can usually be managed without transfusion. Intravenous dexamethasone can reduce the mortality of severe typhoid, which is characterized by delirium, obtundation, stupor, coma, or shock *(126,127)* (Table 2). Hydrocortisone, given in a dose of either 100 mg or 400 mg, 6 hourly for 12 doses, was not effective *(128)*.

Typhoid in pregnancy can be safely treated with β-lactam antibiotics *(129)*. Despite safety concerns, there have been several case reports of the successful use of fluoroquinolones *(130)*.

Relapse cases should be treated the same way as the initial infection. The majority of intestinal carriers can be cured by a prolonged course of antibiotics. Depending on the susceptibility of the organisms, oral ampicillin or amoxicillin 100 mg/kg body weight per day with probenicid 30 mg/kg body weight per day; trimethoprim-sulfamethoxazole two tablets twice daily for 3 mo; ciprofloxacin 750 mg twice a day; or norfloxacin 400 mg twice a day for 28 d have given cure rates of approx 80% *(131,132)*. In the presence of gallstones, antibiotic therapy as well as cholecystectomy may be required. Patients with chronic urinary carriage related to *Schistosoma haematobium* should be treated for the schistosomiasis before treatment for the *S. typhi*.

4.2. Salmonella *Enteritis*

The most important therapy of gastroenteritis caused by *Salmonella* is the replacement of fluid and electrolyte losses, usually by oral rehydration solutions. Severe cases may require intravenous fluids. Antimotility drugs should be restricted to very mild cases and should be avoided in children and the elderly and if there is fever, mucus, or blood in the stools. Antimicrobial therapy is not routinely required *(1,5,133,134)*. Short-course or single-dose regimens with oral amoxicillin, trimethoprim-sulfamethoxazole, or fluoroquinolones have not consistently decreased the duration of symptoms or eliminated stool carriage *(133)*. Some studies have noted higher rates of bacteriological relapse in those treated with antimicrobials *(135)*.

Patients who require hospitalization, who are severely ill, who have signs of systemic sepsis, or who have risk factors for severe or complicated disease should receive empirical antibiotics *(134,136)* (Table 2). An oral or intravenous antimicrobial should be administered for 3 to 5 d or until the patient is afebrile. Longer courses of treatment may lead to an increased risk of relapse or chronic carriage. In adults and in children older than 2 yr, an oral fluoroquinolone is the treatment of choice. Third-generation cephalosporins would generally be used in children younger than 2 yr. Ampicillin, trimethoprim-sulfamethoxazole, ceftriaxone, or cefotaxime are suitable alternatives, depending on the severity of the illness. Cefixime and azithromycin have not proved effective *(137)*. Antimicrobial therapy with a fluoroquinolone has been used in the control of outbreaks in institutions *(138)*, although the results have not always been favorable *(139)*.

Patients with bacteremia or focal infections require therapy with a fluoroquinolone or third-generation cephalosporin until susceptibility patterns are known *(121)*. The duration of treatment depends on the clinical problem, with focal infections often requiring tailored therapy *(1,5)*. Simple bacteremia is usually treated for 7 to 10 d; patients with pulmonary, biliary, and soft tissue infection require 2 wk of therapy; central nervous system infections should be treated for 3 wk; bone and joint infections need 4 to 6 wk of treatment; and endocarditis requires 6 wk of treatment. Infected aneurysms and other endovascular infections usually require surgical resection, including prosthetic grafts when possible, bypassing the infected area, as well as at least 6 wk of antimicrobial therapy *(140)*. Patients with an infected prosthetic graft that cannot be resected require suppressive oral therapy for life. Failure to drain the collection may lead to the emergence of resistance because of poor penetration of the antimicrobial into the site of infection. Patients with HIV infection and invasive salmonellosis treatment need therapy to eradicate the infection and to prevent recurrence. If available, fluoroquinolones are probably the optimal drug and should be used for at least 2 wk *(1,9,13)*. Those who relapse require long-term suppressive therapy.

5. CLINICAL AND PUBLIC HEALTH IMPACT OF RESISTANCE

Whether multiresistant *Salmonella* infections are associated with more severe disease is debated. In children in Pakistan, MDR typhoid infections were associated with more severe clinical illness and higher rates of toxicity, hepatomegaly, hypotension, and death *(141)*. The number of bacteria circulating in the blood of typhoid patients in Vietnam was significantly higher in MDR infection compared with those infections that were fully susceptible *(142)*.

A report from Denmark found excess mortality associated with drug-resistant *S. typhimurium (143)*. In a matched cohort study, the death rate over the 2-yr period following infection was compared with community controls. Those infected with a pansusceptible isolate were 2.3 times more likely to die in the 2-yr period following infection. Those infected with an R-ACSSuT isolate had a 4.8-fold increased risk of death, and for those infected with an isolate with low-level fluoroquinolone resistance, the risk was 10.3-fold higher. *Salmonella typhimurium* DT104 has been associated with more serious disease with high rates of hospitalization *(26)*, although in another study the proportion of bacteremic strains in the United Kingdom was no different from other comparable phage types and serotypes *(144)*.

The insertion of resistance genes into a *Salmonella* virulence plasmid could provide a genetic basis for linking increased severity to resistance, but it is an uncommon occurrence *(112)*. Resolution of this question is complicated by the difficulty of distinguishing poor outcome because of the increased virulence of resistant bacteria or because of the poor response to treatment.

Unrelated antimicrobial use may lead to an increase in the number of infections caused by susceptible and multiresistant salmonellae by causing a transient decrease in the resistance to noncommensal bacteria and increasing the likelihood of infection on exposure to a gastrointestinal pathogen *(22,145,146)*. The additional "selective effect" of antimicrobial resistance has been calculated to result in a more than threefold increase in vulnerability to infection by an antimicrobial-resistant pathogen among individuals receiving antibiotics for an unrelated reason. This has been estimated to lead to 29,379 additional nontyphi *Salmonella* infections in the United States each year, including 342 hospitalizations and 12 deaths *(145)*.

There have been significant outbreaks caused by multiresistant *Salmonella*. Many outbreaks were described in the Indian subcontinent and Southeast Asia when MDR typhoid first appeared in the late 1980s and early 1990s *(1,2)*. In recent years, there have been outbreaks caused by *S. typhi* resistant to nalidixic acid in Tajikistan and Vietnam *(51,52,147)*. An outbreak of typhoid with such strains in Tajikistan in 1997 involved 8000 people in a 6-mo period and caused 150 deaths *(147)*.

Hospital outbreaks with nontyphi salmonellae, particularly involving neonatal units, have occurred in North African countries, Turkey, South America, and India

(6,7,73,148). In a pediatric hospital in Buenos Aires, Argentina, in 1990, of 75 children with multiply resistant *Salmonella* gastroenteritis, the infection was nosocomially acquired in two-thirds of children *(6)*. Six children developed enterocolitis, with two leading to bowel perforation; one had a pulmonary abscess; eight were bacteremic; and four children died (5.3%). In an outbreak of *S. infantis* expressing an ESBL in a neonatal unit in Rio de Janeiro, Brazil, 140 infants with positive cultures were identified *(7)*. Compared with controls, infection was associated with a longer hospital stay, higher costs, and an almost ninefold greater risk of death in the neonatal period.

6. CONCLUSIONS

Resistance to multiple antimicrobial agents is increasing in *S. typhi* and *S. paratyphi* and in many nontyphi serotypes. Plasmid-mediated resistance to chloramphenicol, ampicillin, and cotrimoxazole is widespread. In some serotypes, such as *S. typhimurium* DT104, resistance has moved from the plasmid to the chromosome. Resistance to extended-spectrum cephalosporins and fluoroquinolones is emerging and in some areas is already common. Such strains are causing epidemics and in some areas have become endemic. The widespread emergence of full fluoroquinolone or extended-spectrum cephalosporin resistance in typhoidal and nontyphoidal *Salmonella* serotypes will make treatment difficult and expensive. There is a risk that effectively untreatable *Salmonella* infections may emerge, particularly in resource-poor countries, where available antimicrobials are limited.

Active surveillance of resistance, prudent use of antibiotics in humans and animals, adequate infection control in hospitals, and improvements in food hygiene and in the supply of clean water and sanitation in affected areas are important components required to control this problem. For typhoid and invasive nontyphi salmonellosis, new antibiotics, and perhaps established antibiotics in combinations, are needed in the face of mounting resistance. In areas where the level of resistance in typhoid fever is becoming critical, the cost-effectiveness of mass vaccination needs to be reconsidered seriously *(2,149)*. A new conjugate Vi vaccine may well have a role in that it is likely to be effective in preschool children, who are at significant risk of typhoid fever in endemic areas *(150)*.

REFERENCES

1. Miller S, Pegues D. *Salmonella* species, including *Salmonella typhi*. In: Mandell G, Bennett J, Dolin R (eds.). Principles and Practice of Infectious Diseases. Philadelphia, PA: Churchill Livingstone, 2000, pp. 2344–2362.
2. Parry CM, Hien TT, Dougan G, White NJ, Farrar JJ. Typhoid fever. N Engl J Med 2002; 347:1770–1782.
3. Ackers M-L, Puhr ND, Tauxe RV, Mintz ED. Laboratory-based surveillance of *Salmonella* serotype *typhi* infections in the United States. JAMA 2000; 283:2668–2673.
4. Threlfall EJ, Skinner JA, Ward LR. Detection of decreased susceptibility to ciprofloxacin in *Salmonella enterica* serotypes *typhi* and *paratyphi A*. J Antimicrob Chemother 2001; 48:740–741.
5. Hohmann EL. Nontyphoidal salmonellosis. Clin Infect Dis 2001; 32:263–269.
6. Maiorini E, López EL, Morrow AL, et al. Multiply resistant nontyphoidal *Salmonella* gastroenteritis in children. Pediatr Infect Dis J 1993; 12:139–145.
7. Pessoa-Silva CL, Toscano CM, Moreira BM, et al. Infection due to extended-spectrum

β-lactamase-producing *Salmonella enterica* subsp *enterica* serotype *infantis* in a neonatal unit. J Pediatr 2002; 141:381–387.
8. Lepage P, Bogaerts J, Van Goethem C, et al. Multiresistant *Salmonella typhimurium* systemic infection in Rwanda. Clinical features and treatment with cefotaxime. J Antimicrob Chemother 1990; 26(suppl. A):53–57.
9. Gordon MA, Banda HT, Gondwe M, et al. Non-typhoidal *Salmonella* bacteraemia among HIV-infected Malawian adults: high mortality and frequent recrudescence. AIDS 2002; 16:1633–1641.
10. Buchwald DS, Blaser MJ. A review of human salmonellosis: II. Duration of excretion following infection with nontyphi *Salmonella*. Rev Infect Dis 1984; 6:345–356.
11. Ramos JM, García-Corbeira P, Aguado JM, Arjona R, Alés JM, Soriano F. Clinical significance of primary versus secondary bacteraemia due to nontyphoid *Salmonella* in patients without AIDS. Clin Infect Dis 1994; 19:777–780.
12. Shimoni Z, Pitlik S, Leibovici L, et al. Nontyphoid *Salmonella* bacteremia: age-related differences in clinical presentation, bacteriology, and outcome. Clin Infect Dis 1999; 28: 822–827.
13. Jacobson MA, Hahan SM, Gerberding JL, Lee B, Sande MA. Ciprofloxacin for *Salmonella* bacteremia in the acquired immunodeficiency syndrome (AIDS). Ann Intern Med 1989; 110:1027–1029.
14. Cohen P, O'Brien T, Schoenbaum S, et al. The risk of endothelial infection in adults with *Salmonella* bacteremia. Ann Intern Med 1978; 89:931–932.
15. Rahaman M, Ahmad A, Shoma S. Decline in epidemic of multidrug resistant *Salmonella typhi* is not associated with increased incidence of antibiotic-susceptible strain in Bangladesh. Epidemiol Infect 2002; 129:29–34.
16. Rodrigues C, Shenai S, Mehta A. Enteric fever in Mumbai, India: the good news and the bad news. Clin Infect Dis 2003; 36:535.
17. Wafsy MO, Frenck R, Ismail TF, Mansour H, Malone JL, Mahoney FJ. Trends of multiple drug resistance among *Salmonella* serotype *typhi* isolates during a 14-year period in Egypt. Clin Infect Dis 2002; 35:1265–1268.
18. Parkhill J, Dougan G, James KD, et al. Complete genome sequence of a multiple drug resistant *Salmonella enterica* serovar *typhi* CT18. Nature 2001; 413:848–852.
19. Shanahan PMA, Jesudason MV, Thomson CJ, Amyes SGB. Molecular analysis and identification of antibiotic resistance genes in clinical isolates of *Salmonella typhi* from India. J Clin Microbiol 1998; 36:1595 1600.
20. Shanahan PMA, Karamat KA, Thomson CJ, Amyes SGB. Characterization of multi-drug resistant *Salmonella typhi* isolated from Pakistan. Epidemiol Infect 2000; 124:9–16.
21. Threlfall EJ. Antimicrobial drug resistance in *Salmonella*: problems and perspectives in food- and water-borne infections. FEMS Microbiol Rev 2002; 26:141–148.
22. Spika JS, Waterman SH, Hoo GW, et al. Chloramphenicol-resistant *Salmonella newport* traced through hamburger to dairy farms. A major persisting source of human salmonellosis in California. N Engl J Med 1987; 316:565–570.
23. Threlfall EJ. Multiresistant *Salmonella typhimurium* DT104: a truly international clone. J Antimicrob Chemother 2000; 46:7–10.
24. Lindsay EA, Lawson AJ, Walker RA, et al. Molecular characterisation of a multiresistant strain of *Salmonella enterica* serotype *typhimurium* DT204b responsible for an international outbreak of salmonellosis: importance of electronic exchange of gel data for outbreak investigations. Emerg Infect Dis 2002; 8:732–734.
25. Kariuki S, Gilks C, Kimara J, Muyodi J, Waiyaki P, Hart CA. Analysis of *Salmonella enterica* serotype *typhimurium* by phage typing, antimicrobial susceptibility and pulsed-field gel electrophoresis. J Med Microbiol 1999; 48:1037–1042.
26. Wall PG, Morgan D, Lamden K, Griffen M, Threlfall EJ, Rowe B. A case control study of infection with an epidemic strain of multiresistant *Salmonella typhimurium* DT104 in England and Wales. Commun Dis Rep CDR Rev 1994; 4:R130–R135.

27. Glynn MK, Bopp C, Dewitt W, Dabney P, Mokhtar M, Angulo FJ. Emergence of multidrug-resistant *Salmonella enterica* serotype *typhimurium* DT104 infections in the United States. N Engl J Med 1998; 338:1333–1338.
28. Ribot EM, Wierzba RK, Angulo FJ, Barrett TJ. *Salmonella enterica* serotype *typhimurium* DT104 isolated from humans, United States, 1985, 1990, and 1995. Emerg Infect Dis 2002; 8:387–391.
29. Ng LK, Mulvey MR, Maartin I, Peters GA, Johnson W. Genetic characterisation of antimicrobial resistance in Canadian isolates of *Salmonella* serovar *typhimurium* DT104. Antimicrob Agents Chemother 1999; 43:3019–3021.
30. Markogiannakis A, Tassios PT, Lambiri M, et al. Multiple clones within multidrug-resistant *Salmonella enterica* serotype *typhimurium* phage type DT104. J Clin Microbiol 2000; 38:1269–1271.
31. Boyd D, Cloeckaert A, Chaslus-Danela E, Mulvey MR. Characterization of variant Salmonella genomic island 1 multidrug resistance regions from serovars *typhimurium* DT104 and *agona*. Antimicrob Agents Chemother 2002; 46:1714–1722.
32. Briggs CE, Fratamico PM. Molecular characterisation of an antibiotic resistance gene cluster of *Salmonella typhimurium* DT104. Antimicrob Agents Chemother 1999; 43:846–849.
33. Ridley A, Threlfall EJ. Molecular epidemiology of antibiotic resistance genes in multiresistant *Salmonella typhimurium* DT104. Microb Drug Resist 1998; 2:113–118.
34. Lawson AJ, Dassama MU, Ward LR, Threlfall EJ. Multiply resistant (MR) *Salmonella enterica* serotype *typhimurium* DT 12 and DT 120: a case of MR DT 104 in disguise? Emerg Infect Dis 2002; 8:434–436.
35. Meunier D, Boyd D, Mulvey MR, et al. *Salmonella enterica* serotype *typhimurium* DT 104 antibiotic resistance genomic island 1 in serotype *paratyphi B*. Emerg Infect Dis 2002; 8:430–433.
36. Mølbak K, Baggesen DL, Aarestrup FM, et al. An outbreak of multidrug-resistant, quinolone-resistant *Salmonella enterica* serotype *typhimurium* DT104. N Engl J Med 1999; 341:1420–1425.
37. Hien TT, Bethell DB, Hoa NTT, et al. Short course of ofloxacin for treatment of multidrug-resistant typhoid. Clin Infect Dis 1995; 20:917–923.
38. Piddock LJV. Fluoroquinolone resistance in *Salmonella* serovars isolated from humans and food animals. FEMS Microbiol Rev 2002; 26:3–16.
39. Brown JC, Thomson CJ, Aymes SGB. Mutations of the *gyr*A gene of clinical isolates of *Salmonella typhimurium* and three other *Salmonella* species leading to decreased susceptibilities to the 4-quinolone drugs. J Antimicrob Chemother 1996; 37:351–356.
40. Brown JC, Shanahan PMA, Jesudason MV, Thomson CJ, Aymes SGB. Mutations responsible for reduced susceptibility to 4-quinolones in clinical isolates of multi-resistant *Salmonella typhi* in India. J Antimicrob Chemother 1996; 37:891–900.
41. Chiu CH, Wu TL, Su LH, et al. The emergence in Taiwan of fluoroquinolone resistance in *Salmonella enterica* serotype *choleraesuis*. N Engl J Med 2002; 346:413–419.
42. Eaves DJ, Liebana E, Woodward MJ, Piddock LJV. Detection of *gyr*A mutations in quinolone-resistant *Salmonella enterica* by denaturing high-performance liquid chromatography. J Clin Microbiol 2002; 40:4121–4125.
43. Griggs DJ, Gensberg K, Piddock LJ. Mutations in *gyr*A gene of quinolone-resistant *Salmonella* serotypes isolated from human and animals. Antimicrob Agents Chemother 1996; 40:1009–1013.
44. Heisig P. High-level fluoroquinolone resistance in a *Salmonella typhimurium* isolate due to alterations in both *gyr*A and *gyr*B genes. J Antimicrob Chemother 1993; 32:367–377.
45. Hirose K, Hashimoto A, Tamura K, et al. DNA sequence analysis of DNA gyrase and DNA topoisomerase IV quinolone resistance-determining regions of *Salmonella enterica* serovar *typhi* and *paratyphi A*. Antimicrob Agents Chemother 2002; 46:3249–3252.
46. Wain J, Hoa NTT, Chinh NT, et al. Quinolone-resistant *Salmonella typhi* in Viet Nam:

molecular basis of resistance and clinical response to treatment. Clin Infect Dis 1997; 25:1404–1410.
47. Walker RA, Saunders N, Lawson AJ, et al. Use of a LightCycler *gyr*A mutation assay for rapid identification of mutations conferring decreased susceptibility to ciprofloxacin in multiresistant *Salmonella enterica* serotype *typhimurium* DT104 isolates. J Clin Microbiol 2001; 39:1443–1448.
48. Aarestrup FM, Wiuff C, Mølbak K, Threlfall EJ. Is it time to change fluoroquinolone breakpoints for *Salmonella* spp? Antimicrob Agents Chemother 2003; 47:827–829.
49. Hakanen A, Kotilainen P, Jalava J, Siitonen A, Huovinen P. Detection of decreased fluoroquinolone susceptibility in salmonellas and validation of nalidixic acid screening test. J Clin Microbiol 1999; 37:3572–3577.
50. Chandel DS, Chaudhry R. Enteric fever treatment failures. Emerg Infect Dis 2001; 7:761–762.
51. Murdoch DA, Banatvala N, Bone A, Shoismatulloev BI, Ward LR, Threlfall EJ. Epidemic ciprofloxacin-resistant *Salmonella typhi* in Tajikistan. Lancet 1998; 351:339.
52. Parry C, Wain J, Chinh NT, Vinh H, Farrar J. Quinolone-resistant *Salmonella typhi* in Vietnam. Lancet 1998; 351:1289.
53. Hakanen A, Kotilainen P, Huovinen P, Helenius H, Siitonen A. Reduced fluoroquinolone susceptibility in *Salmonella enterica* serotypes in travellers returning from Southeast Asia. Emerg Infect Dis 2001; 7:996–1003.
54. Herikstad H, Hayes P, Mokhtar M, Fracaro ML, Threlfall EJ, Angulo FJ. Emerging quinolone-resistant *Salmonella* in the United States. Emerg Infect Dis 1997; 3:371–372.
55. Heurtin-Le Corre C, Donnio P-Y, Perrin M, Travert M-F, Avril J-L. Increasing incidence and comparison of nalidixic acid-resistant *Salmonella enterica* subsp *enterica* serotype *typhimurium* isolates from human and animals. J Clin Microbiol 1999; 37:266–269.
56. Mølbak K, Gerner-Smidt, Wegener HC. Increasing quinolone resistance in *Salmonella enterica* serotype *enteritidis*. Emerg Infect Dis 2002; 8:514–515.
57. Turnidge JD, Bell JM. Reduced quinolone susceptibility is common in *Salmonella* species from the Asia-Pacific region. Results from the SENTRY Asia Pacific surveillance programme, 2001. In: Program and Abstracts of the 42nd Interscience Conference of Antimicrobial Agents and Chemotherapy. San Diego, CA: American Society of Microbiology, 2002; Abstract C2-1284:106.
58. Baucheron S, Imberechts H, Cahslus-Dancla E, Clockaert A. The AcrB multidrug transporter plays a major role in high-level fluoroquinolone resistance in *Salmonella enterica* serovar *typhimurium* phage type DT204. Microb Drug Resist 2002; 8:281–289.
59. Lontie M, Verhaegen J, Chasseur-Libotte M-L, Verbist L. *Salmonella typhimurium* serovar *copenhagen* highly resistant to fluoroquinolones. J Antimicrob Chemother 1994; 34:845–846.
60. Mehta G, Randhawa VS, Mohapatra NP. Intermediate susceptibility to ciprofloxacin in *Salmonella typhi* strains in India. Eur J Clin Microbiol 2001; 20:760–761.
61. Nakaya H, Yasuhara A, Yoshimura K, Oshihoi Y, Izumiya H, Watanabe H. Life-threatening infantile diarrhoea from fluoroquinolone resistant *Salmonella enterica typhimurium* with mutations in both *gyr*A and *par*C. Emerg Infect Dis 2003; 9:255–257.
62. Archambaud M, Gerbaud G, Labau E, Marty N, Courvalin P. Possible in-vivo transfer of β-lactamase TEM-3 from *Klebsiella pneumoniae* to *Salmonella kedougou*. J Antimicrob Chemother 1991; 27:427–436.
63. AitMhand R, Soukri A, Moustaoui N, et al. Plasmid-mediated TEM-3 extended-spectrum β-lactamase production in *Salmonella typhimurium* in Casablanca. J Antimicrob Chemother 2002; 49:169–172.
64. Morisini MI, Blazquez J, Negri MC, Canton R, Loza E, Baquero F. Characterisation of a nosocomial outbreak involving an epidemic plasmid encoding for TEM-27 in *Salmonella enterica* subspecies *enterica* serotype *othmarschen*. J Infect Dis 1996; 174:1015–1020.

65. Vahaboglu H, Fuzi M, Cetin S, et al. Characterisation of extended-spectrum β-lactamase (TEM-52)-producing strains of *Salmonella enterica* serovar *typhimurium* with diverse resistance phenotypes. J Clin Microbiol 2001; 39:791–793.
66. Ben Redjeb S, Ben Yaghlane H, Boujnah A, Philippon A, Labia R. Synergy between clavulanic acid and newer β-lactams on nine clinical isolates of *Klebsiella pneumoniae, Escherichia coli* and *Salmonella typhimurium* resistant to third generation cephalosporins. J Antimicrob Chemother 1988; 21:263–266.
67. Garbarg-Chenon A, Vu Thien H, Labia R, et al. Characterisation of plasmid coding for resistance to broad-spectrum cephalosporins in *Salmonella typhimurium*. Drugs Exp Clin Res 1989; 15:145–150.
68. Rossi A, Lopardo H, Woloj M, et al. Non-typhoid *Salmonella* spp resistant to cefotaxime. J Antimicrob Chemother 1995; 36:697–702.
69. Hammami A, Arlet G, Ben Redjeb S, et al. Nosocomial outbreak of acute gastroenteritis in a neonatal intensive care unit in Tunisia caused by multiply drug resistant *Salmonella wein* producing SHV-2 β-lactamase. Eur J Clin Microbiol Infect Dis 1991; 10:641–646.
70. Baraniak A, Sadowy E, Hryniewicz W, Gniadkowski M. Two different extended-spectrum β lactamases (ESBLs) in one of the first ESBL-producing *Salmonella* isolates in Poland. J Clin Microbiol 2002; 40:1095–1097.
71. Mulvey MR, Soule G, Boyd D, et al. Characterization of the first extended-spectrum β-lactamase producing *Salmonella* isolate identified in Canada. J Clin Microbiol 2003; 41: 460–462.
72. Mathai D, Toleman MA, Walsh TR, Jones RN. Molecular determination of β-lactamases (BL) types found in *Salmonella* spp isolated in India: report for the MYSTIC programme (2001). In: Program and Abstracts of the 42nd Interscience Conference of Antimicrobial Agents and Chemotherapy. San Diego, CA: American Society of Microbiology, 2002; Abstract C2-1276:104.
73. Revathi G, Shannon KP, Stapleton PD, Jain BK, French GL. An outbreak of extended-spectrum β-lactamase-producing *Salmonella seftenberg* in a burns ward. J Hosp Infect 1998; 40:295–302.
74. Miriagou V, Filip R, Coman G, Tzouvelekis LS. Expanded-spectrum cephalosporin-resistant *Salmonella* strains in Romania. J Clin Microbiol 2002; 40:4334–4336.
75. Hanson ND, Moland ES, Hossain A, Neville SA, Gosbell IB, Thomson KS. Unusual *Salmonella enterica* serotype *typhimurium* isolate producing CMY-7, SHV-9 and OXA-30 β-lactamases. J Antimicrob Chemother 2002; 49:1011–1014.
76. Cardinale E, Colbachini P, Perrier-Gros-Claude JD, Gassama A, Aidara-Kane A. Dual emergence in food and humans of a novel multiresistant serotype of *Salmonella* in Senegal: *Salmonella enterica* subsp *enterica* serotype 35:c:1,2. J Clin Microbiol 2001; 39:2373–2374.
77. Villa L, Mammina C, Miriagou V, et al. Multidrug and broad-spectrum cephalosporin resistance among *Salmonella enterica* serotype *enteritidis* clinical isolates in southern Italy. J Clin Microbiol 2002; 40:2662–2665.
78. Poupart MC, Chanal C, Sirot D, Labia R, Sirot J. Identification of CTX-2, a novel cefotaximase from a *Salmonella mbandaka* isolate. Antimicrob Agents Chemother 1991; 35:1498–1500.
79. Di Conza J, Ayala JA, Power P, Mollerach M, Gutkind G. Novel Class 1 integron (InS21) carrying blaCTX-M-2 in *Salmonella enterica* serovar *infantis*. Antimicrob Agents Chemother 2002; 46:2257–2261.
80. Orman BE, Piñeiro SA, Arduino S, et al. Evolution of multiresistance in nontyphoid *Salmonella* serovars from 1984 to 1998 in Argentina. Antimicrob Agents Chemother 2002; 46:3963–3970.
81. Tassios PT, Gazouli M, Tzelepi E, et al. Spread of *Salmonella typhimurium* clone resistant to expanded-spectrum cephalosporins in three European countries. J Clin Microbiol 1999; 37:3774–3777.

82. Su LH, Chiu CH, Chu C, Wang MH, Chia JH, Wu TL. In vivo acquisition of ceftriaxone resistance in *Salmonella enterica* serotype *anatum*. Antimicrob Agents Chemother 2003; 47:563–567.
83. Gazouli M, Tzelepi E, Sidorenko SV, Tzouvelekis LS. Sequence of the gene encoding a plasmid-mediated cefotaxime-hydrolyzing class A β-lactamase (CTX-M-4): involvement of serine 237 in cephalosporin hydrolysis. Antimicrob Agents Chemother 1998; 42:1259–1262.
84. Gazouli M, Tzelepi E, Markogiannakis A, Legakis NJ, Tzouvelekis LS. Two novel plasmid-mediated cefotaxime-hydrolyzing β-lactamases (CTX-M-5 and CTX-M-6) from *Salmonella typhimurium*. FEMS Microbiol Lett 1998; 165:289–293.
85. Bradford PA, Yang Y, Sahm D, Grope I, Gardovska D, Storch G. CTX-M-5, a novel cefotaxime hydrolyzing β-lactamase from an outbreak of *Salmonella typhimurium* in Latvia. Antimicrob Agents Chemother 1998; 42:1980–1984.
86. Simarro E, Navarro F, Ruiz J, Miró E, Gómez J, Mirelis B. *Salmonella enterica* serovar Virchow with CTX-M-like β-lactamase in Spain. J Clin Microbiol 2000; 38:4676–4678.
87. Vahaboglu H, Dodanli S, Eroglu C, et al. Characterisation of multiple-antibiotic-resistant *Salmonella typhimurium* strains: Molecular epidemiology of PER-1 producing isolates and evidence for nosocomial plasmid exchange by a clone. J Clin Microbiol 1996; 34:2942–2946.
88. Bauernfeind A, Stemplinger I, Jungwirth R, et al. Characterization of β-lactamase gene $bla_{PER\text{-}2}$, which encodes an extended-spectrum class A β-lactamase. Antimicrob Agents Chemother 1996; 40:616–620.
89. Fey PD, Safranek TJ, Rupp ME, et al. Ceftriaxone-resistant salmonella infection acquired by a child from cattle. N Engl J Med 2000; 342:1242–1249.
90. Winokur PL, Brueggemann A, DeSalvo DL, et al. Animal and human multidrug-resistant cephalosporin-resistant *Salmonella* isolates expressing a plasmid mediated CMY-2 AmpC β-lactamase. Antimicrob Agents Chemother 2000; 44:2777–2783.
91. Rankin SC, Aceto H, Cassidy J, et al. Molecular characterization of cephalosporin-resistant *Salmonella enterica* serotype *newport* isolates from animals in Pennsylvania. J Clin Microbiol 2002; 40:4679–4684.
92. Koeck JL, Arlet G, Philippon A, et al. A plasmid-mediated CMY-2 β-lactamase from an Algerian clinical isolate of *Salmonella seftenberg*. FEMS Microbiol Lett 1997; 152:255–260.
93. Armand-Lefevre L, Leflon-Guibout V, Bredin J, et al. Imipenem resistance in *Salmonella enterica* serovar *wein* related to porin loss and CMY-4 β-lactamase production. Antimicrob Agents Chemother 2003; 47:1165–1168.
94. Verdet C, Arlet G, Barnaud G, Lagragnge PH, Philippon A. A novel integron in *Salmonella enterica* serovar *enteritidis*, carrying the $bla_{DHA\text{-}1}$ gene and its regulator gene *amp*R, originated from *Morganella morganii*. Antimicrob Agent Chemother 2000; 44:222–225.
95. Gaillot O, Clément C, Simonet M, Philippon A. Novel transferable β-lactam resistance with cephalosporinase characteristics in *Salmonella enteritidis*. J Antimicrob Chemother 1997; 39:85–87.
96. Winokur PL, Canton R, Casellas JM, Legakis N. Variations in the prevalence of strains expressing extended-spectrum β-lactamase phenotype and characterization of isolates from Europe, the Americas and the western Pacific regions. Clin Infect Dis 2001; 32:S94–S103.
97. Dunne EE, Fey PD, Kludt P, et al. Emergence of domestically-acquired ceftriaxone-resistant *Salmonella* infections associated with AmpC β-lactamase. JAMA 2000; 284:3151–3156.
98. Threlfall EJ, Skinner JA, Graham A, Ward LR, Smith HR. Resistance to ceftriaxone and cefotaxime in non-typhoidal *Salmonella enterica* in England and Wales. J Antimicrob Chemother 2000; 46:860–862.
99. Otkun M, Erdem B, Akata F, et al. Antibiotic resistance patterns and plasmid profiles of *Salmonella typhimurium* isolates in Turkey. Eur J Clin Microbiol Infect Dis 2001; 20:206–209.

100. Bhutta ZA, Farooqui BJ, Sturm AW. Eradication of a multiple drug resistant *Salmonella paratyphi A* causing meningitis with ciprofloxacin. J Infect 1992; 25:215–219.
101. Saha SK, Taukder SY, Islam M, Saha S. A highly ceftriaxone-resistant *Salmonella typhi* in Bangladesh. Pediatr Infect Dis J 1999; 18:387.
102. Datta N, Richards H, Datta C. *Salmonella typhi* in vivo acquires resistance to both chloramphenicol and cotrimoxazole. Lancet 1981; 1:1181–1183.
103. Schwalbe R. Hoge CW, Morris JG, O'Halon PN, Crawford RA, Gilligan PH. In vivo selection for transmissible drug resistance in *Salmonella typhi* during antimicrobial therapy. Antimicrob Agents Chemother 1990; 34:161–163.
104. Davis MA, Hancock DD, Besser TE. Multiresistant clones of *Salmonella enterica*: the importance of dissemination. J Lab Clin Med 2002; 140:135–141.
105. Llanes C, Kirchgesner V, Plesiat P. Propagation of TEM- and PSE-type β-lactamases among amoxycillin-resistant *Salmonella* spp isolated in France. Antimicrob Agents Chemother 1999; 43:2430–2436.
106. Mirza S, Kariuki S, Mamun KZ, Beeching NJ, Hart CA. Analysis of plasmid and chromosomal DNA of multidrug-resistant *Salmonella enterica* serovar *typhi* from Asia. J Clin Microbiol 2000; 38:1449–1452.
107. Thong K-L, Bhutta ZA, Pang T. Multidrug-resistant strains of *Salmonella enterica* serotype *typhi* are genetically homogenous and coexist with antibiotic-sensitive strains as distinct, independent clones. Int J Infect Dis 2000; 4:194–197.
108. Ling JM, Zhou G-M, Woo THS, French GL. Antimicrobial susceptibilities and β-lactamase production of Hong Kong isolates of gastroenteric salmonellae and *Salmonella typhi*. J Antimicrob Chemother 1991; 28:877–885.
109. Balis E, Vatopoulos AC, Kanelopoulou M, et al. Indications of in vivo transfer of an epidemic R plasmid from *Salmonella enteritidis* to *Escherichia coli* of the normal human gut flora. J Clin Microbiol 1996; 34:977–979.
110. Nastasi A, Mammina C. Presence of class I integrons in multidrug-resistant, low-prevalence *Salmonella* serotypes, Italy. Emerg Infect Dis 2001; 7:455–458.
111. Carattoli A, Villa L, Pezzella C, Bordi E, Visca P. Expanding drug resistance through integron acquisition by IncF1 plasmids of *Salmonella enterica typhimurium*. Emerg Infect Dis 2000; 7:444–447.
112. Guerra B, Soto S, Helmuth R, Mendoza MC. Characterization of a self-transferable plasmid from *Salmonella enterica* serotype *typhimurium* clinical isolates carrying two integron-borne gene cassettes together with virulence and drug resistance genes. Antimicrob Agents Chemother 2002; 46:2977–2981.
113. Cohen ML, Tauxe RV. Drug-resistant *Salmonella* in the United States: an epidemiological perspective. Science 1986; 234:964–969.
114. Girgis NI, Butler T, Frenck RW, et al. Azithromycin versus ciprofloxacin for treatment of uncomplicated typhoid fever in a randomized trial in Egypt that includes patients with multidrug resistance. Antimicrob Agents Chemother 1999; 43:1441–1444.
115. Phuong CXT, Kneen R, Nguyen TA, Truong DL, White NJ, Parry CM. Dong Nai Typhoid Study Group. A comparative study of ofloxacin and cefixime for treatment of typhoid fever in children. Pediatr Infect Dis J 1999; 18:245–248.
116. Bethell DB, Hien TT, Phi LT, et al. Effects on growth of single short courses of fluoroquinolones. Arch Dis Child 1996; 74:44–46.
117. Doherty CP, Saha SK, Cutting WAM. Typhoid fever, ciprofloxacin and growth in young children. Ann Trop Paediatr 2000; 20:297–303.
118. Kubin R. Safety and efficacy of ciprofloxacin in paediatric patients. Infection 1993; 21:413–421.
119. Yee CL, Duffy C, Gerbino PG, Stryker S, Noel GJ. Tendon or joint disorders in children after treatment with fluoroquinolones or azithromycin. Pediatr Infect Dis J 2002; 21:525–529.

120. Chinh NT, Parry CM, Ly NT, et al. A randomized controlled comparison of azithromycin and ofloxacin for treatment of multidrug-resistant or nalidixic acid-resistant enteric fever. Antimicrob Agents Chemother 2000; 44:1855–1859.
121. Soe GB, Overturf GD. Treatment of typhoid fever and other systemic salmonelloses with cefotaxime, ceftriaxone, cefoperazone, and other newer cephalosporins. Rev Infect Dis 1987; 9:719–736.
122. Bhutta ZA, Khan IA, Molla AM. Therapy of multidrug-resistant typhoid fever with oral cefixime versus intravenous ceftriaxone. Pediatr Infect Dis J 1994; 13:990–994.
123. Frenck RW Jr, Nakhla I, Sultan Y. Azithromycin versus ceftriaxone for the treatment of uncomplicated typhoid fever in children. J Infect Dis 2000; 31:1134–1138.
124. Dutta P, Rasaily R, Saha MR, et al. Ciprofloxacin for treatment of severe typhoid fever in children. Antimicrob Agents Chemother 1993; 37:1197–1199.
125. Bitar R, Tarpley J. Intestinal perforation in typhoid fever: a historical and state-of-the-art review. Rev Infect Dis 1985; 7:257–271.
126. Hoffman SL, Punjabi NH, Kumala S, et al. Reduction of mortality in chloramphenicol-treated severe typhoid fever by high dose dexamethasone. N Engl J Med 1984:310:82–88.
127. Punjabi NH, Hoffman SL, Edman DC, et al. Treatment of severe typhoid fever in children with high dose dexamethasone. Pediatr Infect Dis J 1988; 7:598–600.
128. Rogerson SJ, Spooner VJ, Smith TA, Richens J. Hydrocortisone in chloramphenicol-treated severe typhoid fever in Papua New Guinea. Trans R Soc Trop Med Hyg 1991; 85:113–116.
129. Seoud M, Saade G, Uwaydah M, Azoury R. Typhoid fever in pregnancy. Obstet Gynecol 1988; 71:711–714.
130. Leung D, Venkatesan P, Boswell T, Innes JA, Wood MJ. Treatment of typhoid in pregnancy. Lancet 1995; 346:648.
131. Ferreccio C, Morris JG, Valdiviseo C, et al. Efficacy of ciprofloxacin in the treatment of chronic typhoid carriers. J Infect Dis 1988; 157:1235–1239.
132. Gotuzzo E, Guerra JG, Benavente L, et al. Use of norfloxacin to treat typhoid carriers. J Infect Dis 1988; 157:1221–1225.
133. Sirinavin S, Garner P. Antibiotics for treating *Salmonella* gut infections. Cochrane Database Syst Rev 2000; 2:CD001167.
134. Wiström J, Norrby SR. Fluoroquinolones and bacterial enteritis, when and for whom? J Antimicrob Chemother 1995; 36:23–39.
135. Nelson JD, Kusmiesz H, Jackson LH, Woodman E. Treatment of *Salmonella* gastroenteritis with ampicillin, amoxycillin or placebo. Pediatrics 1980; 65:1125–1130.
136. Dryden MS, Gabb RJE, Wright SK. Empirical treatment of severe acute community-acquired gastroenteritis with ciprofloxacin. Clin Infect Dis 1996; 22:1019–1025.
137. Chiu C, Lin TY, Ou JT. A clinical trial comparing oral azithromycin, cefixime and no antibiotics in the treatment of acute uncomplicated *Salmonella* enteritis in children. J Paediatr Child Health 1999; 35:372–374.
138. Lightfoot NF, Ahamad F, Cowden J. Management of institutional outbreaks of *Salmonella* gastroenteritis. J Antimicrob Chemother 1990; 26(suppl. F):37–46.
139. Neill MA, Opal SM, Heelan J, et al. Failure of ciprofloxacin to eradicate convalescent faecal excretion after acute salmonellosis: experience during an outbreak in health care workers. Ann Intern Med 1991; 114:195–199.
140. Wang J-H, Liu Y-C, Yen M-Y, et al. Mycotic aneurysm due to non-typhi *Salmonella*: report of 16 cases. Clin Infect Dis 1996; 23:743–747.
141. Bhutta ZA. Impact of age and drug resistance on mortality in typhoid fever. Arch Dis Child 1996; 75:214–217.
142. Wain J, Diep TS, Ho VA, et al. Quantitative bacteriology of the blood in typhoid fever; relationship to clinical features, transmissibility and antibiotic resistance. J Clin Microbiol 1998; 36:1683–1687.

143. Helms M, Vastrup P, Gerner-Smidt P, Molbak K. Excess mortality associated with antimicrobial drug-resistant *Salmonella typhimurium*. Emerg Infect Dis 2002; 8:490–495.
144. Threlfall EJ, Ward LR, Rowe B. Multiresistant *Salmonella typhimurium* DT104 and bacteraemia. Lancet 1998; 352:287–288.
145. Barza M, Travers K. Excess infections due to antimicrobial resistance: The "Attributable Fraction." Clin Infect Dis 2002; 34(suppl. 3):S126–S130.
146. Riley LW, Cohen ML, Seals JE, et al. Importance of host factors in human salmonellosis caused by multiresistant strains of *Salmonella*. J Infect Dis 1984; 149:878–883.
147. Mermin JH, Villar R, Carpenter J, et al. A massive epidemic of multidrug-resistant typhoid fever in Tajikistan associated with the consumption of municipal water. J Infect Dis 1999; 179:1416–1422.
148. Riley LW, Ceballos BSO, Trabulsi LR, Fernades de Toledo MR, Blake PA. The significance of hospitals as reservoirs for endemic multiresistant *Salmonella typhimurium* causing infection in urban Brazilian children. J Infect Dis 1984; 150:236–241.
149. Tarr PE, Kuppens L, Jones TC, Ivanoff B, Aparin PG, Heymann DL. Considerations regarding mass vaccination against typhoid fever as an adjunct to sanitation and public health measures: potential use in an epidemic in Tajikistan. Am J Trop Med Hyg 1999; 61:163–170.
150. Lin FYC, Ho VA, Khiem HB, et al. The efficacy of a *Salmonella typhi* Vi conjugate vaccine in 2-to-5-year-old children. N Engl J Med 2001; 344:1263–1269.

12
Management of Melioidosis

Andrew J. H. Simpson

1. INTRODUCTION

Melioidosis is an infection caused by the motile aerobic Gram-negative bacterium *Burkholderia* (formerly *Pseudomonas*) *pseudomallei*. In the endemic areas of Southeast Asia and northern Australia, it may be a leading cause of community-acquired septicemia *(1)*. Mortality rates in severe disease are high, and it is therefore an important public health problem, although probably under-recognized in some countries *(2)*. Although melioidosis is not often seen in other parts of the world, imported cases in tourists have been described *(3)*, and the number of such cases is likely to rise with increasing access to international travel.

As many of the agents used for empirical treatment of community-acquired septicemias at best have suboptimal activity against *B. pseudomallei*, awareness of this disease among clinicians is vitally important if mortality is to be minimized. Furthermore, both *B. pseudomallei* and the closely related organism *Burkholderia mallei* (the cause of glanders) are considered potential biological warfare/bioterrorism agents and are listed by the US Centers for Disease Control and Prevention (CDC) as Category B agents.

2. EPIDEMIOLOGY

Burkholderia pseudomallei is an environmental saprophyte and is found in wet soils, particularly rice paddies. The disease was first described in Burma *(4)* and subsequently has been described in many countries of Southeast Asia, as well as in northern parts of Australia *(1,5–8)*. Most cases are in patients who live in rural locations or who are occupationally exposed to soil *(9)*. The majority of cases have been described in Thailand and Australia, with smaller numbers in Malaysia *(10)* and Singapore *(11)*. Sporadic cases have been described elsewhere, mainly in the tropics, but imported cases are increasingly reported in developed countries *(3,12)*.

3. CLINICAL PRESENTATION

Symptomatic melioidosis is a pyogenic, often systemic, infection characterized by abscess formation (commonly in the lungs, liver, spleen, and parotid gland), pneumonia, and septicemia *(1,7,13–15)*. It has similarities to the equine disease glanders, which

From: *Management of Multiple Drug-Resistant Infections*
Edited by: S. H. Gillespie © Humana Press Inc., Totowa, NJ

is caused by *B. mallei (4)*. It is thought that acquisition of the organism is usually through small abrasions, but ingestion or inhalation may also be important.

The majority of infections are probably asymptomatic, and many residents of endemic areas will have serological evidence of exposure at some time *(16,17)*. Patients with underlying diabetes mellitus, renal disease, or alcoholism are at increased risk of infection *(7,18)*. Melioidosis can occur at any age, although there are peaks in childhood and above the age of 40 yr *(9)*.

Local abscesses (e.g., in the skin) may occur, but disseminated infection is more usual. Any organ system may be involved, and clinical presentations may be highly diverse. Acute septicemia (often with shock), disseminated disease, and pneumonia (either primary or secondary to disseminated infection) are the most common presentations *(1,7)*. Visceral and soft tissue abscesses are also common. Osteomyelitis, septic arthritis, and encephalomyelitis are well described *(7)*. Approximately 60% of patients admitted to hospitals will have positive blood cultures *(14,15)*, which is of prognostic importance *(19)*, and 50% will have evidence of lung involvement *(1)*. Chronic suppurative infections also occur, and the disease may be mistaken for tuberculosis. The overall in-hospital mortality is approx 40% despite recent advances in antibiotic treatment *(15)*. Relapse is common, and both the primary illness and subsequent relapse may present following long latent periods *(20–22)*.

4. DIAGNOSIS

The great variety of presentations of melioidosis and the variable incubation period mean that clinical diagnosis of the disease is impracticable, even in endemic areas where clinical suspicion will be highest. A history of previous travel to an endemic area may raise the possibility of the diagnosis. Definitive diagnosis therefore relies on isolation of the organism from clinical specimens such as blood, sputum, urine, or pus. The organism is not difficult to isolate using appropriate culture media and reagents *(23–25)*. Selective broth enrichment media increase the diagnostic sensitivity *(26)*.

Considerable effort should be made to obtain suitable specimens, particularly aspirates of visceral or subcutaneous abscesses. Abdominal imaging is indicated in confirmed cases to exclude liver or splenic abscesses *(13)*. Throat swab culture is useful, particularly in cases with respiratory involvement where sputum is not produced *(27)*. There does not appear to be a carrier state *(16,27)*, so isolation of *B. pseudomallei* from nonsterile sites should be taken as evidence of infection. Cultural methods are slow, and speed of isolation remains a problem. Rapid identification of the organism in blood cultures or on solid culture media has been improved using specific latex agglutination tests *(28,29)*.

Direct demonstration of *B. pseudomallei* in clinical samples by a specific immunofluorescence test has been used successfully and allows a rapid presumptive diagnosis *(30)*.

Serological tests are problematic. Antibody detection tests have been available for some time, but are of limited use for diagnostic purposes in an endemic area *(16,31)*. Detection of immunoglobulin M (IgM) antibodies has improved the utility of these tests, but is not used widely *(32)*. Antigen detection tests have potentially greater value. Several such tests have been described for urine samples, using enzyme-linked immunosorbent assay (ELISA) or latex agglutination, but again they are not widely available *(33,34)*. Other tests for detection of serum antigen have been described, but have not been clinically evaluated *(35)*.

Several molecular tests, such as polymerase chain reaction (PCR), have been described, but none have become established for diagnosis yet *(36,37)*. Combinations of molecular and serological tests have a high negative predictive value and may prove useful for excluding a diagnosis of melioidosis *(38)*.

5. ANTIBIOTIC SUSCEPTIBILITY

Burkholderia pseudomallei is intrinsically resistant to many antibiotics. It is resistant in vitro to penicillins *(39)*, aminopenicillins *(40,41)*, and many early cephalosporins, including cefuroxime *(42,43)*. It is resistant to macrolides *(44)*, lincosamides (such as clindamycin) *(45)*, and rifampicin *(46,47)*. *Burkholderia pseudomallei* is intrinsically resistant to most aminoglycosides (e.g., gentamicin and amikacin) *(7,48)*. Some strains appear sensitive to kanamycin, but it is unclear whether this is clinically useful *(39)*. Most clinical experience with kanamycin was obtained over two decades ago, and it is rarely, if ever, used now *(49)*. Rare wild isolates are susceptible to macrolides and aminoglycosides because of a deficiency in the efflux mechanism *(50)*.

Burkholderia pseudomallei is generally susceptible in vitro to third-generation cephalosporins such as the antipseudomonal agent ceftazidime *(40,51)*. Cefotaxime and ceftriaxone are marginally less active than ceftazidime in vitro *(43)*, and clinical experience has shown that they are much less effective therapeutic agents *(52)*. Cefpirome and cefixime also have activity in vitro *(53)*, as does cefoperazone when combined with the β-lactamase inhibitor sulbactam *(54)*.

Burkholderia pseudomallei is susceptible to the antipseudomonal ureidopenicillins (piperacillin and, to a lesser extent, ticarcillin) *(43,55)* and ureidopenicillin plus β-lactamase inhibitor combinations, such as piperacillin-tazobactam and ticarcillin-clavulanic acid. The combination of amoxicillin and clavulanic acid (coamoxiclav, Augmentin) *(56)* is also active. Carbapenems (imipenem and meropenem) are highly active against *B. pseudomallei* *(46,57,58)*.

Burkholderia pseudomallei is susceptible to both chloramphenicol *(43,46)* and the antifolate inhibitor combination trimethoprim-sulfamethoxazole (cotrimoxazole, TMP-SXT) *(59)*, both of which are used extensively for oral treatment of melioidosis. However, testing of susceptibility to TMP-SXT is unreliable unless minimum inhibitory concentration (MIC) methods are used *(43,60)*; as a result, older reports of susceptibility rates cannot necessarily be considered reliable. *Burkholderia pseudomallei* is only moderately susceptible to fluoroquinolones such as ciprofloxacin *(61)*, as well as the newer agents such as moxifloxacin and gatifloxacin *(62)*. This is disappointing because the fluoroquinolones have good activity against many *Pseudomonas* species and achieve good intracellular concentrations, so they make theoretically attractive agents for melioidosis therapy. *Burkholderia pseudomallei* is unusual among pseudomonads in that it is also susceptible to tetracyclines *(41,46)*. Strains isolated in Hong Kong *(41)*, Malaysia *(63)*, and Australia *(58)* appear to have similar susceptibility patterns as those from Thailand *(43)*.

The β-lactams and fluoroquinolones are bactericidal against *B. pseudomallei* *(43)*. In contrast, chloramphenicol, tetracyclines, trimethoprim, and sulfamethoxazole are bacteriostatic and antagonistic *(51)*. In one study, ciprofloxacin combined with azithromycin was bactericidal *(64)*. The carbapenems and fluoroquinolones also exert a postantibiotic effect against *B. pseudomallei (65)*. In time-kill experiments, the carbapenems are the most active agents, achieving much faster killing than does ceftazidime *(57)*, and they retain activity against ceftazidime-resistant strains.

Acquired resistance was relatively common when the "conventional" bacteristatic four-drug regimen (chloramphenicol, doxycycline, and TMP-SXT) was used for acute therapy (occurring in approx 7% of infections). This rate has dropped considerably with the switch to β-lactams for acute disease. Resistance to the β-lactams can also arise during therapy *(66)*, and a specific ceftazidimase has been identified *(66)*, as well as broader spectrum β-lactamases, that can be inhibited by clavulanic acid *(67)*. Specific carbapenemases have not yet been described in *B. pseudomallei* (although they are present in related bacteria such as *Burkholderia cepacia*), but class D β-lactamases with activity against imipenem have been characterized *(68)*.

6. TREATMENT OF MELIOIDOSIS

6.1. Parenteral Treatment

6.1.1. Antibiotic Management

As discussed in Section 5, *B. pseudomallei* is resistant to many of the first-line agents used in hospitals worldwide to treat community-acquired septicemias (i.e., penicillin-aminoglycoside combinations). In endemic areas, therefore, many patients may receive ineffective empirical therapy. Quadruple or "conventional" therapy with intravenous chloramphenicol (100–150 mg/kg body weight per day), doxycycline (4–6 mg/kg body weight per day), and TMP-SXT (8–12 and 40–60 mg/kg body weight per day, respectively) or variations of this regimen with additional kanamycin were the mainstay of therapy for many years in Thailand *(49,69)*. However, these regimens were associated with an unacceptably high mortality, approx 70–80% in septicemic melioidosis, and are potentially toxic and antagonistic.

Unfortunately, there are still few reported comparative treatment trials in melioidosis. This is partly because of the fact that it is predominantly a disease affecting rural agricultural workers in remote parts of the world, in whom pharmaceutical company interest is minimal, but it is also related to the high cost of the currently available active drugs *(15,70)*. An additional problem is that only two or three centers in Thailand are capable of conducting well-powered clinical studies because of the relatively few cases elsewhere.

The first open, prospective, randomized trial was conducted in northeast Thailand and compared high-dose intravenous ceftazidime (120 mg/kg body weight per day) with conventional therapy in severe disease *(69)*. The study enrolled 161 patients, of whom only 65 were subsequently proven to have melioidosis (although 54 of these were septicemic). Despite the small number of patients, mortality was 50% lower in the ceftazidime arm, to less than 40% in patients who survived for a minimum of 48 h. There were no differences in mortality during the first 48 h of treatment, a feature that also is common to subsequent trials.

A similar trial by a different group compared conventional therapy with a combination of intravenous ceftazidime (100 mg/kg body weight per day) and TMP-SXT (8 and 40 mg/kg body weight per day, respectively) for a minimum of 10 d *(71)*. This trial achieved results similar to the first *(69)*, again from relatively few patients (64 with culture-proven severe melioidosis).

As a result of the above two trials, ceftazidime-containing regimens became the acute treatment of choice for severe melioidosis. Debate continued over the combination with TMP-SXT because of the theoretical possibility of antagonism of the action of ceftazidime *(51)*. Clinical evidence of such an effect is lacking. There have not been any reported trials of intravenous ceftazidime versus this combination of ceftazidime and TMP-SXT, although such trials are being conducted in Thailand. Ceftazidime, however, can be administered with cost savings by constant infusion rather than by bolus dosing every 8 h *(72)*.

Three randomized trials of other agents in acute severe melioidosis were reported subsequently *(14,15,73)*. In the first, ceftazidime was compared with high-dose intravenous coamoxiclav (160 mg/kg body weight per day) *(14)*, following an open trial that suggested the effectiveness of coamoxiclav *(74)*. In the comparative trial, the overall mortality was 47% in both groups (although there was a higher treatment failure rate for coamoxiclav). The authors concluded that coamoxiclav was an effective acute treatment, but that ceftazidime remained the drug of choice.

The next trial, by the same group, compared ceftazidime with intravenous imipenem (50 mg/kg body weight per day) *(15)*. Mortality in the two study arms was similar, although the study was terminated prematurely (despite having already enrolled 214 patients with a positive culture); hence, it is not known whether a mortality difference would have emerged. However, it would appear that imipenem is effective for treatment. Meropenem, another carbapenem antibiotic, has not been subjected to clinical trial in melioidosis, but following the imipenem trial discussed above *(15)*, was used successfully for acute treatment of melioidosis in Australia, including relapsed cases *(7,75)*. It has also been used successfully in combination with TMP-SXT *(7)* in a small number of cases.

Cefoperazone, at 25 mg/kg body weight per day, in combination with sulbactam plus cotrimoxazole, was as effective as ceftazidime plus TMP-SXT *(73,76)* in a further trial. Mortality in both arms was lower than that reported in other studies, but the most ill patients (those likely to die within 24 h) were excluded from the study. This study has also been criticized for a lack of power to determine equivalent efficacy *(77)*. Further data are needed before cefoperazone-sulbactam can be recommended.

As a result of all these trials, ceftazidime (with or without TMP-SXT) has been established as the treatment of choice for severe melioidosis *(78)*, with carbapenems as alternatives. Amoxicillin-clavulanate is a satisfactory empirical treatment for sepsis in endemic areas. The role of antibiotic combinations in improving efficacy is still unclear. Prevention of antibiotic resistance by use of combinations is not relevant to management of individual cases because patients acquire their infections from the environment. More trials are needed.

Other antibiotics with good in vitro activity have not been formally assessed in acute melioidosis. Such agents include piperacillin and the ureidopenicillin plus β-lactamase inhibitor combinations, piperacillin-tazobactam (Tazocin) and ticarcillin-clavulanic acid (Timentin). There is very little documented experience with these agents, even in the form of case reports. Despite the documented use of the fluoroquinolones as oral agents for maintenance therapy, experience with their use in acute disease is very limited, probably because of their marginal in vitro activity. However, combinations of a carbapenem and ciprofloxacin have been used successfully in two intractable cases *(79,80)*.

Other cephalosporins are widely available and are often used for community-acquired sepsis. However, in a retrospective review of 1353 treated melioidosis patients, the mortality associated with initial (i.e., empirical) treatment with ceftriaxone or cefotaxime was nearly double that with ceftazidime. This provides strong evidence against the use of these cephalosporins for treating melioidosis *(81)*.

The therapeutic response is usually slow regardless of antibiotic used. Most patients will be pyrexial for more than a week after starting appropriate therapy, which can be alarming for inexperienced clinicians *(14,15,69)*. Persistence of fever after several days does not necessarily imply treatment failure. At least 10–14 d of parenteral therapy should be given and continued until there is clear evidence of a clinical response; this may take several weeks in severe cases.

6.1.2. Empirical Treatment

Patients presenting in an endemic area, or who have traveled from an endemic area, with conditions consistent with a diagnosis of melioidosis require early treatment that will cover infection with *B. pseudomallei*. If the diagnosis is not clear, then broad-spectrum agents that have activity, such as coamoxiclav or a carbapenem, are indicated. If the diagnosis is confirmed, either continuation with a carbapenem or a switch to ceftazidime should be instituted.

Coamoxiclav has the advantage of a broader antibacterial spectrum than ceftazidime and hence may be more appropriate as empirical therapy for community-acquired septicemias in endemic areas.

6.1.3. Allergy to β-Lactams

If allergy to β-lactams causes problems during treatment, a switch to an alternative agent (e.g., from ceftazidime to a carbapenem) may be all that is required. In cases of genuine life-threatening allergy to all β-lactam agents, the only remaining option may be to treat with the conventional regimen (chloramphenicol, doxycycline, and TMP-SXT), with all drugs given intravenously and in high doses *(69)*, despite the associated high mortality. The risk of a severe reaction to treatment has to be balanced against this disease-associated mortality.

6.1.4. Augmentative Therapies

Appropriate supportive measures should be instituted in acutely ill patients, with prompt resuscitation and transfer to intensive care facilities. Isolation of patients is not necessary; nosocomial infection appears to be an extremely rare event *(82,83)*, but appropriate measures for decontamination of medical equipment must be instituted. Surgical drainage of abscesses, particularly hepatic or splenic, is indicated when possible, although these abscesses may be multiple.

Nonantibiotic therapeutic modalities are of interest in the management of sepsis of any etiology. Few such agents have been tested in melioidosis, although if substantial reductions in the mortality from melioidosis are to be achieved, it could be argued that it is likely to result from the successful introduction of such an agent.

Lexipafant (a platelet-activating factor receptor antagonist) was subjected to a placebo-controlled clinical trial in 131 patients with all-cause sepsis in Thailand; 55% of the patients with positive blood cultures had melioidosis *(84)*. For patients with positive blood cultures, the mortality in the lexipafant group was lower at 28 d, but did not achieve statistical significance ($p = 0.09$). However, there were relatively few patients with positive blood cultures in each arm of the study (34 vs. 32), and it is tempting to speculate on the outcome of the trial if more patients had been recruited.

Granulocyte colony-stimulating factor (G-CSF) *(85)* has been examined in an open trial in Australia in patients with community-acquired septic shock. Although very few patients with melioidosis were included, survival was a remarkable 100%, compared to 5% of historical controls. Further work is being conducted on the use of G-CSF in acute melioidosis, and the results are eagerly awaited. Current practice in Darwin, Australia is to administer G-CSF to all patients with melioidosis who present in septic shock *(7)*.

Other agents, such as antithrombin and activated human recombinant protein C, are also being considered for trial in melioidosis patients following previous multicenter trials in all-cause sepsis *(86,87)*. Activated protein C in particular appears a very promising agent for treatment of sepsis.

6.1.5. Relapsed Infections

Relapse is a common occurrence in melioidosis, despite apparent compliance with maintenance therapy, and should be treated as for first episodes *(20,75)*. All patients should be offered long-term oral therapy after the acute episode to limit relapse because both the mortality and morbidity in relapsed cases are similar to those in first episodes *(20)*. It has therefore been recommended that patients receive follow-up for life *(88)*. Usually, the antimicrobial susceptibility pattern of the relapse isolate is unchanged compared to the previous episode. However, the development of resistance while on treatment has been described for all the commonly used agents *(43)*.

6.2. Maintenance or Oral Treatment

There are very few reports of studies of oral treatment in nonsevere melioidosis. However, there are several reported studies of oral maintenance therapy, following successful intravenous treatment of severe disease, to prevent relapse. Superficial abscesses can be treated effectively with drainage and shorter courses of antibiotics than following systemic infection. Parotid abscesses may respond well to careful incision and drainage plus oral antibiotic treatment (usually amoxicillin-clavulanate for 8–12 wk) *(89)*.

Following successful acute treatment of melioidosis, there remains a substantial risk of relapse, with similar morbidity and mortality to first episodes *(20)*. Prolonged maintenance therapy is necessary to limit this *(20)*. The precise location of organisms causing relapse is unclear, but *B. pseudomallei* can survive within macrophages and other phagocytic cells *(90–93)*, so agents that achieve good intracellular penetration may be advantageous.

Most experience has been gained with oral conventional combination antibiotics, that is, chloramphenicol (for 4 to 8 wk), doxycycline, and TMP-SXT (continued for up to 20 wk). Treatment courses of 8 wk have been associated with a relapse rate of 23% *(20,94)*, but 20-wk courses have reduced this to less than 10%. This conventional combination as oral therapy was compared with oral coamoxiclav (plus additional amoxicillin) in one randomized study *(94)*. Chloramphenicol was given for 8 wk. Compliance problems were considerable. Relapse rates after 20 wk of therapy were 4 and 16%, respectively. The authors concluded that coamoxiclav was safer and better tolerated, but possibly less effective. Coamoxiclav is preferred to the conventional regimen in children or in pregnancy.

Failure of compliance with complex regimens remains a major risk factor for relapse *(20)*, so single agents are preferable for oral therapy, ideally taken once or twice per day to improve compliance. Both the conventional and coamoxiclav regimens in the above study *(94)* involved many capsules or tablets per day. An open study of fluoroquinolone therapy (ciprofloxacin or ofloxacin given twice per day) has been completed. These agents are attractive due to their good intracellular penetration (despite concerns about their in vitro activity), but were clearly unsatisfactory, with a relapse rate approaching 30% despite prolonged treatment *(95)*. Although new fluoroquinolones such as moxifloxacin are now being licensed, so far there are no data to suggest that they will be any better than ciprofloxacin or ofloxacin. Unfortunately, therefore, the fluoroquinolones, as single agents, should be considered third-line drugs at best.

Combined azithromycin and ciprofloxacin has been reported to have good activity in vitro *(64)*, and following this report, a small comparative clinical trial was conducted. The results were again disappointing, with the combination of azithromycin and ciprofloxacin proving no better than a fluoroquinolone alone *(96)*. This trial, however, did provide some evidence for efficacy of the combination of doxycycline and TMP-SXT, given for 20 wk, for maintenance therapy. This combination had not been examined previously in vivo. Partly as a result, further trials are now being conducted in Thailand to determine if chloramphenicol is a necessary component of the conventional regimen or whether combined doxycycline and TMP-SXT have equivalent activity.

Doxycycline is the most active of the four-drug combination in vitro, but monotherapy with doxycycline proved significantly inferior to the four-drug conventional regimen in a comparative study involving over 100 patients *(97)*. One-quarter of the doxycycline-treated patients relapsed (11 patients), compared to only 1 patient in the combination arm of the study. Similar failures of eradication with doxycycline monotherapy have occurred in Australia *(58,75)*. As a result, doxycycline cannot be recommended and, like the fluoroquinolones, should be reserved for difficult cases for which there are no alternatives.

Cotrimoxazole maintenance monotherapy has not yet been investigated in a formal randomized clinical trial, but considerable experience with its use is being gained in Australia. Only 1 relapse in a series of 60 patients given TMP-SXT oral therapy has been reported *(7)*. Further investigation is obviously warranted.

The best simple, nontoxic regimens for the maintenance treatment of melioidosis have still to be elucidated. New oral antibiotics are also needed, but there are no obvious candidate drugs at present. In the meantime, however, untested agents and untried combinations are probably best avoided *(98)*.

7. PROPHYLAXIS

Human-to-human transmission of *B. pseudomallei* appears to be very rare *(83,99)*. Prophylaxis is not advised in contacts of known cases or for attendant health care staff.

Very little is known about prophylaxis of laboratory-acquired infections. A case may be made for offering secondary prophylaxis in certain circumstances, for example, following a laboratory accident involving cultures of the organism. An oral agent such as coamoxiclav would seem suitable in such a situation, but there are no data available on dose or duration *(100)*.

Animal data suggest that ciprofloxacin and doxycycline are effective in preventing or attenuating infection with *B. pseudomallei* if administered within 24 h of challenge *(101)*. Despite the absence of human prophylaxis data and their lack of efficacy in established human infections, both agents have been recommended for prophylaxis in the case of a deliberate release *(102)*. However, this recommendation may be influenced by the activity these drugs also possess against other potential deliberate-release agents, such as *Yersinia pestis* (plague) and *Bacillus anthracis* (anthrax), and the need to keep stocks of a limited number of drugs with broad activity to cover such emergencies.

8. CONCLUSIONS

Melioidosis remains a rare disease outside the endemic areas of Southeast Asia and Australia. Severe disease carries high mortality, but both a lack of clinical suspicion and diagnostic difficulty may delay diagnosis. Ceftazidime or a carbapenem are the first-line agents for acute severe melioidosis, and coamoxiclav (Augmentin) is a suitable alternative. High-dose intravenous treatment should continue for at least 10 d and until there has been a clinical response. Oral maintenance therapy is then required, ideally for 20 wk. Currently recommended regimes are either the four-drug antibiotic combination of chloramphenicol, doxycycline, and cotrimoxazole (TMP-SXT) or coamoxiclav alone. TMP-SXT alone or the three-drug combination of doxycycline and TMP-SXT appear promising as oral therapies, but further research is needed. The optimum intravenous and oral antibiotic therapy of melioidosis remains to be determined.

REFERENCES

1. Chaowagul W, White NJ, Dance DAB, et al. Melioidosis: a major cause of community-acquired septicemia in northeastern Thailand. J Infect Dis 1989; 159:890–899.
2. Dance DAB. Melioidosis. Curr Opin Infect Dis 2002; 15:127–132.
3. Dance DAB, Smith MD, Aucken HM, Pitt TL. Imported melioidosis in England and Wales. Lancet 1999; 353:208.
4. Whitmore A. An account of a glanders-like disease occurring in Rangoon. J Hyg 1913; 13:1–34.
5. Dance DAB. Melioidosis as an emerging global problem. Acta Trop 2000; 74:115–119.
6. Currie BJ, Fisher DA, Howard DM, et al. The epidemiology of melioidosis in Australia and Papua New Guinea. Acta Trop 2000; 74:121–127.
7. Currie BJ, Fisher DA, Howard DM, et al. Endemic melioidosis in tropical northern Australia: a 10-year prospective study and review of the literature. Clin Infect Dis 2000; 31: 981–986.
8. Dance DAB. Melioidosis: the tip of the iceberg? Clin Microbiol Rev 1991; 4:52–60.
9. Suputtamongkol Y, Hall AJ, Dance DAB, et al. The epidemiology of melioidosis in Ubon Ratchatani, northeast Thailand. Int J Epidemiol 1994; 23:1082–1090.
10. Puthucheary SD, Parasakthi N, Lee MK. Septicaemic melioidosis: a review of 50 cases from Malaysia. Trans R Soc Trop Med Hyg 1992; 86:683–685.
11. Heng BH, Goh KT, Yap EH, Loh H, Yeo M. Epidemiological surveillance of melioidosis in Singapore. Ann Acad Med Singapore 1998; 27:478–484.

12. Wilks D, Jacobson SK, Lever AM, Farrington M. Fatal melioidosis in a tourist returning from Thailand. J Infect 1994; 29:87–90.
13. Vatcharapreechasakul T, Suputtamongkol Y, Dance DAB, Chaowagul W, White NJ. *Pseudomonas pseudomallei* liver abscesses: a clinical, laboratory, and ultrasonographic study. Clin Infect Dis 1992; 14:412–417.
14. Suputtamongkol Y, Rajchanuwong A, Chaowagul W, et al. Ceftazidime versus amoxicillin/clavulanate in the treatment of severe melioidosis. Clin Infect Dis 1994; 19:846–853.
15. Simpson AJH, Suputtamongkol Y, Smith MD, et al. Comparison of imipenem and ceftazidime as therapy for severe melioidosis. Clin Infect Dis 1999; 29:381–387.
16. Kanaphun P, Thirawattanasuk N, Suputtamongkol Y, et al. Serology and carriage of *Pseudomonas pseudomallei*: a prospective study in 1000 hospitalized children in northeast Thailand. J Infect Dis 1993; 167:230–233.
17. Ashdown LR, Guard RW. The prevalence of human melioidosis in Northern Queensland. Am J Trop Med Hyg 1984; 33:474–478.
18. Suputtamongkol Y, Chaowagul W, Chetchotisakd P, et al. Risk factors for melioidosis and bacteremic melioidosis. Clin Infect Dis 1999; 29:408–413.
19. Walsh AL, Smith MD, Wuthiekanun V, et al. Prognostic significance of quantitative bacteremia in septicemic melioidosis. Clin Infect Dis 1995; 21:1498–1500.
20. Chaowagul W, Suputtamongkol Y, Dance DAB, Rajchanuvong A, Pattara-Arechachai J, White NJ. Relapse in melioidosis: incidence and risk factors. J Infect Dis 1993; 168:1181–1185.
21. Morrison RE, Lamb AS, Craig DB, Johnson WM. Melioidosis: a reminder. Am J Med 1988; 84:965–967.
22. Chodimella U, Hoppes WL, Whalen S, Ognibene AJ, Rutecki GW. Septicemia and suppuration in a Vietnam veteran. Hosp Pract (Off Ed) 1997; 32:219–221.
23. Walsh AL, Wuthiekanun V. The laboratory diagnosis of melioidosis. Br J Biomed Sci 1996; 53:249–253.
24. Dance DAB, Wuthiekanun V, Naigowit P, White NJ. Identification of *Pseudomonas pseudomallei* in clinical practice: use of simple screening tests and API 20NE. J Clin Pathol 1989; 42:645–648.
25. Wuthiekanun V, Dance DAB, Wattanagoon Y, Supputtamongkol Y, Chaowagul W, White NJ. The use of selective media for the isolation of *Pseudomonas pseudomallei* in clinical practice. J Med Microbiol 1990; 33:121–126.
26. Walsh AL, Wuthiekanun V, Smith MD, Suputtamongkol Y, White NJ. Selective broths for the isolation of *Pseudomonas pseudomallei* from clinical samples. Trans R Soc Trop Med Hyg 1995; 89:124.
27. Wuthiekanun V, Suputtamongkol Y, Simpson AJH, Kanaphun P, White NJ. Value of throat swab in diagnosis of melioidosis. J Clin Microbiol 2001; 39:3801–3802.
28. Dharakul T, Songsivilai S, Smithikarn S, Thepthai C, Leelaporn A. Rapid identification of *Burkholderia pseudomallei* in blood cultures by latex agglutination using lipopolysaccharide-specific monoclonal antibody. Am J Trop Med Hyg 1999; 61:658–662.
29. Smith MD, Wuthiekanun V, Walsh AL, Pitt TL. Latex agglutination test for identification of *Pseudomonas pseudomallei*. J Clin Pathol 1993; 46:374–375.
30. Walsh AL, Smith MD, Wuthiekanun V, et al. Immunofluorescence microscopy for the rapid diagnosis of melioidosis. J Clin Pathol 1994; 47:377–379.
31. Ashdown LR. Demonstration of human antibodies to *Pseudomonas pseudomallei* by indirect fluorescent antibody staining. Pathology 1981; 13:597–601.
32. Kunakorn M, Boonma P, Khupulsup K, Petchclai B. Enzyme-linked immunosorbent assay for immunoglobulin M specific antibody for the diagnosis of melioidosis. J Clin Microbiol 1990; 28:1249–1253.
33. Desakorn V, Smith MD, Wuthiekanun V, et al. Detection of *Pseudomonas pseudomallei* antigen in urine for the diagnosis of melioidosis. Am J Trop Med Hyg 1994; 51:627–633.

34. Smith MD, Wuthiekanun V, Walsh AL, et al. Latex agglutination for rapid detection of *Pseudomonas pseudomallei* antigen in urine of patients with melioidosis. J Clin Pathol 1995; 48:174–176.
35. Sirisinha S, Anuntagool N, Dharakul T, et al. Recent developments in laboratory diagnosis of melioidosis. Acta Trop 2000; 74:235–245.
36. Kunakorn M, Raksakait K, Sethaudom C, Sermswan RW, Dharakul T. Comparison of three PCR primer sets for diagnosis of septicemic melioidosis. Acta Trop 2000; 74:247–251.
37. Sura T, Smith MD, Cowan GM, Walsh AL, White NJ, Krishna S. Polymerase chain reaction for the detection of *Burkholderia pseudomallei*. Diagn Microbiol Infect Dis 1997; 29:121–127.
38. Sermswan RW, Wongratanacheewin S, Anuntagool N, Sirisinha S. Comparison of the polymerase chain reaction and serologic tests for diagnosis of septicemic melioidosis. Am J Trop Med Hyg 2000; 63:146–149.
39. Eickhoff TC, Bennett JV, Hayes PS, Feeley J. *Pseudomonas pseudomallei*: susceptibility to chemotherapeutic agents. J Infect Dis 1970; 121:95–102.
40. Ashdown LR. In vitro activities of the newer β-lactam and quinolone antimicrobial agents against *Pseudomonas pseudomallei*. Antimicrob Agents Chemother 1988; 32:1435–1436.
41. Chau PY, Ng WS, Leung YK, Lolekha S. In vitro susceptibility of strains of *Pseudomonas pseudomallei* isolated in Thailand and Hong Kong to some newer β-lactam antibiotics and quinolone derivatives. J Infect Dis 1986; 153:167–170.
42. Ashdown LR, Frettingham RJ. In vitro activity of various cephalosporins against *Pseudomonas pseudomallei*. J Infect Dis 1984; 150:779–780.
43. Dance DAB, Wuthiekanun V, Chaowagul W, White NJ. The antimicrobial susceptibility of *Pseudomonas pseudomallei*. Emergence of resistance in vitro and during treatment. J Antimicrob Chemother 1989; 24:295–309.
44. Simpson AJH, White NJ, Wuthiekanun V. Aminoglycoside and macrolide resistance in *Burkholderia pseudomallei*. Antimicrob Agents Chemother 1999; 43:2332.
45. Hall WH, Manion RE. Antibiotic susceptibility of *Pseudomonas pseudomallei*. Antimicrob Agents Chemother 1973; 4:193–195.
46. Yamamoto T, Naigowit P, Dejsirilert S, et al. In vitro susceptibilities of *Pseudomonas pseudomallei* to 27 antimicrobial agents. Antimicrob Agents Chemother 1990; 34:2027–2029.
47. Fisher MW, Hillegas AB, Nazeeri PL. Susceptibility in vitro and in vivo of *Pseudomonas pseudomallei* to rifampin and tetracyclines. Appl Microbiol 1971; 22:13–16.
48. McEniry DW, Gillespie SH, Felmingham D. Susceptibility of *Pseudomonas pseudomallei* to new β-lactam and aminoglycoside antibiotics. J Antimicrob Chemother 1988; 21:171–175.
49. Leelarasamee A, Bovornkitti S. Melioidosis: review and update. Rev Infect Dis 1989; 11:413–425.
50. Simpson AJH, White NJ, Wuthiekanun V. Aminoglycoside and macrolide resistance in *Burkholderia pseudomallei*. Antimicrob Agents Chemother 1999; 43:2332.
51. Dance DAB, Wuthiekanun V, Chaowagul W, White NJ. Interactions in vitro between agents used to treat melioidosis. J Antimicrob Chemother 1989; 24:311–316.
52. Chaowagul W, Simpson AJH, Suputtamongkol Y, White NJ. Empirical cephalosporin treatment of melioidosis. Clin Infect Dis 1999; 28:1328.
53. Seymour-Murray J, Norton R, Ashhurst-Smith C. Comparative in vitro susceptibility of *Burkholderia pseudomallei* to cefpirome, ceftazidime and cefepime. Pathology 1997; 29:329–330.
54. Koay AS, Rohani MY, Cheong YM. In-vitro susceptibility of *Burkholderia pseudomallei* to cefoperazone-sulbactam combination. Med J Malaysia 1997; 52:158–160.
55. Sookpranee T, Sookpranee M, Mellencamp MA, Preheim LC. *Pseudomonas pseudomallei*, a common pathogen in Thailand that is resistant to the bactericidal effects of many antibiotics. Antimicrob Agents Chemother 1991; 35:484–489.

56. Dance DAB, Wuthiekanun V, Chaowagul W, White NJ. The activity of amoxycillin/clavulanic acid against *Pseudomonas pseudomallei*. J Antimicrob Chemother 1989; 24:1012–1014.
57. Smith MD, Wuthiekanun V, Walsh AL, White NJ. In-vitro activity of carbapenem antibiotics against β-lactam susceptible and resistant strains of *Burkholderia pseudomallei*. J Antimicrob Chemother 1996; 37:611–615.
58. Jenney AWJ, Lum G, Fisher DA, Currie BJ. Antibiotic susceptibility of *Burkholderia pseudomallei* from tropical northern Australia and implications for therapy of melioidosis. Int J Antimicrob Agents 2001; 17:109–113.
59. Bassett DCJ. The sensitivity of *Pseudomonas pseudomallei* to trimethoprim and sulphamethoxazole in vitro. J Clin Pathol 1971; 24:798–800.
60. Piliouras P, Ulett GC, Ashhurst-Smith C, Hirst RG, Norton RE. A comparison of antibiotic susceptibility testing methods for cotrimoxazole with *Burkholderia pseudomallei*. Int J Antimicrob Agents 2002; 19:427–429.
61. Winton MD, Everett ED, Dolan SA. Activities of five new fluoroquinolones against *Pseudomonas pseudomallei*. Antimicrob Agents Chemother 1988; 32:928–929.
62. Ho PL, Cheung TKM, Kinoshita R, Tse CWS, Yuen KY, Chau PY. Activity of five fluoroquinolones against 71 isolates of *Burkholderia pseudomallei*. J Antimicrob Chemother 2002; 49:1042–1044.
63. Puthucheary SD, Parasakthi N. Antimicrobial susceptibility of *Pseudomonas pseudomallei*. J Antimicrob Chemother 1987; 20:921–922.
64. Vorachit M, Chongtrakool P, Arkomsean S, Boonsong S. Antimicrobial resistance in *Burkholderia pseudomallei*. Acta Trop 2000; 74:139–144.
65. Walsh AL, Smith MD, Wuthiekanun V, White NJ. Postantibiotic effects and *Burkholderia (Pseudomonas) pseudomallei*: evaluation of current treatment. Antimicrob Agents Chemother 1995; 39:2356–2358.
66. Godfrey AJ, Wong S, Dance DAB, Chaowagul W, Bryan LE. *Pseudomonas pseudomallei* resistance to β-lactam antibiotics due to alterations in the chromosomally encoded β-lactamase. Antimicrob Agents Chemother 1991; 35:1635–1640.
67. Dance DAB, Wuthiekanun V, Chaowagul W, Suputtamongkol Y, White NJ. Development of resistance to ceftazidime and co-amoxiclav in *Pseudomonas pseudomallei*. J Antimicrob Chemother 1991; 28:321–324.
68. Niumsup P, Wuthiekanun V. Cloning of the class D β-lactamase gene from *Burkholderia pseudomallei* and studies on its expression in ceftazidime-susceptible and -resistant strains. J Antimicrob Chemother 2002; 50:445–455.
69. White NJ, Dance DAB, Chaowagul W, Wattanagoon Y, Wuthiekanun V, Pitakwatchara N. Halving of mortality of severe melioidosis by ceftazidime. Lancet 1989; ii:697–701.
70. Phetsouvanh P, Phongmany S, Newton P, et al. Melioidosis and Pandora's box in the Lao People's Democratic Republic. Clin Infect Dis 2001; 32:653–654.
71. Sookpranee M, Boonma P, Susaengrat W, Bhuripanyo K, Punyagupta S. Multicenter prospective randomized trial comparing ceftazidime plus co-trimoxazole with chloramphenicol plus doxycycline and co-trimoxazole for treatment of severe melioidosis. Antimicrob Agents Chemother 1992; 36:158–162.
72. Angus BJ, Smith MD, Suputtamongkol Y, et al. Pharmacokinetic-pharmacodynamic evaluation of ceftazidime continuous infusion versus intermittent bolus injection in septicaemic melioidosis. Br J Clin Pharmacol 2000; 50:184–191.
73. Chetchotisakd P, Porramatikul S, Mootsikapun P, Anunnatsiri S, Thinkhamrop B. Randomized, double-blind, controlled study of cefoperazone-sulbactam plus cotrimoxazole versus ceftazidime plus cotrimoxazole for the treatment of severe melioidosis. Clin Infect Dis 2001; 33:29–34.
74. Suputtamongkol Y, Dance DAB, Chaowagul W, Wattanagoon Y, Wuthiekanun V, White NJ. Amoxycillin-clavulanic acid treatment of melioidosis. Trans R Soc Trop Med Hyg 1991; 85:672–675.

75. Currie BJ, Fisher DA, Anstey NM, Jacups SP. Melioidosis: acute and chronic disease, relapse and re-activation. Trans R Soc Trop Med Hyg 2000; 94:301–304.
76. Thamprajamchit S, Chetchotisakd P, Thinkhamrop B. Cefoperazone/sulbactam + co-trimoxazole versus ceftazidime + co-trimoxazole in the treatment of severe melioidosis: a randomized, double-blind, controlled study. J Med Assoc Thai 1998; 81:265–271.
77. Apisarnthanarak A, Little JR. The role of cefoperazone-sulbactam for treatment of severe melioidosis. Clin Infect Dis 2002; 34:721–723.
78. Samuel M, Ti TY. Interventions for treating melioidosis. Cochrane Database Syst Rev 2001; 2:CD001263.
79. Patel RK, Smith MD, Rimmer D, Hanid MA. Melioidosis: problems in treatment. J Infect 1998; 36:132–133.
80. Inglis TJ, Golledge CL, Clair A, Harvey J. Case report: recovery from persistent septicemic melioidosis. Am J Trop Med Hyg 2001; 65:76–82.
81. Chaowagul W, Simpson AJH, Suputtamongkol Y, White NJ. Empirical cephalosporin treatment of melioidosis. Clin Infect Dis 1999; 28:1328.
82. Ashdown LR. Nosocomial infection due to *Pseudomonas pseudomallei*: two cases and an epidemiologic study. Rev Infect Dis 1979; 1:891–894.
83. Kunakorn M, Jayanetra P, Tanphaichitra D. Man-to-man transmission of melioidosis. Lancet 1991; 337:1290–1291.
84. Suputtamongkol Y, Intaranongpai S, Smith MD, et al. A double-blind placebo-controlled study of an infusion of lexipafant (platelet-activating factor receptor antagonist) in patients with severe sepsis. Antimicrob Agents Chemother 2000; 44:693–696.
85. Stephens DP, Fisher DA, Currie BJ. An audit of the use of granulocyte colony-stimulating factor in septic shock. Intern Med J 2002; 32:143–148.
86. Bernard GR, Vincent J-L, Laterre P-F, et al. Efficacy and safety of recombinant human activated protein C for severe sepsis. N Engl J Med 2001; 344:699–709.
87. Warren BL, Eid A, Singer P, et al. High-dose antithrombin III in severe sepsis: a randomized controlled trial. JAMA 2001; 286:1869–1878.
88. Chaowagul W. Recent advances in the treatment of severe melioidosis. Acta Trop 2000; 74:133–137.
89. Dance DAB, Davis TME, Wattanagoon Y, et al. Acute suppurative parotitis caused by *Pseudomonas pseudomallei* in children. J Infect Dis 1989; 159:654–660.
90. Jones AL, Beveridge TJ, Woods DE. Intracellular survival of *Burkholderia pseudomallei*. Infect Immun 1996; 64:782–790.
91. Pruksachartvuthi S, Aswapokee N, Thankerngpol K. Survival of *Pseudomonas pseudomallei* in human phagocytes. J Med Microbiol 1990; 31:109–114.
92. Utaisincharoen P, Tangthawornchaikul N, Kespichayawattana W, Chaisuriya P, Sirisinha S. *Burkholderia pseudomallei* interferes with inducible nitric oxide synthase (iNOS) production: a possible mechanism of evading macrophage killing. Microbiol Immunol 2001; 45:307–313.
93. Harley VS, Dance DAB, Drasar BS, Tovey G. Effects of *Burkholderia pseudomallei* and other *Burkholderia* species on eukaryotic cells in tissue culture. Microbios 1998; 96:71–93.
94. Rajchanuvong A, Chaowagul W, Suputtamongkol Y, Smith MD, Dance DAB, White NJ. A prospective comparison of co-amoxiclav and the combination of chloramphenicol, doxycycline, and co-trimoxazole for the oral maintenance treatment of melioidosis. Trans R Soc Trop Med Hyg 1995; 89:546–549.
95. Chaowagul W, Suputtamongkul Y, Smith MD, White NJ. Oral fluoroquinolones for maintenance treatment of melioidosis. Trans R Soc Trop Med Hyg 1997; 91:599–601.
96. Chetchotisakd P, Chaowagul W, Mootsikapun P, Budhsarawong D, Thinkamrop B. Maintenance therapy of melioidosis with ciprofloxacin plus azithromycin compared with cotrimoxazole plus doxycycline. Am J Trop Med Hyg 2001; 64:24–27.
97. Chaowagul W, Simpson AJH, Suputtamongkol Y, Smith MD, Angus BJ, White NJ. A

comparison of chloramphenicol, trimethoprim-sulfamethoxazole, and doxycycline with doxycycline alone as maintenance therapy for melioidosis. Clin Infect Dis 1999; 29:375–380.
98. Simpson AJH, White NJ. Combination antibiotic therapy for severe melioidosis. Clin Infect Dis 1999; 28:410.
99. McCormick JB, Sexton DJ, McMurray JG, Carey E, Hayes P, Feldman RA. Human-to-human transmission of *Pseudomonas pseudomallei.* Ann Intern Med 1975; 83:512–513.
100. Dance DAB, Suputtamongkol Y, Chaowagul W, White NJ. Prophylaxis for contacts of melioidosis. J Infect 1990; 21:222–223.
101. Russell P, Eley SM, Ellis J, et al. Comparison of efficacy of ciprofloxacin and doxycycline against experimental melioidosis and glanders. J Antimicrob Chemother 2000; 45: 813–818.
102. Health Protection Agency Interim Guideline for Action in the Event of a Deliberate Release of Glanders and Melrodosis, version 2.2. London: HPA. Available at www.hpa.org.uk/infections/topics-az/deliberate_release_static/glanders/glanders_meliodosishomepage.htm. Accessed September 19, 2003.

III

Mycobacteria

13

The Molecular Epidemiology of MDR-TB

Paul D. van Helden, Robin M. Warren, Pieter Uys, Gian D. van der Spuy, and Thomas C. Victor

1. INTRODUCTION

For those involved in infectious disease medicine, it seems that, to paraphrase an old adage, there are three certain things in life: taxes, death, and drug resistance. The variation in drug resistance detected in isolates of well-known bacteria (e.g., *Pneumococcus*) between different nations with different prescribing policies is well known. This is perhaps not surprising because the treatment of most infectious bacterial diseases is by monotherapy. Thus, logically, one might not expect much drug resistance in *Mycobacterium tuberculosis* (tuberculosis, TB) because the therapy for TB involves 2–4 different drugs administered simultaneously, and the risk of developing resistance for multiple drugs is additively small, as outlined in Section 3.2.

That TB evolves drug resistance easily was noted within months of the introduction of single drugs (e.g., streptomycin or isoniazid) to treat it. This is a potentially serious scenario because it is estimated that one-third of the global population is infected with *M. tuberculosis*; thus, the total burden of disease is very large. Under these circumstances, even low levels of resistance pose a potentially serious problem for TB control, particularly given the MDR (multidrug resistant) nature of resistance in *M. tuberculosis*. The World Health Organization (WHO) estimates of MDR-TB in new cases vary widely (Table 1), but may even exceed 14% in some regions *(1–4)*. Thus, the global burden of drug-resistant TB cases will be in the order of hundreds of thousands of cases in any year.

It is known that episodes of TB in different patients are not necessarily caused by only one strain of that bacterium. The ability to sensitively genotype bacteria, particularly *Mycobacterium tuberculosis*, has shown that the global epidemiology of TB is propagated by hundreds or possibly thousands of different strains of the organism. The ability to type strains brings a new dimension to the study of epidemiology and this branch of science, known as molecular epidemiology, can add value to traditional epidemiology. The applications of molecular techniques for the study of MDR-TB are discussed in this chapter.

From: *Management of Multiple Drug-Resistant Infections*
Edited by: S. H. Gillespie © Humana Press Inc., Totowa, NJ

Table 1
Estimates of Drug Resistance in New Tuberculosis Cases

Country	Population	Estimated incidence (all cases/ 100,000 population)	Global rank (by estimated number of cases)	Estimated adult (15–49-yr-old) TB cases HIV+ (%)	Estimated multidrug resistance (new cases)
Zimbabwe	12,627,277	584	21	67	1.9
Cambodia	13,104,030	572	20	20	4.2
South Africa	43,309,197	526	9	60	1.5
Mozambique	18,292,382	433	19	48	3.5
Ethiopia	62,907,788	397	6	42	2.3
Uganda	23,300,162	351	17	35	0.5
Afghanistan	21,764,955	321	22	0.0	7.3
DRC*	50,948,236	320	11	24	1.5
Vietnam	78,136,913	189	13	1.4	2.3
India	1,008,937,356	184	1	4.0	3.4
Russian Federation	145,491,666	132	10	1.0	6.0
Brazil	170,406,280	68	15	3.3	0.9

Source: From refs. *1–4* and www.who.int/gtb.
*Democratic Republic of Congo.

2. MOLECULAR EPIDEMIOLOGY

2.1. *Basic Principles and Uses*

Traditional epidemiological methods provide insight into the dynamics of diseases such as tuberculosis, but have relied on a number of assumptions. The application of molecular techniques to the study of epidemiology has allowed us to re-examine the clinical dogmas, ask new questions, and be less reliant on assumptions.

Mycobacterium tuberculosis has a transposable element known as IS*6110* that occurs at various loci and at variable copy numbers in the genome *(5)*. This element has proved useful in genotyping isolates of *M. tuberculosis* and classifying them into strains and strain families (groups of isolates of >65% similarity) *(6–10)*. Other repeat elements have also been used to genotype *M. tuberculosis*; these include the PGRS element *(11–13)* and spoligotyping elements *(14,15)*.

Spoligotyping is based on polymerase chain reaction (PCR), offers the possibility of typing directly from sputum, and detects the presence (or absence) of 43 unique direct variable repeat (DVR) sequences by line-blot hybridization. Strains are differentiated based on the presence of specific variable repeat sequences. Although the discriminatory power of the spoligotyping method is generally regarded as lower than that of the internationally standardized restriction fragment length polymorphism (RFLP) method *(16)*, spoligotyping remains an important tool to genotype clinical isolates in different epidemiological settings *(17–21)*. A similar, but potentially more discriminatory, technique known as multiple interspersed repeat units (MIRU) typing may become a technique for the future *(22)* because it could also be used on sputum samples.

2.2. Application of Typing Techniques

Strain typing methodology has been used to demonstrate the transmission of one isolate (strain) from one individual to others in many different settings in which a matched (identical) genotype indicates transmission *(12,23,24)*. Genotyping and spoligotyping data have been used to monitor the spread of specific strains within defined geographical regions *(19)* and between different countries *(20)*. They can also be used to define episodes of TB as relapse or reinfection *(21)*. Unmatched (unique) isolates are regarded as reactivation cases (but may also be imported isolates, as frequently seen in immigrants newly arrived from high-incidence societies).

In any given setting, the relative proportion of matched isolates (the extent of clustering) gives an indication of the relative contribution of transmission in TB disease dynamics. In this regard, it is important to note that there are essentially two components in any TB epidemic: recent transmission, which leads to disease, and historical transmission, which leads to disease years (or decades) later, known as a reactivation disease. It is generally regarded that transmission events that lead to active disease episodes within 2 yr after transmission are regarded as recent transmission events *(12,23,24)*. The relative proportion of these two components can be estimated as a function of the proportion of matched isolates (clusters) versus unmatched isolates (uniques) over the given time period (e.g., 2 yr).

The relative proportions of these two components of TB can be useful in monitoring the course of the epidemic and designing the most effective intervention strategies for any given environment. For example, public health measures to combat TB in high-incidence societies in which most disease occurs from transmission in younger persons *(25)* should be very different from societies in which the majority of cases occur in immigrants or the elderly. Molecular epidemiology provides for the first time a tool to quantitate these components *(9,26)*: By quantifying the relative proportion of isolates that occur in clusters to the total isolates in circulation in that community, the quantitative estimate of recent transmission from molecular epidemiology studies is obtained. Estimates of recent transmission are perhaps unexpectedly low, with quantitative estimates varying from approx 16 to 50% *(27)*.

2.3. Defining Identical Isolates

There is not always a clear understanding of which method should be used to calculate these proportions (using cluster analysis) and what the interpretation of the answer is or should be *(27,28)*. The *n* method simply sums all strains that have at least 1 other match as a proportion of total strains and provides an estimate of the number of people included or excluded from transmission chains. The *n*–1 method sums all strains with at least 1 match minus the number of clusters of matched strains as a proportion of total strains. The –1 component subtracts a source case for each cluster. This estimate quantifies transmitted primary disease and, by difference, those caused by reactivation.

Problems may be encountered with either method, such as incomplete sampling *(29)*, which will usually lead to an underestimate of transmission; a bias in patient selection, which could increase or decrease clustering; or lack of indication that, in a high-incidence community, there is not necessarily only one source case for a cluster of identical strains. Finally, no adjustment for evolutionary change *(30,31)* is made in strain genotype matching, which will result in underestimation of transmission. The period that should be used for this calculation is also subject to interpretation. Clearly, at the extremes of a very short period (a few weeks) or a long period (decades), assuming no evolution of genotype, in all likelihood 0 or 100% transmission would be measured, respectively. Periods of 2 yr are commonly used for this estimate, but there are arguments that up to 5 yr may be more appropriate *(9,27,29,32)*.

Using approx 5 yr as a period and making no allowances for the evolution of strains (or immigration), cluster analysis showed that at least 75% of affected individuals (of all ages) in a high-incidence society are probably involved in transmission chains *(9,28)*, whereas this will be lower, but may still be a major component of disease, in low-incidence societies *(29)*. Allowing for evolution, arguably another 15% should be added to the estimate even over this short period (*30*; 2003, our unpublished results).

This methodology has shown transmission chains extend even to elderly persons *(26–28)*, for whom transmission was not previously thought common. Even in low-incidence societies, there is considerable ongoing transmission; given that the current published estimates are very likely considerably lower than the true situation, it follows that much effort at the public health level should be devoted to breaking transmission chains.

If we can achieve this, the incidence of disease should steadily decline, even if reactivation disease occurs decades after infection. The disease will (theoretically) disappear, especially if there is treatment available, as the cohort of infected children matures to adulthood, gradually ages, and dies. The key lies in devising strategies that can break these transmission chains in different societies. If we fail to break transmission chains, then not only will the current epidemic continue, but also each reactivation case will propagate the epidemic. This concept applies to both drug-sensitive and drug-resistant cases *(33)*.

3. DRUG RESISTANCE

3.1. Drug Resistance Detection

Traditional drug susceptibility tests (by phenotype) require a positive culture for diagnosis, followed by subcultures that are exposed to drugs. This procedure can take 6–10 wk on solid media using conventional techniques or 15 d when liquid-based culture methods such as the BACTEC system are used *(34–37)*. Thus, diagnosis of MDR-TB is a relatively slow process that can be further retarded as a function of the "index of suspicion." Without a high index of suspicion, a very long "time to diagnosis" will result because of a delay in a request for laboratory tests. In addition to these problems, culture testing poses significant technical problems associated with the standardization: establishing appropriate inoculum volume, stability of the compounds in different culture media, and the reproducibility of results *(38,39)*. The slow diagnosis of drug resistance may thus be a major contributor to chains of transmission of MDR-TB, allowing more infection events to take place from MDR cases than from susceptible cases (Fig. 1).

Accelerated culture-based susceptibility testing is possible using recombinant phages *(40)*. These assays could be semiautomated, having a relatively high throughput, with substantially reduced culture time. However, they are still sensitive to some of the problems inherent in traditional culture testing; require live, cultured bacteria; and do not define bacterial strains by genotype.

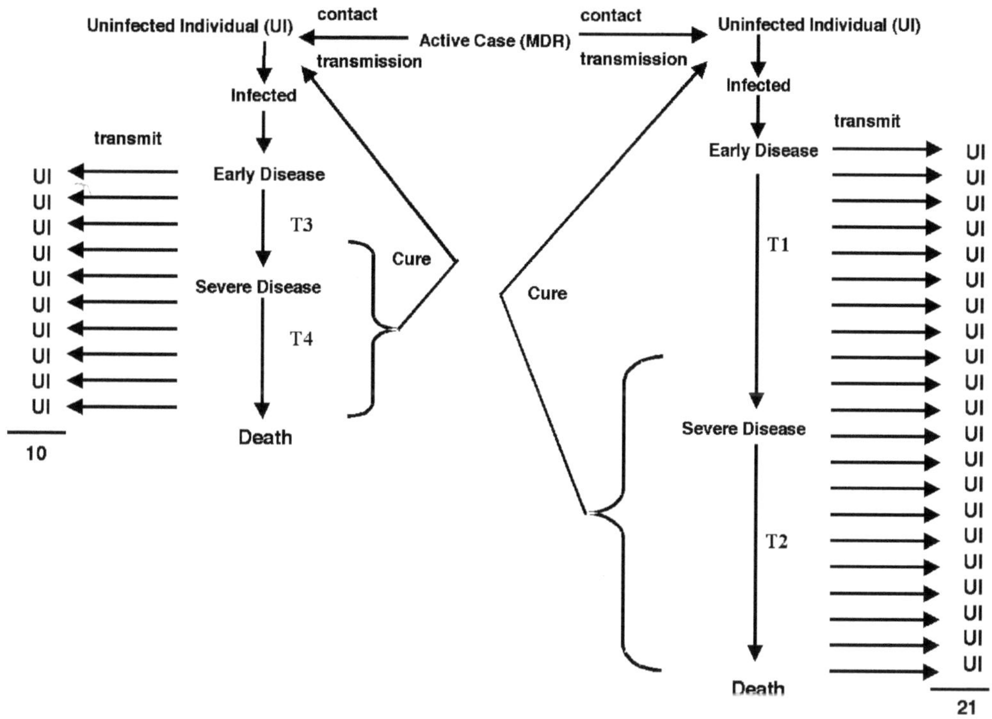

Fig. 1. Disease progression in tuberculosis. Delayed diagnosis in MDR-TB cases could lead to more transmission events and thus perpetuate or advance the MDR epidemic. In this case, T1 + T2 > T3 + T4 because of a delay in diagnosis of MDR-TB and delay in implementation of appropriate chemotherapy or other control measures. (T represents time.)

It is now known that resistance to antibiotics is because of a number of mutations in specific genes of the *M. tuberculosis* genome *(41)*. Thus far, mutations in 11 genes have been linked to resistance to anti-TB drugs. These genes are *kat*G, *inh*A, *aph*C, *kas*A, *ndh* for isoniazid (INH) resistance, *rpo*B for rifampicin (Rif) resistance, *rps*L and *rrs* for streptomycin (SM) resistance, *emb* for ethambutol (EMB) resistance, *pnc*A for pyrazinamide (PZA) resistance, and *gyr* for fluoroquinolone resistance (Table 2).

The mutations identified in these genes have been associated with drug resistance based largely on their absence in drug-susceptible isolates. Multiple drug resistance occurs when a particular isolate has mutations in different genes. However, not all mutations identified produce a resistance phenotype. Three polymorphisms—*kat*G463 *(43)*, *gyr*A95 *(59,61)*, and *rrs*491 *(59)*—that are not associated with drug resistance in *M. tuberculosis* have been described thus far, and these have been used to study the evolution of *M. tuberculosis (61)*. The molecular mechanisms of drug resistance in a small proportion of clinical isolates are yet unknown, but may include transient induction of genes encoding efflux pumps *(62)* or genes with natural polymorphisms that may provide low-level resistance to certain drugs *(63)*.

Several PCR-based strategies have been designed to detect these mutations, including DNA sequencing, dideoxy fingerprinting, heteroduplex analysis, RFLP, single-strand conformation polymorphism (SSCP), molecular beacon analysis, and the use of probes. The method must be able to differentiate between wild-type and mutant

Table 2
Molecular Diagnostics in *Mycobacterium tuberculosis* Drug Resistance

Antibiotic	Locus	Product	Proportion of clinical isolates with mutations associated with resistance (%)	Codon most often associated with resistance	Polymorphisms not encoding drug resistance	Reference
Isoniazid	*kat*G	Catalase-peroxidase	55–75	*kat*G315 (approx 60%)	*kat*G463	*42–46*
	*inh*A	Ketoacyl reductase	5–10			*47, 48*
	*ahp*C	Alkylhydro-peroxidase	6–13			*49, 50*
	*kas*A	β-ketoacyl synthase	5–20			*42, 51*
	ndh	NADH dehy-drogenase	10			*52*
Rifampicin	*rpo*B	β-subunit of RNA polymerase	90–98	*rpo*B531 (approx 40%), *rpo*B526 (approx 35%), *rpo*B516 (approx 10%)		*9, 42, 47, 51–56*
Ethambutol	*emb*B	Polymerization of arabinose into arabino-galactan	70–80	*emb*B306 (approx 85%)		*42, 57, 58*
Streptomycin	*rrs*	16S rRNA	54–60	*rrs*513 (approx 8%)	*rrs*491	*42, 46, 59*
	*rps*L	Ribosomal protein S12	8–12	*rps*L43 (approx 55%)		*42, 46, 59*
Pyrazinamide	*pnc*A	Pyrazinamidase	approx 70			*42, 59, 60*
Fluoro-quinolones	*gyr*A	A subunit of DNA gyrase	approx 100		*gyr*A95	*59, 61*

Abbr: NADH, nicotinamide adenine dinucleotide.

sequences. These methods were developed to accelerate diagnosis of drug-resistant TB. However, these methods are not always universally applicable: For example, not all mutations result in the gain or loss of a restriction enzyme site, therefore limiting the use of RFLP as a general method to screen for mutations that confer resistance. Other screening procedures that depend on DNA mobility shifts (e.g., PCR-SSCP) are often used, but are technically demanding and are not sufficiently sensitive because mutations are not always detected. PCR amplification followed by DNA sequencing is possibly the most widely used technique for the identification of mutations, but is not readily available in routine laboratories and therefore is not currently suitable for large numbers of samples.

PCR-based screening methods, which allow batch analysis of samples via dot-blot hybridization, offer a potential solution *(64)*. These methods are based on PCR amplification of target genes associated with drug resistance in *M. tuberculosis*, followed by selective hybridization under stringent conditions with allele-specific probes. The method is reproducible, not technically demanding, and can take 2 normal working days to obtain results from the start of amplification (done in batches of 30–40 samples) to the final autoradiography step of the dot-blot hybridization (done in batches of up to 150 samples, including controls). In various studies (using molecular techniques), the sensitivities and specificities varied between 58 and 100% for the different drugs under investigation (*see* references in Table 2).

The molecular diagnostic methods may offer significant advantages over traditional phenotyping. However, they have one major limitation: they may lack sensitivity. Drug resistance develops because of natural selection *(64–66)*, and mixed drug-resistant (mutant sequence) and susceptible (wild-type sequence) populations of mycobacteria may therefore coexist in the same episode of disease. It will be difficult to identify mutants within an overwhelming pool of wild-type sequences at early stages of acquisition of resistance, whereas culture-based techniques may do so. Certain methods based on PCR amplification only will be affected as they do not selectively amplify the mutant allele.

Other limitations are that different assays (sometimes involving more than one gene per drug) are necessary for each drug tested, and not all of the molecular mechanisms leading to drug resistance in clinical isolates are known. Therefore, identification of a resistance-associated mutation is clinically informative, whereas lack of a mutation in the target sequence must be interpreted with caution. Also, false-positive results can occur because of amplicon (previously amplified PCR products) contamination. Last, culture-based susceptibility testing can determine the minimum inhibitory concentration (MIC) for the different drugs, whereas molecular results only suggest a relationship between the type of a mutation and the level of resistance (MIC) *(46)*.

When the performance (sensitivity, specificity, repeatability) of molecular prediction of drug resistance was compared to culture susceptibility testing, the molecular method was assessed to provide a high degree of reproducibility, whereas reproducibility of results from the traditional culture method was variable. Guidelines concerning how to deal with these discrepant results are available *(42,52,64–66)*.

3.2. *Integrating Drug Susceptibility Analysis With Molecular Epidemiology*

To understand the molecular epidemiology of MDR-TB, that of TB as a whole should be considered first because MDR-TB is a subset of this population. For example, there is an assumption that multiple-case households necessarily represent household transmission when there is skin test conversion or an active case without molecular analysis. However, the close scrutiny of strain typing shows that, in high-incidence societies, at least 50% of TB cases in multiple-case households are because of transmission from the community and not from within the home *(67)*. This has major implications for intervention studies because it does not necessarily imply that prophylactic treatment of household members is justified in an environment of limited resources. However, adult–adult transmission rates may occur at lower frequency than adult–child cases *(68)*.

Irrespective of the tools used to identify the source of drug resistance in *M. tuberculosis*, it is evident that there are two major sources of drug-resistant *M. tuberculosis*: acquired resistance and primary or transmitted resistance. It is essential to note that second or subsequent episodes of TB can be caused by relapse or reinfection *(69–71)*. Repeat episodes of disease are traditionally referred to as *relapse* cases and are regarded as patients who have not been bacteriologically sterilized during treatment. This assumption arose from the observation that patients could have recurring bouts of tuberculosis even prior to the era of antibiotics and because, in the early days of antibiotics when the treatment course was too short or before multiple drugs were used, many repeat cases were observed; there are very few seen if chemotherapy consists of 6 mo of therapy using 2–4 drugs in combination *(69)*. However, repeat episodes of TB can be caused by reinfection, for which the risk must be proportional to the incidence of disease in that population. It has been shown that reinfection may be relatively common *(70,71)*.

It follows that, in a situation of reinfection or multiple infection, a proportion of individuals are likely to be infected with more than one strain simultaneously. Autopsy and other culture-based studies have shown this to be the case *(72,73)*, and it is possible that a sensitive and an underlying MDR strain may be present simultaneously in a given patient. This patient may initially appear to be "cured" (of the sensitive strain) and then "relapse" (with MDR-TB).

Clinical drug resistance to TB can also develop because of selection and are classified as acquired resistance when drug-resistant mutants are selected as a result of ineffective treatment or as primary resistance, such as when a patient is infected by a source case with a resistant strain *(64)*. Mutations that confer resistance to anti-TB drugs occur spontaneously, with an estimated frequency of 3.5×10^{-6} for INH and 3.1×10^{-8} for Rif, for example. The risk of developing resistance to INH and RIF under optimal treatment conditions is 9×10^{-14} *(66)*. Acquired MDR (resistance to at least INH and RIF) will thus occur mainly when treatment is not optimal, whereas primary cases may occur even under conditions of compliance. It therefore is not surprising that most surveillance studies report that the proportion of individuals with drug-resistant episodes of tuberculosis is lower in primary compared to repeat episodes of disease *(74,75)*. The assumption is therefore made that resistance has developed (been acquired) in these individuals with repeat episodes of TB. However, surveillance results (although valuable) should be interpreted with caution since

1. These results are seldom sufficiently accurate to be certain of classification of patients into primary or repeat cases.
2. Traditional phenotype testing has a number of technical problems.
3. There is a bias toward analyzing repeat episodes of disease more carefully.
4. Patients with low-level resistance may appear to be cured, but are not rendered bacteriologically sterile.
5. Patients may not complete the course of treatment and not have culture-based and sensitivity testing done on a primary episode, but may return some months later, be classified with a second episode of disease, and have sensitivity testing done only at this stage.

Additional problems may occur because there are usually fewer repeat episodes, data are usually based on files, patients are not all given a standard interview at diagnosis, and there is little quality control of clinical information *(76)*. All of this may result in the illness of a number of patients falling into wrong categories. Furthermore, and perhaps most important, the data on primary resistance (first disease episode) may be used as a marker of transmitted drug resistance. In this case, and given that this is likely to be the minimum estimate, estimates of subsequent drug-resistant cases will include transmission cases for which the proportion is at least the same as primary episodes, and the balance of cases will be acquired disease.

Thus, it may be reasoned as follows: If (for a given population size), initial resistance presents as 10 cases and subsequent episodes as 26 cases with the relative risk (RR) for repeat episodes 2.6 *(74)*, then the subtotal of cases caused by transmission in primary and subsequent episodes is 20/36 or 56%. This estimate for a specific area is close to that measured by molecular epidemiology in the same high-incidence area *(65)*. A global estimate using data from a limited number of mixed countries *(1,2,75)* using the same approach suggested that approx 43% of MDR-TB is the result of transmission.

Given the problems inherent in such surveys, these should be regarded as minimum estimates, particularly because it has been shown that the clinical estimation of primary or acquired disease may be quite inaccurate *(65)*. In at least one survey, the same level of resistance was found in new and repeat cases of TB *(77)*, suggesting that transmission is possibly the only source of drug-resistant TB in that region.

More recent evidence for transmission of MDR-TB came from a follow-up study of over 300 patients from 72 clinics in the area surrounding greater Metropolitan Cape Town, South Africa, where we showed that over 30% of the patients with drug-resistant isolates of *M. tuberculosis* were infected by isolates from one of two strain families, and that in approximately only 7% (by spoligotype analysis) of these patients, a unique isolate was identified (Victor T, Streicher L, van der Spuy G, Warren R, and van Helden P, 2002; unpublished results). It was not possible to know whether individuals with these unique strains were in fact infected elsewhere and moved into the area subsequently. Furthermore, studies in childhood cases, for which resistance is by definition almost certainly primary and based on contact with adult MDR cases in a household, demonstrate clearly the transmission of drug-resistant isolates of *M. tuberculosis (68)*.

Other evidence for transmission as a major source of MDR-TB includes reports of nosocomial outbreaks of MDR-TB in institutions such as hospitals *(78–81)* and prisons *(82)* in the United States, Europe, and developing countries *(83,84)*. Infection followed by active MDR-TB in health care workers after exposure to patients with MDR-TB *(85–87)* and outbreaks within communities have also been reported *(88–90)*. The most extensive MDR-TB outbreak identified, documented, and reported to date occurred in 267 patients from New York who were infected by Beijing/W isolates *(91)*. However, in regions with poor surveillance and where MDR-TB incidence is high *(92)*, larger outbreaks may have occurred, but were not necessarily recognized as such.

Much, if not all of our recent detailed understanding of the dynamics of such outbreaks comes from a combination analysis using phenotyping, mutation analysis, and genotyping. The last two are particularly important. Some of the problems inherent in using one technique (even one as accurate and defining as molecular analysis) are illustrated in Fig. 2, which illustrates the difficulty of distinguishing one isolate from another by phenotype analysis, although mutation and spoligotype together can be highly

	A	B	C	D	E	F
Phenotype	INH STR	INH STR Rif	INH STR Rif	INH STR Rif	INH STR Rif	INH STR Rif
Genotype	*katG*315 gc→ca *rpsL*43 a→g	*katG*315 gc→ca *RpsL*43 a→g *rpoB*531 c→t	*katG*315 gc→ca *rpsL*43 a→g *rpoB*526 c→t	*katG*315 g→c *rrs*513 a→t *rpoB*531 c→t	*katG*315 gc→ca *rpsL*43 a→g *rpoB*531 c→t	*katG*315 gc→ca *rpsL*43 a→g *rpoB*516 a→t
Spoligotype	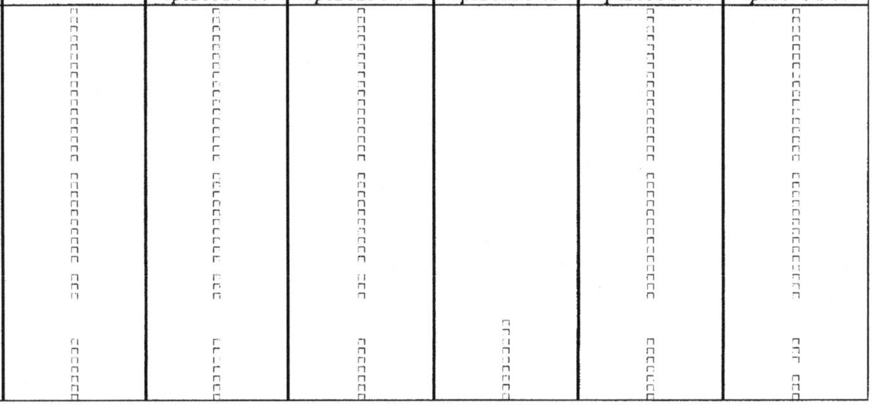					

Fig. 2. Phenotype and genotype analysis of drug resistance in *M. tuberculosis* together with spoligotyping of clinical MDR-TB strains. Lanes A–C illustrate that phenotype and spoligotype will not differentiate these three strains; lanes B–F show that phenotype cannot distinguish these five isolates from each other. A combination of mutation analysis and spoligotype is adequate to identify all six as distinct.

informative. Conclusions drawn from the phenotype of these six isolates could be very different from those drawn using molecular data.

Using such technology, it has been shown that certain strains, such as the Beijing/W type *(93)*, may be most prevalent in some areas, and that certain mutations are most common in those areas *(42,65,90)*. This knowledge could be used to devise rapid screening tests (which may be region targeted) that, even if not 100% sensitive or specific, may yield enough data to make a difference to treatment and the disease burden.

4. VIRULENCE, FITNESS, LATENCY, AND MDR-TB INCIDENCE

As discussed above, there are some *M. tuberculosis* strain families (a collection of strains with >65% similar genotype) that occur in areas geographically distant *(42,88,90,93–95)*. Often, these strains are responsible for a considerable proportion of disease episodes in those regions *(9,93–96)*. This and other observations has led to the notion that some strains may be more virulent than others *(97–99)*, although it must be cautioned that simple abundance *(96)* is not necessarily an indicator of virulence *(100)*.

One of the most obvious phenotypes of bacteria is drug resistance. Although it has been argued that the acquisition of multidrug resistance may render the bacterium less virulent, this may be of lesser consequence than other factors because diagnosis of these MDR strains usually takes far longer than of sensitive strains, allowing infection and transmission chains to continue for longer than for sensitive stains *(101–103)*. Furthermore, careful in vitro analysis suggested that at least one of the most common *kat*G mutations (S315T) produces active catalase-peroxidase, and that little or no loss of virulence results from this mutation *(102)*. In the case of MDR-TB, the calculation of reproductive fitness varies according to region *(101)*. This may be simply because these regions have quite different success rates in dealing with this problem, and estimates of fitness may not reflect any intrinsic change in virulence or "fitness"; rather, the estimates of high fitness levels may reflect a failure of the program in various locations. This suggests that transmission and spread of drug-resistant strains may be at least equivalent to sensitive isolates, which has important implications for control.

The nature of the different strains of *M. tuberculosis* may also be viewed as a matrix, with each strain having a function for transmission and potential for pathology *(103)*. One of these functions may include potential for latency. Evidence that bacteria may indeed remain latent in an individual for up to three decades *(104)* and that these bacterial strains may be infrequent can provide target organisms to study that may potentially be of a "transmitter" phenotype *(9,99)* or a "latent" phenotype *(104)*.

Although not yet proven, latent organisms may well be the source of acquired drug-resistant organisms, experiencing antibiotic selection pressure, but not being killed at the time of exposure to antibiotics because of altered metabolism. The current research in this field is therefore important, as are drugs that can target this state.

5. FUTURE

Molecular epidemiology and mutation analysis for a MDR-TB diagnosis are remarkable tools that have provided many new insights into the disease dynamics of tuberculosis. They have allowed us to ask intriguing new questions and provided tools that can be used to help design and measure the efficacy of new intervention strategies. Because these are not yet fully mature technologies, it affords us the opportunity for research growth and exciting new research angles.

Ultimately, it may be that a simple PCR-based genotyping assay (e.g., MIRU) together with an amplification refractory mutation system (ARMS) PCR protocol for common mutations conferring drug resistance and automated for large-scale assay may be adequate for prediction of 70–90% of MDR-TB strains in any given area. A 70% diagnosis together with 70–80% cure rate may ultimately provide an acceptable solution for the scourge of TB in general and MDR-TB in particular.

Alternatively, the next generation of molecular methods for the prediction of drug resistance in *M. tuberculosis* may consist of matrix hybridization formats such as DNA oligonucleotide arrays on slides or silicon micron chips, particularly if these systems can be fully automated and reused. This may be particularly useful for mutations in the *rpo*B gene, which can serve as a marker for MDR-TB *(41,42)* and for the multiple loci that are involved in INH resistance (Table 1). Selection of a limited number of target mutations that enable the detection of the majority of drug resistance would be useful in this strategy. It is essential that developments for new techniques must consider the fact that the majority of drug-resistant cases occur in resource-poor countries; therefore, the methodologies must be cheap and robust. Diagnosis is only one component in the control of TB, and it is essential that treatment be complemented with the correct diagnosis.

If one considers the progression from infection to disease in tuberculosis (Fig. 1), then it is evident that once a certain stage of disease (infectiousness) is reached, transmission to other individuals can occur. A proportion of these individuals will progress to active disease; thus, by reducing the number of infected individuals, the number of

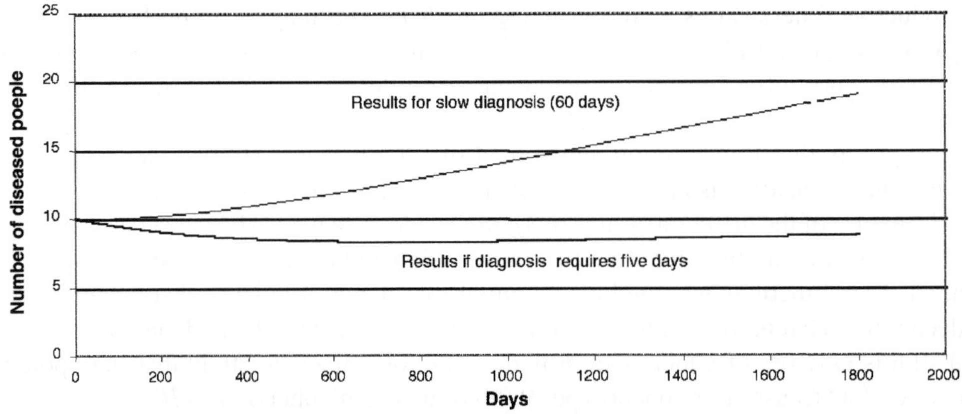

Fig. 3. Mathematical model for estimating MDR-TB cases based on a population of 10,000 with 10 initial MDR cases given different diagnostic procedures: slow (current) 60-d diagnosis and rapid 5-d diagnosis.

active cases will decrease. In the case of MDR-TB, because evidence suggests that much of the burden of disease is from transmission, the most obvious way to reduce this burden is to reduce transmission. The most effective way to do this is to effect diagnosis of TB, specifically MDR-TB, as early as possible.

Simple mathematical modeling (P. Uys, 2002; unpublished analysis) of the impact of delayed diagnosis compared to rapid diagnosis (Fig. 3) shows that the MDR-TB epidemic can be stabilized by a drastic reduction in diagnosis time. We believe that, using molecular diagnostics, time to diagnosis can be reduced; by adding molecular epidemiological tools, outbreak and transmission chains can be identified. In this way, resources can be more effectively targeted to reduce the burden of MDR-TB.

ACKNOWLEDGMENTS

We acknowledge GlaxoSmithKline Action TB, IAEA (International Atomic Energy Agency), and Sequella Foundation for funding our research; E. Streicher and A. Lambrechts for assistance with the figures and manuscript preparation; and the TB team for excellent collaborative work.

REFERENCES

1. Dye C, Espinal MA, Watt CJ, Mbiaga C, Williams BG. Worldwide incidence of multidrug-resistant tuberculosis. J Infect Dis 2002; 185:1197–1202.
2. Dye C, Scheele S, Dolin P, Pathania V, Raviglione MC. Consensus statement. Global burden of tuberculosis: estimated incidence, prevalence, and mortality by country. WHO Global Surveillance and Monitoring Project. JAMA 1999; 282:677–686.
3. Raviglione MC, Snider DE Jr, Kochi A. Global epidemiology of tuberculosis. Morbidity and mortality of a worldwide epidemic. JAMA 1995; 273:220–226.
4. Nunn P, Felten M. Surveillance of resistance to antituberculosis drugs in developing countries. Tuber Lung Dis 1994; 75:163–167.
5. Thierry D, Brisson-Noel A, Vincent-Levy-Frebault V, Nguyen S, Guesdon JL, Gicquel B. Characterization of a *Mycobacterium tuberculosis* insertion sequence, IS*6110*, and its application in diagnosis. J Clin Microbiol 1990; 28:2668–2673.
6. van Embden JD, Cave MD, Crawford JT, et al. Strain identification of *Mycobacterium*

tuberculosis by DNA fingerprinting: recommendations for a standardized methodology. J Clin Microbiol 1993; 31:406–409.

7. Hermans PW, Messadi F, Guebrexabher H, et al. Analysis of the population structure of *Mycobacterium tuberculosis* in Ethiopia, Tunisia, and The Netherlands: usefulness of DNA typing for global tuberculosis epidemiology. J Infect Dis 1995; 171:1504–1513.
8. van Soolingen DL, Qian PE, de Haas JT, et al. Predominance of a single genotype of *Mycobacterium tuberculosis* in countries of east Asia. J Clin Microbiol 1995; 33:3234–3238.
9. Warren RM, Richardson M, van der Spuy GD, et al. DNA fingerprinting and molecular epidemiology of tuberculosis: use and interpretation in an epidemic setting. Electrophoresis 1999; 20:1807–1812.
10. Warren RM, Sampson SL, Richardson M, et al. Mapping of IS*6110* flanking regions in clinical isolates of *M. tuberculosis* demonstrates genome plasticity. Mol Microbiol 2000; 37:1405–1416.
11. van Soolingen D, de Haas PE, Hermans PW, Groenen PM, van Embden JD. Comparison of various repetitive DNA elements as genetic markers for strain differentiation and epidemiology of *Mycobacterium tuberculosis*. J Clin Microbiol 1993; 31:1987–1995.
12. Warren RM, Richardson M, Sampson S, et al. Genotyping of *Mycobacterium tuberculosis* with additional markers enhances accuracy in epidemiological studies. J Clin Microbiol 1996; 34:2219–2224.
13. Chaves F, Yang Z, el Hajj H, et al. Usefulness of the secondary probe pTBN12 in DNA fingerprinting of *Mycobacterium tuberculosis*. J Clin Microbiol 1996; 34:1118–1123.
14. Groenen PM, Bunschoten AE, van Soolingen D, van Embden JD. Nature of DNA polymorphism in the direct repeat cluster of *Mycobacterium tuberculosis*; application for strain differentiation by a novel typing method. Mol Microbiol 1993; 10:1057–1065.
15. Kamerbeek J, Schouls L, Kolk A, et al. Simultaneous detection and strain differentiation of *Mycobacterium tuberculosis* for diagnosis and epidemiology. J Clin Microbiol 1997; 35: 907–914.
16. Kremer K, van Soolingen D, Frothingham R, et al. Comparison of methods based on different molecular epidemiological markers for typing of *Mycobacterium tuberculosis* complex strains: interlaboratory study of discriminatory power and reproducibility. J Clin Microbiol 1999; 37:2607–2618.
17. Cronin WA, Golub JE, Magder LS, et al. Epidemiologic usefulness of spoligotyping for secondary typing of *Mycobacterium tuberculosis* isolates with low copy numbers of IS*6110*. J Clin Microbiol 2001; 39:3709–3711.
18. Bauer J, Andersen AB, Kremer K, Miorner H. Usefulness of spoligotyping to discriminate IS*6110* low-copy-number *Mycobacterium tuberculosis* complex strains cultured in Denmark. J Clin Microbiol 1999; 37:2602–2606.
19. Sola C, Devallois A, Horgen L, et al. Tuberculosis in the Caribbean: using spacer oligonucleotide typing to understand strain origin and transmission. Emerg Infect Dis 1999; 5: 404–414.
20. Sola C, Filliol I, Gutierrez MC, Mokrousov I, Vincent V, Rastogi N. Spoligotype database of *Mycobacterium tuberculosis*: biogeographic distribution of shared types and epidemiologic and phylogenetic perspectives. Emerg Infect Dis 2001; 7:390–396.
21. Warren RM, Streicher EM, Charalambous S, et al. Use of spoligotyping for accurate classification of recurrent tuberculosis. J Clin Microbiol 2002; 40:3851–3853.
22. Supply P, Mazars E, Lesjean S, Vincent V, Gicquel B, Locht C. Variable human minisatellite-like regions in the *Mycobacterium tuberculosis* genome. Mol Microbiol 2000; 36:762–771.
23. Alland D, Kalkut GE, Moss AR, et al. Transmission of tuberculosis in New York City. An analysis by DNA fingerprinting and conventional epidemiologic methods. N Engl J Med 1994; 330:1710–1716.

24. Small PM, Hopewell PC, Singh SP, et al. The epidemiology of tuberculosis in San Francisco. A population-based study using conventional and molecular methods. N Engl J Med 1994; 330:1703–1709.
25. Rieder HL. Epidemiologic Basis of Tuberculosis Control. Paris: International Union Against Tuberculosis and Lung Disease, 1999.
26. Van Soolingen D, Borgdorff MW, de Haas PE, et al. Molecular epidemiology of tuberculosis in the Netherlands: a nationwide study from 1993 through 1997. J Infect Dis 1999; 180:726–736.
27. Van Soolingen D. Molecular epidemiology of tuberculosis and other mycobacterial infections: main methodologies and achievements. J Intern Med 2001; 249:1–26.
28. Murray M, Alland D. Methodological problems in the molecular epidemiology of tuberculosis. Am J Epidemiol 2002; 155:565–571.
29. Glynn JR, Vannycky E, Fine PE. Influence of sampling on estimates of clustering and recent transmission of *Mycobacterium tuberculosis* derived from DNA fingerprinting techniques. Am J Epidemiol 1999; 149:366–371.
30. Warren RM, van der Spuy GD, Richardson M, et al. Evolution of the IS*6110*-based restriction fragment length polymorphism pattern during the transmission of *Mycobacterium tuberculosis*. J Clin Microbiol 2002; 40:1277–1282.
31. Warren RM, van der Spuy GD, Richardson M, et al. Calculation of the stability of the IS*6110* banding pattern in patients with persistent *M. tuberculosis* disease. J Clin Microbiol 2002; 40:1705–1708.
32. Glynn JR, Bauer J, de Boer AS, et al. Interpreting DNA fingerprint clusters of *Mycobacterium tuberculosis*. European concerted action on molecular epidemiology and control of tuberculosis. Int J Tuberc Lung Dis 1999; 3:1055–1060.
33. van Helden PD. Molecular epidemiology of TB: challenging dogmas and asking new questions. IUBMB Life 2002; 53:219–223.
34. Rastogi N, Goh KS, David HL. Drug susceptibility testing in tuberculosis: a comparison of the proportion methods using Lowenstein-Jensen, Middlebrook 7H10 and 7H11 agar media and a radiometric method. Res Microbiol 1989; 140:405–417.
35. Siddiqi SH, Hawkins JE, Laszlo A. Interlaboratory drug susceptibility testing of *Mycobacterium tuberculosis* by a radiometric procedure and two conventional methods. J Clin Microbiol 1985; 22:919–923.
36. Snider DE Jr, Good RC, Kilburn JO, et al. Rapid drug-susceptibility testing of *Mycobacterium tuberculosis*. Am Rev Respir Dis 1981; 123:402–406.
37. Tarrand JJ, Groschel DH. Evaluation of the BACTEC radiometric method for detection of 1% resistant populations of *Mycobacterium tuberculosis*. J Clin Microbiol 1985; 21: 941–946.
38. Victor TC, Warren R, Butt JL, et al. Genome and MIC stability in *Mycobacterium tuberculosis* and indications for continuation of use of isoniazid in multidrug-resistant tuberculosis. J Med Microbiol 1997; 46:847–857.
39. Martin-Casabona N, Xairo MD, Gonzalez T, Rossello J, Arcalis L. Rapid method for testing susceptibility of *Mycobacterium tuberculosis* by using DNA probes. J Clin Microbiol 1997; 35:2521–2525.
40. Takiff H, Heifets L. In search of rapid diagnosis and drug-resistance detection tools: is the FAST Plaque TB test the answer? Int J Tuberc Lung Dis 2002; 6:560–561.
41. Victor TC, van Helden PD, Warren R. Prediction of drug resistance in *M. tuberculosis*: molecular mechanisms, tools, and applications. IUBMB Life 2002; 53:231–237.
42. van Rie A, Warren R, Mshanga I, et al. Analysis for a limited number of gene codons can predict drug resistance of *Mycobacterium tuberculosis* in a high-incidence community. J Clin Microbiol 2001; 39:636–641.
43. van Doorn HR, Kuijper EJ, van der Ende A, et al. The susceptibility of *Mycobacterium*

tuberculosis to isoniazid and the Arg→Leu mutation at codon 463 of *kat*G are not associated. J Clin Microbiol 2001; 39:1591–1594.
44. Heym B, Alzari PM, Honore N, Cole ST. Missense mutations in the catalase-peroxidase gene, *kat*G, are associated with isoniazid resistance in *Mycobacterium tuberculosis*. Mol Microbiol 1995; 15:235–245.
45. Victor TC, Pretorius GS, Felix JV, Jordaan AM, van Helden PD, Eisenach KD. *kat*G mutations in isoniazid-resistant strains of *Mycobacterium tuberculosis* are not infrequent. Antimicrob Agents Chemother 1996; 40:1572.
46. Victor TC, Warren R, Butt JL, et al. Genome and MIC stability in *Mycobacterium tuberculosis* and indications for continuation of use of isoniazid in multidrug-resistant tuberculosis. J Med Microbiol 1997; 46:847–857.
47. Telenti A, Imboden P, Marchesi F, et al. Detection of rifampicin-resistance mutations in *Mycobacterium tuberculosis*. Lancet 1993; 341:647–650.
48. Rouse DA, Li Z, Bai GH, Morris SL. Characterization of the *kat*G and *inh*A genes of isoniazid-resistant clinical isolates of *Mycobacterium tuberculosis*. Antimicrob Agents Chemother 1995; 39:2472–2477.
49. Sreevatsan S, Pan X, Zhang Y, Deretic V, Musser JM. Analysis of the *oxy*R-*ahp*C region in isoniazid-resistant and -susceptible *Mycobacterium tuberculosis* complex organisms recovered from diseased humans and animals in diverse localities. Antimicrob Agents Chemother 1997; 41:600–606.
50. Mdluli K, Slayden RA, Zhu Y, et al. Inhibition of a *Mycobacterium tuberculosis* β-ketoacyl ACP synthase by isoniazid. Science 1998:280:1607–1610.
51. Lee AS, Teo AS, Wong SY. Novel mutations in *ndh* in isoniazid-resistant *Mycobacterium tuberculosis* isolates. Antimicrob Agents Chemother 2001; 45:2157–2159.
52. Telenti A, Honore N, Bernasconi C, et al. Genotypic assessment of isoniazid and rifampin resistance in *Mycobacterium tuberculosis*: a blind study at reference laboratory level. J Clin Microbiol 1997; 35:719–723.
53. Williams DL, Waguespack C, Eisenach K, et al. Characterization of rifampin-resistance in pathogenic mycobacteria. Antimicrob Agents Chemother 1994; 38:2380–2386.
54. Rossauc R, Traore H, De Beenhouwer H, et al. Evaluation of the INNO-LiPA Rif TB assay, a reverse hybridization assay for the simultaneous detection of *Mycobacterium tuberculosis* complex and its resistance to rifampin. Antimicrob Agents Chemother 1997; 41:2093–2098.
55. Piatek AS, Tyagi S, Pol AC, et al. Molecular beacon sequence analysis for detecting drug resistance in *Mycobacterium tuberculosis*. Nat Biotechnol 1998; 16:359–363.
56. Kapur V, Li LL, Iordanescu S, et al. Characterization by automated DNA sequencing of mutations in the gene (*rpo*B) encoding the RNA polymerase β subunit in rifampin-resistant *Mycobacterium tuberculosis* strains from New York City and Texas. J Clin Microbiol 1994; 32:1095–1098.
57. Sreevatsan S, Stockbauer KE, Pan X, et al. Ethambutol resistance in *Mycobacterium tuberculosis*: critical role of *emb*B mutations. Antimicrob Agents Chemother 1997; 41: 1677–1681.
58. Ramaswamy SV, Amin AG, Goksel S, et al. Molecular genetic analysis of nucleotide polymorphisms associated with ethambutol resistance in human isolates of *Mycobacterium tuberculosis*. Antimicrob Agents Chemother 2000; 44:326–336.
59. Victor TC, van Rie A, Jordaan AM, et al. Sequence polymorphism in the *rrs* gene of *Mycobacterium tuberculosis* is deeply rooted within an evolutionary clade and is not associated with streptomycin resistance. J Clin Microbiol 2000; 39:4184–4186.
60. Hirano K, Takahashi M, Kazumi Y, Fukasawa Y, Abe C. Mutation in *pnc*A is a major mechanism of pyrazinamide resistance in *Mycobacterium tuberculosis*. Tuber Lung Dis 1997; 78:117–122.

61. Sreevatsan S, Pan X, Stockbauer KE, et al. Restricted structural gene polymorphism in the *Mycobacterium tuberculosis* complex indicates evolutionarily recent global dissemination. Proc Natl Acad Sci USA 1997; 94:9869–9874.
62. Viveiros M, Portugal I, Bettencourt R, et al. Isoniazid transient high level resistance in *Mycobacterium tuberculosis*. Antimicrob Agents Chemother 2002; 46:2804–2810.
63. Upton AM, Mushtaq A, Victor TC, et al. Arylamine *N*-acetyltransferase of *Mycobacterium tuberculosis* is a polymorphic enzyme and a site of isoniazid metabolism. Mol Microbiol 2001; 42:309–317.
64. Victor TC, Jordaan AM, van Rie A, et al. Detection of mutations in drug resistance genes of *Mycobacterium tuberculosis* by a dot-blot hybridization strategy. Tuber Lung Dis 1999; 79:343–348.
65. van Rie A, Warren R, Richardson M, et al. Classification of drug-resistant tuberculosis in an epidemic area. Lancet 2000; 356:22–25.
66. Dooley SW, Simone PM. The extent and management of drug-resistant tuberculosis: the American experience. Clinical tuberculosis. London: Chapman and Hall, 1994, pp. 171–189.
67. Classen CN, Warren R, Richardson M, et al. Impact of social interactions in the community on the transmission of tuberculosis in a high incidence area. Thorax 1999; 54:136–140.
68. Schaaf HS, Gie RP, Kennedy M, Beyers N, Hesseling PB, Donald PR. Evaluation of young children in contact with adult multidrug-resistant pulmonary tuberculosis: a 30-mo follow-up. Pediatrics 2002; 109:765–771.
69. Fox W, Ellard GA, Mitchison DA. Studies on the treatment of tuberculosis undertaken by the British Medical Research Council Tuberculosis Units, 1946–1986, with relevant subsequent publications. Int J Tuberc Lung Dis 1999:3:S231–S279.
70. Van Rie A, Warren RM, Richardson M, et al. Exogenous reinfection is a common cause of tuberculosis recurrence after cure. N Engl J Med 1999; 341:1174–1179.
71. Sonnenberg P, Murray J, Glynn JR, Shearer S, Kambashi B, Godfrey-Faussett P. HIV-1 and recurrence, relapse, and reinfection of tuberculosis after cure: a cohort study in South African mineworkers. Lancet 2001; 358:1687–1693.
72. Du Plessis DG, Warren R, Richardson M, Joubert JJ, van Helden PD. Demonstration of reinfection and reactivation in HIV-negative autopsied cases of secondary tuberculosis: multilesional genotyping of *Mycobacterium tuberculosis* utilizing IS*6110* and other repetitive element-based DNA fingerprinting. Tuberculosis 2001; 81:211–220.
73. Richardson M, Carroll NM, Engelke E, et al. Multiple *M. tuberculosis* strains in early cultures from patients in a high incidence community setting. J Clin Microbiol 2002; 40: 2750–2754.
74. Weyer K, Groenewalt P, Zwarenstein M, Lombard CJ. Tuberculosis drug resistance in the Western Cape. S Afr Med J 1995; 85:499–504.
75. Espinal MA, Laserson K, Camacho M, et al. Determinants of drug-resistant tuberculosis: analysis of 11 countries. Int J Tuberc Lung Dis 2001; 5:885–886.
76. Chaulet P. Measuring the prevalence of *Mycobacterium tuberculosis* resistance is not that easy: the interest and limits of a retrospective survey. Int J Tuberc Lung Dis 2001; 5:1077.
77. Al-Marri MRHA. Patterns of mycobacterial resistance to four anti-tuberculosis drugs in pulmonary tuberculosis patients in the State of Qatar after the implementation of DOTS and a limited expatriate screening programme. Int J Tuberc Lung Dis 2001; 5:1116–1121.
78. Bifani PJ, Plikaytis BB, Kapur V, et al. Origin and interstate spread of a New York City multidrug-resistant *Mycobacterium tuberculosis* clone family. JAMA 1996; 275:452–457.
79. Coronado VG, Beck-Sague CM, Hutton MD, et al. Transmission of multidrug-resistant *Mycobacterium tuberculosis* among persons with human immunodeficiency virus infection in an urban hospital: epidemiologic and restriction fragment length polymorphism analysis. J Infect Dis 1993; 168:1052–1055.
80. Edlin BR, Tokars JI, Grieco MH, et al. An outbreak of multidrug-resistant tuberculosis

among hospitalized patients with the acquired immunodeficiency syndrome. N Engl J Med 1992; 326:1514–1521.
81. Fischl MA, Uttamchandani RB, Daikos GL, et al. An outbreak of tuberculosis caused by multiple-drug-resistant tubercle bacilli among patients with HIV infection. Ann Intern Med 1992; 117:177–183.
82. Valway SE, Richards SB, Kovacovich J, Greifinger RB, Crawford JT, Dooley SW. Outbreak of multi-drug-resistant tuberculosis in a New York State prison, 1991. Am J Epidemiol 1994; 140:113–122.
83. Rullan JV, Herrera D, Cano R, et al. Nosocomial transmission of multidrug-resistant *Mycobacterium tuberculosis* in Spain. Emerg Infect Dis 1996; 2:125–129.
84. Ritacco V, Di Lonardo M, Reniero A, et al. Nosocomial spread of human immunodeficiency virus-related multidrug-resistant tuberculosis in Buenos Aires. J Infect Dis 1997; 176:637–642.
85. Beck-Sague C, Dooley SW, Hutton MD, et al. Hospital outbreak of multidrug-resistant *Mycobacterium tuberculosis* infections. Factors in transmission to staff and HIV-infected patients. JAMA 1997; 268:1280–1286.
86. Pearson ML, Jereb JA, Frieden TR, et al. Nosocomial transmission of multidrug-resistant *Mycobacterium tuberculosis*. A risk to patients and health care workers. Ann Intern Med 1992; 117:191–196.
87. Jereb JA, Klevens RM, Privett TD, et al. Tuberculosis in health care workers at a hospital with an outbreak of multidrug-resistant *Mycobacterium tuberculosis*. Arch Intern Med 1995; 155:854–859.
88. Agerton T, Valway S, Gore B, et al. Transmission of a highly drug-resistant strain (strain W1) of *Mycobacterium tuberculosis*. Community outbreak and nosocomial transmission via a contaminated bronchoscope. JAMA 1997; 278:1073–1077.
89. Shafer RW, Small PM, Larkin C, et al. Temporal trends and transmission patterns during the emergence of multidrug-resistant tuberculosis in New York City: a molecular epidemiologic assessment. J Infect Dis 1995; 171:170–176.
90. van Rie A, Warren RM, Beyers N, et al. Transmission of a multidrug resistant *Mycobacterium tuberculosis* strain resembling "strain W" among noninstitutionalized, human immunodeficiency virus-seronegative patients. J Infect Dis 1999; 180:1608–1615.
91. Frieden TR, Sherman LF, Maw KL, et al. A multi-institutional outbreak of highly drug-resistant tuberculosis: epidemiology and clinical outcomes. JAMA 1996; 276:1229–1235.
92. Viljanen MK, Vyshnevskiy BI, Otten TF, et al. Survey of drug-resistant tuberculosis in northwestern Russia from 1984 through 1994. Eur J Clin Microbiol Infect Dis 1998; 17:177–183.
93. Glynn JR, Whiteley J, Bifani PJ, Kremer K, van Soolingen D. Worldwide occurrence of Beijing/W strains of *Mycobacterium tuberculosis*: a systematic review. Emerg Infect Dis 2002; 8:843–849.
94. van Helden PD, Warren RM, Victor TC, van der Spuy G, Richardson M, Hoal-van Helden E. Strains of *Mycobacterium tuberculosis*. Trends Microbiol 2002; 10:167–168.
95. Bifani PJ, Mathema B, Kurepina NE, Kreiswirth BN. Global dissemination of the *Mycobacterium tuberculosis* W-Beijing family strains. Trends Microbiol 2002; 10:45–52.
96. Warren RM, Sampson SL, Richardson M, et al. Mapping of IS*6110* flanking regions in clinical isolates of *M. tuberculosis* demonstrates genome plasticity. Mol Microbiol 2000; 37:1405–1416.
97. Hoal-van Helden EG, Hon D, Lewis L-A, Beyers N, van Helden PD. Mycobacterial growth in human macrophages: variation according to donor, inoculum and bacterial strain. Cell Biol Int 2001; 25:77–81.
98. Hoal-van Helden EG, Stanton L-A, Warren R, Richardson R, van Helden PD. Diversity of in vitro cytokine responses by human macrophages to infection by *Mycobacterium tuberculosis* strains. Cell Biol Int 2001; 25:83–90.

99. Van Crevel R, Nelwan RHH, de Lenne W, et al. *Mycobacterium tuberculosis* Beijing genotype strains associated with febrile response to treatment. Emerg Infect Dis 2001; 7:880–883.
100. Day NPJ, Moore CE, Enright MC, et al. A link between virulence and ecological abundance in natural population of *Staphylococcus aureus*. Science 2002; 295:971.
101. Dye C, Williams BG, Espinal MA, Raviglione MC. Erasing the world's slow stain: strategies to beat multidrug-resistant tuberculosis. Science 2002; 295:2042–2046.
102. Pym AS, Saint-Joanis B, Cole ST. Effect of *kat*G mutations on the virulence of *Mycobacterium tuberculosis* and the implication for transmission in humans. Infect Immun 2002; 70:4955–4960.
103. van Helden PD. Bacterial genetics and strain variation. In: Novartis Foundation Symposium No. 217: Genetics and Tuberculosis. New York: Wiley, 1998, pp. 178–194.
104. Lillebaek T, Dirksen A, Baess I, Strunge B, Thomsen VØ, Andersen AB. Molecular evidence of endogenous reactivation of *Mycobacterium tuberculosis* after 33 yr of latent infection. J Infect Dis 2002; 185:401–404.

14

The Management of Multiple Drug-Resistant Tuberculosis

Sanjay Bhagani and Marc Lipman

1. INTRODUCTION

Tuberculosis (TB) will not go away. The decline that has occurred in rates in high-income countries because of chemotherapy *(1)* has now been reversed; TB remains the leading cause of death worldwide. Between 1998 and 2030, there are expected to be 225 million new cases of TB and 79 million deaths attributable to the disease *(2)*. It is inevitable that the number of drug-resistant cases will also increase. This has serious implications for TB control, especially in low-income countries *(3)*.

The situation is compounded if TB is allowed to become simultaneously resistant to the two most effective drugs used in its treatment, isoniazid (INH) and rifampicin (Rif). Irrespective of the presence or absence of other drug sensitivities, this is defined as multidrug resistant TB (MDR-TB). Worldwide, 50 million people are thought to be infected with MDR-TB *(4)*. Of the approx 9 million new TB cases each year, an estimated 3.1% are infected with an MDR strain *(5)*. This chapter focuses on the clinical implications, diagnosis, and current management of patients with MDR-TB.

2. IMPLICATIONS OF DRUG RESISTANCE

The development of active TB after infection with resistant strains is defined as *primary resistance*. However, *secondary* or *acquired* resistance is much more common and arises when insufficient or inadequate treatment is given because of noncompliance, malabsorption, or inadequate drug prescription. This leads to the selection of spontaneously resistant strains. Acquired resistance can only develop in patients who have received at least 4 wk of anti-TB treatment *(6)*. The term *initial* resistance is used when a history of prior anti-TB chemotherapy use is unknown *(7)*.

The anti-TB drugs INH and Rif, together with pyrazinamide (PZA) and ethambutol (EMB) or streptomycin (SM), are widely used as effective and affordable short-course chemotherapy (SCC) regimens *(8)*. With or without directly observed therapy (DOTS, directly observed therapy, short course), these have resulted in cure rates of more than 90%. Drug-resistant strains rarely emerge with adequate short-course regimens *(9,10)*. Where INH and Rif are lost to drug resistance (i.e., MDR-TB), outcomes in terms of

From: *Management of Multiple Drug-Resistant Infections*
Edited by: S. H. Gillespie © Humana Press Inc., Totowa, NJ

morbidity and mortality are much worse *(11,12)*. A case-control study from the French national tuberculosis database indicated a 59% failure rate (including a 20% loss to follow-up) over a 5-yr period, with median survival of 31 mo *(13)*. In South Africa, a mortality rate of approx 25% was reported at 5 yr among 42 patients with MDR-TB treated in an urban setting *(14)*. The outlook is even worse in patients co-infected with human immunodeficiency virus (HIV) *(15)*.

The public health implication of MDR-TB is possibly more concerning. As drug resistance develops rapidly (in weeks), inadequate treatment or nonadherence to therapy will result in transmission of drug-resistant strains within the community. This is especially likely when individuals live close to each other. It has contributed to outbreaks in prisons *(16,17)* and in hospitals in Europe *(18–21)* and the United States *(13,22)*. Of note, the patients in these outbreaks had very high rates of HIV infection (between 20 and 100%) and the mortality rate was significant (60 to 89%). The time between TB diagnosis and death was 4 to 16 wk *(23)*.

Public health measures to prevent the spread of MDR-TB or to control and reverse an existing problem are not cheap. The cost of one multi-institutional outbreak of MDR-TB in New York was estimated to be in excess of $25 million when calculated based on in-hospital costs alone *(24)*.

2.1. Case History

A 23-yr-old HIV-negative Afro-Caribbean male was diagnosed with drug-sensitive, smear-negative pulmonary TB and started on Rif, INH, EMB, and PZA together with vitamin B_6 supplements. Clinic attendance was poor, and the patient was lost to follow-up until he was traced 9 mo later because his sister developed TB. He was recommenced on supervised triple (Rif, INH, and PZA) therapy, but left the country and did not return until the next year, by which time his chest radiograph had deteriorated, and his smear was positive. He had not taken treatment and was given quadruple therapy for sensitive disease. Compliance (despite DOT) was poor; at mo 9, he was still smear positive and had now developed resistance to INH, Rif, and PZA. He was started on EMB, ciprofloxacin, intramuscular streptomycin (SM), clarithromycin, para-aminosalicylic acid (PAS), and prothionamide. He did not tolerate the PAS, developed a drug fever thought to be caused by the SM, and was switched to amikacin. He continued to prove difficult to treat and often absconded from the hospital, to which he had now been admitted. Over the next 15 mo, he became progressively more drug resistant, until he was only sensitive to (or able to tolerate) EMB, clarithromycin, and ciprofloxacin. His disease progressed, and he died of respiratory failure. For the last months of his life, he also had profound sensory-neural deafness and peripheral neuropathy, most probably because of his drug treatments.

3. WHEN TO SUSPECT DRUG-RESISTANT TUBERCULOSIS

A high index of suspicion is the cornerstone of early identification of a patient with drug-resistant tuberculosis. This should set in motion the process of early microbiological diagnosis, appropriate isolation of the patient, initiation of drug and other therapies, and public health actions to identify contacts and prevent further community and nosocomial spread of infection. A number of risk factors have been defined for MDR-TB, although they may be absent in a significant number of cases. The single most important indicator is if an individual (either consciously or unconsciously) is taking or receiving an inadequate level of treatment on a sustained basis.

3.1. Geographical Origin of Infection and Ethnicity of the Patient

There is an uneven global distribution of MDR-TB. According to the World Health Organization (WHO), 70% of all new MDR-TB cases occur in just 10 countries *(4,25)*. Drug resistance surveys in 58 countries during 1996–1999 revealed that the highest rate of resistance to any drug for patients with newly diagnosed tuberculosis was in Estonia (36.9%) *(5)*. The median incidence of multidrug resistance was only 1.0% overall, although it was much greater than this in Estonia (14.1%), Henan Province in China (10.8%), Latvia (9.0%), the Russian oblasts of Ivanovo (9.0%) and Tomsk (6.5%), Zheijang Province in China (4.5%), and Iran (5.0%).

In the United Kingdom, from 1993 to 1999, 6.1% of all TB isolates were resistant to one or more drugs, with a MDR-TB rate of 1.2% *(26)*. Resistance and MDR rates were higher among patients resident in London (1.7% MDR-TB) than in the rest of the United Kingdom (0.9% MDR-TB). Furthermore, in London, the data suggested a higher proportion of resistance among foreign-born patients and those of African, Oriental, and Indian subcontinent ethnic origin. This confirms previous findings of higher levels of drug-resistant tuberculosis within specific communities in the United Kingdom *(27,28)*.

3.2. Previous/Recently Failed or Failing Standard Tuberculosis Treatment

Although most national treatment guidelines *(29,30)* suggest susceptibility testing as a guide to therapy, this is not routinely available in most resource-poor settings where the majority of the world's tuberculosis is treated. Thus, the three- or four-drug SCC with INH/Rif together with PZA and EMB or SM are part of the standard treatment regimen in most of the world. The rationale for these regimens, their high cure rates, and their low relapse rates were established in studies in East Africa and Hong Kong in the 1980s *(31)*.

Treatment failure either because of nonresponse (i.e., persistently smear-positive sputum despite 6 mo of treatment) or from poor compliance, drug absorption, or drug availability is highly suggestive of drug-resistant infection *(32)*. The recurrence of positive mycobacterial cultures after previous sputum conversion should also suggest acquired drug resistance. In the United Kingdom, previous TB treatment was associated with an odds ratio of 3.1 (95% confidence interval [CI] 1.8–5.3) for the likelihood of drug resistance *(33)*.

3.3. Close Contacts of Drug-Resistant Subjects and Association With HIV Infection

The spread of tuberculosis in conditions of poverty and overcrowding is well known. In similar circumstances, a high prevalence of MDR-TB has been documented in prison inmates in Azerbhaijan *(17)* and Russia *(18)*. Two outbreaks of hospital-associated drug-resistant tuberculosis have been reported in the United Kingdom *(19,22)*.

The higher incidence of infection among HIV-positive contacts deserves further discussion. The impaired cellular immunity associated with HIV disease increases enormously the risk of asymptomatic (latent) infection with *M. tuberculosis* developing into clinically manifest TB. HIV-uninfected subjects with latent TB have an overall estimated lifetime risk of approx 10%. This increases to an *annual* risk of up to 10% in areas where TB and HIV co-infection is widespread. Studies in Malawi have indicated that almost three-quarters of patients with TB may be HIV positive *(34)*. Although HIV infection does not appear to contribute directly to the development of MDR-TB *(35)*, the potential exists for immunosuppressed individuals to become infected with less-virulent strains, which could include MDR-TB variants *(23)*. Further, it is likely that the association between HIV and MDR-TB reported in New York arose from confounders such as injecting drug use and homelessness *(36)*. In the United Kingdom, HIV-positive status has been associated with an odds ratio of 4.3 (95% CI 1.9–9.8) for the likelihood of drug-resistant TB *(33)*. The numbers were too small to assess using multivariate analysis whether the same applied to MDR-TB.

3.4. *Other Factors*

In a UK-wide study performed between 1993 and 1999, patients with pulmonary smear-positive disease were at an overall greater risk of drug-resistant TB. Men generally tended to have higher levels of drug resistance, with a significantly higher proportion of MDR-TB compared to women *(26)*. These findings could either result from direct reduced treatment adherence or because of other risk factors associated with male sex (homelessness, alcohol misuse, and HIV infection).

4. MAKING THE DIAGNOSIS: DETECTION OF DRUG RESISTANCE

Once clinical suspicion of drug-resistant tuberculosis has arisen, rapid detection and sensitivity testing need to be instituted. TB microscopic diagnosis has changed little since the development of acid-fast staining techniques, described by Koch in 1882. Direct microscopy is rapid, but requires concentrations above 5×10^3 organisms per milliliter and does not indicate viability or drug resistance. The development of automated liquid culture systems improve time to detection of growth to 12–18 d and have resulted in faster susceptibility testing results *(37)*.

Molecular diagnostic methods have revolutionized rapid testing for drug resistance. Results are available within 24 h of receipt of a suitable specimen. This has been made possible by the identification of the relevant genes and mutations involved in mycobacterial drug resistance. The simplest drug-resistant mutation to analyze has been to Rif. Of all clinical isolates resistant to Rif, 95% have a mutation in an 81-basepair region of the *rpo*B gene encoding the β-chain of the DNA-dependent RNA polymerase *(38)*. As approx 90% of all Rif-resistant isolates in the United Kingdom are also resistant to INH, a positive result for Rif resistance is a strong indicator of MDR-TB. INH resistance is much more complex, however, because at least four genes are implicated *(39)*.

There are several options for the genotypic detection of resistance mutations: DNA sequencing, which is time consuming and impractical for routine use; polymerase chain reaction (PCR); single-strand conformation polymorphism (PCR-SSCP) *(40)*; heteroduplex analysis; restriction enzyme analysis *(41)*; and solid-phase hybridization methods *(42)*. A solid-phase hybridization assay, the line-probe assay (LiPA, Innogenetics, Belgium) for the detection of the Rif-resistant mutation is commercially available. This system has been in use in the United Kingdom and has, on average, 90% correlation with standard culture and sensitivity methods, both for cultures and primary specimens *(43)*. One appraisal of the LiPA kit showed there was 91.7% correlation with standard methods when used on culture specimens, 90.2% correlation on primary specimens, and 91.7% correlation on smear-positive sputum specimens. This rapid detection system allowed drug resistance detection on average 27.6 d earlier for smear-positive sputum specimens, 27.7 d earlier for all primary specimens, and 19.1 d earlier for cultures *(43)*.

5. THERAPY

5.1. General Guidance

Treatment of MDR-TB is complex, time consuming, and demanding for all involved. At a community level, the best approach to treatment is prevention through optimum management of all drug-sensitive and monoresistant cases, thus minimizing the number of secondary/acquired MDR-TB. In practice, an individual who is well on the way to MDR status (given a history of nonadherence) or already has confirmed resistance is often encountered. In the United Kingdom, the advice is that such treatment should only be carried out by physicians with substantial experience in managing complex resistant cases, only in hospitals with appropriate isolation facilities, and in close liaison with Mycobacterial Reference Units *(29)*.

5.2. Drug Regimens and Duration of Therapy

There are two situations to consider in the choice of a treatment regimen: patients for whom drug resistance is suspected or known, but susceptibility testing is not avail able; and patients for whom sensitivities to a wide range of drugs are at hand. A modification to the first scenario in high-income countries is when Rif-resistance LiPA testing has been performed, and this has suggested MDR-TB, but there is a delay in obtaining full drug sensitivities.

Every effort should be made to obtain a clear history of previous drug treatments as well as some estimate of patient compliance. Previous failed therapy for more than 1 mo is usually associated with diminished efficacy with all the drugs in that regimen *(44)*. A new treatment combination when drug sensitivities are unknown should always include at least five, but as many as six or seven, drugs, of which three should, if possible, be new to the patient *(45)*. Therapy often needs to be initiated in the hospital to permit observation for toxicity and intolerance and to allow for changes in regimen if needed.

Determination of peak and trough serum concentrations may be used to optimize therapy and avoid side effects because the bioavailability and clearance of most drugs are not predictable *(46)*. In patients with HIV infection, particular care should be taken to document adequate levels of both antituberculous and antiretroviral drugs because of the risk of malabsorption *(47)* and drug interactions. The choice of drugs used in the treatment combination should take into account local TB resistance patterns if possible.

The treatment of patients for whom drug susceptibilities are available is somewhat more straightforward. Therapy should start with five or more drugs to which the organism is susceptible *(48)*. Treatment must be closely monitored because of the potential toxicity of second-line agents, but more importantly, full adherence is essential to prevent the further emergence of drug resistance. It is our experience that individuals who do not wish to take medication will often achieve this whether or not they are apparently "supervised." However, as discussed in Section 5.9, a directly observed approach to drug therapy must be regarded as the standard of care.

Data on the duration of therapy are largely based on empiricism *(11,45,48)*. The current recommendations are to continue with five or more drugs until sputum (or other body site) cultures become negative. Treatment is then maintained with at least three drugs to which the organism is susceptible for a minimum of 9 additional months and perhaps up to 24 mo or more. It is important to continue obtaining samples for culture as the pattern of resistance may evolve when new or unproven drug therapies (with potential patient toxicity) are added.

In practice, prolonged treatment with many toxic drugs is often difficult. The clinician may be forced to stop treatment after the shortest "curative" time (i.e., time for negative cultures plus another 6 to 9 mo) and then closely monitor the patient.

5.2.1. Case History

A 51-yr-old HIV-positive Caucasian male was diagnosed as having pulmonary MDR-TB as part of an outbreak within a health center. His initial TB isolate was resistant to INH, Rif, and PZA, and he was started on EMB, ciprofloxacin, prothionamide, clofazimine, and antiretroviral HIV medication. He also had a history of depressive psychosis and was maintained on an antipsychotic agent. He responded to treatment, and smear and culture were negative at mo 12. He continued his drugs for a planned further 24 mo.

At this point, he was producing minimal amounts of sputum and felt well. However, his culture grew TB resistant to INH, Rif, PZA, EMB, clofazamine, and prothionamide. He was switched to a regimen containing ciprofloxacin, clarithromycin, injectable amikacin, cycloserine, and PAS (drugs to which he was sensitive on in vitro testing). This resulted in rapid reversion of his cultures to negative. The cycloserine led to a major depressive episode, which recurred on rechallenge. PAS was unobtainable after 12 mo (no further manufacture), and he had some hearing loss from the amikacin despite careful dose monitoring. His general health is stable, there is no current evidence of active TB, and the decision has been made by his treating clinicians to stop his therapy (mo 18 of retreatment) and monitor for recurrence. His future options are limited.

5.3. Specific Drug Treatments

There are a number of second-line or reserve antituberculosis drugs available *(45)*. Generally, these do not have the antimycobacterial potency of standard first-line treatments, which should be included in a treatment regimen if there is evidence of sensitivity to them. Second-line drugs are summarized in Table 1.

The aminoglycosides (SM, amikacin, kanamycin) are only available in injectable form and can be administered either intramuscularly or intravenously. Amikacin and kanamycin are structurally similar, and there is usually cross-resistance between them; however, resistance between these drugs and SM is rare. Capreomycin, another injectable antituberculous drug, is structurally different and usually has no cross-resistance with amikacin, kanamycin, or SM.

Ofloxacin and ciprofloxacin are fluoroquinolones that are proving useful in retreatment and MDR treatment regimens. Ofloxacin has shown excellent activity in animal models *(49)* and in clinical studies of treatment regimens for MDR-TB *(50,51)*. The minimal inhibitory concentrations of both ofloxacin and ciprofloxacin are low for strains not previously exposed to these drugs *(52)*, and it is possible to use ofloxacin

Table 1
Commonly Used Second-Line Antituberculous Drugs and Their Side Effects

Drug	Usual dose	Side effects
Aminoglycosides, streptomycin, kanamycin, Amikacin	15 mg/kg body weight per day iv or im	Sensory-neuronal hearing loss, renal failure, ataxia, proteinuria, serum electrolyte disturbances
Capreomycin	15 mg/kg body weight per day iv or im	Hearing loss, renal failure, electrolyte disturbances, hypersensitivity reactions
Ofloxacin	400 mg twice daily	Nausea and vomiting, headache, anxiety, vasculitic reactions
Ciprofloxacin	750 mg twice daily	Vasculitis, tremor, nephritis, nausea and vomiting
Ethionamide	250 mg three times daily	Nausea and vomiting, abdominal pain, metallic taste, diarrhea, hepatitis
Para-aminosalicylic acid	3 g four times daily	Abdominal pain, diarrhea, nausea and vomiting, rash
Cycloserine	250 mg twice daily	Psychosis, mood disturbances, seizures
Clarithromycin	500 mg twice daily	Nausea and vomiting, diarrhea

once daily. Moxifloxacin has even better antimycobacterial activity and ultimately may supplant both of the other fluoroquinolones in clinical practice *(53)*.

PAS and ethionamide are relatively poorly tolerated. The high pill burden of PAS makes it an unattractive option, and it is currently unavailable. Treatment with either should be initiated slowly and dosages increased cautiously. Ethionamide has a very short half-life and is often considered the weakest of the TB drugs *(46)*. It is very poorly tolerated, with gastrointestinal side effects occurring almost universally, together with a bitter metallic taste that often causes profound anorexia. Its propyl derivative prothionamide offers little advantage.

Cycloserine is relatively well tolerated in terms of gastrointestinal side effects, but has potential for substantial and severe central nervous system toxicity. High serum concentrations may precipitate focal or generalized seizures as well as psychotic or suicidal ideation. High-dose pyridoxine (vitamin B_6) is often given with cycloserine in the hope of preventing neurological toxicity, but its value has not been proven *(45)*.

Other oral medications that have been used in MDR-TB include thiacetazone, clofazimine, the macrolides (clarithromycin and azithromycin), and amoxicillin-clavulanate *(54)*. Thiacetazone has modest tuberculostatic activity, but its side effects include severe erythema multiforme, especially in patients with HIV infection *(55)*. There are reports of potential efficacy of amoxicillin-clavulanate, but minimal inhibitory concentrations for most strains are very high *(54)*.

5.4. Surgical Intervention

Surgical procedures were the mainstay of anti-TB therapy prior to the introduction of antibiotics. Surgery for pulmonary TB may be considered for selected MDR-TB cases if chemotherapy with second-line drugs is not working sufficiently well. This may be particularly useful in pulmonary cavitation, for which drug penetration may be poor, resulting in continued bacillary multiplication. Indications for surgical treatment of MDR-TB include persistent cavitation, destruction of one lobe or one lung, failure to convert to culture negativity, previous relapses, and a high or potential risk of relapse. All of these are provided there are no contraindications to a pneumonectomy or lobectomy and patients often have severe bilateral disease *(56)*.

Bacteriological cure rates above 90% after surgery and in combination with adequate chemotherapy have been reported from experienced centers *(57–60)*. Treatment with anti-TB therapy needs to be continued for an appropriate length of time after surgery, usually 18–24 mo. The timing of surgery is often difficult because a balance must be struck between the need to achieve adequate bacteriological control prior to a major surgical procedure and not allowing the patient to deteriorate any further on a failing regimen. Close cooperation between surgical and medical staff (including careful nutritional assessment) is essential for a successful outcome.

5.5. Treatment Outcomes

In patients receiving second-line drug treatments, outcomes are variable and depend on a variety of factors. Goble et al. *(11)* reviewed the clinical course of 171 patients in New York with pulmonary MDR-TB treated with individually tailored regimens. There were 22 patients lost to follow-up, and 15 others were not analyzed. Of the 134 patients for whom results were available, sputum conversion was reported in 87 cases (65%), while 47 (35%) remained culture positive; 63 patients (46%) died, with 37 deaths directly attributed to TB. Goble and coworkers concluded that even the best available treatment is often unsuccessful. In that study, resistance to five or more drugs was an important predictor of treatment failure.

In a study by Tahaoglu et al. *(61)*, 158 patients with MDR-TB were evaluated; 36 (23%) had adjunctive surgery. Only 13 (8%) patients were categorized as having treatment failure. A good outcome was associated with younger age and no history of previous exposure to fluoroquinolones. In a nationwide case-control study from France *(12)*, factors related to a worse outcome were HIV co-infection, treatment with fewer than two active drugs, and lack of knowledge of MDR status at the time of diagnosis. Even in HIV co-infected patients, treatment outcomes may be improved by starting therapy promptly with at least two drugs to which the isolate is susceptible *(62)*.

Taking the results from four studies *(56)* with available susceptibilities, the overall sputum conversion rates ranged from 51 to 95%, treatment success ranged from 44 to 77%, and an associated mortality ranged between 0 and 37%. In some patients, a complete cure may not be achievable. For these individuals, it may be possible to control clinical disease and mycobacterial multiplication with intermittent courses of carefully selected drug regimens.

5.6. New and Experimental Therapies

Antimicrobial oxazolidinones such as linezolid *(53)*, as well as phenothiazine drugs (e.g., thioridazine), exhibit in vitro activity against MDR-TB. When put into experimental culture systems, they are found at high concentrations in human macrophages phagocytosing *M. tuberculosis (63)*. These drugs may prove a cheap and effective addition to the current regimens. Immunotherapy with *Mycobacterium vaccae* has recently been shown to improve the cure rates when combined with appropriate chemotherapy *(64)*. This approach in the immunocompetent patient shows promise and awaits further study in randomized clinical trials. Other immune-based methods include boosting the natural immune responses with cytokines involved in clearing TB infection. Studies are under way with, among others, interleukin-2, interleukin-12, interferon-γ, interferon-α, and granulocyte-macrophage colony-stimulating factor *(65,66)*.

6. CONTACT SCREENING AND CHEMOPROPHYLAXIS

Contact tracing and case finding are important public health measures. They can detect associated clinical cases, those cases with latent infection, and the infectious source in an outbreak. If MDR-TB is suspected, appropriate rapid confirmation of the diagnosis should be performed before a large contact-tracing exercise is planned or undertaken *(67)*. MDR-TB is no more infectious than drug-sensitive forms. However, there are clear implications for contacts who either are infected or are at such high risk that they require chemoprophylaxis (e.g., HIV-positive close contacts).

INH, Rif, and PZA are the only drugs with proven efficacy for the prevention of active disease in latently infected patients *(67–70)*. Given that both INH and Rif will be ineffective, options for preventive chemotherapy of MDR-TB are potentially problematic. A Delphi technique survey in 1992 resulted in clear support for PZA and ofloxacin or ciprofloxacin as chemoprophylaxis for high-risk contacts of patients with MDR-TB *(71)*. Centers for Disease Control and Prevention guidelines recommend treatment with EMB and PZA or, alternatively, ofloxacin or ciprofloxacin and pyrazinamide *(72)*. Decisions regarding choice of chemoprophylaxis should be made in close liaison with the microbiology laboratory where susceptibility testing occurred. Drug treatment should be given for a minimum of 6 mo.

7. THE COST OF TREATING MULTIDRUG-RESISTANT TUBERCULOSIS

Drug-resistant tuberculosis requires more than good clinical care *(73)*. There are cost implications for individual patient treatments, spending on public health measures to prevent the spread of MDR-TB, and at a national level, the cost associated with the lost productivity of infected persons and the responsibility of care for their families and dependents *(74,75)*.

Within an institution, the costs associated with the provision and staffing of negative-pressure rooms, laboratory charges for susceptibility testing and toxicity monitoring, as well as the costs associated with the use of expensive second-line drugs must be taken into account. In one London hospital, the minimum mean cost of caring for an HIV-negative patient with "uncomplicated" pulmonary MDR-TB was estimated at over £60,000 ($90,000), 10 times more than for a patient with drug-sensitive disease *(76)*. A study commissioned by the Regional Public Health Office estimated that, in London, 2.5% of culture-confirmed MDR-TB cases accounted for 20% of the total health care spending on TB *(77)*.

8. TREATMENT OF MULTIDRUG-RESISTANT TUBERCULOSIS: DIRECTLY OBSERVED THERAPY, SHORT COURSE PLUS, A GLOBAL STRATEGY

The DOTS strategy recommended by WHO *(78)* comprises five key elements: (1) fully supervised treatment with a standard short-course regimen, (2) case detection with special attention to the use of sputum microscopy, (3) reliable drug provision, (4) effective monitoring of TB control programs, and (5) government commitment to TB control. In the absence of facilities for culture and antimicrobial susceptibility testing, the detection of MDR-TB is algorithmic and becomes a diagnosis of exclusion *(32)*.

The increasing prevalence of drug-resistant TB has resulted in modification of the DOTS strategy, taking into account the need for access to reliable susceptibility testing to detect cases of MDR-TB and the use of second-line drugs. These elements have been incorporated into the "DOTS-plus" strategy *(79)*.

Some successful MDR-TB treatment programs in Peru, the Republic of Korea, and the United States have used individually tailored treatment regimens based on susceptibility testing *(80,81)*. These treatment strategies require ready access to sophisticated laboratories and medical personnel versed in interpreting the results and prescribing tailored expensive regimens *(82)*.

Other programs have successfully used standardized treatment regimens containing second-line drugs. Suarez et al. demonstrated the feasibility and cost-effectiveness of this in Peru *(83)*. They used an 18-mo regimen consisting of kanamycin (for 3 mo only) with ciprofloxacin, ethionamide, PZA, and EMB. They achieved a cure rate of 46%, which is comparable to response rates in the United States *(11)*. However, as the authors noted, this study was largely applicable to middle-income countries where high cure and compliance rates with first-line drugs are achieved, prevalence of HIV is low, and ambulatory care is used and accessible.

In reality, for a global DOTS-plus strategy to be effective, there needs to be a worldwide commitment to increasing the access to well-designed treatment programs and efforts made to reduce the costs of laboratory testing and second-line drugs.

9. PATIENT ISOLATION

Patients with suspected MDR-TB may require assessment and initiation of treatment in the hospital *(48)*. This is ideally achieved with the cooperation of the patient, the patient's relatives, and the patient's primary care physicians. Occasionally, where this is not forthcoming, in the United Kingdom the Sections 37, 38, and 35 of the Public Health Act allow compulsory admission, detention, and examination of the patient *(67,84)*. It should be noted that this can only be applied in the context of infectious (smear-positive) tuberculosis of the respiratory tract. Under these sections, the patient cannot be forced to take medication, and the Act has to be balanced against the patient's individual rights.

Within the hospital setting, guidelines for appropriate isolation—as laid down by the Joint Tuberculosis Committee of the British Thoracic Society *(67)*—can be summarized as follows:

1. All patients with suspected or known MDR-TB should be admitted to a negative-pressure ventilation room. If such facilities are not available locally, the patient should be transferred to a hospital where such facilities, plus expertise in the diagnosis and management of MDR-TB, are available.

2. Staff and visitors to the room should wear appropriate dust/mist masks while in the negative-pressure room.
3. The decision to discharge the patient must be discussed with the hospital infection control team, the local microbiologist, and public health officials.
4. Before discharge from the hospital, secure arrangements for the supervision and administration of antituberculosis therapy should have been made and agreed with the patient and caregivers.
5. All treatment, either as an inpatient or as an outpatient, should be fully supervised unless there are exceptional circumstances.

10. CONCLUSIONS

MDR-TB is an escalating global threat that has implications both for communities and for the individual. The best treatment is prevention. This is achieved by initiating, managing, and sustaining national TB programs with high cure rates. At a patient level, routine risk assessment and good laboratory facilities are the key to a prompt diagnosis. Early and carefully chosen second-line drug therapy is crucial for a favorable outcome. The successful management of the individual patient is both complex and costly and requires an expert multidisciplinary team approach and patient cooperation. Without the last, any strategy is bound to fail.

REFERENCES

1. Harris HW. Chemotherapy of tuberculosis: the beginning. In: Rom WN, Garay SM (eds.). Tuberculosis. Boston, MA: Little Brown, 1996, pp. 745–749.
2. Murray C, Saloman JA. Modelling the impact of global tuberculosis strategies. Proc Natl Acad Sci U S A 1998; 95:13,881–13,886.
3. Snider DE, Castro DK. The global threat of drug-resistant tuberculosis. N Engl J Med 1998; 338:1689–1690.
4. World Health Organization. IUATLD Global Project on Anti-tuberculosis Drug Resistance Surveillance. Anti-tuberculosis Drug Resistance in the World. Report no. 2. Prevalence and Trends (2000). Geneva: World Health Organization, 2000. Publication No. WHO/CDS/TB/2000.278. Geneva, Communicable Diseases.
5. Espinal MA, Laszlo A, Simenson L, et al. Global trends in resistance to antituberculosis drugs. N Engl J Med 2001; 344:1294–1303.
6. Pablos-Mendez A, Lazlo A, Bustreo F. Anti-tuberculosis Drug Resistance in the World. Geneva, Switzerland: World Health Organization, 1997. WHO/GTP/97.229.
7. Crofton J, Chaulet P, Maher D. Guidelines for the Management of Drug-Resistant Tuberculosis. Geneva, Switzerland: World Health Organization, 1997. WHO/TB 96.210 (Rev. 1).
8. Yew W. Directly observed therapy, short course: the best way to prevent MDR-TB. Chemotherapy 1999; 45(suppl. 12):26–33.
9. Espinal MA, Laszlo A, Simonsen L, et al. Global trends in resistance to antituberculosis drugs. N Engl J Med 1993; 328:521–526.
10. Lambregts-van Weezenbeek CSB, Veen J. Control of drug resistant tuberculosis. Tuber Lung Dis 1995; 76:455–459.
11. Goble M, Iseman MD, Madsen LA, Waite D, Ackerson L, and Horsburgh CR, Jr. Treatment of 171 patients with pulmonary tuberculosis resistant to isoniazid and rifampicin. N Engl J Med 1993; 328:527–532.
12. Fament-Sailloue M, Robert J, Jarlier V, Grosset J. Outcome of multi-drug resistant tuberculosis in France. A nationwide case-cohort study. Am J Resp Crit Care Med 1999; 160: 587–593.
13. Pitchenik AE, Burr J, Laufer M, et al. Outbreak of drug-resistant tuberculosis at an AIDS centre. Lancet 1990; 336:440–441.

14. Van Rie A, Gie RP, Enarson D, Beyers N. The outcome of MDR-TB patients in an urban area of South Africa. Int J Tuberc Lung Dis 1999; 3(suppl. 1):s84–s85.
15. Fischl MA, Daikos GL, Uttamchandani RB, et al. Clinical presentation and outcome of patients with HIV infection and tuberculosis caused by multiple-drug resistant bacilli. Ann Intern Med 1992; 117:184–190.
16. Portaels F, Rigouts L, Bastian I. Addressing multi-drug resistant tuberculosis in penitentiary hospitals and the general population of the former Soviet Union. Int J Tuberc Lung Dis 1999; 3:582–588.
17. Pfyffer GE, Sraessle A, van Gorkum T, et al. Multidrug-resistant tuberculosis in prison inmates, Azerbhaijan. Emerg Infect Dis 2001; 7:855–861.
18. Hannan MM, Peres H, Maltez F, et al. Investigation and control of a large outbreak of multi-drug resistant tuberculosis at a central Lisbon hospital. J Hosp Infect 2001; 72:91–97.
19. Moro ML, Errante I, Infuso A, et al. Effectiveness of infection control measures in controlling a nosocomial outbreak of multidrug-resistant tuberculosis among HIV patients in Italy. Int J Tuberc Lung Dis 2000; 41:61–68.
20. Breathnach AS, De Ruiter A, Holdsworth GM, et al. An outbreak of multi-drug-resistant tuberculosis in a London teaching hospital. J Hosp Infect 1998; 92:111–117.
21. Coronado VG, Beck-Sague CM, Hutton MD, et al. Transmission of multidrug-resistant *Mycobacterium tuberculosis* among persons with human immunodeficiency virus infection in an urban hospital: epidemiological and restriction fragment length polymorphism analysis. J Infect 1993; 1684:1052–1055.
22. Centers for Disease Control and Prevention. Outbreak of multidrug-resistant tuberculosis at a hospital—New York City, 1991. MMWR Morb Mortal Wkly Rep 1993; 4222:427, 433–434.
23. Pozniak A. Multidrug-resistant tuberculosis and HIV infection. Ann N Y Acad Sci 2001; 953:192–198.
24. Frieden TR, Sherman LF, Lay Maw K, et al. A multi-institutional outbreak of highly drug-resistant tuberculosis. JAMA 1996; 276:1229–1235.
25. Pablos-Mendez A, Raviglione MC, Laszlo A, et al. Global surveillance for antituberculosis drug resistance, 1994–1997. N Engl J Med 1998; 344:1294–1303.
26. Djuretic T, Herbert J, Drobniewski F, et al. Antibiotic resistant tuberculosis in the United Kingdom: 1993–1999. Thorax 2002; 57:477–482.
27. Ormerod P. Tuberculosis and immigration. Br J Hosp Med 1996; 56:209.
28. McCarthy OR. Asian immigrant tuberculosis: the effect of visiting Asia. Br J Dis Chest 1984; 78:248–253.
29. Joint Tuberculosis Committee of the British Thoracic Society. Chemotherapy and management of tuberculosis in the United Kingdom: recommendations. Thorax 1998; 53:536–548.
30. American Thoracic Society. Treatment of tuberculosis and tuberculosis infections in adults and children. Am J Respir Crit Care Med 1994; 149:1359–1374.
31. Hong Kong Chest Service/British Medical Research Council. Five-year follow-up of a controlled trial of five 6-month regimens of chemotherapy for pulmonary tuberculosis. Am Rev Resp Dis 1987; 136:1339–1342.
32. World Health Organization. Treatment of Tuberculosis: Guidelines for National Programmes. 2nd ed, Geneva, Switzerland: WHO, 1997. WHO/TB/97.220.
33. Hayward AC, Bennett DE, Herbert J, et al. Risk factors for drug resistance in patients with tuberculosis in England and Wales 1993–1994. Thorax 1996; 51(suppl. 3):S32.
34. Harries AD, Maher D, Muula B, Nyangula D. An audit of HIV serostatus in tuberculosis patients, Blantyre, Malawi. Tuber Lung Dis 1995; 76:413–417.
35. Espinal MA, Laserson K, Comacho M, et al. Determinants of drug-resistant tuberculosis: analysis of 11 countries. Int J Tuberc Lung Dis 2001; 10:887–893.
36. Frieden TR, Sterling T, Pablos-Mendez A, Kilburn JO, Cauthen GM, Dooley SW. The emergence of drug-resistant tuberculosis in New York City. N Engl J Med 1993; 328:521–526.
37. Caws M, Drobniewski FA. Molecular techniques in the diagnosis of *Mycobacterium tuberculosis* and the detection of resistance. Ann N Y Acad Sci 2001; 953:138–145.

38. Telenti A, Imboden P, Marchesi F. Detection of rifampicin-resistance mutations in *Mycobacterium tuberculosis*. Lancet 1993; 341:647–649.
39. Quemard AJC, Sacchetini A, Dessen C, et al. Enzymatic characterization of the target for isonization in *Mycobacterium tuberculosis*. Biochemistry 1995; 34:8235–8241.
40. Telenti A, Marchesi F, Balz M. Rapid identification of *Mycobacteria* to species level by polymerase chain reaction and restriction enzyme analysis. J Clin Microbiol 1993; 31:175–178.
41. Rossaur R, Traore H, De Beenhouwer H, et al. Evaluation of INNO-Lipa Rif. TB assay, a reverse hybridisation assay for the simultaneous detection of *Mycobacterium tuberculosis* complex and its resistance to rifampin. Antimicrob Agents Chemother 1997; 41:2093–2098.
42. Carriere C, Riska PF, Zimhony O, et al. Conditionally replicating luciferase reporter phages: improved sensitivity for rapid detection and assessment of drug susceptibility of *Mycobacterium tuberculosis*. J Clin Microbiol 1997; 35:3232–3239.
43. Drobniewski FA, Watterson SA, Wilson SM, Harris GS. A clinical, microbiological and economic analysis of a national service for the rapid diagnosis of tuberculosis and rifampicin resistance in *Mycobacterium tuberculosis*. J Med Microbiol 2000; 49:271–278.
44. Costello HD, Cras GJ, Snider DE Jr. Drug resistance among previously treated tuberculosis patients, a brief report. Am Rev Respir Dis 1980; 121:313–316.
45. Iseman MD. Treatment of multidrug-resistant tuberculosis. N Engl J Med 1993; 329:784–791.
46. Heifets LB, Lindhom-Levy PJ. Bacteriostatic and bacteriocidal activity of ciprofloxacin and ofloxacin against *Mycobacterium tuberculosis* and *Mycobacterium avium*–complex. Tubercle 1987; 68:267–276.
47. Berning SE, Huitt GA, Iseman MD, Peloquin CA. Malabsorption of antituberculosis medication by patients with AIDS. N Engl J Med 1992; 327:1817–1818.
48. Ormerod P. The clinical management of the drug-resistant patient. Ann N Y Acad Sci 2001; 953:185–191.
49. Tsukumara M. Antituberculosis activity of ofloxacin (DL8280) on experimental tuberculosis in mice. Am Rev Respir Dis 1985; 132:915.
50. Marentra KN. Quinolones and multidrug-resistant tuberculosis. Chemotherapy 1999; 45(suppl. 2):12–18.
51. Mangunnegoro H, Hudoyo A. Efficacy of low-dose ofloxacin in the treatment of multidrug-resistant tuberculosis in Indonesia. Chemotherapy 1999; 45(suppl. 2):19–25.
52. Peloquin C. Pharmacological issues in the treatment of tuberculosis. Ann N Y Acad Sci 2001; 93:157–163.
53. Rodriguez JC, Ruiz M, and Royo G. In vitro activity of moxifloxacin, levofloxacin, gatifloxacin, and linezolid against mycobacterium tuberculosis. Int J Antimicrob Agents 2002;20:464–467.
54. Nadler JP, Berger J, Nord JA, Cofsky R, and Saxena, M. Amoxycillin–clavulanic acid for treating drug-resistant *Mycobacterium tuberculosis*. Chest 1991; 99:1025–1026.
55. Nunn P, Kibuga D, Gathua S, et al. Cutaneous hypersensitivity reactions due to thiacetezone in HIV-1 seropositive patients treated for tuberculosis. Lancet 1991; 337:627–630.
56. Loddenkemper R, Sagebiel D, Brendel A. Strategies against multi-drug resistant tuberculosis. Eur Respir J 2002; 20(suppl. 36):66s–77s.
57. Muthuswamy P, Chechani V, Barker W. Surgical management of pulmonary tuberculosis. Am Rev Respir Dis 1992; 145(suppl. 4):A816.
58. Van Leuven M, de Groot M, Shean K, von Oppellum, and Wilcox PA. Pulmonary resection as an adjunct in the treatment of multiple drug-resistant tuberculosis. Ann Thorac Surg 1997; 63:1368–1373.
59. Chiang CY, Yu MC, Bai KL, Suo J, Lin TP, and Lee YC. Pulmonary resection in the treatment of patients with pulmonary multidrug-resistant tuberculosis in Taiwan. Int J Tuberc Lung Dis 2001;5: 272–277.
60. Pomerantz BJ, Cleveland JC, Olson HK, Pomerantz M. Pulmonary resection for multidrug resistant tuberculosis. J Thorac Cardiovasc Surg 2001; 121:448–453.

61. Tahaoglu K, Torun T, Sevim T, et al. The treatment of multidrug-resistant tuberculosis in Turkey. N Engl J Med 2001; 345:170–174.
62. Turett GS, Telzak EE, Torian VL, et al. Improved outcomes for patients with multidrug-resistant tuberculosis. Clin Infect Dis 1995; 21:1238–1244.
63. Amaral L, Kristiansen JE, Viveros M, and Antouguia J. Activity of phenothiazines against antibiotic-resistant *Mycobacterium tuberculosis*: a review supporting further studies that may elucidate the potential use of thioridazine as anti-tuberculosis therapy. J Antimicrob Chemother 2001; 47:505–511.
64. Stanford JL, Stanford CA, Grange JM, Lan NN, and Gtemadi A. Does immunotherapy with heat-killed *Mycobacterium vaccae* offer hope for the treatment of multi-drug resistant pulmonary tuberculosis? Respir Med 2001; 95:435–436.
65. Holland SM. Cytokine therapy of mycobacterial infections. Adv Intern Med 2001; 45:505–511.
66. Kristiansen JE, Amaral L. The potential management of resistant infections with non-antibiotics. J Antimicrob Chemother 1997; 40:319–327.
67. Joint Tuberculosis Committee of the British Thoracic Society. Control and prevention of tuberculosis in the United Kingdom: Code of Practice 2000. Thorax 2000; 55:887–901.
68. Dillon J, Dickinson JM, Sole K, et al. Preventive chemotherapy of tuberculosis in Cornell model mice with combinations of rifampicin, isoniazid and pyrazinamide. Antimicrob Agents Chemother 1996; 40:552–555.
69. Halsey NA, Coberly JS, Desormeaux J, et al. Randomised trial of isoniazid versus rifampin and pyrazinamide for prevention of tuberculosis in HIV-1 infection. Lancet 1998; 351:786–792.
70. Mwinga A, Hosp M, Godfrey-Faussett P, et al. Twice weekly tuberculosis preventive therapy in HIV infection in Zambia. AIDS 1998; 12:2447–2457.
71. Gallagher CT, Passannante MR, Reichman LB. Preventive therapy for multi-drug resistant tuberculosis (MDR-TB): a Delphi survey. Am Rev Respir Dis 1992; 145(suppl.): A812.
72. Management of persons exposed to multidrug-resistant tuberculosis. MMWR Morb Mortal Wkly Rep 1992; 41:61–71.
73. Moore-Gillon J. Multidrug-resistant tuberculosis—this is the cost. Ann N Y Acad Sci 2001; 953:233–240.
74. Rajeswari R, Balasubramanian R, Muniyandi M, Geetharamanis Theresa X, and Venkatasan P. Socio-economic impact of tuberculosis on patients and family in India. Int J Tuberc Lung Dis 1999; 3:869–877.
75. Kamolratanaku P, Sawert H, Kongsin S, et al. Economic impact of tuberculosis at the household level. Int J Tuberc Lung Dis 1999; 3:596–602.
76. White VLC, Moore-Gillon J. Resource implications of multidrug-resistant tuberculosis. Thorax 2000; 55:962–963.
77. NHS. Tuberculosis Control in London—the Need for a Change. NHS Executive, December 1998. (NT 980004).
78. World Health Organization. Tuberculosis Programme: Framework for Effective Tuberculosis Control. Geneva, Switzerland: World Health Organisation, 1994. WHO/TB/94.179.
79. Farmer PE, Kim JY. Community-based approaches to the control of multidrug-resistant tuberculosis: introducing "DOTS-plus," BMJ 1998; 317:671–674.
80. Park SK, Kim CT, Sond SD. Outcome of therapy in 107 patients with pulmonary tuberculosis resistant to isoniazid and rifampicin. Int J Tuberc Lung Dis 1998; 2:877–884.
81. Farmer P. The dilemma of MDRTB in the global era. Int J Tuberc Lung Dis 1998; 2:869–876.
82. Bastian I, Rigouts A, Van Deun A, Porteals F. Directly observed treatment, short-course strategy and multidrug-resistant tuberculosis: are any modifications required? Bull WHO 2000; 78:238–251.
83. Suarez PG, Floyd K, Portocarrero J, et al. Feasibility and cost-effectiveness of standardised second-line drug treatment for chronic tuberculosis patients: a national cohort study in Peru. Lancet 2002; 359:1980–1989.
84. Public Health (Control of Disease) Act 1984, §35, 37, 38.

15

Management of Infection With Nontuberculosis Mycobacteria

Stephen H. Gillespie

1. INTRODUCTION

The nontuberculosis mycobacteria are often naturally resistant to the conventional antibiotics and to antituberculosis drugs *(1–3)*. In addition, providing advice for the treatment of nontuberculosis is complicated by the variable and changing designations of these organisms, the heterogeneity of the clinical syndromes and patients, and the relative lack of controlled clinical trials *(1,2)*. This chapter discusses the management of these difficult infections.

1.1. Nomenclature

The clinical importance of *Mycobacterium tuberculosis* as a major cause of death has meant that microbiologists have rightly focused on this organism. The remaining *Mycobacterium* species, which appeared to lack the potential to cause infection in healthy individuals, were often dismissed as "anonymous" or "atypical" *(4)*. This approach was neither accurate nor clinically helpful. As environmental organisms, their low pathogenic potential and failure to produce diseases that resemble tuberculosis is expected. Thus, the term *nontuberculosis mycobacterium* (NTM) is preferred *(2)*.

Now that conventional and molecular taxonomic techniques have been applied to this group of organisms, clinicians will increasingly be able to identify the invading mycobacteria accurately and to detect previously unrecognized species. As the pathogenic potential of each species is more accurately defined, it will become easier to choose the most appropriate drugs and management strategies.

1.2. Epidemiology

Mycobacteria are organisms that mainly live in the inanimate environment or as colonizers of humans and animals *(5)*. In one sense, it is the pathogenic species *M. tuberculosis* and *Mycobacterium leprae* that are atypical in that they lack an environmental reservoir. Most other species of the *Mycobacterium* genus are found in the environment and can be isolated from soil, water, and carriage sites in animals and humans *(6)*.

The number of cases of NTM infection has been increasing throughout the world *(7)*. The reasons for this are varied, but are important and need to be considered to

From: *Management of Multiple Drug-Resistant Infections*
Edited by: S. H. Gillespie © Humana Press Inc., Totowa, NJ

understand the interaction of the epidemiology of NTM and therapeutic strategies. There has been a genuine increase in the number of cases because of changes in medical practice that provide opportunities for colonization and infection, for example, colonization of intravenous long lines with rapidly growing mycobacteria *(8)*. The increase in the number of patients who are receiving immunosuppressive therapy also provides opportunities for NTM to cause disease. The human immunodeficiency virus (HIV) epidemic brought about an enormous increase in the number of *Mycobacterium avium-intracellulare* cases *(9,10)*.

The number of cases has also been increasing because the diagnostic methods employed for mycobacteria have improved significantly over the last 20 yr *(11)*. In addition, simpler identification techniques, including molecular methods, have simplified diagnosis sufficiently that it is no longer the province of a reference laboratory. This has led to increased recognition, which has helped define the patterns of disease caused by different species and in the description of many new species *(12–14)*.

1.3. Scope of the Chapter

This chapter discusses the diagnosis and management of the NTM that are difficult to treat by virtue of their natural resistance to antibiotics. The major clinical syndromes discussed include bacteremia with *M. avium-intracellulare*, cervical lymphadenopathy and pulmonary infection with NTM, and infection with rapidly growing mycobacteria.

2. DIAGNOSIS OF NONTUBERCULOSIS MYCOBACTERIA

The isolation of *M. tuberculosis* from a specimen is sufficient to indicate a diagnosis of tuberculosis. The only other possible explanation of this finding is cross-contamination of the specimen either in the clinical setting or in the laboratory. The diagnostic problem is more difficult for NTM. As many of these organisms can form part of the normal flora or represent environmental contaminants, a single isolate is often not sufficient to make a diagnosis *(1,2)*.

2.1. Pulmonary Disease

The radiological appearances of NTM pulmonary disease exhibit subtle differences from that of tuberculosis. Cavities, when present, are thin walled, and there is less surrounding infiltrate. Spread is more contiguous with more marked involvement of the pleura. Occasionally, NTM may cause a single pulmonary nodule. An important part of confirming a diagnosis of NTM infection is to exclude potential confounding diagnoses, such as tuberculosis and lung malignancy. As *Mycobacterium kansasii, Mycobacterium xenopi, Mycobacterium malmoense*, and the rapid growers can form part of the normal flora, multiple isolates of an NTM are required from sputum or bronchial washings obtained at different times to support a positive diagnosis *(10)*. More weight is to be placed on single specimens that are also smear positive *(1,2)*. Alternatively, a single isolate from a biopsy specimen is diagnostic provided it is supported by compatible histology *(2)*.

Sputum is usually an adequate specimen with which to obtain a positive diagnosis of infection with *M. kansasii, M. xenopi,* and *M. malmoense*. In contrast, in HIV-seronegative individuals infected with *M. avium-intracellulare*, sputum is insensitive, and a more aggressive approach using bronchial lavage should be adopted *(15)*.

2.2. Lymphadenitis

The most important part of diagnosis of lymphadenitis is to exclude tuberculosis. The diagnosis depends on granulomata in a biopsy of lymph glands in the context of a negative tuberculin test. A single isolate from a biopsy specimen is sufficient to make the diagnosis, although yields may be less than 50% of cases *(16,17)*. This in part may be because of the methods employed and the presence of fastidious mycobacterial species such as *Mycobacterium haemophilum* and *Mycobacterium genavense*.

2.3. Cutaneous Infection

The presence of rapidly growing mycobacteria in skin specimens must be evaluated carefully. Multiple isolates are required in clinical circumstances that support the diagnosis, for example, the presence of a plastic catheter or prosthetic device. Alternatively, individual cases may form part of known outbreaks with contaminated injections or prostheses. For *Mycobacterium ulcerans* and *Mycobacterium marinum*, the situation is often simpler as these species are likely to be isolated from patients with characteristic cutaneous lesions, making diagnosis easy. The management of these specific cutaneous infections is not discussed further.

2.4. Disseminated Infection in HIV-Infected Individuals

Disseminated infection with *M. avium-intracellulare* is usually only found in patients with advanced HIV infection who have not received antiretroviral therapy or have failed to take it. The CD count is usually low (<50), and the patient has clinical signs of advanced disease *(18)*. Patients are usually febrile and wasted and with significant anemia. Alkaline phosphatase is often elevated as hepatic involvement by *M. avium-intracellulare* is common. Usually, a single isolate from the blood is sufficient to confirm the diagnosis of disseminated *M. avium-intracellulare* infection *(1,2)*.

2.5. Role of Susceptibility Testing

The role of susceptibility testing in treatment choice for NTMs is controversial. There are many older studies that indicate that in vitro susceptibility test results do not correlate well with clinical outcome *(19,20)*. A more recent study of *M. avium* complex, *M. malmoense*, and *M. xenopi* found only one significant correlation of resistance and treatment failure for *M. xenopi (21)*. Similarly, a study of *M. avium-intracellulare* infection in HIV-seronegative patients found no correlation between the in vitro susceptibility and outcome *(22)*. However, such relationships are difficult to demonstrate unequivocally because all therapeutic regimens are with multiple drugs, and most centers only have a few patients, with the effect that these studies lack statistical power. One study of 256 patients showed a significant association ($p < 0.001$) between partial or no in vitro resistance to 1 mg/L of isoniazid and the time required for conversion of sputum from culture positive to negative, whereas complete resistance to isoniazid had a statistically significant adverse effect *(23)*. Others have found susceptibility testing for rapid growers valuable for planning chemotherapy *(24)*. Also, patients who responded to treatment for pulmonary *M. avium-intracellulare* received significantly more drugs to which their isolate was susceptible *(25)*.

Much of the contradiction provided by these articles may be because mycobacterial susceptibility tests are designed for use with *M. tuberculosis*. NTM may be inhibited with antibiotic concentrations achievable in serum, but at concentrations higher than that required for tuberculosis. Thus, in vitro test results based on a breakpoint for tuberculosis will produce false resistance for an isolate of NTM *(21,22)*. The use of methods that provide minimum inhibitory concentration (MIC) data will enable regimens to be constructed specifically for NTM that take into account the achievable concentrations of antibiotics *(26,27)*.

3. MANAGEMENT OF *MYCOBACTERIUM KANSASII* INFECTION

3.1. Pulmonary Infections

Mycobacterium kansasii is an important pulmonary pathogen with a tendency to affect older male patients with pre-existent pulmonary disease. Mortality rates are high, but this is often because of the severe underlying conditions that coexist in these patients *(28)*. All authorities agree that it is the inclusion of rifampicin that is responsible for favorable outcomes of culture conversion in almost all patients within 4 mo. On the other hand, resistance to this agent or its absence in the regimen underlies many of the reported examples of treatment failure *(23,29,30)*. With regimens that contain rifampicin, relapse rates are typically low, with figures of between 2.5 and 9% *(23,28)*.

The current American Thoracic Society (ATS) recommendation for treatment of pulmonary disease caused by *M. kansasii* in adults is the regimen of isoniazid (300 mg), rifampin (600 mg), and ethambutol (25 mg/kg body weight for the first 2 mo, then 15 mg/kg body weight) given daily for 18 mo and with at least 12 mo of negative sputum cultures. In patients who are unable to tolerate one of these three drugs, clarithromycin would seem a reasonable alternative, but its effectiveness has not been established by clinical trials (*see* below). Pyrazinamide has no role to play in therapy for *M. kansasii* infections because all isolates are resistant *(2)*.

A prospective clinical trial performed by the British Thoracic Society (BTS) in 173 patients with two sputum cultures positive for NTM showed that *M. kansasii* pulmonary infection responded well to 9 mo of treatment with rifampicin and ethambutol, but patients who contract this disease have a high mortality rate from other causes. Isoniazid did not appear to be a necessary part of the regimen *(28)*. Consequently, the BTS recommend that 9 mo of rifampicin and ethambutol is adequate treatment for most patients, but when there is evidence of compromising conditions, treatment can be extended to 15–24 mo *(1)*. The use of intermittent drug regimens or short-course therapy has not been studied sufficiently for advice to be given.

In patients who have an inadequate response or who are unable to tolerate the standard agents, prothionamide (1 g/d orally) and streptomycin (0.75–1 g/d im) could be added *(1)*, but both are associated with frequent adverse events. Both clarithromycin and fluoroquinolones are highly active against *M. kansasii* and are likely to be beneficial *(3,31)*, although there is no clinical trial data available. These agents have proved useful in the treatment of *M. avium-intracellulare* infection (*see* Section 6.1.1.) and may be useful as part of the regimen.

Rifampicin resistance among *M. kansasii* appears to be increasing in part because of the HIV epidemic. Although rifampicin is the most important drug in the treatment of *M. kansasii* infection if patients are treated with a regimen that includes three drugs to which the infecting organism is susceptible a good outcome is likely. Many of these regimens include clarithromycin and ciprofloxacin *(26)*.

3.2. Extrapulmonary Infection

The treatment of extrapulmonary disease should probably be similar to the pulmonary regimens. For lymphadenopathy, excision is recommended as this is the optimal treatment for *M. avium-intracellulare* infection, the most common cause (*see* Section 6.1.2.) *(1,2)*.

4. MANAGEMENT OF *MYCOBACTERIUM MALMOENSE* DISEASE

4.1. Pulmonary Disease

Retrospective studies have shown that patients treated for 18–24 mo with regimens that included rifampicin and ethambutol did better than those treated with other regimens or who had shorter durations of treatment *(32)*. The addition of second- or third-line drugs increased the rate at which adverse events were reported without improving the outcome. Surgery has an important role to play for those who are suitable for operation, and chemotherapy should be continued afterward for at least 18 mo. A clinical trial of chemotherapy in *M. malmoense* infection showed that treatment of *M. malmoense* with rifampicin and ethambutol for 2 yr is preferable to a regimen that contains isoniazid, although there was a nonsignificant reduction in the relapse rate for the three-drug regimen. However, there was a higher death rate for the three-drug regimen *(1)*.

Macrolides and quinolones are active in vitro *(3,31)*, and there are some anecdotal reports of treatment response when these agents are used in the management of patients who are very susceptible to infection *(33)*. New clinical trials have been designed and are under way to evaluate the role of macrolides and quinolones in therapeutic regimens and to detect the value of immunizing with *Mycobacterium vaccae (1)*.

4.2. Mycobacterium malmoense Extrapulmonary Disease

Lymphadenitis is the most common form of *M. malmoense* extrapulmonary disease, and this syndrome should be treated with excision. Otherwise, extrapulmonary disease should be treated in the same way as pulmonary disease.

5. MANAGEMENT OF *MYCOBACTERIUM XENOPI* DISEASE

5.1. Pulmonary Disease

Mycobacterium xenopi poses many diagnostic and therapeutic problems. In some patients, *M. xenopi* may act as a colonizer without causing disease *(34–36)*. Therefore, it will be present in multiple specimens, thus passing the test for "significance," although in many such cases it is not responsible for clinical symptoms. In addition, infection with *M. xenopi* is normally indolent, with disease developing over a number of years *(32)*. Thus, an isolate in an apparently asymptomatic patient cannot be lightly dismissed, especially in HIV-infected individuals. To overcome the diagnostic difficulty, it has been proposed that the criteria for diagnosis of *M. xenopi* infection be two sputum isolations in the absence of other likely causes of symptoms *(37)*.

Early studies have suggested that regimens should contain rifampicin and isoniazid together with ethambutol or streptomycin *(32,38)*. A clinical trial suggested that a regimen of rifampicin and ethambutol is optimal, although there is a trend to a higher cure rate when isoniazid is added, but the complication rate is increased *(39)*. In view of the higher complication rate with added isoniazid, guidelines suggest that this drug should be included only if treatment fails to render the sputum culture negative *(1)*.

Macrolides and quinolones may have an important role in the treatment of *M. xenopi* infections as they are active in vitro and in animal models *(3,31,40)*. There are anecdotal reports of the value of these agents *(33)*. Clinical trial data are not yet available to inform therapeutic choice, but these could rationally be added to treatment of patients who fail to respond.

The results of medical therapy can be poor, with a 5-yr mortality of up to 57% (although a minority of these deaths were directly attributed to mycobacterial infection) *(39)*. Pulmonary resection is often necessary as an adjunct to treatment *(41)*. Pulmonary resection should be considered in patients who are failing on therapy, but who otherwise have good pulmonary function and whose disease is localized. When these criteria are applied, sputum conversion is complete in all but the patients who have incomplete resection *(42)*.

6. MANAGEMENT OF *MYCOBACTERIUM AVIUM-INTRACELLULARE* DISEASE

Infection with *M. avium-intracellulare* was once rare and was found as sporadic disease and in severely immunocompromised patients *(2,10)*. This situation was transformed by the HIV epidemic, in which disseminated *M. avium-intracellulare* infection and bacteremia were common late complications, usually when the CD4 count fell below 50. Management of *M. avium-intracellulare* infection is so influenced by the severity of HIV infection, it is considered separately.

6.1. *HIV-Seronegative Patients*

6.1.1. *Mycobacterium avium-intracellulare Pulmonary Disease*

Pulmonary disease caused by *M. avium* complex in HIV-seronegative patients usually occurs in those with concomitant chronic lung disease or deficient cellular immunity, and its prevalence is increasing *(10)*. The predisposing conditions include pneumoconiosis and silicosis because of chronic and long-term exposure to occupational dusts (e.g., from coal mining and farming) *(43)*. For example, in one study, 73% of patients had pre-existing pulmonary disease, 38% smoked, and 33% reported alcohol abuse.

The prognosis in *M. avium* complex pulmonary infections was strongly correlated with the underlying condition *(44)*. Older studies of treatment and the natural history of disease showed that patients who are symptomatic have progressive disease that is difficult to treat, whereas many of those who were asymptomatic at the time of isolation went on to develop invasive disease *(20)*.

Isolated pulmonary disease in otherwise healthy women has been described *(45)*. Surveys suggest that approximately half of these patients fail therapy *(15)*.

Treatment with three drugs, including rifampicin and isoniazid, coupled with either streptomycin or ethambutol were thought to give the best results *(20)*. A clinical trial of treatment of *M. avium-intracellulare* pulmonary infection in HIV-seronegative patients suggested that the optimum treatment regimen is with rifampicin and ethambutol, and that isoniazid reduced the failure and relapse rate *(39)*. Five-year follow-up of patients treated with this regimen showed that 15% of patients failed therapy, and 14% relapsed *(46)*.

The activity of clarithromycin and quinolones suggests that they may have a role to play, and clinical trials are under way to evaluate this *(39)*. Open trials suggested that sputum conversion rates greater than 75% can be achieved with regimens that include a macrolide *(47–49)*. Thus, although no comparative clinical trials have yet been reported, macrolides should probably now always be included in regimens used to treat *M. avium-intracellulare* infections in immunocompetent patients. Intermittent therapy (three times a week) is also reported to have a similar conversion rate *(50)*.

A recent article may give some insight into the reasons for the high relapse rate. Study of the organisms obtained from patients treated with clarithromycin who had suffered late relapses after 4 consecutive months of negative culture showed that the majority of these isolates were different from the original infecting strain. This suggests that many late relapses are caused by reinfection from this common environmental organism among patients who are highly predisposed to infection *(49)*.

Some authorities suggest that rifabutin should be the rifamycin of choice for treatment of *M. avium-intracellulare* infection because of its greater in vitro activity. However, this drug has a different adverse event profile, and only comparative clinical trials can tell whether the additional activity is gained without increased adverse events.

6.1.2. Management of Lymphadenitis

Mycobacterium avium-intracellulare is the commonest cause of cervical lymphadenopathy in children in countries where tuberculosis has been controlled *(51)*. Surgical excision is essential for diagnosis as the yield from fine-needle aspiration is not complete, and there is a considerable risk of sinus formation *(2)*. Optimal treatment of this condition is surgical excision, which has a lower reoperation rate than incision and drainage, curettage, or aspiration *(17)*. Relapse and sinus formation are rare, occurring in less than 5% of cases *(16,52)*. Antimicrobial chemotherapy appears to be unnecessary *(2)*, although there are reports of successful management with clarithromycin monotherapy *(53)*.

6.2. HIV-Seropositive Patients

6.2.1. Management of Disseminated Infection in HIV-Seropositive Patients

Disseminated *M. avium-intracellulare* infection is a late complication of HIV infection. Since the introduction of highly active antiretroviral therapy (HAART), it has become much less common in developed countries, occurring in patients who are untreated or who have been unable to tolerate therapy. The optimal regimen has not yet been established, partly because patients with this infection are at a very late stage of HIV disease for which the clinical course is complicated by other opportunistic infections and the consequence of HIV itself. In the era of HAART, the management of disseminated *M. avium-intracellulare* infection is underwritten by therapeutic efforts to reduce the HIV viral load, increase the CD4 count, and bring about reversal of the immune deficit.

Antibiotics have an important role in reducing bacteremia, and the antibiotics able to do that include macrolides such as clarithromycin and azithromycin, quinolones such as ciprofloxacin, and rifabutin, a rifamycin. The macrolides are highly active and are the cornerstones of all regimens. They are capable of reducing the count of bacteria in the blood when given alone *(54,55)*. Monotherapy results in the rapid emergence of resistance; thus, combination therapy should be chosen.

Clinical trials have supported the superiority of clarithromycin, ethambutol, and rifabutin over rifampicin, ethambutol, clofazimine, and ciprofloxacin *(56)*. A comparative trial suggested that lower doses of rifabutin (300 mg daily) together with ethambutol are more effective than a four-drug regimen of rifampicin, ethambutol, clofazimine, and ciprofloxacin, still retaining much of the activity of clarithromycin (1000 mg twice daily) and rifabutin (600 mg daily) doses *(56)*.

6.2.2. Prophylaxis of Mycobacterium avium-intracellulare

Prophylaxis is necessary to prevent infection in patients with late-stage HIV infection with low CD4 count. Macrolides have been shown to be more effective than rifabutin, which also is an effective agent, but is associated with a higher rate of intolerance *(57,58)*. Ultimately, the choice of prophylactic agent will depend on the choice of HAART because rifabutin interacts with protease inhibitors, and patients differ considerably in their ability to tolerate drugs *(59)*.

7. MANAGEMENT OF INFECTION WITH RAPID GROWERS

7.1. Pulmonary Disease

More than 80% of cases of pulmonary disease are caused by *M. abscessus*, which is the naturally most resistant member of the group of organisms *(60)*. Treatment of *M. abscessus* infections is often disappointing. Treatment can bring about clinical improvement, but cure is rare. When surgery is technically possible, it is recommended *(1)*. Susceptibility testing of rapidly growing mycobacteria is thought to give a good guide to treatment, and regimens should be constructed based on susceptibility test results *(24)*. Regimens should probably include rifampicin (450 mg if the patient weighs less than 50 kg, 600 mg if the patient weighs more than 50 kg), ethambutol (15 mg/kg body weight), and clarithromycin (500 mg twice daily). There are reports of the value of fluoroquinolones, sulfonamides, amikacin, cefoxitin, and penems in treatment *(1,24,61)*.

7.2. Extrapulmonary Disease

Many cases of infection by rapid growers occur in the context of an infected prosthetic device, for example, intravenous canullae or other implants. Successful therapy of these catheter-related infections involves removal of the catheter and antimicrobial therapy, usually for 2 to 4 mo. Although disease caused by *M. fortuitum* may resolve if the catheter is removed, reinsertion of another catheter in a similar location without drug therapy usually results in disease recurrence (as in the above case) *(8)*. Adjunctive therapy should be with ciprofloxacin, amikacin, and clarithromycin for up to 4 mo. When there is a tunneled line that also has a tissue infection, then treatment may need to be extended for 6 mo *(12)*.

Postinjection abscesses should be treated by surgical drainage and clarithromycin for between 3 and 6 mo. This advice comes as a result of the experience obtained from a series of outbreaks *(62,63)*.

Wound infections are one of the most common manifestations of infection with rapidly growing mycobacteria. Infections have often been associated with augmentation mammoplasty and other plastic surgery procedures *(12,64,65)*. Therapy depends of the removal of any infected foreign material, followed by 6 mo of chemotherapy *(66,67)*.

Clarithromycin is the main choice, with other drugs added to prevent the emergence of resistance *(68)*.

Disseminated cutaneous infection is mainly with *M. abscessus*, usually in patients who are compromised by renal failure or corticosteroid therapy *(69)*. This is one of the most common presentations of nonpulmonary infection with rapidly growing organisms *(12)*. Treatment includes drainage of any abscesses coupled with clarithromycin for 6 mo and with another agent to which the isolate is susceptible during the first 2 mo *(68)*.

8. SUMMARY

Infections with NTM continue to pose significant diagnostic and therapeutic problems for clinicians. Infection often occurs in the context of other serious disease, which may influence the outcome more than the infective process. Diagnosis can be difficult, but modern laboratory methods are improving rapidly. For several important infections, clinical trial information is helping to inform clinicians *(39)*. The results of trials currently under way to elucidate the activity of quinolones and macrolides may soon improve the evidence base for defining more effective regimens.

REFERENCES

1. Joint Tuberculosis Committee. Management of opportunist mycobacterial infections: Joint Tuberculosis Committee guidelines 1997. Thorax 2000; 55:210–218.
2. American Thoracic Society. Diagnosis and treatment of disease caused by nontuberculous mycobacteria. Am J Respir Crit Care Med 1997; 156:S1–S25.
3. Gillespie SH, Morrissey I, Everett D. A comparison of the bactericidal activity of quinolone antibiotics in a *Mycobacterium fortuitum* model. J Med Microbiol 2001; 50:565–570.
4. Runyon EH. Anonymous mycobacteria in pulmonary disease. Med Clin North Am 1957; 43:273–290.
5. O'Brien RJ, Geiter LJ, Snider DE Jr. The epidemiology of nontuberculous mycobacterial diseases in the United States. Results from a national survey. Am Rev Respir Dis 1987; 135:1007–1014.
6. Kirschner RA Jr, Parker BC, Falkinham JO III. Epidemiology of infection by nontuberculous mycobacteria. *Mycobacterium avium, Mycobacterium intracellulare*, and *Mycobacterium scrofulaceum* in acid, brown-water swamps of the southeastern United States and their association with environmental variables. Am Rev Respir Dis 1992; 145(2, pt. 1):271–275.
7. Lambden K, Watson J, Knerer G, Ryan MJ, Jenkins PA. Opportunist mycobacteria in England and Wales: 1982 to 1994. Commun Dis Rep CDR Rev 1996; 6:R147–R151.
8. McWhinney PH, Yates M, Prentice HG, Thrussell M, Gillespie SH, Kibbler CC. Infection caused by *Mycobacterium chelonae*: a diagnostic and therapeutic problem in the neutropenic patient. Clin Infect Dis 1992; 14:1208–1212.
9. Tortoli E, Bartoloni A, Bottger EC, et al. Burden of unidentifiable mycobacteria in a reference laboratory. J Clin Microbiol 2001; 39:4058–4065.
10. Falkinham JO III. Epidemiology of infection by nontuberculous mycobacteria. Clin Microbiol Rev 1996; 9:177–215.
11. Hale YM, Pfyffer GE, Salfinger M. Laboratory diagnosis of mycobacterial infections: new tools and lessons learned. Clin Infect Dis 2001; 33:834–846.
12. Brown-Elliott BA, Wallace RJ Jr. Clinical and taxonomic status of pathogenic nonpigmented or late-pigmenting rapidly growing mycobacteria. Clin Microbiol Rev 2002; 15:716–746.
13. Tortoli E, Bartoloni A, Erba ML, et al. Human infections due to *Mycobacterium lentiflavum*. J Clin Microbiol 2002; 40:728–729.

14. Turenne C, Chedore P, Wolfe J, Jamieson F, May K, Kabani A. Phenotypic and molecular characterization of clinical isolates of *Mycobacterium elephantis* from human specimens. J Clin Microbiol 2002; 40:1230–1236.
15. Huang JH, Kao PN, Adi V, Ruoss SJ. *Mycobacterium avium-intracellulare* pulmonary infection in HIV-negative patients without pre-existing lung disease: diagnostic and management limitations. Chest 1999; 115:1033–1040.
16. Danielides V, Patrikakos G, Moerman M, Bonte K, Dhooge C, Vermeersch H. Diagnosis, management and surgical treatment of non-tuberculous mycobacterial head and neck infection in children. ORL J Otorhinolaryngol Relat Spec 2002; 64:284–289.
17. Flint D, Mahadevan M, Barber C, Grayson D, Small R. Cervical lymphadenitis due to non-tuberculous mycobacteria: surgical treatment and review. Int J Pediatr Otorhinolaryngol 2000; 53:187–194.
18. Dautzenberg B, Olliaro P, Ruf B, et al. Rifabutin versus placebo in combination with three drugs in the treatment of non-tuberculous mycobacterial infection in patients with AIDS. Clin Infect Dis 1996; 22:705–708.
19. Pfeutze KM, Nuchprayoon CV, Berg GS, Pamintuan R. Present status of open negative cavities due to photochromogenic mycobacteria among co-operative patients. Am Rev Respir Dis 1966; 94:467–470.
20. Hunter AM, Campbell IA, Jenkins PA, Smith PA. Treatment of pulmonary infection caused by mycobacteria of *Mycobacterium avium-intracellulare* complex. Thorax 1981; 36:326–329.
21. Heginbothom ML. The relationship between the in vitro drug susceptibility of opportunist mycobacteria and their in vivo response to treatment. Int J Tuberc Lung Dis 2001; 5:539–545.
22. Jenkins PA, Banks J, Campbell IA, Gelder CM, Prescott RJ, Smith AP. Pulmonary disease caused by *Mycobacterium avium-intracellulare* in HIV sero-negative patients: a 5 year follow-up of patients receiving standardised treatment. Int J Tuberc Lung Dis 2002; 6:628–625.
23. Ahn CH, Lowell JR, Ahn SS, Ahn S, Hurst GA. Chemotherapy for pulmonary disease due to *Mycobacterium kansasii*: efficacies of some individual drugs. Rev Infect Dis 1981; 3:1028–1034.
24. Wallace RJ Jr, Swenson JM, Silcox VA, Bullen MG. Treatment of non-pulmonary infections due to *Mycobacterium fortuitum* and *Mycobacterium chelonei* on the basis of in vitro susceptibilities. J Infect Dis 1985; 152:200–214.
25. Horsburgh CR Jr, Mason UG III, Heifets LB, Southwick K, Labrecque J, Iseman MD. Response to therapy of pulmonary *Mycobacterium avium-intracellulare* infection correlates with results of in vitro susceptibility testing. Am Rev Respir Dis 1987; 135:418–421.
26. Wallace RJ Jr, Dunbar D, Brown BA, et al. Rifampin-resistant *Mycobacterium kansasii.* Clin Infect Dis 1994; 18:736–743.
27. Rastogi N, Goh KS, Guillou N, Labrousse V. Spectrum of drugs against atypical mycobacteria: how valid is the current practice of drug susceptibility testing and the choice of drugs? Zentralbl Bakteriol 1992; 277:474–484.
28. Jenkins PA, Banks J, Campbell IA, Smith AP. *Mycobacterium kansasii* pulmonary infection: a prospective study of the results of 9 months of treatment with rifampicin and ethambutol. Research Committee, British Thoracic Society. Thorax 1994; 49:442–445.
29. Banks J, Hunter AM, Campbell IA, Jenkins PA, Smith AP. Pulmonary infection with *Mycobacterium kansasii* in Wales, 1970–9: review of treatment and response. Thorax 1984; 39: 376–382.
30. Pezzia W, Raleigh JW, Bailey MC, Toth EA, Silverblatt J. Treatment of pulmonary disease due to *Mycobacterium kansasii*: recent experience with rifampin. Rev Infect Dis 1981; 3:1035–1039.
31. Yew WW, Piddock LJ, Li MS, Lyon D, Chan CY, Cheng AF. In-vitro activity of quinolones and macrolides against mycobacteria. J Antimicrob Chemother 1994; 34:343–351.
32. Banks J, Hunter AM, Campbell IA, Jenkins PA, Smith AP. Pulmonary infection with *Mycobacterium xenopi*: review of treatment and response. Thorax 1984; 39:376–382.

33. Scmitt H, Schnitzler N, Riehl J, Adam G, Siebert H-G, Haase G. Successful treatment of pulmonary *Mycobacterium xenopi* infection in a natural killer cell-deficient patient with clarithromycin, rifabutin, and sparfloxacin. Clin Infect Dis 1999; 29:120–124.
34. Smith MJ, Citron KM. Clinical review of pulmonary disease caused by *Mycobacterium xenopi*. Thorax 1983; 38:373–377.
35. Jiva TM, Jacoby HM, Weymouth LA, Kaminski DA, Portmore AC. *Mycobacterium xenopi*: innocent bystander or emerging pathogen? Clin Infect Dis 1997; 24:226–232.
36. Simor AE, Salit IE, Vellend H. The role of *Mycobacterium xenopi* in human disease. Am Rev Respir Dis 1984; 129:435–438.
37. Juffermans NP, Verbon A, Danner SA, Kuijper EJ, Speelman P. *Mycobacterium xenopi* in HIV-infected patients: an emerging pathogen. AIDS 1998; 12:1661–1666.
38. Costrini AM, Mahler DA, Gross WM, Hawkins JE, Yesner R, D'Esopo ND. Clinical and roentgenographic features of nosocomial pulmonary disease due to *Mycobacterium xenopi*. Am Rev Respir Dis 1981; 123:104–109.
39. Research Committee BTS. First randomised trial of treatments for pulmonary disease caused by *M. avium intracellulare, M. malmoense*, and *M. xenopi* in HIV negative patients: rifampicin, ethambutol and isoniazid versus rifampicin and ethambutol. Thorax 2001; 56:167–172.
40. Lounis N, Truffot-Pernot C, Bentoucha A, Robert J, Ji B, Grosset J. Efficacies of clarithromycin regimens against *Mycobacterium xenopi* in mice. Antimicrob Agents Chemother 2001; 45:3229–3230.
41. Parrot RG, Grosset JH. Post-surgical outcome of 57 patients with *Mycobacterium xenopi* pulmonary infection. Tubercle 1988; 69:47–55.
42. Lang-Lazdunski L, Offredo C, Pimpec-Barthes F, Danel C, Dujon A, Riquet M. Pulmonary resection for *Mycobacterium xenopi* pulmonary infection. Ann Thorac Surg 2001; 72:1877–1882.
43. Schaefer WB, Birn KJ, Jenkins PA, Marks J. Infection with the avian-Battey group of mycobacteria in England and Wales. BMJ 1969; 2:412–415.
44. Contreras MA, Cheung OT, Sanders DE, Goldstein RS. Pulmonary infection with nontuberculous mycobacteria. Am Rev Respir Dis 1988; 137:149–152.
45. Prince DS, Peterson DD, Steiner RM, et al. Infection with *Mycobacterium avium* complex in patients without predisposing conditions. N Engl J Med 1989; 321:863–868.
46. Pulmonary disease caused by *Mycobacterium avium-intracellulare* in HIV-negative patients: 5-year follow-up of patients receiving standardised treatment. Int J Tuberc Lung Dis 2002; 6:628–634.
47. Griffith DE, Brown BA, Murphy DT, Girard WM, Couch L, Wallace RJ Jr. Initial (6-month) results of three-times-weekly azithromycin in treatment regimens for *Mycobacterium avium* complex lung disease in human immunodeficiency virus-negative patients. J Infect Dis 1998; 178:121–126.
48. Wallace RJ Jr, Brown BA, Griffith DE, et al. Initial clarithromycin monotherapy for *Mycobacterium avium-intracellulare* complex lung disease. Am J Respir Crit Care Med 1994; 149:1335–1341.
49. Wallace RJ Jr, Zhang Y, Brown-Elliott BA, et al. Repeat positive cultures in *Mycobacterium intracellulare* lung disease after macrolide therapy represent new infections in patients with nodular bronchiectasis. J Infect Dis 2003; 186:266–273.
50. Griffith DE, Brown BA, Cegielski P, Murphy DT, Wallace RJ Jr. Early results (at 6 months) with intermittent clarithromycin-including regimens for lung disease due to *Mycobacterium avium* complex. Clin Infect Dis 2000; 30:288–292.
51. Grange JM, Yates MD, Pozniak A. Bacteriologically confirmed non-tuberculous mycobacterial lymphadenitis in southeast England: a recent increase in the number of cases. Arch Dis Child 1995; 72:516–517.
52. Rahal A, Abela A, Arcand PH, Quintal MC, Lebel MH, Tapiero BF. Nontuberculous mycobacterial adenitis of the head and neck in children: experience from a tertiary care pediatric center. Laryngoscope 2001; 111:1791–1796.

53. Tunkel DE, Romaneschi KB. Surgical treatment of cervicofacial nontuberculous mycobacterial adenitis in children. Laryngoscope 1995; 105:1024–1028.
54. Dautzenberg B, Saint MT, Meyohas MC, et al. Clarithromycin and other antimicrobial agents in the treatment of disseminated *Mycobacterium avium* infections in patients with acquired immunodeficiency syndrome. Arch Intern Med 1993; 153:368–372.
55. Hoy J, Mijch A, Sandland M, Grayson L, Lucas R, Dwyer B. Quadruple-drug therapy for *Mycobacterium avium-intracellulare* bacteremia in AIDS patients. J Infect Dis 1990; 161: 801–805.
56. Shafran SD, Singer J, Zarowny DP, et al. A comparison of two regimens for the treatment of *Mycobacterium avium* complex bacteremia in AIDS: rifabutin, ethambutol, and clarithromycin versus rifampin, ethambutol, clofazimine, and ciprofloxacin. Canadian HIV Trials Network Protocol 010 Study Group. N Engl J Med 1996; 335:377–383.
57. Phillips P, Chan K, Hogg R, et al. Azithromycin prophylaxis for *Mycobacterium avium* complex during the era of highly active antiretroviral therapy: evaluation of a provincial program. Clin Infect Dis 2002; 34:371–378.
58. Havlir DV, Dube MP, Sattler FR, et al. Prophylaxis against disseminated *Mycobacterium avium* complex with weekly azithromycin, daily rifabutin, or both. California Collaborative Treatment Group. N Engl J Med 1996; 335:392–398.
59. Cohn SE, Kammann E, Williams P, Currier JS, Chesney MA. Association of adherence to *Mycobacterium avium* complex prophylaxis and antiretroviral therapy with clinical outcomes in acquired immunodeficiency syndrome. Clin Infect Dis 2002; 34:1129–1136.
60. Griffith DE, Girard WM, Wallace RJ Jr. Clinical features of pulmonary disease caused by rapidly growing mycobacteria. An analysis of 154 patients. Am Rev Respir Dis 1993; 147: 1271–1278.
61. Tanaka E, Kimoto T, Tsuyuguchi K, Suzuki K, Amitani R. Successful treatment with faropenem and clarithromycin of pulmonary *Mycobacterium abscessus* infection. J Infect Chemother 2002; 8:252–255.
62. Galil K, Miller LA, Yakrus MA, et al. Abscesses due to *Mycobacterium abscessus* linked to injection of unapproved alternative medication. Emerg Infect Dis 1999; 5:681–687.
63. Villanueva A, Calderon RV, Vargas BA, et al. Report on an outbreak of post-injection abscesses due to *Mycobacterium abscessus*, including management with surgery and clarithromycin therapy and comparison of strains by random amplified polymorphic DNA polymerase chain reaction. Clin Infect Dis 1997; 24:1147–1153.
64. Clegg HW, Foster MT, Sanders WE Jr, Baine WB. Infection due to organisms of the *Mycobacterium fortuitum* complex after augmentation mammoplasty: clinical and epidemiologic features. J Infect Dis 1983; 147:427–433.
65. Bolan G, Reingold AL, Carson LA, et al. Infections with *Mycobacterium chelonei* in patients receiving dialysis and using processed hemodialyzers. J Infect Dis 1985; 152: 1013–1019.
66. Morris-Jones R, Fletcher C, Morris-Jones S, Brown T, Hilton RM, Hay R. *Mycobacterium abscessus*: a cutaneous infection in a patient on renal replacement therapy. Clin Exp Dermatol 2001; 26:415–418.
67. Ozluer SM, De'Ambrosis BJ. *Mycobacterium abscessus* wound infection. Australas J Dermatol 2001; 42:26–29.
68. Wallace RJ Jr, Tanner D, Brennan PJ, Brown BA. Clinical trial of clarithromycin for cutaneous (disseminated) infection due to *Mycobacterium chelonae*. Ann Intern Med 1993; 119:482–486.
69. Wallace RJ Jr. The clinical presentation, diagnosis, and therapy of cutaneous and pulmonary infections due to the rapidly growing mycobacteria, *M. fortuitum* and *M. chelonae*. Clin Chest Med 1989; 10:419–429.

IV

Fungal and Parasitic Infections

16

Management of Resistant *Candida* Infections

Sanya Clements and Christopher C. Kibbler

1. INTRODUCTION

The incidence of superficial and deep fungal infections has been steadily increasing during the last two decades because of an increased number of patients at risk for invasive fungal infections. Advances in therapeutic technology, the use of aggressive chemotherapy and immunosupression regimens, and the insertion of increasing numbers of intravascular devices account for this steady rise. Nosocomial candidiasis has risen more than threefold in the last decade, and *Candida* species are now the fourth most common cause of bloodstream infection in the United States *(1)*. Systemic and deep organ fungal infections have become the leading causes of death among patients with hematological malignancies and among transplant recipients *(2)*. Patients with acquired immunodeficiency syndrome (AIDS) are particularly at risk for fungal infections. Resistance of *Candida* species to antifungal agents has arisen because of a combination of the increased number of patients at risk, increased antifungal drug usage, and altered epidemiology of *Candida* infections.

New antifungal agents, namely, the echinocandins and the new triazoles, have now become available and have given clinicians alternative agents for treatment of invasive fungal infections. It is important to consider therapy with these new agents in the light of the current understanding of the mechanisms of resistance and the settings in which they arise if their usefulness is to be preserved.

In this chapter, the epidemiology of resistance of *Candida* infections, the correlation between in vitro susceptibility testing and clinical outcome, the risk factors for development of resistance, the clinical implications of antifungal resistance, and the guidelines on management of infections with resistant *Candida* species in commonly encountered clinical settings are reviewed.

2. MECHANISM OF ACTION OF ANTIFUNGAL DRUGS

Antifungal drugs can be divided into four classes because of their mechanism of action: polyenes, azoles, fluoropyrimidines, and echinocandins.

2.1. *Polyenes*

The most important polyene is amphotericin B. It binds to ergosterol, the primary fungal cell membrane sterol, altering membrane permeability. The drug can also cause

From: *Management of Multiple Drug-Resistant Infections*
Edited by: S. H. Gillespie © Humana Press Inc., Totowa, NJ

oxidative damage to fungal cells. Reformulating amphotericin B in association with lipids has reduced clinical toxicity of amphotericin B, especially nephrotoxicity.

2.2. *Azoles*

The azoles include fluconazole, itraconazole, ketoconazole, and the newer agents voriconazole, posaconazole, and ravuconazole. They inhibit ergosterol synthesis through their action on the cytochrome P450-dependent enzyme lanosterol 14 α-demethylase. Differences among azoles are primarily in their pharmacokinetics, although there are also some differences in their antifungal spectrum. Voriconazole, a synthetic triazole derivative of fluconazole, has activity against many yeasts and filamentous fungi. Voriconazole also inhibits 24-methylene dihydrolanosterol demethylation of certain yeasts and filamentous fungi. This explains the extended spectrum of activity. It has activity against *Candida* species that are fluconazole resistant, including *Candida krusei* and *Candida glabrata.*

2.3 *Fluoropyrimidines*

Flucytosine (5-fluorocytosine, 5-FC) is a synthetic fluorinated pyrimidine. It is transported into susceptible fungal cells by the action of cytosine permease and is then converted by cytosine deaminase to fluorouracil. It is this molecule that is incorporated into RNA in place of uracil, resulting in mistranslation. In addition, it blocks thymidylate synthetase, an essential enzyme for DNA synthesis, causing inhibition of DNA synthesis. Excessive concentrations can cause toxicity, particularly myelosuppression, as a consequence of these mechanisms.

2.4. *Echinocandins*

Caspofungin, micafungin, and anidulafungin are members of a new class of antifungal agents that inhibit fungal cell wall synthesis by noncompetitive blockade of the enzyme (1,3)-β-D-glucan synthase, preventing the formation of (1,3)-β-D-glucan, an essential component of the fungal cell wall. This leads to formation of a weakened wall and to its subsequent lysis.

3. MECHANISM OF RESISTANCE OF *CANDIDA* TO ANTIFUNGAL AGENTS

Understanding antifungal drug resistance is fundamental to developing effective prophylactic and therapeutic strategies to avoid the emergence of resistant fungi. Antifungal drug resistance can be the result of replacement of a susceptible strain with a more resistant strain or species or the alteration of an endogenous strain (by gene mutation) to a resistant phenotype.

At the molecular level, resistance of *Candida* spp to azoles has been most extensively studied. It can be the result of an alteration of the target enzyme, the cytochrome P-450 lanosterol 14-α-demethylase, either by overexpression or by point mutations in its encoding gene (ERG11). A second major mechanism is the failure of azole antifungal agents to accumulate inside the yeast cell as a consequence of enhanced drug efflux. This mechanism is mediated by two types of multidrug efflux transporters, the major facilitators (encoded by MDR genes) and those belonging to the ATP-binding cassette superfamily (ABC transporters, encoded by CDR genes). A striking difference is that upregulation of CDR genes confers resistance to multiple azoles, whereas upregulation of the MDR1 gene alone leads to fluconazole resistance only *(3–6)*.

In *Candida albicans* isolates highly resistant to fluconazole, many different mechanisms of resistance operate simultaneously, with efflux pumps commonly both deregulated and overexpressed *(6,7)*. In general, overexpression of the genes encoding for the efflux pumps is detected in 85% of cases, mutations in the gene encoding for the enzyme lanosterol 14-α-demethylase in 65%, and overexpression of this gene in 35% *(7)*.

In contrast to the findings with *C. albicans* and *C. glabrata*, high-level resistance to fluconazole and itraconazole has been observed in *C. krusei* isolates without concomitant resistance to ravuconazole and voriconazole *(8)*. These findings imply different mechanisms of resistance to azoles in *C. krusei* compared with other *Candida* spp. The mechanism of amphotericin B resistance appears to be an alteration or a decrease in ergosterol in the cell membrane.

Primary resistance of *Candida* spp to flucytosine is usually the result of downregulation of cytosine permease, leading to poor uptake of the drug; secondary resistance in *C. albicans* is primarily because of a decrease in the activity of the uracil phosphoribosyl transferase, preventing the metabolism of flucytosine to toxic metabolites of pyrimidine biosynthesis *(6)*.

3.1. Definitions of Resistance

Traditionally, resistance has been classified as primary, secondary, or clinical. An organism that is resistant to a drug prior to exposure is described as having *primary* or *intrinsic resistance*. *Secondary* or *acquired resistance* develops in response to exposure to an antifungal agent. *Clinical resistance* is defined as treatment failure despite microbial susceptibility in vitro.

Treatment failure, a less-ambiguous term than clinical resistance, can arise because an agent fails to reach an infected site in sufficient quantity, because the patient's immune system is unable to eradicate a fungus, or because of the presence of intravenous catheters, noncompliance, drug interactions, or undrained abscesses *(9,10)*. Abscess drainage, recovery from neutropenia, and removal of intravascular catheters can significantly alter the course of infection. The situation when an infecting fungus shows resistance to an agent in vitro, but the patient responds clinically to treatment with that agent, can arise because the patient's immune system can eradicate the infection or because the antifungal agent reaches the infected site in sufficient concentrations to inhibit or kill the fungus.

3.2. Antifungal Susceptibility Testing

Determination of susceptibility to antifungals in vitro has lagged behind that of antibacterial agents, mainly because of lack of standardized susceptibility testing, leading to marked interlaboratory variation. For this reason, susceptibility testing has not been used previously as a guide for antifungal therapy.

However, antifungal susceptibility testing has evolved rapidly during the last decade. The Subcommittee on Antifungal Susceptibility Testing of the National Committee for Clinical Laboratory Standards (NCCLS) first proposed a reference method, M27-P, for antifungal susceptibility testing with yeasts in 1992. The final approved method, M27-A, was published in 1997 *(11)* and gives detailed recommendations for culture medium,

Table 1
Interpretive Breakpoints for *Candida* spp for Fluconazole, Itraconazole, and Flucytosine

	Range of MICs (μg/mL) per category		
Antifungal agent	Susceptible (S)	Susceptible-dose dependent (S-DD)	Resistant (R)
Fluconazole	≤8	16–32	≥64
Itraconazole	≤0.125	0.25–0.5	≥1
Flucytosine	≤4	8–16 (intermediate)	≥32

Source: Data from refs. *9* and *11*.

yeast inoculum size, incubation time, and end point measurement. This method has dramatically reduced variability between laboratories. It has enabled minimum inhibitory concentrations (MICs) to be correlated with clinical outcome.

However, M27-A methodology has its limitations and susceptibility testing is not an infallible guide to treatment of fungal diseases. Trailing growth phenomenon seen when determining the susceptibilities of *Candida* isolates to the azole antifungal agents makes consistent end point determination difficult *(12)*. The breakpoint MIC that determines when an isolate is designated resistant to an antifungal is far from clear-cut. NCCLS resistance breakpoints are based on data relating treatment outcomes to antifungal MICs and indicate the MIC at which clinical responses showed a marked fall off. Although about 100 patients with candidemia were included in the analysis, these breakpoints have been extrapolated mainly from outcomes in patients with AIDS with oropharyngeal candidiasis (OPC) *(9)*. Data for itraconazole breakpoints are limited to mucosal disease. Interpretive breakpoints of resistance with this standard method currently exist only for fluconazole, itraconazole, and flucytosine (Table 1). A new category was also introduced, susceptible-dose dependent (S-DD). This indicates that treatment with a dosage higher than usual might be required and emphasizes the need to maximize drug dose and delivery.

NCCLS M27-A methodology has a limited ability to identify *Candida* isolates resistant to amphotericin B. In a study of candidemia in non-neutropenic patients, all amphotericin B MICs were 1.0 μg/mL or less, so clinical failures were all associated with the isolates with low MICs *(13)*.

The insensitivity of MICs in predicting outcome stems from the inability of the standardized testing method to yield a wide range of amphotericin B MICs, limiting the ability to identify isolates likely to cause therapeutic failure *(14)*. A study by Nguyen et al. *(15)* demonstrated that breakpoint minimal lethal concentrations (MLCs) and MICs of 1 μg/mL or more of amphotericin at 48 h can accurately predict microbiological failure of amphotericin B therapy for *Candida* species. Only 5% of isolates exhibited MICs of 1 μg/mL or more. MLC range was significantly broader, and methods based on this may be preferred. Rex et al. also found that using alternative media (antibiotic medium 3 broth) more readily identifies isolates resistant to amphotericin B *(14)*.

Several studies have suggested the potential value of the Etest (AB Biodisk, Solna, Sweden) as a convenient alternative and reproducible method for testing the susceptibilities of yeasts *(16–18)*. It is less labor intensive and much simpler to set up than broth dilution methods, but some isolates are difficult to read because of growth of minute colonies within the inhibition ellipse. Some studies have found that the Etest method yielded a wider distribution of amphotericin B MICs, and that Etest is a potentially useful method of identifying *Candida* isolates resistant to amphotericin B *(19–21)*.

Results of a British Society of Antimicrobial Chemotherapy (BSAC) Working Party on Antifungal Therapy have demonstrated that that Etest is suitable for testing *Candida* spp against amphotericin B or flucytosine. It would appear that the Etest is less reliable for the azoles, and isolates that appear to demonstrate resistance should be retested with well-established reference methods *(22)*.

Comparison of NCCLS M27-A and EUCAST (European Committee on Antibiotic Susceptibility Testing) microdilution procedures for antifungal testing of *Candida* spp against amphotericin B, flucytosine, fluconazole, and itraconazole have shown a 92% overall agreement *(23)*. There is not yet a consensus on the application of susceptibility testing to the most recently licensed antifungal agents (caspofungin, voriconazole), so future efforts are directed toward establishing and validating interpretive breakpoints for amphotericin B, the new triazoles, and echinocandins.

3.3. *Correlation of In Vitro Testing With Clinical Outcome*

The development of standardized susceptibility testing has vastly improved the correlation between in vitro test results and clinical outcome and is increasingly used as an adjunct to the treatment of fungal infections.

Rex and Pfaller *(24)* summarized the key principles of susceptibility testing as follows:

1. Host factors are often more important than a susceptibility test result in determining the outcome.
2. Susceptibility of a microorganism in vitro does not predict successful therapy.
3. Resistance in vitro should often predict therapeutic failure.
4. MIC values must be interpreted in the light of pharmacodynamic analysis.

Current data regarding the predictive utility of susceptibility testing for the fungi are consistent with the "90–60" rule that infections caused by susceptible isolates respond to appropriate therapy about 90% of the time, whereas infections caused by resistant isolates respond about 60% of the time.

Clinical response in OPC in patients with AIDS correlates well with in vitro susceptibility determinations by NCCLS methods. The data to support an in vitro–in vivo correlation for antifungal susceptibility studies are not as strong for candidemia or deep-seated candidiasis as those for OPC *(9)*. Testing of *Candida* spp against fluconazole is associated with predictive values that approximate the 90–60 rule *(24)*. This applies to both mucosal and invasive disease, although supportive data are stronger for mucosal disease. For reasons discussed in Section 3.2, there is poor correlation of amphotericin B susceptibility tests with outcome.

4. RESISTANCE OF *CANDIDA* SPECIES TO TRADITIONAL ANTIFUNGAL AGENTS

4.1. *Resistance to Azoles*

Resistance of *Candida* species to azole compounds has emerged in AIDS patients with OPC. Population surveillance in the United States, Canada, Latin America, and

Europe showed a low frequency (0–1%) of fluconazole and itraconazole resistance in bloodstream isolates of *C. albicans (25–29)*. The data recently reviewed by Sanglard and Odds showed that the principal cause of candidemia, *C. albicans*, has not yet globally acquired significant azole resistance *(10)*.

Candida krusei is intrinsically resistant to fluconazole and has higher MICs to itraconazole, in the susceptible dose dependent to resistant range. *Candida glabrata* isolates generally exhibit bimodal susceptibility to azoles, with some isolates demonstrating azole resistance and others susceptibility. The surveillance study by Safdar et al. *(30)* found significant differences in susceptibility profiles to azole agents of *C. glabrata* depending on patient population. They found that centers caring for patients with human immunodeficiency virus (HIV) infection or with an underlying malignancy may have higher frequencies of fluconazole- and itraconazole-resistant *C. glabrata* strains associated with either colonization or invasive disease. The study found an overall 10.7% resistance to fluconazole and an S-DD of 9.8%. Of the isolates, 15.2% were resistant to itraconazole, and there was a 42% S-DD. A review of several candidemia surveillance programs found fluconazole resistance in approx 10% of *C. glabrata* bloodstream isolates *(27)*. Although *C. glabrata* showed less fluconazole resistance in the SENTRY international program from 1997 to 1999, continued surveillance is needed to confirm this trend *(31)*. In a UK study the majority of *C. glabrata* isolates responsible for candidemia were sensitive to fluconazole *(29)*. Fluconazole-resistant *C. glabrata* isolates are almost always resistant to itraconazole.

Some strains of *Candida tropicalis* exhibit azole resistance, although generally the MIC_{90} for this species indicates susceptibility. Apparent in vitro resistance may be explained by the strong tendency of the species to produce trailing growth (*see* Section 3.2).

Other nonalbicans species such as *Candida parapsilosis* and *Candida lusitaniae* are usually susceptible to fluconazole and itraconazole *(26)*.

4.2. Resistance to Polyenes

Resistance to amphotericin B can be intrinsic or acquired. Many, but not all, *C. lusitaniae* and some *Candida guilliermondii* isolates demonstrate primary resistance to amphotericin B. The exact frequency of this event is uncertain.

Fortunately, secondary resistance to amphotericin B remains limited *(32)*. The *Candida* species *C. albicans, C. tropicalis, C. parapsilosis*, and *C. dubliniensis* appear to remain susceptible to amphotericin B, although as discussed in Section 3.2, NCCLS M27-A methodology does not reliably identify isolates resistant to amphotericin B. Strains of *C. albicans* acquiring resistance to amphotericin B have been described, but occur rarely *(33)*. *Candida glabrata* and *C. krusei* are usually considered susceptible to amphotericin B, but they tend to have higher MICs to polyenes than *C. albicans* and may require maximal doses of amphotericin B. Most rational therapy for infections caused by these species (*C. lusitaniae, C. glabrata, C. krusei,* and *C. guilliermondii*) with a higher propensity than other *Candida* spp to possess or develop resistance to amphotericin B is based on awareness of this possibility and cautious use of susceptibility testing *(34)*.

4.3. Resistance to Flucytosine

Much of the data concerning primary resistance to flucytosine among *Candida* spp has been derived from studies conducted in the 1970s and 1980s, prior to introduction of standardized NCCLS method. Primary resistance among *C. albicans* has been

Table 2
Patient Groups at Increased Risk of Resistance Emerging

Patient groups	Resistance problems
HIV	*C. albicans* and azole resistance, especially fluconazole, seen in late-stage disease; nonalbicans species are less of a problem
Hematological malignancies	Primarily problem with fluconazole resistance in nonalbicans species; polyene resistance described, but remains rare
Intensive care unit/surgical	Resistance is a rare cause of treatment failure and appears uncommon; *C. albicans* is the most common isolate in this group of patients
Recurrent vulvo-vaginal candidiasis (RVVC)	Resistance is a rare cause of RVVC and is almost always associated with nonalbicans species, particularly *C. glabrata*; *C. albicans* resistance is very rare

reported to range from 6.5% in Europe to 33% in the United States, mainly associated with serotype B isolates. Surveys based on method M27-A do not corroborate these high rates of primary flucytosine resistance. Studies have found a very low level of primary resistance among virtually all *Candida* spp except for *C. krusei (26,35,36)*. Pfaller et al. *(36)* tested 8803 clinical *Candida* isolates against flucytosine using NCCLS methodology and found that percentage susceptible of each species was as follows: 99% *C. glabrata*, 99% *C. parapsilosis*, 100% *C. dubliniensis*, 100% *C. guilliermondii*, 97% *Candida albicans*, and 92% *C. tropicalis*. Notably, *C. krusei* was the least susceptible species (5% susceptible, 67% intermediate, and 28% resistant). In a study by Barchiesi et al., 82% of *C. glabrata* isolates were susceptible to flucytosine, but this study evaluated a small number of clinical isolates *(35)*.

Candida spp rapidly acquire resistance to flucytosine when used as monotherapy, with 30% of the patients developing secondary resistance. For this reason, flucytosine has been used almost always in combination with other antifungal agents.

Clinicians are often hesitant to use flucytosine because of concerns about toxicity and either primary or secondary resistance. With revised susceptibility patterns and dosing regimens, this drug could be a useful adjunct in the treatment of serious and resistant *Candida* infections.

5. RISK FACTORS ASSOCIATED WITH ANTIFUNGAL DRUG RESISTANCE

In many studies of OPC in HIV infection, one of the most important host factors for development of resistance is profound immunosuppression and previous exposure to antifungal agents *(37,38)*. In the majority of patients, mutation of a previously susceptible strain of *C. albicans* to a resistant strain appears to have occurred. In patients with hematological malignancy, the situation seems to be different. Although not all reports agree, the use of fluconazole prophylaxis in this setting seems to be associated with emergence of nonalbicans species, notably *C. glabrata* and *C. krusei*.

Fluconazole prophylaxis does not seem to increase the incidence of resistance in *C. albicans* in this patient population. It is thought that suppression of the more common *Candida* pathogens with prophylaxis may permit other *Candida* species, which are naturally resistant, to emerge as systemic pathogens. *Candida krusei*, an organism intrinsically resistant to fluconazole, has become more prevalent in some centers, associated with the introduction of fluconazole prophylaxis *(39–42)*, although in most cases the incidence of *C. krusei* infections has remained stable *(43)*. Similarly, some centers have found an increase in infections caused by *C. glabrata* in association with fluconazole prophylaxis *(42,44)*. There has also been a decrease in incidence of infections caused by *C. tropicalis* and *C. lusitaniae* associated with fluconazole prophylaxis *(42)*. *Candida albicans* and *C. parapsilosis* infections occur more commonly in patients with a normal neutrophil count, whereas *C. krusei* and *C. tropicalis* are associated more with neutropenia.

There have been no reports of the selection of resistant species with prophylactic itraconazole. Itraconazole is thought to be less likely to lead to the emergence of resistance because of its broader spectrum of activity.

Some authors have postulated that, although the species causing candidemia have changed, with an increase in nonalbicans species this may be secondary to greater marrow and mucosal toxicity caused by current chemotherapy and radiotherapy regimens, which permits "less-virulent" *Candida* species to invade *(45)*.

Factors leading to intermittent drug levels, such as reduced compliance or drug interactions, may increase the risk of resistance. Compliance can potentially be a problem with itraconazole oral solution (because of its unpalatable flavor).

Failure to deal with the source of infection may also lead to development of resistance. The association among prostheses, formation of biofilms, and antimicrobial resistance is well documented. Evidence suggests that *Candida* biofilms dramatically reduce susceptibility to antifungal drugs *(46)* and may explain the persistence of infection despite antifungal therapy. Affected devices generally need to be removed to achieve a successful outcome.

Dosing and the duration of therapy may be implicated in the emergence of antifungal resistance. It is still not established whether lower doses used for longer periods of time do lead to antifungal resistance and whether using higher doses for shorter periods would prevent it *(47)*.

Combination therapy has been known to reduce the emergence of resistance in the case of flucytosine, and it has been increasingly proposed that this concept could apply to other antifungal agents. However, combination antifungal therapy is expensive, and its use needs to be based on convincing evidence.

As over-the-counter azole antifungal agents are now widely available for treatment of vulvovaginal candidiasis (VVC), there is potential for drug resistance to increase. However, there is no evidence that this is occurring *(48,49)*.

6. RECOMMENDATIONS FOR USE OF ANTIFUNGAL SUSCEPTIBILITY TESTING IN THE CLINICAL LABORATORY

Antifungal susceptibility testing is not recommended on a routine basis. It would create a considerable workload for a laboratory, and it does not influence the management of patients in many situations. Knowledge of the local antibiogram for *Candida* spp in conjunction with an accurate identification to species level are usually completely satisfactory. Identification of *Candida* to species level can be obtained in less

Table 3
Nature of Antifungal Resistance in *Candida* Species

- Antifungal resistance remains at a low level in both mucosal and invasive infections.
- Clinical failure is often caused by factors other than antifungal resistance of the causative organism.
- Most clinical problems of resistance have been with azole antifungals.
- The mechanisms responsible vary between different strains of the same species and between different species; they may be combined in the same organism.
- Azole resistance in *C. albicans* is most commonly seen in HIV infections, where in the neutropenic setting, reduced susceptibility is usually because of infection with a non-albicans species.

than 24 h with some of the newer identification systems. All *Candida* isolates from the bloodstream or other sterile sites, including continuous ambulatory peritoneal dialysis (CAPD) and bronchoscopy fluids and intravenous line tips, should be identified to species level. In patients who are at high risk of invasive fungal infections, such as patients undergoing chemotherapy, neutropenic patients, and patients in the intensive care unit, identification of colonizing *Candida* to species level is very helpful in guiding empirical therapy should the need arise.

Testing susceptibility of invasive (bloodstream or other sterile site) isolates of *Candida* should be performed on *C. albicans* isolates from patients with persistent candidemia or progressive disseminated candidiasis, despite fluconazole therapy, and on nonalbicans *Candida* isolates from patients with candidemia or invasive disease *(50)*. Whether susceptibility testing should also be performed on all isolates of *C. albicans* from blood cultures is controversial as azole resistance in this setting is rare.

Periodic batch antifungal susceptibility testing of *Candida* spp obtained from hospitalized patients could be performed to establish an antibiogram of an institution that is helpful during selection of empirical therapy *(50,51)*.

Susceptibility testing of isolates from patients with AIDS and refractory OPC is recommended *(51)*. In this group of patients, there is a good correlation between MICs and clinical outcome, and the knowledge that a patient's therapy is failing despite the fact that the MICs of the *Candida* spp are low may point to problems with compliance, drug absorption, or drug interactions. Typical incidence would be in a patient whose therapy with a moderate or high dose of an azole antifungal agent is failing.

Many studies suggest that identification and susceptibility testing need not be routinely performed and should be reserved only for the minority of patients with complicated VVC who fail to respond to conventional therapy despite good compliance because some nonalbicans species are less susceptible to azoles *(52–54)*.

When resistance is documented, therapy should be guided by susceptibility testing, but there should be awareness that in vitro susceptibility does not always correlate with clinical outcome. Susceptibility testing would therefore be rarely indicated, especially in cases of *C. albicans* vaginitis.

7. REFRACTORY OROPHARYNGEAL AND ESOPHAGEAL CANDIDIASIS IN HIV-INFECTED PATIENTS

7.1. Incidence of Refractory Esophageal and Oropharyngeal Candidiasis

Diagnosis of refractory disease is made when persistent or progressive disease is observed after adequate treatment with an antifungal agent. It is important to distinguish between clinical failure because of in vitro resistance and clinical failure because of host factors, drug interactions, and absorption or compliance problems. Fluconazole-resistant OPC has become a significant management problem, mainly in patients with advanced AIDS. It is thought that the annual incidence of clinical failures of fluconazole in OPC is around 5% *(38,55,56)*, even though initial retrospective reports suggested this incidence was significantly higher. There are limited data on the incidence of non-fluconazole-associated drug failures. Refractory disease is almost always associated with in vitro resistance. The most important risk factors for development of resistance are profound immunosuppression and prior exposure to antifungal agents.

7.2. Nonalbicans Species and Oropharyngeal Candidiasis

Clinically resistant OPC is most commonly associated with *C. albicans*. Nonalbicans species *C. parapsilosis, C. tropicalis, C. krusei,* and *C. glabrata* have been implicated in mucosal infections and refractory disease, but at much lower rates than *C. albicans (55)*. Infections with mixed *Candida* species can also occur.

Some authors have questioned the role of nonalbicans species in oropharyngeal infections, postulating that these infections occur with increased frequency in patients treated with azoles, but are rarely responsible for clinically significant disease *(55)*. However, others have suggested that nonalbicans species are clinically significant in OPC, with *C. glabrata* and *C. krusei* the most common nonalbicans species isolated *(57)*. Itraconazole solution 200 mg/d for 7 d was an effective alternative agent in the treatment of infections caused by isolates of *C. glabrata* and *C. krusei* that demonstrated in vitro susceptibility to itraconazole *(57)*.

The newly described species *C. dubliniensis* has been increasingly implicated in OPC in HIV-infected patients, but may be underreported because of its close resemblance to *C. albicans*. Most *C. dubliniensis* isolates are susceptible to fluconazole, but in vitro resistance can be easily induced.

7.3. Refractory Oropharyngeal Candidiasis and Highly Active Antiretroviral Therapy

Following the introduction of highly active antiretroviral therapy (HAART), the prevalence of OPC and fluconazole resistance is declining among isolates of *C. albicans* isolated from HIV-infected patients *(58)*. Besides the effect of HAART on immunorestoration, recent experimental data have shown that some antiretroviral protease inhibitors can interfere with *Candida* infection by inhibiting the fungal secretory aspartyl proteinases (SAPs), which have a pathogenic role in mucosal invasion *(59)*.

Tacconelli et al. compared susceptibility patterns of oral *Candida* isolates in the HAART era with data obtained in the pre-HAART era and showed a significant reduction of resistance rates to itraconazole and fluconazole, from 37 to 7% *(60)*. Whether this reduction of resistance is secondary to decreased usage of fluconazole remains to be seen. These data also demonstrate that most cases of HIV-associated OPC observed in the HAART era are caused by azole-susceptible strains of *C. albicans*. A study by Barchiesi and coworkers found that the majority of patients on HAART harbor strains of *C. albicans* susceptible to fluconazole (93% sensitive and 7% S-DD) *(61)*.

7.4. *Management of Refractory Esophageal/Oropharyngeal Candidiasis*

The optimal approach to fluconazole-refractory OPC is not known. If failure of treatment occurs, a number of factors need to be considered. First, cultures need to be obtained to establish whether the diagnosis of recurrent fungal infection is correct. It is important to ascertain whether there are any potential drug interactions or compliance or absorption problems. Identification of *Candida* to the species level and sensitivity testing is the next step.

The use of high-dose fluconazole (400 mg to 800 mg) has been recommended for the treatment of refractory OPC after initial failure of lower dose fluconazole *(62,63)*, even when *Candida* isolates show decreased susceptibility to fluconazole (S-DD range).

If this approach fails, itraconazole oral suspension (200 mg/d) can be tried, and it has been reported effective, with a 50–60% response rate, in several trials in patients with refractory OPC *(64,65)*.

Current Infectious Diseases Society of America guidelines include amphotericin B 100 mg/mL oral solution as a potentially effective option at a dose of 1 mL four times daily for the treatment of OPC *(34)*. However, there is little published experience with oral amphotericin B *(66,67)*, and it has limited efficacy for treatment of fluconazole-resistant OPC.

Intravenous amphotericin B has been effective salvage therapy in azole-refractory OPC. Usually, patients respond to doses of 0.3–0.5 mg/kg body weight per day, but this dose may need to be increased to 1 mg/kg body weight per day *(56)*. The duration of treatment is based on response, but 7–10 d for OPC and 3 wk for esophageal disease are typically required. Clinical failures with parenteral amphotericin B are rare. Other reported approaches to treatment failures have included the use of fluconazole with flucytosine.

Adjunctive immune therapy (such as granulocyte-macrophage colony-stimulating factor, GM-CSF) and introduction of HAART therapy may be of value in refractory OPC. Small studies have found GM-CSF to be beneficial as adjunctive therapy to fluconazole in the management of fluconazole-resistant OPC *(68)*. HAART is probably the single most important factor in preventing refractory OPC.

Despite the efficacy of initial treatment, relapse rates are high among patients with refractory disease, and these patients require maintenance therapy, usually with itraconazole or amphotericin B oral solutions, to prevent recurrences. It is not clear which dose should be given. The relapse of fluconazole-resistant OPC occurs in approx 50% of patients *(38)*.

7.5. *New Antifungal Agents and Oropharyngeal Candidiasis*

7.5.1. Caspofungin

Caspofungin (50 mg/d) has been found as safe and effective as fluconazole (200 mg/d) for patients with advanced HIV infection and documented *Candida* esophagitis *(69)*. In a phase II comparative study, caspofungin appeared to be at least as efficacious and better tolerated than amphotericin B for management of OPC and esophageal candidiasis *(70)*. Patients with history of azole-resistant infections were underrepresented in this trial. In a report by Kartsonis et al., caspofungin appeared to be efficacious therapy for some patients with esophageal candidiasis who were clinically refractory to fluconazole or infected with *Candida* spp with reduced susceptibility to fluconazole in vitro. The aim of this study was to determine the effect of treatment with caspofungin on esophageal candidiasis in patients with clinical or laboratory evidence of decreased susceptibility to fluconazole *(71)*.

Caspofungin may provide an equally effective, but less-toxic, alternative to conventional amphotericin B therapy for HIV-infected patients with azole-refractory *Candida* esophagitis. Its ultimate role in clinical practice remains to be determined, as do the optimal doses for treatment of OPC and esophageal candidiasis.

7.5.2. Voriconazole

Voriconazole (200 mg twice daily) was shown to be at least as effective as fluconazole (400 mg on d 1, followed by 200 mg daily) in the treatment of esophageal candidiasis in immunocompromised patients, including those with advanced AIDS *(72)*. Side effects were more common with voriconazole, with transient and reversible visual disturbances affecting 23% of patients.

A small study by Hegener et al. found that switching therapy from fluconazole to voriconazole 200 mg twice daily was effective in patients with advanced AIDS and fluconazole-resistant OPC *(73)*. Further trials will determine whether voriconazole should be considered an effective alternative therapy in refractory OPC.

8. MANAGEMENT OF RESISTANT CANDIDEMIA

Almost all patients with documented candidemia should be treated with systemic antifungal agents. Intravascular catheters should be changed or removed in both neutropenic and non-neutropenic patients whenever this is feasible. In neutropenic patients, the role of the gut as a source for disseminated candidiasis is evident, but it is difficult to determine whether the gut or the catheter is the primary source of candidemia. Removal of central venous catheters was associated with significant reduction in mortality in a number of studies *(29,74)*. In one study, retention of central venous catheters significantly increased the mortality from 15.7 to 48.8%, and this was particularly evident in infections with *C. glabrata (29)*.

Without adequate therapy, endophthalmitis, endocarditis, osteomyelitis, and other severe disseminated forms of candidiasis may complicate candidemia. Therapy should probably be continued for 2 wk after the last positive culture and resolution of signs and symptoms of infection and until the resolution of neutropenia *(75)*. Patients with evidence of acute or chronic disseminated candidosis (CDC) require longer therapy for treatment of organ involvement and eventual cure (*see* Section 8.9.). Evaluation of the patient should consist of repeated cultures and clinical examinations for manifestations of disseminated disease.

8.1. Candida albicans

Data show a low level of azole resistance of bloodstream isolates of *C. albicans* (0–1%), and resistance to azoles in this setting does not seem to be increasing despite increase

Table 4
Typical Antifungal Susceptibility Patterns for *Candida* spp Based on MIC_{90}

Candida spp	Fluconazole	Itraconazole	Flucytosine	Amphotericin B	Caspofungin	Voriconazole
C. albicans	S	S	**S-R**[a]	S	S	S
C. glabrata	**S-DD/R**	**S-DD/R**	S	**S/I**	S	**Higher MICs**
C. krusei	**R**	**S-DD/R**	**I/R**	**S/I**	S	S
C. parapsilosis	S	S	S	S	**Higher MICs**	S
C. lusitaniae	S	S	**S/R**	**S/R**[b]		S
C. guilliermondii	S	S	S	**S/R**[b]	**Higher MICs**	S
C. tropicalis	S	S	S	S	S	S[c]

Source: Adapted from refs. *10, 25, 36, 50, 86, 100, 101.*
Bold type denotes increased likelihood of elevated MICs.
[a]Serotype B.
[b]Some isolates demonstrate primary resistance to amphotericin B.
[c]Bimodal distribution in some studies *(8,33).*

in use of fluconazole prophylaxis (Table 4). Initial treatment with fluconazole is therefore appropriate.

8.2. Candida parapsilosis

Candida parapsilosis is most commonly associated with prosthetic devices and parenteral nutrition. *Candida parapsilosis* is recognized as a major causative agent of candidemia in neonatal intensive care units. It is usually sensitive to azoles and polyenes, which are appropriate for initial therapy. There are reports of increased MICs to caspofungin compared with *C. albicans* species, but how this relates to clinical outcome is not known at present.

8.3. Candida krusei

Candida krusei is more commonly associated with hematological malignancy than with solid tumors. In one case series, the overall mortality associated with *C. krusei* fungemia reached 49%, compared with 28% in *C. albicans* fungemia *(76).*

Infections caused by *C. krusei* should not be treated with fluconazole or itraconazole because of the high likelihood of resistance to these agents. *Candida krusei* is generally susceptible to amphotericin B, but the MICs to polyenes tend to be higher than for *C. albicans* and may require maximal doses of amphotericin B. *Candida krusei* is generally resistant to flucytosine.

Available data suggest that amphotericin B at 1.0 mg/kg body weight per day is the preferred agent. Voriconazole has excellent in vitro activity against *C. krusei,* so the newer azoles may become preferred therapy for this resistant pathogen. In vitro data suggest that caspofungin may also be a valuable agent for treatment of *C. krusei.*

8.4. Candida glabrata

Candida glabrata infections occur in patients with hematological malignancies and with solid tumors. The general mortality rate associated with *C. glabrata* bloodstream infections was 49% in a retrospective series of 139 cases *(77).* For infections caused by

C. glabrata, fluconazole dose-dependent responses may be observed. Because *C. glabrata* can have reduced susceptibility to both azoles and amphotericin B, there is no clear consensus on empirical treatment for *C. glabrata* bloodstream infections. Most authorities would recommend a higher dose of amphotericin B, at 0.7 mg/kg body weight per day, as initial therapy *(75,78)* until the susceptibility tests indicate that the isolate is susceptible to fluconazole *(79)*. Fluconazole at 12 mg/kg body weight per day (800 mg for a 70-kg patient) also appears suitable, particularly in patients who are less critically ill *(34)*.

8.5. Candida lusitaniae

Candida lusitaniae is an uncommon pathogen, and some strains are resistant to amphotericin B, so fluconazole at 6 mg/kg body weight per day is the preferred empirical therapy for this species *(34)*. A literature review of infections caused by *C. lusitaniae* in the 1990s found 21.7% of isolates resistant to amphotericin, but the clinical responses to amphotericin did not seem to correlate with in vitro resistance. Survival among patients with fungemia was high (95% of treated patients) *(80)*. This contrasts with studies in the late 1980s, which reported 53–78% mortality in patients with *C. lusitaniae* fungemia. In a report of 12 cases, Minari et al. found that *C. lusitaniae* fungemia had a poor response to amphotericin B despite apparent susceptibility of this pathogen to amphotericin B in vitro *(81)*.

Because of the lack of correlation of in vitro resistance and clinical outcome in this setting, it is not clear what the best treatment for *C. lusitaniae* is. The majority of isolates are sensitive to fluconazole, and in one review, there was no difference in the outcome in patients treated with amphotericin or fluconazole *(80)*.

8.6. Candida tropicalis

Disseminated disease is common with *C. tropicalis* and dissemination to the skin associated with septic shock is a common presentation. *Candida tropicalis* is associated with hematological malignancy and is associated with high overall mortality. Studies found the crude mortality in *C. tropicalis* fungemia to range from 44 *(74)* to 56% *(82)*. Breakthrough candidemia while patients are on treatment or prophylaxis has an even worse prognosis.

The SENTRY surveillance study found 96% of bloodstream isolates of *C. tropicalis* susceptible to fluconazole *(25)*. A study using an animal model of invasive candidiasis suggested that the maximum tolerated dose of liposomal amphotericin B should be used in the treatment of fluconazole-resistant *C. tropicalis* infections *(83)*. *Candida tropicalis* is usually sensitive to flucytosine, so this agent could be used in combination therapy with amphotericin B in severe infections not responding to monotherapy.

8.7. Recommended Doses of Antifungal Agents for Treatment of Candidemia

8.7.1. Fluconazole

Both human and animal data suggest that S-DD isolates may be treated successfully with a fluconazole dose of 12 mg/kg body weight per day *(9)*. An international consensus conference was held in 1995, and there was general agreement that doses higher than normal (400 mg/d) should be given to neutropenic patients, with the recommendation for a daily adult dose of 800 mg. Patients who are unstable or with impaired gastrointestinal absorption should receive intravenous fluconazole. A recent study showed that there is no benefit in combining fluconazole with amphotericin B, although there is additional toxicity as a consequence.

8.7.2. Itraconazole

Intravenous itraconazole has been studied only as a treatment for mucosal infections. The intravenous formulation of itraconazole is given at 200 mg twice daily for four doses (2 d), followed by 200 mg daily. Formal studies of intravenous itraconazole as therapy for invasive candidiasis have not been completed.

8.7.3. Amphotericin B

Doses of amphotericin B have been in the range 0.3–1.0 mg/kg body weight per day, although the optimal dose, in terms of both efficacy and toxicity, has not been clearly established. When amphotericin B is used to treat infections caused by *C. glabrata* or *C. krusei,* doses approaching or exceeding 1 mg/kg body weight per day may be needed, especially in profoundly immunocompromised hosts *(34)*. The optimal dose for liposomal formulation of amphotericin B for *Candida* infections is unclear, but doses of 3–5 mg/kg body weight would appear suitable for treatment of candidemia *(34)*. The lipid formulations of amphotericin B offer less toxicity, but no clear outcome advantages for the treatment of *Candida* infections.

8.7.4. Flucytosine

The addition of flucytosine (100–150 mg/kg body weight per day) to amphotericin B is appropriate for those slow to respond to amphotericin B and those with extensive disseminated disease. If the organism is later found to be resistant to flucytosine, the drug should be discontinued *(78)*. The use of flucytosine requires monitoring of serum concentrations. Peak serum levels should be maintained at 70–80 mg/L and trough levels at 25–30 mg/L.

8.8. New Antifungal Agents and Their Role in the Management of Candidemia

8.8.1. New Triazoles

Voriconazole is a new triazole antifungal agent that has potent in vitro activity against many isolates of *Candida* spp. It is significantly more effective than fluconazole in inhibiting ergosterol synthesis in *C. krusei*, consistent with the increased antifungal potency of voriconazole against this species *(84)*. The results of in vitro studies showed that *C. albicans* is the most susceptible species to voriconazole (MIC_{90} of 0.06 μg/mL), and *C. glabrata* is the least susceptible (MIC_{90} of 2.0 μg/mL). Voriconazole is more active than itraconazole and fluconazole against *C. albicans, C. parapsilosis, C. tropicalis*, and *C. krusei* (8,85–87). A study by Pfaller et al. *(8)* found that 98% of *C. krusei* isolates were susceptible to voriconazole and ravuconazole (MIC $\leq$ 1 μg/mL) irrespective of their level of resistance to itraconazole. Among the six antifungal agents tested (fluconazole, itraconazole, amphotericin B, flucytosine, ravuconazole, and voriconazole), only ravuconazole and voriconazole were reliably active against *C. krusei*. Increased antifungal activity of voriconazole against *C. krusei* compared with amphotericin has also been shown in animal models *(88)*. In vitro results for *C. tropicalis* varied among different studies, from low to high MICs *(8,87)*.

Because breakpoints have not been established for the new triazoles, detailed discussion of resistance is not possible. However, in isolates of *C. albicans* and *C. glabrata* that showed resistance to both fluconazole and itraconazole (RR phenotype), the MICs for voriconazole were also elevated *(8,85,86)*. This would suggest cross-resistance that is likely to be mediated by one or more efflux mechanism. Isolates that are resistant to fluconazole alone (RS phenotype) tend to have low voriconazole MICs.

Although NCCLS methods can be used to determine the antifungal activity of voriconazole, interpretation criteria have not yet been determined, so the translation of in vitro activity into clinical efficacy is awaited.

As yet, there have been no published clinical trials comparing voriconazole with traditional antifungal agents in the treatment of candidemia, although one such study has just been completed. Despite the possibility of cross-resistance, this agent has a potential role in managing invasive infections in cases of toxicity with traditional antifungal agents or antifungal resistance, particularly in infections caused by *C. krusei*.

8.8.2. Echinocandins

It is expected that all three echinocandins will be effective in most serious *Candida* infections. In vitro testing of fluconazole-resistant clinical isolates of *Candida* spp against anidulafungin, amphotericin B, and itraconazole has shown that anidulafungin was more potent than either itraconazole or amphotericin B against *C. albicans, C. glabrata, C. krusei,* and *C. tropicalis (89,90)*. Echinocandins are significantly less active against *C. parapsilosis* and *C. guilliermondii* compared with all other common pathogenic species (MICs typically 1–2 mg/L compared with 0.001 mg/L) *(90,91)*. Caspofungin seems to be highly active against azole-susceptible and azole-resistant isolates of *C. albicans* regardless of the underlying molecular mechanism of resistance *(92)*.

Efforts to induce caspofungin resistance in *C. albicans* by serial passage in the presence of the agent in vitro failed in one study, suggesting that the potential for development of resistance to the echinocandins is low *(93)*.

A recently completed randomized, double-blind study comparing caspofungin (70 mg loading dose followed by 50 mg/d) and amphotericin B for invasive candidiasis clearly demonstrated that caspofungin is at least as effective an agent for treatment of invasive candidiasis, but less toxic *(94)*. Among patients with nonalbicans species, outcome was similar for both agents. Only 11% of the enrolled patients had neutropenia at baseline, so the outcome data for these patients need to be interpreted with caution. This study also found that MICs of echinocandins tend to be higher for *C. parapsilosis* than other *Candida* species. At present, it is unclear whether higher doses of caspofungin may be needed in treatment of infections with *C. parapsilosis* to prevent persistent fungemia. It is also unknown how the efficacy of caspofungin compares with lipid-associated amphotericin or fluconazole. Further clinical studies are needed to correlate the excellent in vitro activity of echinocandins against *Candida* spp with clinical outcome.

Given that these agents act on a cell wall target rather than the cell membrane, it has been suggested that combination with other agents might be synergistic. However, there is currently no clinical evidence to support this.

8.9. Management of Chronic Disseminated Candidiasis

Chronic disseminated candidiasis (also referred to as hepatosplenic candidiasis) occurs in a small subgroup of patients with hematological malignancies. Chemotherapy and the subsequent neutropenia are associated with the development of CDC. It usually becomes apparent following the recovery of the bone marrow. Lesions can be seen in the liver, spleen, kidneys, and lungs on ultrasound or computerized tomographic (CT) scanning.

Treatment of CDC requires prolonged administration of antifungal agents, and recommendations for treatment include intravenous amphotericin B (0.6–0.7 mg/kg body weight per day), lipid-associated amphotericin B, or oral fluconazole (6 mg/kg body weight per day). Amphotericin B may be used in acutely ill patients or patients with refractory disease. Addition of flucytosine in combination with one of these agents is recommended for more refractory infections *(34)*. Therapy should be continued until resolution of lesions (usually between 4 and 6 mo) *(95)*. Some experts would recommend an initial 1- to 2-wk course of amphotericin B for all patients, followed by a prolonged course of fluconazole. Others would recommend use of fluconazole only in microbiologically documented infections *(95)*. This is based on observation of a change in epidemiology of *Candida* spp infections, with an increase in nonalbicans species.

Cases of CDC resistant to amphotericin B have been reported, but are rare *(96,97)*. New antifungal agents caspofungin and voriconazole may have a role in treatment of CDC. Successful treatment with caspofungin of a patient with CDC resistant to liposomal amphotericin B has been reported *(96)*. There is also anecdotal evidence for the benefit of adjunctive therapy with GM-CSF and interferon gamma in the management of this condition *(98,99)*.

8.10. Recurrent Vulvovaginal Candidiasis

The majority of women with *Candida* vaginitis suffer from uncomplicated vaginitis characterized by sporadic mild-to-moderate attacks. In complicated *Candida* vaginitis, attacks are more severe, are recurrent, or are caused by nonalbicans species.

Candida albicans is the causative agent of 80–92% of episodes of VVC. Both VVC and recurrent vulvovaginal candidiasis (RVVC) are most commonly caused by *C. albicans*. Among nonalbicans species, *C. glabrata* is most commonly isolated and accounts for 5% of infections. Less commonly, *C. krusei* and *C. guilliermondii* are implicated.

RVVC is defined as four or more episodes of VVC infection per year. Approximately 5% of the women who have experienced one or more attacks of VVC will develop RVVC. Strain typing methods have shown that women with recurrent infection usually harbor the same strains of *C. albicans* (48,102).

There are many controversies surrounding the pathogenesis of RVVC and the potential importance of immunopathogenesis in some cases, but this discussion is beyond the scope of this chapter.

8.10.1. Resistance of Candida albicans *in Vaginal Candidiasis and Its Role in Recurrent Vulvovaginal Candidiasis*

Episodes of RVVC caused by *C. albicans* are rarely if ever attributable to azole antifungal resistance. Only a very few isolated cases have been reported in the literature *(103)*. Other factors, such as poor compliance or mixed infections, are much more frequent reasons for a poor clinical or mycological response. Drug resistance needs to be considered if yeasts other than *C. albicans* are the causative agents.

Despite widespread use of antifungal drugs, there is no evidence that this has led to resistance to either fluconazole or clotrimazole or selection for nonalbicans species in immunocompetent patients with recurrent infection *(48,104)*.

8.10.2. Vaginal Candidiasis Caused by Candida glabrata

There are no clear guidelines for management of vaginitis caused by *C. glabrata*. The clinical response of patients with *C. glabrata* vaginitis to conventional azole therapy is largely unknown. Published data on management of *C. glabrata* vaginitis represents a population of patients seen in specialized clinics only after they have failed to respond to a large number of topical and azole agents.

Treatment failure is common in patients with vaginitis caused by *C. glabrata*, which is less susceptible to azoles, and with vaginitis caused by *C. krusei,* which is intrinsically resistant to fluconazole. In vitro studies showed that MICs for *C. glabrata* are lower with butoconazole, miconazole, and clotrimazole. Itraconazole and ketoconazole showed moderate activity, and fluconazole was less active. Despite this activity in vitro, azole therapy does not predictably eradicate *C. glabrata* in vivo.

In a study by Sobel and Chaim, the treatment of *C. glabrata* with vaginal boric acid (600 mg/day for 14 d) resulted in clinical improvement or cure in 81% and mycological eradication in 77% of patients. The clinical response and mycological eradication rates associated with topical and systemic azoles were 50% *(105)*. Many of the patients who remained culture positive had recurrence of vulvovaginal symptoms. These patients were then re-treated with boric acid and given a maintenance regimen of boric acid *(105)*.

However, the safety of this regimen is unknown, and there is still limited experience of its efficacy *(106)*. There are anecdotal reports of successful treatment of *C. glabrata* vaginitis with topical flucytosine and amphotericin B *(107)*. For patients who fail to respond to boric acid, topical flucytosine prescribed once a day for 14 d has been recommended. Most patients achieve clinical response to flucytosine, and *C. glabrata* is highly sensitive to this drug. A maintenance regimen with flucytosine is not recommended because of local toxicity and the potential for development of resistance *(79)*. The value of oral itraconazole as definitive therapy for *C. glabrata* vaginitis is largely unknown.

There are very scanty data on recommended regimens for treatment of *C. krusei* vaginitis, although there are reports of successful treatment with topical boric acid *(108)*.

8.10.3. Maintenance Regimens for Recurrent Vulvovaginal Candidiasis

After any possible causal factors are identified and controlled, initial therapy with 2 wk of topical or oral azole should be followed by a maintenance regimen for 6 mo. Unfortunately, the identifiable risk factors, such as diabetes or immunosuppressive therapy, are apparent in only a minority of patients with RVVC *(54)*.

Several studies have confirmed the success of maintenance regimens with oral ketoconazole, oral itraconazole, and topical clotrimazole in significantly reducing the frequency of symptomatic episodes of vaginitis, but there is an absence of controlled studies comparing the efficacy of various drug regimens in RVVC. A randomized controlled study in HIV-positive women found that 200 mg fluconazole weekly was effective in preventing oropharyngeal and vaginal candidiasis *(109)*. Regimens in current use for treatment of RVVC are empirical and not all are based on randomized controlled trials.

Some of the recommended regimens (all unlicensed) include *(110)*

1. 100 mg fluconazole once weekly for 6 mo
2. 500 mg clotrimazole vaginal pessary once weekly for 6 mo *(111)*
3. 400 mg itraconazole (as two divided doses on one day) every month for 6 mo *(112)*

In patients with recurrent, but not severe, disease, more prolonged therapy (i.e., two sequential 150-mg doses of fluconazole given 3 d apart) did not enhance eradication rates achieved with single-dose fluconazole. In patients with severe *Candida* vaginitis infected with *C. albicans*, the two-dose fluconazole regimen was found to achieve superior clinical and mycological eradication *(113)*. Whether initial prolonged therapy reduced the rates of recurrence remains to be validated.

9. ADJUNCTIVE IMMUNE THERAPY

Antifungal therapy can be ineffective in the setting of immune suppression. Host immunomodulation is an area explored for a number of years to improve response to antifungal agents. Immune therapy can be nonspecific or specific. Cytokines such as granulocyte colony-stimulating factor (G-CSF), GM-CSF, macrophage colony-stimulating factor (M-CSF), and interferon gamma are examples of nonspecific immunotherapy. Monoclonal antibodies are examples of specific immunotherapy directed at the pathogen. A study in animal models showed that antibodies against certain cell surface antigens of *C. albicans* help the host resist disseminated candidiasis *(114)*.

Cytokines have shown promising results in vitro when used in combination with antifungal agents. Clinical experience with immunotherapy for invasive fungal infections is still limited, and the beneficial adjunctive role of cytokines in treating refractory mycoses is supported only by anecdotal case reports and small studies *(98,99)*.

The next step in evaluating cytokines and monoclonal antibodies as adjunct therapy for fungal infections will require randomized controlled studies. These agents are expensive and have the potential for inducing side effects; therefore, they should not be extensively used without further investigation. Unfortunately, at least one attempt to conduct randomized, placebo-controlled studies on GM-CSF failed to recruit sufficient patients and was abandoned.

Currently, G-CSF or GM-CSF is recommended for persistently neutropenic patients who have proven invasive candidiasis *(34)*. These recommendations have been made in the absence of data from clinical trials, and consensus was based on evidence that, in addition to accelerating recovery from neutropenia, colony-stimulating factors may enhance the activity of neutrophils and macrophages against *Candida* species.

10. INFECTION CONTROL AND ANTIFUNGAL RESISTANCE

To control the spread of resistant *Candida* species, infection control measures should be implemented in the same way as when controlling infections with resistant bacterial pathogens.

Table 5
Management of Antifungal Resistance in *Candida* Infections

- Identification to species level should be performed on all isolated from sterile fluids (including blood cultures), mucosal isolates from HIV-infected patients, and in cases of recurrent or persistent VVC.
- Antifungal susceptibility testing is probably not required for the management of many cases of invasive candidosis; it is recommended in the setting of nonalbicans candidemia persistent fungemia or clinical failure of invasive candidiasis, in refractory mucosal candidiasis in AIDS patients, and in cases of RVVC.
- Fluconazole remains suitable for the treatment of most cases of candidemia.
- The newly licensed agents voriconazole and caspofungin are suitable for managing these infections in cases of antifungal resistance or toxicity with traditional antifungals.

Although the source of invasive candidosis is usually endogenous, acquisition of exogenous organisms has been reported in intensive care units *(115)* and neonatal units. *Candida parapsilosis* is a frequently implicated species in outbreaks in neonatal intensive care units *(116,117)*, but outbreaks with other *Candida* species have also been described *(118,119)*. Colonization with *C. parapsilosis* has been shown to occur either by horizontal transmission from nurses or by cross-infection between infants through the hands of health care workers. Outbreaks can also occur via contaminated intravenous fluids and biomaterials.

There is no evidence that source isolation of patients is required to prevent transmission of *Candida* species, but at least one study has demonstrated the carriage of an epidemic strain on the hands of health care workers and the termination of an outbreak in association with stringent hand hygiene practices. It seems likely that the practice of good standards of infection control measures aimed at preventing transmission of other organisms in high-risk units will help prevent the insidious spread of resistant *Candida* species.

11. CONCLUSION

Management of antifungal resistance in candida infections is summarized in Table 5.

REFERENCES

1. Edmond MB, Wallace SE, McClish DK, et al. Nosocomial bloodstream infections in the United States Hospitals: a 3-year analysis. Clin Infect Dis 1999; 29:239–244.
2. Denning DW. Invasive aspergillosis. Clin Infect Dis 1998; 26:781–805.
3. Lopez-Ribot JL, McAtee RK, Lee LN, et al. Distinct patterns of gene expression associated with development of fluconazole resistance in serial *Candida albicans* isolates from human immunodeficiency virus–infected patients with oropharyngeal candidiasis. Antimicrob Agents Chemother 1998; 42:2932–2937.
4. Sanglard D, Kuchler K, Ischer F, et al. Mechanisms of resistance to azole antifungal agents in *Candida albicans* isolates from AIDS patients involve specific multidrug transporters. Antimicrob Agents Chemother 1995; 39:2378–2386.
5. White TC. Increased mRNA levels of ERG16, CDR, and MDR1 correlate with increases in azole resistance in *Candida albicans* isolates from a patient infected with human immunodeficiency virus. Antimicrob Agents Chemother 1997; 41:1482–1487.

6. White TC, Marr KA, Bowden AR. Clinical, cellular and molecular factors that contribute to antifungal drug resistance. Clin Microb Rev 1998; 11:382–402.
7. Perea S, Lopez-Ribot JL, Kirkpatrick WR, et al. Prevalence of molecular mechanisms of resistance to azole antifungal agents in *Candida albicans* strains displaying high-level fluconazole resistance isolated from human immunodeficiency virus–infected patients. Antimicrob Agents Chemother 2001; 45:2676–2684.
8. Pfaller MA, Messer SA, Hollis RJ, et al. In vitro activities of ravuconazole and voriconazole compared with those of four approved systemic antifungal agents against 6970 clinical isolates of *Candida* spp. Antimicrob Agents Chemother 2002; 46:1723–1727.
9. Rex JH, Pfaller MA, Galgiani JN, et al. Subcommittee on antifungal susceptibility testing of the National Committee for Clinical Laboratory Standards. Development of interpretive breakpoints for antifungal susceptibility testing: conceptual framework and analysis of in vitro–in vivo correlation data for fluconazole, itraconazole and *Candida* infections. Clin Infect Dis 1997; 24:235–247.
10. Sanglard D, Odds F. Resistance of *Candida* species to antifungal agents: molecular mechanisms and clinical consequences. Lancet Infect Dis February 2002:73–85.
11. National Committee for Clinical Laboratory Standards. Reference Method for Broth Dilution Antifungal Susceptibility Testing of Yeasts; Approved Standard. Wayne, PA: National Committee for Clinical Laboratory Standards, 1997. NCCLS document M27-A.
12. Rex JH, Pfaller MA, Walsh TJ, et al. Antifungal susceptibility testing: practical aspects and current challenges. Clin Microb Rev 2001; 14:643–658.
13. Rex JH, Pfaller MA, Barry AL, et al. Antifungal susceptibility testing of isolates from a randomised, multicentre trial of fluconazole versus amphotericin B as treatment of nonneutropenic patients with candidemia. NIAID Mycoses Study Group and the Candidamia Study Group. Antimicrob Agents Chemother 1995; 39:40–44.
14. Rex JH, Cooper WG, Merz JN, et al. Detection of amphotericin B resistant *Candida* isolates in a broth-based system. Antimicrob Agents Chemother 1995; 39:906–909.
15. Nguyen MH, Clancy JC, Yu VL, et al. Do in vitro susceptibility data predict the microbiologic response to amphotericin B? Results of a prospective study of patients with *Candida* fungemia. J Infect Dis 1998; 177:425–430.
16. Espinel-Ingroff A, Pfaller MA, Erwin ME, et al. Interlaboratory evaluation of E test method for testing antifungal susceptibilities of pathogenic yeast to five antifungal agents by using Casitone agar and solidified RPMI 1640 medium with 2% glucose. J Clin Microbiol 1996; 34:848–852.
17. Pfaller MA, Messer SA, Karlsson A, et al. Evaluation of the Etest method for determining fluconazole susceptibilities of 402 clinical yeast isolates by using three different agar media. J Clin Microbiol 1998; 36:2586–2589.
18. Arendrup M, Lundgren B, Jensen IM, et al. Comparison of Etest and a tablet diffusion test with the NCCLS broth microdilution method for fluconazole and amphotericin B susceptibility testing of *Candida* isolates. J Antimicrob Chemother 2001; 47:521–526.
19. Clancy CJ, Nguyen MH. Correlation between in vitro susceptibility determined by Etest and response to therapy with amphotericin B: results from a multicentre prospective study of candidemia. Antimicrob Agents Chemother 1999; 43:1289–1290.
20. Peyron F, Favel A, Nguyen AM, et al. Improved detection of amphotericin B resistant isolates of *Candida lusitaniae* by Etest. J Clin Microbiol 2001; 39:399–342.
21. Pfaller MA, Messer SA, Bolstrom A. Evaluation of Etest for determining in vitro susceptibility of yeast isolates to amphotericin B—enhanced ability to detect amphotericin B resistant *Candida* isolates. Diagn Microbiol Infect Dis 1998; 32:223–227.
22. Warnock DW, Johnson EM, Rogers TR. Multi-centre evaluation of the Etest method for antifungal drug susceptibility testing of *Candida* spp and *Cryptococcus neoformans*. BSAC Working Party on Antifungal Chemotherapy. J Antimicrob Chemother 1998; 42:321–331.
23. Cuenca-Estrella M, Lee-Yang W, Meral A, et al. Comparative evaluation of NCCLS M27-A and EUCAST Broth microdilution procedures for antifungal susceptibility testing of *Candida* species. Antimicrob Agents Chemother 2002: 46:3644–3647.

24. Rex JH, Pfaller MA. Has antifungal susceptibility come of age? Clin Infect Dis 2002; 35: 982–989.
25. Pfaller MA, Diekema DJ, Jones RN, et al. Trends in antifungal susceptibility of *Candida* spp isolated from pediatric and adult patients with bloodstream infections: SENTRY Antimicrobial Surveillance Program, 1997 to 2000. J Clin Microbiol 2002; 40:852–856.
26. Hoban DJ, Zhanel GG, Karlowsky JA. In vitro susceptibilities of *Candida* and *Cryptococcus neoformans* isolates from blood cultures of neutropenic patients. Antimicrob Agents Chemother 1999; 43:1463–1464.
27. Pfaller MA, Diekema DJ. Role of sentinel surveillance of candidemia: trends in species distribution and antifungal susceptibility. J Clin Microbiol 2002; 40:3551–3557.
28. St-Germain G, Laverdiere M, Pelletier R, et al. Prevalence and antifungal susceptibility of 442 *Candida* isolates from blood and other normally sterile sites: results of a 2-year (1996–1998) multicenter surveillance study in Quebec, Canada. J Clin Microbiol 2001; 39:949–953.
29. Kibbler CC, Seaton S, Barnes RA, et al. Management and outcome of bloodstream infections due to *Candida* species in England and Wales. J Hosp Infect 2003; 54:18–24.
30. Safdar A, Chaturvedi V, Koll BS, et al. Prospective, multicenter surveillance study of *Candida glabrata*: fluconazole and itraconazole susceptibility profiles in bloodstream, invasive, and colonising strains and differences between isolates from three urban teaching hospital in New York City (*Candida* susceptibility trends study, 1998 to 1999). Antimicrob Agents Chemother 2002; 46:3268–3272.
31. Pfaller MA, Diekema DJ, Jones N, et al. International surveillance of bloodstream infections due to *Candida* species: frequency of occurrence and in vitro susceptibilities to fluconazole, ravuconazole, and voriconazole of isolates collected from 1997 through 1999 in the SENTRY antimicrobial surveillance program. J Clin Microbiol 2001; 36:3254–3259.
32. Ellis D. Amphotericin B: spectrum and resistance. Antimicrob Agents Chemother 2002; 49:7–10.
33. Nolte FS, Parkinson T, Falconer DJ, et al. Isolation and characterisation of fluconazole and amphotericin B resistant *Candida albicans* from blood of two patients with leukemia. Antimicrob Agents Chemother 1997; 41:196–199.
34. Rex JH, Walsh TJ, Sobel JD, et al. Practice guidelines for the treatment of candidiasis. Guidelines from the Infectious Diseases Society of America. Clin Infect Dis 2000; 30:662–678.
35. Barchiesi F, Arzeni D, Caselli F, et al. Primary resistance to flucytosine among clinical isolates of *Candida* spp. J Antimicrob Chemother 2000; 45:408–409.
36. Pfaller MA, Messer SA, Boyken L, et al. In vitro activities of 5-fluorocytosine against 8803 clinical isolates of *Candida* spp: global assessment of primary resistance using National Committee for Clinical Laboratory Standards Susceptibility Testing methods. Antimicrob Agents Chemother 2002; 46:3518–3521.
37. Maenza JR, Keruly JC, Moore RD, et al. Risk factors for fluconazole-resistant candidiasis in human immunodeficiency virus-infected patients. J Infect Dis 1996; 173:219–225.
38. Fichtenbaum CJ, Koletar S, Yiannoutsos C, et al. Refractory mucosal candidiasis in advanced human immunodeficiency virus infection. Clin Infect Dis 2000; 30:749–756.
39. Viscoli C, Girmenia C, Marinus A, et al. Candidemia in cancer patients: a prospective, multicenter surveillance study by the Invasive Fungal Infection Group (IFIG) of the European Organization for Research and Treatment of Cancer (EORTC). Clin Infect Dis 1999; 28:1070–1079.
40. Wingard JR, Merz WG, Rinaldi MG, et al. Increase in *Candida krusei* infection among patients with bone marrow transplantation and neutropenia treated prophylactically with fluconazole. N Engl J Med 1991; 325:1274–1277.
41. Hope W, Morton A, Eisen DP. Increase in prevalence of nosocomial non-*Candida albicans* candidaemia and the association of *C. krusei* with fluconazole use. J Hosp Infect 2002; 50:56–65.

42. Abi-Said D, Anaissie E, Uzun O, et al. The epidemiology of hematogenous candidiasis caused by different *Candida* species. Clin Infect Dis 1997; 24:1122–1128.
43. Trick WE, Fridkin SK, Edwards JR, et al. Secular trend of hospital-acquired candidaemia among intensive care unit patients in the United States during 1989–1999. Clin Infect Dis 2002; 35:627–630.
44. Nguyen MH, Peacock JE, Morris AJ, et al. The changing face of candidemia: emergence of non-*Candida albicans* species and antifungal resistance. Am J Med 1996; 100:617–623.
45. Paterson PJ, Whinney PHM, Potter M, Kibbler CC, et al. The combination of oral amphotericin B with azoles prevents the emergence of resistant *Candida* species in neutropenic patients. Br J Haem 2001; 112:175–180.
46. Chandra JC, Kuhn D, Mukherjee PK, et al. Biofilm formation by the fungal pathogen *Candida albicans*: development, architecture and drug resistance. J Bacteriol 2001; 183:5385–5394.
47. Denning DW. Can we prevent azole resistance in fungi? Lancet 1995; 346:454.
48. El-Din SS, Reynolds MT, Ashbee HR, et al. An investigation into the pathogenesis of vulvo-vaginal candidiosis. Sex Transm Infect 2001; 77:179–183.
49. Mathema B, Cross E, Dun E, et al. Prevalence of vaginal colonization by drug-resistant *Candida* species in college-age women with previous exposure to over the counter azole antifungal. Clin Infect Dis 2001; 33:23–27.
50. Dismukes W. Introduction to antifungal drugs. Guidelines from the Infectious Diseases Society of America. Clin Infect Dis 2000; 30:653–657.
51. Pfaller MA, Rex JH, Rinaldi MG. Antifungal susceptibility testing: technical advances and potential clinical applications. Clin Infect Dis 1997; 24:776–784.
52. Sobel JD. Vaginitis. N Engl J Med 1997; 337:1896–1903.
53. Denning DW. Fortnightly review: management of genital candidiasis. Working Group of the British Society for Medical Mycology. BMJ 1995; 310:1241–1244.
54. Sobel JD. Pathogenesis and treatment of recurrent vulvovaginal candidiasis. Clin Infect Dis 1992; 14(suppl. 1):S148–S153.
55. Baily GG, Pery FM, Denning DW, et al. Fluconazole-resistant candidiosis in an HIV cohort. AIDS 1994; 8:787–792.
56. Fichtenbaum CJ, Powderly WG. Refractory mucosal candidiasis in patients with human immunodeficiency virus infection. Clin Infect Dis 1998; 26:556–565.
57. Cartledge JD, Midgley J, Gazzard BG. Non-albicans oral candidiosis in HIV-positive patients. J Antimicrob Chemother 1999; 43:419–422.
58. Martins MD, Lozano-Chiu M, Rex JH. Declining rates of oropharyngeal candidiasis and carriage of *Candida albicans* associated with trends toward reduced rates of carriage of fluconazole-resistant *C. albicans* in human immunodeficiency virus–infected patients. Clin Infect Dis 1998; 27:1291–1294.
59. Cassone A, De Bernardis F, Torosantucci A, et al. In vitro and in vivio anticandidal activity of human immunodeficiency virus protease inhibitors. J Infect Dis 1999; 180:448–453.
60. Tacconelli E, Bertagnolio S, Posterar B, et al. Azole susceptibility patterns and genetic relationship among oral *Candida* strains isolated in the era of highly active antiretroviral therapy. J Acquir Immun Defic Syndr 2002; 31:38–44.
61. Barchiesi F, Maracci M, Radi B, et al. Point prevalence, microbiology and fluconazole susceptibility patterns of yeast isolates colonizing the oral cavities of HIV-infected patients in the era of highly active antiretroviral therapy. J Antimicrob Chemother 2002; 50:999–1002.
62. Johnson EM, Warnock DW. Azole drug resistance in yeasts. J Antimicrob Chemother 1995; 36:751–755.
63. Ravenkar SG, Dib OP, Kirkpatrick WR, et al. Clinical evaluation and microbiology of oropharyngeal infection due to fluconazole-resistant *Candida* in human immunodeficiency virus–infected patients. Clin Infect Dis 1998; 26:960–963.
64. Phillips P, Zemcov J, Mahmood W, et al. Itraconazole cyclodextrin solution for

fluconazole-refractory oropharyngeal candidiasis in AIDS: correlation of clinical response with in vitro susceptibility. AIDS 1996; 10:1369–1376.
65. Cartledge JD, Midgley J, Youle M, et al. Itraconazole cyclodextrin solution effective treatment HIV-related candidiosis unresponsive to other azole therapy. J Antimicrob Chemother 1994; 33:1071–1073.
66. Grim SA, Smith KM, Romanelli F, et al. Treatment of azole resistant oropharyngeal candidiasis with topical amphotericin B. Ann Pharmacother 2002; 36:1383–1386.
67. Fichtenbaum CJ, Zackin R, Rajcic N, et al. Amphotericin B oral suspension for fluconazole-refractory oral candidiasis in persons with HIV infection. AIDS 2000; 14:845–852.
68. Vazquez JA, Hidalgo JA, De Bono S. Use of sargramostim (rh-GM-CSF) as adjunctive treatment of fluconazole-refractory oropharyngeal candidiasis in patients with AIDS: a pilot study. HIV Clin Trials 2000; 1:23–29.
69. Villaneuva A, Gotuzzo E, Arathood EG, et al. A randomised double-blind study of caspofungin versus fluconazole for the treatment of esophageal candidiasis. Am J Med 2002; 113:294–299.
70. Arathoon EG, Gotuzzo E, Noriega ML, et al. Randomised, double-blind, multicenter study of caspofungin versus amphotericin B for treatment of oropharyngeal and esophageal candidiasis. Antimicrob Agents Chemother 2002; 46:451–457.
71. Kartsonis N, DiNubile MJ, Bartizal K, et al. Efficacy of caspofungin in the treatment of esophageal candidiasis resistant to fluconazole. J Acquir Immun Defic Syndr 2002; 31:183–197.
72. Ally R, Schurmann D, Kreisel W, et al. A randomised, double-blind, double-dummy, multicenter trial of voriconazole and fluconazole in the treatment of esophageal candidiasis in immunocompromised patients. Clin Infect Dis 2001; 33:1447–1454.
73. Hegener P, Troke PF, Fatkenheuer G, et al. Treatment of fluconazole-resistant candidiasis with voriconazole in patients with AIDS. AIDS 1998; 12:2227–2241.
74. Tortorano MA, Biraghi E, Astolfi A, et al. European Confederation of Medical Mycology (ECMM) prospective survey of candidaemia: report from one Italian region. J Hosp Infect 2002; 51:297–304.
75. Edwards JE. International conference for the development of a consensus on the management and prevention of severe candidal infections. Clin Infect Dis 1997; 25:43–59.
76. Abbas J, Bodey GP, Hanna HA, et al. *Candida krusei* fungaemia. An escalating serious infection in immunocompromised patients. Arch Intern Med 2000; 17:2659–2664.
77. Gumbo T, Isada CM, Hall G, et al. *Candida glabrata* fungemia. Clinical features of 139 patients. Medicine (Baltimore) 1999; 78:220–227.
78. British Society for Antimicrobial Chemotherapy Working Party. Management of deep *Candida* infection in surgical and intensive care unit patients. Intensive Care Med 1994; 20:522–528.
79. Fidel PL Jr, Vazquez JA, Sobel JD. *Candida glabrata*: review of epidemiology, pathogenesis and clinical disease with comparison to *C. albicans*. Clin Microb Rev 1999; 12:80–96.
80. Hawkins JL, Baddour LM. *Candida lusitaniae* infections in the era of fluconazole availability. Clin Infect Dis 2003; 36:14–18.
81. Minari A, Hachem R, Raad I. *Candida lusitaniae*: a cause of breakthrough fungemia in cancer patients. Clin Infect Dis 2001; 32:186–190.
82. Leung AY, Chim CS, Ho PL, et al. *Candida tropicalis* fungaemia in adult patients with haematological malignancies: clinical features and risk factors. J Hosp Infect 2002; 50: 316–319.
83. Warn PA, Morrissey J, Moore CB, et al. In vivo activity of amphotericin B lipid complex in immunocompromised mice against fluconazole-resistant or fluconazole-susceptible *Candida tropicalis*. Antimicrob Agents Chemother 2000; 44:2664–2671.
84. Sanati H, Belanger P, Fratti R, et al. A new triazole, voriconazole (UK-109,496), blocks

sterol biosynthesis in *Candida albicans* and *Candida krusei*. Antimicrob Agents Chemother 1997; 41:2492–2496.

85. Pfaller MA, Messer SA, Hollis RJ, et al. In vitro susceptibilities of *Candida* bloodstream isolates to the new triazole antifungal agents BMS-207147, Sch 56592, and voriconazole. Antimicrob Agents Chemother 1998; 42:3242–3244.
86. Marco F, Pfaller MA, Messer S, et al. In vitro activities of voriconazole (UK-109,496) and four other antifungal agents 394 clinical isolates of *Candida* spp. Antimicrob Agents Chemother 1998; 42:161–163.
87. Pelletier R, Loranger L, Marcotte H, et al. Voriconazole and fluconazole susceptibility of *Candida* isolates. J Med Microbiol 2002; 51:479–483.
88. Ghannoum MA, Okogbule-Wondi I, Bhat N, et al. Antifungal activity of voriconazole, fluconazole and amphotericin B against hematogenous *Candida krusei* infection in neutropenic guinea pig model. J Chemother 1999; 11:34–39.
89. Maesaki S, Hossain MA, Miyazaki Y, et al. Efficacy of FK463, a (1,3)-β-D-glucan synthase inhibitor, in disseminated azole resistant *Candida albicans* infection in mice. Antimicrob Agents Chemother 2000; 44:1728–1730.
90. Cuenca-Estrella M, Mellado E, Diaz-Guerra T, et al. Susceptibility of fluconazole-resistant clinical isolates of *Candida* spp to echinocandin LY 303366, itraconazole and amphotericin B. J Antimicrob Chemother 2000; 46:475–477.
91. Moore CB, Oakley KL, Denning DW. In vitro activity of a new echinocandin, LY303366, and comparison with fluconazole, flucytosine and amphotericin B against *Candida* species. Clin Microbiol Infect 2001; 7:11–16.
92. Bachmann SP. Patterson TF, Lopez-Ribot JL, et al. In vitro activity of caspofungin (MK-0991) against *Candida albicans* clinical isolates displaying different mechanisms of azole resistance. J Clin Microbiol 2002; 40:2228–2230.
93. Bartizal K, Gill CJ, Abruzzo GK, et al. In vitro preclinical evaluation studies with the echinocandin antifungal MK-0991 (L-743,872). Antimicrob Agents Chemother 1997; 41: 2326–2332.
94. Mora-Duarte J, Betts R, Rotstein C, et al. Comparison of caspofungin and amphotericin for invasive candidiasis. N Engl J Med 2002; 347:2020–2029.
95. Pagano L, Mele L, Fianchi L, et al. Chronic disseminated candidiasis in patients with hematologic malignancies. Clinical features and outcome of 29 episodes. Haematologica 2002; 87:535–541.
96. Sora F, Chiusolo P, Piccirillo N, et al. Successful treatment with caspofungin of hepatosplenic candidiasis resistant to liposomal amphotericin B. Clin Infect Dis 2002; 35: 1135–1136.
97. Conly J, Rennier R, Johnson J, et al. Disseminated candidiasis due to amphotericin B-resistant *Candida albicans*. J Infect Dis 1992; 165:761–764.
98. Rokusz L, Liptay L, Kadar K. Successful treatment of chronic disseminated candidiasis with fluconazole and a granulocyte-macrophage colony-stimulating factor combination. Scand J Infect Dis 2001; 33:784–786.
99. Poynton CH, Barnes RA, Rees J. Interferon gamma and granulocyte-macrophage colony stimulating factor for the treatment of hepatosplenic candidiosis in patients with acute leukemia. Clin Infect Dis 1998; 26:239–240.
100. Kontoyiannis D, Lewis R. Antifungal drug resistance of pathogenic fungi. Lancet 2002; 359:1135–1144.
101. Perea S, Patterson TF. Antifungal resistance in pathogenic fungi. Clin Infect Dis 2002; 35: 1073–1080.
102. Vazquez JA, Sobel JD, Demitriou R, et al. Karyotyping of *Candida albicans* isolates obtained longitudinally in women with recurrent vulvovaginal candidiasis. J Infect Dis 1994; 170:1566–1569.

103. Dorrell L, Edwards A. Vulvovaginitis due to fluconazole resistant *Candida albicans* following self treatment with non-prescribed triazoles. Sex Transm Infect 2002; 78:308–312.
104. Walker PP, Reynolds MT, Ashbee HR, et al. Vaginal yeasts in the era of "over the counter" antifungal. Sex Transm Infect 2000; 76:437–438.
105. Sobel JD, Chaim W. Treatment of *Torulopsis glabrata* vaginitis: retrospective review of boric acid therapy. Clin Infect Dis 1997; 24:649–652.
106. Guaschino S, De Deat F, Sartore A, et al. Efficacy of maintenance therapy with topical boric acid comparison with oral itraconazole in the treatment of recurrent vulvovaginal candidiasis. Am J Obstet Gynecol 2001; 184:598–602.
107. White DJ, Habib AR, Vanthuyne A, et al. Combined topical flucytosine and amphotericin B for refractory vaginal *Candida glabrata* infection. Sex Transm Infect 2001; 77:212–213.
108. Singh S, Sobel JD, Bhargava P, et al. Vaginitis due to *Candida krusei*: epidemiology, clinical aspects, and therapy. Clin Infect Dis 2002; 35:1066–1070.
109. Schuman P, Capps L, Peng G, et al. Weekly fluconazole for the prevention of mucosal candidiasis in women with HIV infection. A randomized, double-blind, placebo-controlled trial. Terry Beirn Community Programs for Clinical Research in AIDS. Ann Intern Med 1997; 126:689–196.
110. Fitzgerald MR, Ahmed-Jushuf I, Radcliffe KW, et al. Clinical effectiveness group. Revised UK national guidelines on sexually transmitted infections and closely related conditions 2002. Sex Transm Infect 2002; 78:81–82.
111. Fong IW. The value of chronic suppressive therapy with itraconazole versus clotrimazole in women with recurrent vaginal candidiasis. Genitourin Med 1992; 68:374–377.
112. Spinillo A, Colonna L, Piazzi G, et al. Managing recurrent vulvovaginal candidiasis. Intermittent prevention with itraconazole. J Reprod Med 1997; 42:83–87.
113. Sobel JD, Kapernick PS, Zervos M, et al. Treatment of complicated *Candida* vaginitis: comparison of single and sequential doses of fluconazole. Am J Obstet Gynecol 2001; 185:363–369.
114. Han Y, Cutler JE. Antibody response that protects against disseminated candidiasis. Infect Immun 1995; 63:2714–2719.
115. Burnie JP, Lee W, Williams JD, et al. Control of an outbreak of systemic *Candida albicans*. BMJ (Clin Res Ed) 1985; 291:1091–1093.
116. Lupetti A, Tavanti A, Davini P, et al. Horizontal transmission of *Candida parapsilosis* candidemia in a neonatal intensive care unit. J Clin Microbiol 2002; 40:2363–2369.
117. Huang YC, Lin TY, Leu HS, et al. Outbreak of *Candida parapsilosis* fungemia in neonatal intensive care units: clinical implications and genotyping analysis. Infection 1999; 27: 97–102.
118. Boccia S, Poteraro B, La Sorda M, et al. Genotypic analysis by 27A DNA fingerprinting of *Candida albicans* isolated during an outbreak in neonatal intensive care unit. Infect Control Hosp Epidemiol 2002; 23:281–284.
119. Fowler SL, Rhoton B, Springer SC, et al. Evidence for person to person transmission of *Candida lusitaniae* in a neonatal intensive care unit. Infect Control Hosp Epidemiol 1998; 19:343–345.

17

Management of Infection With Naturally Amphotericin B-Resistant Fungi

Thean Yen Tan and Rosemary A. Barnes

1. INTRODUCTION

There has been a progressive increase in the incidence of invasive fungal infections over the last two decades *(1)*. Most occur in severely immunocompromised patients, such as those with hematological malignancy or undergoing stem cell transplantation. While candidal infections predominate, mortality rates from this infection have progressively decreased. Conversely, infections caused by molds are associated with high mortality and have continued to increase disproportionately. Many centers report that the largest increase is seen with emerging fungi, including *Aspergillus terreus, Aspergillus flavus, Fusarium* spp, and *Scedosporium* spp *(2)*.

Many of these species are considered naturally resistant to amphotericin B *(3)*, and alternative management strategies are required to combat these infections. New antifungal agents, including triazole drugs, echinocandins, and combinations of agents have widened the choice of agents available to treat these problem infections. However, invasive fungal infections are supremely opportunistic, and recovery is determined more by restoration of host defenses than antifungal drug treatment. Biological response modifiers, avoidance of risk factors, adjunctive therapy, and surgery are all clinically relevant in patient management.

2. AMPHOTERICIN B RESISTANCE

Amphotericin B is an amphipathic polyene that binds to sterols in cell membranes. This binding disrupts the integrity of the membrane, supposedly through the formation of pores, resulting in leakage of intracellular potassium, magnesium, sugars, and metabolites and ultimately cell death. The drug binds preferentially to the primary fungal cell membrane sterol, ergosterol, resulting in the intrinsic antifungal activity of amphotericin B. However, binding to other sterols such as cholesterol and human lipoproteins occurs and is associated with significant toxicity, especially nephrotoxicity.

Most pathogenic fungal species contain ergosterol; consequently, amphotericin B has a very broad spectrum of activity. The mechanisms of resistance are not fully understood. Ergosterol-deficient fungi appear resistant *(4)*, and primary resistance has been reported in *Scedosporium* spp, *Trichosporon beigelii, A. terreus, Malassezia furfur*,

From: *Management of Multiple Drug-Resistant Infections*
Edited by: S. H. Gillespie © Humana Press Inc., Totowa, NJ

and *Fusarium* spp, as well as certain species of *Candida* (e.g., *Candida lusitaniae*). Other mechanisms are also involved *(5–10)*, and any fungal species may be resistant. Depletion of fungal ergosterol by prior azole therapy may play a role *(10)*.

In vitro susceptibility testing of fungi is plagued by poor reproducibility, with wide inter- and intralaboratory variation depending on media, pH, inoculum size, and growth conditions. The publication of methodologies by the National Committee for Clinical Laboratory Standards (NCCLS) *(11,12)* has provided a standard, but these broth macrodilution methods are cumbersome and time consuming. Moreover, because of the narrow range of minimum inhibitory concentrations (MICs) in various fungal species, distinguishing resistance from susceptibility is difficult.

Resistance determination is only of value when it correlates with clinical outcome. The relationship between amphotericin B MICs and response to treatment is far from clear *(13,14)*. Various modifications of the NCCLS methodology are approved *(15–21)* and show moderate correlation between MIC or MLC (minimum lethal concentration) and outcome *(22,23)*. However, newer liposomal formulations of amphotericin B are now available. The variation in dosages and heterogeneity of study populations make determining dose–outcome relationships impossible *(24)*.

Few studies on the serum levels and pharmacokinetics of amphotericin B have been performed *(25)*. With conventional amphotericin B deoxycholate, serum trough levels above 2 mg/L are associated with unacceptable toxicities. When compared with reported MICs *(26–29)*, it can be appreciated that therapeutic levels may not be achievable for many species of *Aspergillus* (especially *A. terreus*), *Scedosporium* spp, *T. beigelii, C. lusitaniae*, and *Fusarium* spp. Even with the improved therapeutic index available from the higher dosing regimens of the lipid preparations, the pharmacodynamic profile of amphotericin B, including the area under the MIC curve, is suboptimal when compared to most antibacterial agents.

These confounding factors mean that the concept of amphotericin-resistant fungi may be flawed, and ultimately host factors appear more crucial in determining recovery from invasive infection. In general, true primary in vitro resistance to amphotericin B is uncommon. However, with the changing spectrum of fungal invasive disease, it is increasingly likely that some of the more uncommon filamentous fungi and yeasts will be encountered that have traditionally been associated either with in vitro amphotericin resistance or a poor clinical outcome despite treatment with amphotericin B. These are discussed in more detail in the following paragraphs, and a summary of suggested treatment regimes is listed in Table 1.

3. NATURALLY RESISTANT MOLDS

3.1. Scedosporium *Species*

The genus *Scedosporium* consists of two species: *S. apiospermum* and *S. prolificans*. The sexual stage of *S. apiospermum* is known as *Pseudallescheria boydii*.

3.1.1. Scedosporium prolificans

Scedosporium prolificans is a filamentous fungus that appears to be ubiquitous in the environment. Infection with this organism is increasingly recognized, usually in patients with underlying immunosuppression. Asymptomatic colonization has been described and is probably a function of both host susceptibility and environmental

Table 1
Chemotherapy of Invasive Resistant Fungal Infections

Fungal disease	First-line therapy	Alternative therapy
Scedosporium prolificans	No therapy with documented efficacy	Consider high-dose lipid preparations of amphotericin or combination of itraconazole and terbinafine
Pseudoallescheria infections	Itraconazole or high-dose lipid preparations of amphotericin	Voriconazole
Fusarium spp	Amphotericin or high-dose lipid preparations of amphotericin	Voriconazole or other third-generation triazoles
Aspergillus spp	Amphotericin or high-dose lipid preparations of amphotericin	Voriconazole or other third-generation triazoles; caspofungin
Scopulariopsis brevicaulis	Amphotericin or high-dose lipid preparations of amphotericin	Voriconazole or other third-generation triazoles or terbinafine
Trichosporon spp	Itraconazole or fluconazole	Voriconazole or other third-generation triazoles
Candida spp	Amphotericin or high-dose lipid preparations of amphotericin	Itraconazole or voriconazole or other third-generation triazoles
Zygomycoses	High-dose lipid preparations of amphotericin	

acquisition *(30)*. Most cases of invasive disease have been reported from Spain and Australia, although it remains unclear if this is a true geographic distribution. Invasive disease manifests both as localized *(31)* and disseminated infection. Patients who have undergone hematopoetic stem cell transplantation are particularly at risk for deep-seated infections with this mold; these infections include pneumonia *(32)*, osteoarticular infections, endocarditis, peritonitis, and meningoencephalitis *(33)*. Clinical features of disseminated infection include a high rate of isolation from blood cultures, the presence of skin lesions, and signs of central nervous system involvement *(34)*.

On culture, colonies of *S. prolificans* grow rapidly at 25°C. The texture is moist (yeastlike) initially and later becomes flat with short, gray-to-black mycelial tufts. The reverse of the colony is black. Microscopically, septate hyaline hyphae are visualized, together with numerous conidia and coniaphores (annelides). Annelides are short with inflated bases, sometimes arranged in clusters with tapering tips. Conidia are oval and appear to cluster around the annelide tip.

Localized disease with this organism has responded to surgical debridement and fluconazole therapy *(35)*. Therapy of invasive disease has been limited by the multiresistant nature of the organism. Antifungal susceptibility testing against clinical isolates of this mold has generally demonstrated increased MICs against most available antifungal agents, including amphotericin B *(33,36)*. Of note, the glucan synthesis inhibitor caspofungin *(37)* also demonstrates very limited in vitro activity. Of available antifungal agents, voriconazole may have slightly improved activity *(38)*, although clinical experience to date has been disappointing *(33)*.

One in vitro study suggested that a combination of terbinafine and itraconazole might demonstrate synergistic activity at achievable serum levels *(39)*, although the in vivo response to this combination has not been confirmed. Ultimately, it is likely that resolution of the underlying immunosuppression will be the final determinant of successful clinical resolution of disease, for which there may be a limited role for adjuvants like granulocyte colony-stimulating factor (G-CSF) *(40)*. The significant mortality associated with disease caused by this mold is amply demonstrated by a review of 18 cases of disseminated disease and colonization *(33)*. Of the 6 cases with invasive disease, failure of resolution of underlying neutropenia resulted in a 100% mortality rate (4 of 6 patients).

3.1.2. Scedosporium apiospermum

Scedosporium apiospermum is more commonly described as the telemorph or sexual stage *P. boydii*. This filamentous fungus is found in most environmental sources and has a worldwide distribution. Infections caused by this mold are usually opportunistic and occur in immunosuppressed individuals following hematological malignancies, solid organ transplantation, or acquired immunodeficiency syndrome (AIDS). However, localized disease in immunocompetent adults presenting as lymphadenitis has been reported *(41)*. Invasive disease may manifest as endophthalmitis, endocarditis *(42)*, brain abscesses *(43)*, pneumonia *(44,45)*, and disseminated infection *(46)*. Cerebral infections are thought to be particularly common in patients who have suffered near-drowning incidents *(47)*.

On culture, colonies of *P. boydii* grow rapidly at 25°C, reaching a diameter of 40 mm in a week. The colonies are high and dome shaped, with a cottony texture. From the front, the color changes initially from white to dark gray. From the reverse, it is pale with brownish-black zones. Microscopically, in the asexual stage, the conidiophores form long, slender annelides that are sometimes aggregated into treelike structures. The conidia are pale yellow and oval with a truncated scar at the base.

In vitro testing of *P. boydii* has generally demonstrated resistance to amphotericin B *(36,48)*. The azoles appear to have better in vitro activity against this fungus, with voriconazole in particular demonstrating the lowest MICs *(36,48)*. Reported clinical experience suggests that itraconazole *(41,45)* or voriconazole *(49,50)* may be successfully employed in the treatment of invasive disease. The newer triazoles in development, such as posaconazole *(51)*, may prove more useful in treatment of this infection *(43)*, although more clinical data are required. Concomitant surgical debridement and drainage should always be considered in the treatment of brain abscesses *(43,49)* or other localized collections.

3.2. Fusarium *Species*

Fusarium spp are ubiquitous in the environment and are classified as hyaline septate molds *(52)*. These were originally described as common causes of onychomycosis and now comprise some of the more common invasive fungal isolates from hematology and cancer centers. Risk factors for invasive disease with this organism include neutropenia secondary to stem cell transplantation or chemotherapy, solid organ transplantation, steroid administration, and diabetes. Common primary sites of entry with this mold include the skin and nails, paranasal sinuses, pulmonary system, and indwelling vascular catheters.

Signs and symptoms of disease include a persistent fever in a neutropenic patient, sinusitis, pulmonary infiltrates, or metastatic skin lesions *(53)*. Primary skin lesions are described as cellulitic areas surrounding a site of onychomycosis; metastatic skin lesions range from subcutaneous nodules to ecthyma gangrenosum-like lesions. Invasion of blood vessels is a characteristic feature, and this mold may be recovered from blood cultures in 40–60% of disseminated infections *(53)*. Histopathological demonstration of hyphae in tissue is difficult to distinguish from *Aspergillus* infections, and it may take newly developed polymerase chain reaction (PCR) techniques to establish the diagnosis clearly *(54)*. Differentiating the two infections is clinically important because disseminated fusariosis responds poorly to amphotericin treatment.

Fusarium spp remain one of the most drug-resistant fungal species, with consistently high MICs demonstrated with most of the azoles, including itraconazole. The use of the newer triazoles, such as voriconazole, remains uncertain. In vitro testing of voriconazole against *Fusarium solani* revealed a range of MIC values *(55,56)* and a lack of fungicidal activity when compared with amphotericin B *(56)*. Clinical experience with the use of voriconazole for the treatment of *Fusarium* infections remains limited, although it has been successfully used for the treatment of a localized keratitis *(57)*. None of the currently available glucan synthesis inhibitors, such as caspofungin, demonstrate any useful activity against *Fusarium* spp *(58)*.

Most in vitro evidence suggests that amphotericin B has the best activity against *Fusarium* spp *(58,59)*, although there have been some reports of in vitro amphotericin resistance *(29,60)*. Anecdotal clinical success has been achieved using lipid formulations of amphotericin B *(61–63)* at high doses. The role of granulocyte infusions and granulocyte-macrophage colony-stimulator factor (GM-CSF) may have a role to play in the severely immunosuppressed patient *(64)*. Despite aggressive antifungal therapy, overall mortality rates remain high and may approach 100% in patients who remain persistently neutropenic *(65)*.

3.3. Aspergillus *Species*

Aspergillus is a filamentous fungus widespread throughout the environment, including soil and plant material. Over 185 species have been described. Clinical infection is usually ascribed to 20 species; the most important are *Aspergillus fumigatus* (90%), *A. flavus* (10%), *Aspergillus niger* (2%), *A. terreus* (2%), and *Aspergillus nidulans* (<1%) *(66)*.

Disease caused by *Aspergillus* can be classified into three categories: allergic disease, localized disease, and invasive disease. The incidence of invasive aspergillosis (IA) has been increasing since the late 1990s *(67)*. Risk factors for IA are well documented and include patients with hematological malignancy, solid organ transplant patients, patients with AIDs, and diabetics and other patients receiving prolonged corticosteroid therapy *(68)*. The most common manifestation of IA is with pulmonary disease, although this may vary depending on the patient population *(66)*. Other forms of IA include sinusitis *(69)*, cerebral aspergillosis, disseminated disease, and cutaneous disease (reviewed in ref. *70*).

Although IA incidence appears to be increasing, it is also important to note the gradual shift in the distribution of disease caused by the different species of *Aspergillus*, with an increasing proportion of disease attributable to *A. terreus* and *A. flavus* *(2,67)*. This has implications both for the laboratory identification of *Aspergillus* spp and for the choice of antifungal therapy.

The diagnosis of IA remains problematic and has led to the clinical categorization of patients according to the certainty of diagnosis *(71)*. Definitive proof of infection requires histopathological identification of fungal invasion or culture of the organism from a normally sterile site. Both methods of diagnosis may be difficult to obtain, especially as blood cultures are rarely positive in cases of IA. To improve the early diagnosis of IA, various other tests have been employed, including the use of high-resolution computed tomography scanning, antigen detection (galactomannan or 1-3-β-D-glucan), and the detection of fungal DNA in blood. These have been reviewed elsewhere *(72)*.

Amphotericin B has been the mainstay of treatment in IA, primarily because of its broad spectrum of activity against *Aspergillus*. The introduction of lipid-based preparations of amphotericin B has reduced the incidence of adverse infusion-related events and nephrotoxicity *(73)* associated with this drug, albeit at a financial cost. Primary resistance to amphotericin B in *Aspergillus* spp has not been well documented, and secondary resistance following therapy appears to be uncommon *(74)*.

Historically, in vitro susceptibility testing of aspergillus was hampered by a lack of standardization. Since then, guidelines for antifungal susceptibility testing for molds have been published by the NCCLS *(11)*. However, defined breakpoints for the classification of resistance have yet to be established, although a consensus appears to be emerging *(75)*. Based on previously published susceptibility testing, the MICs of different *Aspergillus* spp appear to lie within a relatively narrow range *(29,56)*, with a relatively low frequency of isolates with high MICs. Some isolates of *A. terreus* have been reported with increased MICs to amphotericin B *(76)*. Interestingly, these isolates are also associated with MLCs that were increased beyond normally achievable serum levels of conventional amphotericin B *(27,76)*, suggesting a lack of fungicidal activity.

Amphotericin resistance in *A. terreus* has been demonstrated in a murine model of disseminated aspergillosis *(77)*. Invasive disease in human hosts with *A. terreus* has been reported to be refractory to treatment with amphotericin and associated with higher mortality *(23,78)*, although the influence of host factors in these reported cases has generally not been examined.

Voriconazole has been demonstrated to have consistently low MICs for most *Aspergillus* species *(29,76)*, including *A. terreus*, although persistently high MLCs would seem to indicate that voriconazole lacks fungicidal activity against *Aspergillus* spp *(27,76)*. The role of voriconazole in the treatment of IA remains to be defined clearly. A recent randomized trial comparing the use of voriconazole versus conventional amphotericin B for the therapy of IA concluded that voriconazole achieved a better outcome than amphotericin B in all patient subgroups *(79)*. However, it is unclear if the superiority of voriconazole would have been maintained if a lipid preparation of amphotericin had been employed as treatment.

Of newer antifungal agents, the echinocandins appear to maintain low MICs against *Aspergillus* spp in general, including *A. terreus (37,80)*. Clinical experience with caspofungin in the treatment of IA remains limited *(81)*, although the use of this agent in combination with amphotericin B may hold promise for the future *(82)*.

Practice guidelines for the treatment of IA have been published by the Infectious Diseases Society of America (IDSA), which recommended that first-line therapy for IA is still amphotericin B or lipid preparations of amphotericin B *(83)*. These guidelines provided little clarification regarding the role of the triazoles and echinocandins in treatment or the role of antifungal susceptibility testing. Current practice probably dictates the commencement of standard therapy with amphotericin B for cases of IA; this therapy may then be altered according to clinical response, dose-limiting toxicity, or subsequent diagnostic laboratory results.

Despite the fact that most *Aspergillus* spp demonstrate in vitro susceptibility to amphotericin B, the mortality associated with IA has been considerable *(84)*, with mortality rates of 50–85% cited. Early diagnosis and treatment of IA appear to improve survival rates *(85)*, while restoration of host immunity plays a crucial role.

3.4. *Zygomycoses*

Zygomycoses are caused by the Mucorales, such as *Rhizomucor* spp, *Rhizopus* spp, *Mucor* spp, *Absidia corymbifera, Cunninghamella berthollettiae*, and members of the families Saksenaceae, Mortierellaceae, and Syncephalastracaea *(86)*. Rhinocerebral disease is the most recognized manifestation in leukemic and diabetic patients, but is rarely reported after transplantation. In this group of patients, sinonasal disease with pain, epistaxis, and congestion is the usual presentation, but pulmonary disease and disseminated disease resembling aspergillosis may occur *(87)*. Burn and trauma patients are at risk of wound infections, and desferrioxamine therapy is a specific risk factor.

Susceptibility testing is not standardized; although no resistance has been reported, outcome is very poor, and infection usually is fatal *(88)*. New antifungal agents have limited activity, and zygomycoses are best treated by lipid preparations of amphotericin B at dosages of 5 mg/kg body weight per day or higher in combination with aggressive surgical debridement *(89)*. Pulmonary zygomycosis also responds better to surgical resection *(90)*.

3.5. Scopulariopsis brevicaulis

Scopulariopsis brevicaulis is a filamentous fungus that is distributed widely in the environment. It is a common cause of onychomycosis, particularly of the toenails. Invasive disease is reported to occur in immunocompromised patients; and these invasions include brain abscesses *(91)*, endocarditis *(92)*, and disseminated disease. Very scanty susceptibility data are available for this organism. MICs for the azoles and flucytosine are consistently high, suggesting a lack of therapeutic activity; amphotericin and voriconazole have variable MICs *(93)*. Terbinafine may be effective for treatment of locally invasive disease *(94)*.

4. NATURALLY RESISTANT YEASTS

4.1. Trichosporon *Species*

Trichosporon is a yeast that is part of normal commensal flora in humans and is present in other animal species and the environment. Discussion about this organism is complicated by the proposed changes in taxonomy and nomenclature *(95)*. Previously, most invasive infections were attributable to two species: *T. beigelii* and *Trichosporon capitatum*. The latter has now been reclassified as *Blastoschizomyces capitatus*. *Trichosporon beigelii* (also known synonymously as *Trichosporon cutaneum*) has now been reclassified into six species, *T. cutaneum, Trichosporon asteroides, Trichosporon ovoides, Trichosporon inkin, Trichosporon asahii*, and *Trichosporon mucoides*. Some questions remain about the new classification scheme; for example, antifungal susceptibilities vary widely among the new species, and it is not known how the previously documented amphotericin resistance of *T. beigelii* applies to all six species. It will also be difficult to correlate previously published data on *T. beigelii* in the literature with the new taxonomic system.

Trichosporon spp are the cause of infections that range from asymptomatic colonization *(96)*, to superficial infections (e.g., of hair shafts, known as white piedra), to disseminated trichosporonosis. Disseminated disease is predominantly an opportunistic infection in immunosuppressed patients, although it has rarely been described in immunocompetent hosts *(97)*. Populations at risk include bone marrow and organ transplant recipients, premature infants *(98)*, and patients with indwelling vascular catheters *(99)*. Infective endocarditis has been described in patients with artificial heart valves *(100,101)*.

Invasive disease usually presents as a pyrexia with fungemia *(102)* and may progress to invasion of other body organs such as the kidney, spleen, eye, and lungs *(103)*. Widespread disease may be associated with cutaneous lesions that appear as scattered red papules. These may ulcerate and reveal fungal elements on biopsy *(104)*. Chronic disseminated infection with *T. asahii* resembling that of chronic disseminated disease caused by *Candida* spp has also been reported *(105)*.

Diagnosis of invasive disease, like that of most other fungal infections, requires clinical suspicion and microbiological confirmation. Blood cultures are frequently positive with this organism. Alternatively, the organism may be cultured from histological or biopsy specimens. Of note, false-positive *Cryptococcal* antigen results from serum may be noted because of interactions of cell wall antigens of this organism with the capsular polysaccharide antigens found in *Cryptococcus neoformans (106)*.

On culture, *Trichosporon* colonies are yeastlike; they rapidly grow with a characteristic wrinkled appearance that becomes more prominent with time. The colonies range from white to a waxy cream color. On cornmeal agar at 25°C after 72 h incubation, *Trichosporon* produces abundant pseudohyphae and true hyaline septate hyphae. The most typical microscopic feature of this genus is production of elongate arthroconidia. On histopathological specimens, the presence of pleomorphic yeast cells together with septate hyphae may be observed.

The antifungal susceptibility of this organism is complicated by the fact that most published work has been performed on *T. beigelii*. It remains unclear how these historical data will translate to the new taxonomic status of *Trichosporon* spp. Antifungal susceptibility testing for amphotericin B is also complicated by the different methodologies used *(101)*. Some clinical isolates of *T. beigelii* have increased amphotericin B MICs and MLCs, suggesting tolerance to this agent *(102)*.

There are laboratory data to suggest that azoles may have improved activity against *Trichosporon* spp *(107)*. The reported MICs for itraconazole appear to be lower than those reported for fluconazole, but there is little clinical evidence to support improved clinical efficacy. Of the new triazoles, posaconozole *(107)* and voriconazole *(108)* appear to have good in vitro activity. In contrast, the echinocandins *(80,107)* appear to have no useful activity against *Trichosporon* spp, and breakthrough infections with *Trichosporon* have been reported when a patient was treated with caspofungin *(109)*.

The optimum antifungal therapy for treatment of trichosporonosis remains to be resolved. It is clear that invasive disease is associated with significant mortality (64%

in one review; *103*), and that resolution of the underlying immunosuppression may be the most important factor in neutropenic patients *(110)*. Neutropenic animal models have shown a lack of efficacy with amphotericin B preparations *(111)*, and this may mirror the relatively unsuccessful use of amphotericin in clinical practice *(110,112)*. On the other hand, both experimental models *(111)* and clinical case reports *(105,112)* support the use of azole therapy such as with itraconazole or fluconazole. The use of the triazole agents such as voriconazole remains untested, although in vitro data appear promising.

4.2. Candida *Species*

In the early 1980s, the majority of candidemia was caused by *Candida albicans*. Since then, an epidemiological shift has occurred toward noncandida species, such as *C. glabrata, C. parapsilosis*, or *C. tropicalis (113)*. Although *C. albicans* has generally remained susceptible to the azoles, this may not necessarily be so for the other described *Candida* species.

The majority of *Candida* species remain susceptible to amphotericin on in vitro testing (summarized in ref. *114*). However, one of the difficulties with detecting amphotericin resistance in yeasts is that no clear consensus has emerged on the most effective antifungal susceptibility testing method for the detection of amphotericin resistance. The use of Etests® (AB Biodisk, Solna, Sweden) has been reported as superior to conventional NCCLS broth microdilution methods *(17,22)*. When using this susceptibility testing method, a 3-yr study of invasive bloodstream yeast isolates reported a 30% amphotericin resistance rate *(113)* when a breakpoint of 1 μg/mL was used. In addition, some striking differences in species susceptibility to amphotericin were noted, with approx 95% of *C. albicans* isolates inhibited by 1 μg/mL compared to only 41% of *C. glabrata* isolates and 0% of *C. krusei* isolates.

However, these data alone provide no information regarding the correlation between the selected breakpoints for resistance and clinical outcome. In addition, it is not known if the reported resistance was primary resistance or acquired resistance following prolonged antifungal therapy. Some *Candida* species have been associated with a propensity to develop resistance following treatment with amphotericin, particularly *C. guilliermondii (115)* and *C. lusitaniae (116)*. Testing of *C. lusitaniae* by NCCLS methods *(117)* and Etest *(118)* has generally failed to demonstrate in vitro resistance.

It is apparent that more work is required to establish the most appropriate susceptibility testing methods for yeasts and to develop accurate clinical breakpoints for the classification of amphotericin resistance. Until such time, current guidelines still suggest the use of amphotericin B to treat invasive candidal infections. However, clinicians should be aware of the possibility of antifungal resistance, particularly when treating infections caused by *C. lusitaniae, C. guilliermondii*, or *C. glabrata*. The selective use of antifungal susceptibility testing may help guide the choice of antifungal therapy in these clinical circumstances *(119)*. The clinical role of the newer antifungal drugs such as the triazole and glucan synthesis inhibitors remains to be elucidated.

5. MANAGEMENT OF INFECTION

Standard approaches to the management of systemic fungal infection are based on the use of amphotericin B, but the continued rise in the incidence of infections, the considerable mortality in immunocompromised patients, and the emergence of resistant species have led to a re-evaluation and the introduction of newer agents and more aggressive treatments. Despite the advances in antifungal therapy, it is important to remember that immunocompromised patients with systemic fungal infection may need a combination of fungicidal drugs, immunomodulation, and surgery.

5.1. Antifungal Drugs

Amphotericin B is a relatively toxic drug, with acute infusion-related side effects and significant renal toxicity. Because dose-limiting toxicity may result in suboptimal therapy, alternative preparations of amphotericin B have been developed. The entrapment of amphotericin B within a lipid carrier formulation has been shown to reduce both immediate infusion-related adverse events and nephrotoxicity. The postulated protective mechanism is thought to derive from increased transfer of the amphotericin B–lipid complex to ergosterol and reduced transfer to human cell membranes. Higher dosing regimens are possible and will achieve a greater therapeutic index, enabling consideration of treatment of "resistant" species.

There are three commercially available lipid formulations of amphotericin B. Amphotericin B lipid complex (Abelcet® or ABLC, Elan Phama Ltd., Stevanage, UK) consists of amphotericin B complexed with lipid bilayers in a "ribbonlike" structure. Amphotericin B colloidal dispersion (Amphocil® or ABCD Cambridge Labs, Newcastle, UK) consists of a lipid complex in a disklike structure. Finally, liposomal amphotericin B (AmBisome® or L-AmB, Gilead Sciences, Cambridge, UK) is the only formulation that contains true liposomal structures. All three lipid formulations differ significantly in their physical attributes; thus, they have different pharmacokinetics and plasma levels. Because of this, dose-to-dose equivalence has not been demonstrated, and dosage recommendations should be followed for each type of preparation used. Following intravenous administration, lipid-complexed formulations achieve higher tissue concentrations in the spleen, liver, and lungs and lower levels in the kidney, heart, and brain compared to the conventional formulation *(120)*.

Clinical data for all three lipid formulations were derived from case reports of treatment of fungal infections in patients intolerant or refractory to conventional amphotericin B *(121)* and clinical trials that compared the use of lipid preparations with conventional amphotericin B for the treatment of confirmed fungal infections (summarized in ref. *122*). A summary of the available data suggests that lipid formulations are of at least equal efficacy to conventional amphotericin B; the reduction in toxicity may allow dose escalation to overcome perceived resistance. There is little consensus on the indications for the initial use of lipid preparations of amphotericin. However, there are some data to suggest that lipid formulations may be a cost-effective alternative when the clinical and financial costs of nephrotoxicity related to amphotericin B are taken into consideration *(123,124)*. Similarly, there is little clear evidence on which invasive fungal infections should be treated with lipid formulations of amphotericin. However, based on the historically poor clinical response to zygomycotic infections, lipid-based preparations of amphotericin B at dosages ranging from 5 to 10 mg/kg body weight per day are probably the treatment of choice for these infections, usually in combination with surgical debridement.

Newer antifungal drugs have been introduced, some of which target novel synthetic pathways in fungi. The first of these compounds are the echinocandins, which inhibit β-(1,3)-glucan synthesis *(125)*. Caspofungin is the first agent in this class to be licensed for use. The spectrum of activity of the echinocandins suggests a limited role in the treatment of nonaspergillus molds *(37)*. The triazole agents such as voriconazole *(126)* and posaconazole represent the second generation of development of existing azoles. As with other members of the azole class, these agents act by inhibition of the cytochrome P450 pathway. Early data suggest that voriconazole demonstrates promising activity, particularly against *Fusarium* and *Scedosporium* spp.

5.2. Combination Therapy

The principle of using synergistic or additive antibiotics in combination in the treatment of bacterial infection is well established, particularly when dealing with serious infection in immunocompromised hosts. Extrapolation of the principle to the treatment of fungal infection appears logical, especially because the number of broad-spectrum antifungal agents available is increasing. Lipid preparations of amphotericin, newer triazole agents, echinocandins, and potentially synergistic combinations incorporating flucytosine or terbinafine have been used successfully. However, not all drugs are fungicidal against all species, and the results of in vitro susceptibility testing do not always accurately reflect clinical outcome. Animal models may show different pharmacokinetics. Decisions must be based on the individual patients, infecting species, and site of infection.

5.2.1. Amphotericin B Plus Flucytosine

There is good evidence to support the use of the combination of amphotericin B plus flucytosine in the treatment of cryptococcal disease; this evidence includes improvements in cure rates and time to sterilization of cerebrospinal fluid when compared to use of amphotericin B alone *(127)* and reduced relapse rates compared to fluconazole *(128)*.

In other fungal infections, data are more limited, and there are few randomized controlled trials. Amphotericin B and flucytosine are often advocated for the treatment of resistant candidal infections in neonates and for *Candida* endocarditis. Despite demonstration of in vitro synergy, good tissue penetration, and activity against resistant *Candida* species (e.g., *C. glabrata* and *C. lusitaniae*), there is little evidence that combinations of flucytosine are more effective than monotherapy *(119,129)*.

Little or no activity of flucytosine against molds can be demonstrated, and although some historical successes are reported *(130)*, the evidence for efficacy is absent *(83)*.

5.2.2. Amphotericin B and Azole Combinations

Theoretical considerations suggest that the combination of a cidal antifungal that binds to ergosterol (e.g., amphotericin B) and a fungistatic agent that reduces ergosterol synthesis (e.g., an azole) could potentially display antagonism through reduction in ergosterol binding sites and reduced polyene activity. In vitro evidence suggests this may be the case, and there is no rational basis for this combination in practice. Standardized methodologies (NCCLS) cannot identify interactions because MICs tend to distribute over a very narrow range, leading to a clustering effect that can mask significant interactions. Etesting methodologies clearly demonstrate inhibition between azoles, including newer triazole agents, and amphotericin B *(131)*. Time-kill studies showed little interaction when the two agents were given simultaneously, but showed antagonism when azole precedes polyene treatment *(132)*. With lipophilic azoles such as ketoconazole and itraconazole, the effect may be marked and prolonged, possibly through adsorption onto the cell surface *(133)*. Animal studies support the in vitro results, with antagonism demonstrated between amphotericin and fluconazole or itraconazole in mouse and rabbit models *(134,135)*.

5.3. Other Combinations

Terbinafine, an allylamine compound, is widely used for the treatment of superficial dermatophyte infections. However, in vitro susceptibility data suggest it may have a broader spectrum of activity and could be useful in the treatment of resistant candidal infection *(136)* and other systemic mycoses *(137)*. Synergy with azoles and amphotericin has been demonstrated *(138)*, and preliminary clinical studies confirm this, but further experience is needed *(139)*. Anecdotal data suggest that this could provide a useful strategy for the treatment of resistant species of fungi.

In vitro studies suggest some synergy between polyenes and echinocandins, but because caspofungin is the only licensed member of the group and has only recently become available for clinical use, information is limited *(82)*.

5.4. Immunomodulation

Patients with systemic infection display marked immune dysfunction. In addition, the immune response may be modulated by the fungus itself and at the level of the antigen-presenting cell.

5.4.1. Cytokines

Protective immune responses to fungal infection are dependant on a Th1-type response that requires the concerted effect of proinflammatory cytokines, including interferon gamma, tumor necrosis factor-α (TNF-α), interleukin-12 (IL-12), and IL-6 in the relative absence of Th2-type cytokines such as IL-4, IL-10, and transforming growth factor β *(140)*. T-cell responses in mice with candidosis are dose dependent: low levels of infection lead to Th1 responses and high levels to Th2 responses. Neutralization of interferon gamma and IL-12 leads to a Th2 response, whereas the addition of recombinant IL-2, soluble IL-4 receptors, or IL-10 monoclonal antibodies is protective *(141)*. Clinical data are limited, but interferon gamma is established as a useful agent in the prevention of fungal and other infections in patients with chronic granulomatous disease *(142)*. It is effective in mouse models of disseminated candidosis *(143)* and has been used in a few anecdotal cases of chronic infection in humans *(144)*.

5.4.2. Growth Factors

The widespread use of growth factors to ameliorate chemotherapy-induced neutropenia has significantly reduced the incidence of febrile neutropenia, although no survival benefit has been demonstrated. In addition to increasing phagocyte numbers, growth factors act as immunomodulators. GM-CSF has the broadest range of activities in terms of stimulating phagocytes and fungicidal killing capacity, followed by macrophage colony-stimulating factor (M-CSF) and granulocyte colony-stimulating factor (G-CSF) *(145)*. Growth factors and antifungal agents (including lipid preparations) may act synergically, and this may convert the fungistatic activity of many azole agents into a fungicidal one *(146)*.

Most studies have involved G-CSF; however, the anti-inflammatory effects of this growth factor, including decreased TNF and IL-12 and increased IL-10 production, may be significant *(147)*. Clinical evidence suggests that G-CSF post-transplantation can induce long-lasting Th2-type responses associated with defective immunity against fungal infection *(148)*. Such treatment could be detrimental in chronic fungal infection.

Growth factors with proinflammatory activity, such as GM-CSF, are more attractive. Other proinflammatory cytokines may have a role *(149)*. Most important, novel therapeutic strategies should consider ways of overcoming the defects in the host immune response *(140)*.

5.4.3. *Granulocyte Transfusions*

The ability to prime unrelated donors with G-CSF has overcome many of the earlier limitations of this treatment *(141)*. Resistant fungal infections may be an indication for such adjunctive therapy *(64)*.

5.4.4. *Surgery*

Historically, surgery has been limited by the concerns regarding perioperative morbidity and mortality associated with the presence of neutropenia and thrombocytopenia in many patients. However, many studies have reported low operative morbidity and improved survival rates, particularly for patients with aspergillosis and zygomycoses *(90,151–152)*.

Even multilobular disease may not be a contraindication to surgery as removal of a dominant focus may improve survival. It is likely that reduction of fungal load is immunomodulatory and can switch immune responses in much the same way as proinflammatory cytokines *(156)*.

6. CONCLUSIONS

Management of invasive fungal infections requires a multidisciplinary approach. Confidence in the predictive value of antifungal susceptibility testing is growing *(158)*, but the opportunist nature of fungal pathogens renders this of only secondary importance. Amphotericin B resistance is just one facet to be considered; ultimately, restoration of host defenses may be more important. Appreciation of the changing trends in fungal pathogens and the forces driving these changes, such as widespread azole prophylaxis, new immunosuppressive regimens, and modalities for transplantation, will increase understanding and inform management of the infections.

REFERENCES

1. Rees JR, Pinner RW, Hajjeh RA, Brandt ME, Reingold AL. The epidemiological features of invasive mycotic infections in the San Francisco Bay area, 1992–1993: results of population-based laboratory active surveillance. Clin Infect Dis 1998; 27:1138–1147.
2. Marr KA, Carter RA, Crippa F, et al. Epidemiology and outcome of mould infections in hematopoietic stem cell transplant recipients. Clin Infect Dis 2002; 34:909–917.
3. White TC, Marr KA, Bowden RA. Clinical, cellular, and molecular factors that contribute to antifungal drug resistance. Clin Microbiol Rev 1998; 11:382–402.
4. Vanden Bossche H, Marichal P, Odds FC. Molecular mechanisms of drug resistance in fungi. Trends Microbiol 1994; 2:393–400.
5. Broughton MC, Bard M, Lees ND. Polyene resistance in ergosterol producing strains of *Candida albicans*. Mycoses 1991; 34:75–83.

6. JosephHorne T, Loeffler RST, Hollomon DW, et al. Amphotericin B resistant isolates of *Cryptococcus neoformans* without alteration in sterol biosynthesis. J Med Vet Mycol 1996; 34:223–225.
7 Seo K, Akiyoshi H, Ohnishi Y. Alteration of cell wall composition leads to amphotericin B resistance in *Aspergillus flavus*. Microbiol Immunol 1999; 43:1017–1025.
8. Younsi M, Ramanandraibe E, Bonaly R, et al. Amphotericin B resistance and membrane fluidity in *Kluyveromyces lactis* strains. Antimicrob Agents Chemother 2000; 44:1911–1916.
9. Kontoiannis D. Why prior fluconazole use is associated with an increased risk of invasive mold infections in immunosuppressed hosts; an alternative hypothesis. Clin Infect Dis 2002; 34:1281–1283.
10. McClenny NB, Fei HH, Baron EJ, et al. Change in colony morphology of *Candida lusitaniae* in association with development of amphotericin B resistance. Antimicrob Agents Chemother 2002; 46:1325–1328.
11. National Committee for Clinical Laboratory Standards. Reference Method for Broth Dilution Antifungal Susceptibility Testing of Conidium-Forming Filamentous Fungi; Proposed Standard. Wayne, PA: National Committee for Clinical Laboratory Standards, 1998. NCCLS document M38-P.
12. National Committee for Clinical Laboratory Standards. Reference Method for Broth Dilution Antifungal Susceptibility Testing of Yeasts; Approved Standard. Wayne, PA: National Committee for Clinical Laboratory Standards, 1998. NCCLS document M27-A.
13. Johnson EM, Oakley KL, Radford SA, et al. Lack of correlation of in vitro amphotericin B susceptibility testing with outcome in a murine model of *Aspergillus* infection. J Antimicrob Chemother 2000; 45:85–93.
14. Nguyen MH, Clancy CJ, Yu VL, et al. Do in vitro susceptibility data predict the microbiologic response to amphotericin B? Results of a prospective study of patients with *Candida* fungemia. J Infect Dis 1998; 177:425–430.
15. Szekely A, Johnson EM, Warnock DW. Comparison of E-test and broth microdilution methods for antifungal drug susceptibility testing of molds. J Clin Microbiol 1999; 37:1480–1483.
16. Peyron F, Favel A, Michel-Nguyen A, et al. Improved detection of amphotericin B-resistant isolates of *Candida lusitaniae* by Etest. J Clin Microbiol 2001; 39:339–342.
17. Pfaller MA, Messer SA, Bolmstrom A. Evaluation of Etest for determining in vitro susceptibility of yeast isolates to amphotericin B. Diagn Microbiol Infect Dis 1998; 32:223–227.
18. Lozano-Chiu M, Lancaster MV, Rex JH. Evaluation of a colorimetric method for detecting amphotericin B–resistant *Candida* isolates. Diagn Microbiol Infect Dis 1998; 31:417–424.
19. Arendrup M, Lundgren B, Jensen IM, et al. Comparison of Etest and a tablet diffusion test with the NCCLS broth microdilution method for fluconazole and amphotericin B susceptibility testing of *Candida* isolates. J Antimicrob Chemother 2001; 47; 521–526.
20. Favel A, Peyron F, De Meo M, et al. Amphotericin B susceptibility testing of *Candida lusitaniae* isolates by flow cytofluorometry: comparison with the Etest and the NCCLS broth macrodilution method. J Antimicrob Chemother 1999; 43:227–232.
21. VanEldere J, Joosten L, Verhaeghe A, et al. Fluconazole and amphotericin B antifungal susceptibility testing by National Committee for Clinical Laboratory Standards broth macrodilution method compared with E-test and semiautomated broth microdilution test. J Clin Microbiol 1996; 34:842–847.
22. Clancy CJ, Nguyen MH. Correlation between in vitro susceptibility determined by Etest and response to therapy with amphotericin B: results from a multicenter prospective study of candidemia. Antimicrob Agents Chemother 1999; 43:1289–1290.
23. Lass-Florl C, Kofler G, Kropshofer G, et al. In-vitro testing of susceptibility to amphotericin B is a reliable predictor of clinical outcome in invasive aspergillosis. J Antimicrob Chemother 1998; 42:497–502.

24. Edwards JE Jr, Bodey GP, Bowden RA, et al. International conference for the development of a consensus on the management and prevention of severe candidal infections. Clin Infect Dis 1997; 25:43–59.
25. Nagata MP, Gentry CA, Hampton EM. Is there a therapeutic or pharmakinetic rationale for amphotericin B dosing in systemic *Candida* infection? Ann Pharmacother 1996; 30:811–818.
26. Espinel-Ingroff A. Comparison of the E-test with the NCCLS M38-P method for antifungal susceptibility testing of common and emerging pathogenic filamentous fungi. J Clin Microbiol 2001; 39:1360–1367.
27. Espinel-Ingroff A. In vitro fungicidal activities of voriconazole, itraconazole, and amphotericin B against opportunistic moniliaceous and dematiaceous fungi. J Clin Microbiol 2001; 39:954–958.
28. Pfaller MA, Messer SA, Hollis RJ, et al. Antifungal activities of posaconazole, ravuconazole, and voriconazole compared to those of itraconazole and amphotericin B against 239 clinical isolates of *Aspergillus* spp and other filamentous fungi: report from SENTRY Antimicrobial Surveillance Program. Antimicrob Agents Chemother 2002; 46: 1032–1037.
29. Arikan S, Lozano-Chiu M, Paetznic V, Nangia S, Rex JH. Microdilution susceptibility testing of amphotericin B, itraconazole, and voriconazole against clinical isolates of *Aspergillus* and *Fusarium* species. J Clin Microbiol 1999; 37:3946–3951.
30. Salkin IF, McGinnis MR, Dykstra MJ, et al. *Scedosporium inflatum*, an emerging pathogen. J Clin Microbiol 1988; 26:498–503.
31. Gillum PS, Gurswamy A, Taira JW. Localized cutaneous infection by *Scedosporium prolificans (inflatum)*. Int J Dermatol 1997; 36:297 299.
32. Berenguer JJ, Rodriguez-Tudela L, Richard C, et al. Deep infections caused by *Scedosporium prolificans*. A report on 16 cases in Spain and a review of the literature. *Scedosporium prolificans* Spanish Study Group. Medicine (Baltimore) 1997; 76:256–265.
33. Idigoras P, Perez-Trallero E, Pineiro L, et al. Disseminated infection and colonization by *Scedosporium prolificans*: a review of 18 cases, 1990–1999. Clin Infect Dis 2001; 32: e158–e165.
34. Maertens J, Lagrou K, Deweerdt H, et al. Disseminated infection by *Scedosporium prolificans*: an emerging fatality amongst haematology patients. Case report and review. Ann Haematol 2000; 79:340–344.
35. Pickles RW, Pacey DE, Muir DB, Herrell WH. Experience with infection by *Scedosporium prolificans* including apparent cure with fluconazole therapy. J Infect 1996; 33:193–197.
36. Cuenca-Estrella M, Ruiz-Díez B, Martínez-Suárez JV, et al. Comparative in-vitro activity of voriconazole (UK-109,496) and six other antifungal agents against clinical isolates of *Scedosporium prolificans* and *Scedosporium apiospermum*. J Antimicrob Chemother 1999; 43:149–151.
37. Del Poeta M, Schell WA, Perfect JR. In vitro antifungal activity of pneumocandin L-743,872 against a variety of clinically important molds. Antimicrob Agents Chemother 1997; 41:1835–1836.
38. Radford SA, Johnson EM, Warnock DW. In vitro studies of activity of voriconazole (UK-109,496), a new triazole antifungal agent, against emerging and less-common mold pathogens. Antimicrob Agents Chemother 1997; 41:841–843.
39. Meletiadis J, Mouton JW, Rodríguez-Tudela JL, et al. In vitro interaction of terbinafine with itraconazole against clinical isolates of *Scedosporium prolificans*. Antimicrob Agents Chemother 2000; 44:470–472.
40. Bouza E, Muñoz P, Vega L, et al. Clinical resolution of *Scedosporium prolificans* fungemia associated with reversal of neutropenia following administration of granulocyte colony-stimulating factor. Clin Infect Dis 1996; 23:192–193.
41. Kiraz N, Gulbas Z, Akgun Y, Uzun O. Lymphadenitis caused by *Scedosporium apiospermum* in an immunocompetent patient. Clin Infect Dis 2001; 32:e59–e61.

42. O'Bryan TA, Browne FA, Schonder JF. *Scedosporium apiospermum (Pseudallescheria boydii)* endocarditis. J Infect 2002; 44:189–192.
43. Mellinghoff IK, Winston DJ, Mukwaya G, Schiller GJ. Treatment of *Scedosporium apiospermum* brain abscesses with posaconazole. Clin Infect Dis 2002; 15; 34:1648–1650.
44. Rollot F, Blanche P, Richaud-Thiriez B, et al. Pneumonia due to *Scedosporium apiospermum* in a patient with HIV infection. Scand J Infect Dis 2000; 32:439.
45. Nomdedeu J, Brunet S, Martino R, et al. Successful treatment of pneumonia due to *Scedosporium apiospermum* with itraconazole: case report. Clin Infect Dis 1993; 16:731–733.
46. Raj R, Frost AE. *Scedosporium apiospermum* fungemia in a lung transplant recipient. Chest 2002; 121:1714–1716.
47. Hachimi-Idrissi SM, Willemsen B, Desprechins A, et al. *Pseudallescheria boydii* and brain abscesses. Pediatr Infect Dis J 1990; 9:737–741.
48. Meletiadis J, Meis JF, Mouton JW, et al. In vitro activities of new and conventional antifungal agents against clinical *Scedosporium* isolates. Antimicrob Agents Chemother 2002; 46:62–68.
49. Nesky MA, McDougal EC, Peacock JE Jr. *Pseudallescheria boydii* brain abscess successfully treated with voriconazole and surgical drainage: case report and literature review of central nervous system pseudallescheriasis. Clin Infect Dis 2000; 31:673–677.
50. Munoz P, Marin M, Tornero P, et al. Successful outcome of *Scedosporium apiospermum* disseminated infection treated with voriconazole in a patient receiving corticosteroid therapy. Clin Infect Dis 2000; 31:1499–1501.
51. Carrillo AJ, Guarro J. In vitro activities of four novel triazoles against *Scedosporium* spp. Antimicrob Agents Chemother 2001; 45:2151–2153.
52. Nelson PE, Dignani MC, Anaissie EJ. Taxonomy, biology, and clinical aspects of *Fusarium* species. Clin Microbiol Rev 1994; 7:479–504.
53. Boutati EI, Anaissie EJ. *Fusarium*, a significant emerging pathogen in patients with hematologic malignancy: 10 years' experience at a cancer center and implications for management. Blood 1997; 90:999–1008.
54. Hue FX, Huerre M, Rouffault MA, de Bievre C. Specific detection of *Fusarium* species in blood and tissues by a PCR technique. J Clin Microbiol 1999; 37:2434–2438.
55. Espinel-Ingroff A. In vitro activity of the new triazole voriconazole (UK-109,496) against opportunistic filamentous and dimorphic fungi and common and emerging yeast pathogens. J Clin Microbiol 1998; 36:198–202.
56. Johnson EM, Szekely A, Warnock DW. In-vitro activity of voriconazole, itraconazole and amphotericin B against filamentous fungi. J Antimicrob Chemother 1998; 42:741–745.
57. Reis A, Sundmacher R, Tintelnot K, Agostini H, Jensen HE, Althaus C. Successful treatment of ocular invasive mould infection (fusariosis) with the new antifungal agent voriconazole. Br J Ophthalmol 2000; 84:932–933.
58. Arikan S, Lozano-Chiu M, Paetznick V, Rex JH. In vitro susceptibility testing methods for caspofungin against *Aspergillus* and *Fusarium* isolates. Antimicrob Agents Chemother 2001; 45:327–330.
59. Rotowa NA, Shadomy HJ, Shadomy S. In vitro activities of polyene and imidazole antifungal agents against unusual opportunistic fungal pathogens. Mycoses 1990; 33:203–211.
60. Reuben A, Anaissie E, Nelson PE, Hashem R, Legrand C, Ho DH, Bodey GP. Antifungal susceptibility of 44 clinical isolates of *Fusarium* species determined by using a broth microdilution method. Antimicrob Agents Chemother 1989; 33:1647–1649.
61. Sampathkumar P, Paya CV. Fusarium infection after solid-organ transplantation. Clin Infect Dis 2001; 32:1237–1240.
62. Walsh TJ, Hiemenz JW, Seibel N, et al. Amphotericin lipid complex in patients with invasive fungal infections: analysis of safety and efficacy in 556 cases. Clin Infect Dis 1998; 26:1383–1396.

63. Cofrancesco E, Boschetti C, Viviani MA, et al. Efficacy of liposomal amphotericin B (AmBisome) in the eradication of *Fusarium* infection in a leukaemic patient. Haematologica 1992; 77:280–283.
64. Spielberger, RT, Falleroni MJ, Coene AJ, Larson RA. Concomitant amphotericin B therapy, granulocyte transfusions, and GM-CSF administration for disseminated infection with *Fusarium* in a granulocytopenic patient. Clin Infect Dis 1993; 16:528–530.
65. Groll AH, Walsh TJ. Uncommon opportunistic fungi: new nosocomial threats. Clin Microbiol Infect 2001; 7(suppl. 2):8–24.
66. Denning DW. *Aspergillus* species. In: Mandel GL, Bennett JE, Dolin R (eds.). Principles and Practice of Infectious Diseases. 5th ed. Philadelphia: Churchill Livingston, 2000, pp. 2674–2685.
67. Singh N. Trends in the epidemiology of opportunistic fungal infections: predisposing factors and the impact of antimicrobial use practices. Clin Infect Dis 2001; 33:1692–1696.
68. Manuel RJ, Kibbler CC. The epidemiology and prevention of invasive aspergillosis. J Hosp Infect 1998; 39:95–109.
69. Iwen PC, Rupp ME, Hinrichs SH. Invasive mold sinusitis: 17 cases in immunocompromised patients and review of the literature. Clin Infect Dis 1997; 24:1178–1184.
70. Denning DW. Invasive aspergillosis. Clin Infect Dis 1998; 26:781–805.
71. Ascioglu S, Rex JH, de Pauw B, et al. Defining opportunistic invasive fungal infections in immunocompromised patients with cancer and hematopoietic stem cell transplants: an international consensus. Clin Infect Dis 2002; 34:7–14.
72. Klont RR, Meis JF, Verweij PE. Critical assessment of issues in the diagnosis of invasive aspergillosis. Clin Microbiol Infect 2001; 7(suppl. 2):32–37.
73. Dupont B. Overview of the lipid formulations of amphotericin B. J Antimicrob Chemother 2002; 49(suppl. S1):31–36.
74. Moosa MY, Alangaden GJ, Manavathu E, Chandrasekar PH. Resistance to amphotericin B does not emerge during treatment for invasive aspergillosis. J Antimicrob Chemother 2002; 49:209–213.
75. Ellis D. Amphotericin B: spectrum and resistance. J Antimicrob Chemother 2002; 49(suppl. S1):7–10.
76. Sutton DA, Sanche SE, Revankar SG, Fothergill AW, Rinaldi MG. In vitro amphotericin B resistance in clinical isolates of *Aspergillus terreus*, with a head-to-head comparison to voriconazole. J Clin Microbiol 1999; 37:2343–2345.
77. Dannaoui E, Borel E, Persat F, Piens MA, Picot S. Amphotericin B resistance of *Aspergillus terreus* in a murine model of disseminated aspergillosis. J Med Microbiol 2000; 49: 601–606.
78. Iwen PC, Rupp ME, Langnas AN, Reed EC, Hinrichs SH. Invasive pulmonary aspergillosis due to *Aspergillus terreus*: 12-year experience and review of the literature. Clin Infect Dis 1998; 26:1092–1097.
79. Herbrecht R, Denning DW, Patterson TF, et al. Voriconazole versus amphotericin B for primary therapy of invasive aspergillosis. N Engl J Med 2002; 347:408–415.
80. Espinel-Ingroff A. Comparison of in vitro activities of the new triazole SCH56592 and the echinocandins MK-0991 (L-743,872) and LY303366 against opportunistic filamentous and dimorphic fungi and yeasts. J Clin Microbiol 1998; 36:2950–2956.
81. Koss T, Bagheri B, Zeana C, Romagnoli MF, Grossman ME. Amphotericin B-resistant *Aspergillus flavus* infection successfully treated with caspofungin, a novel antifungal agent. J Am Acad Dermatol 2002; 46:945–947.
82. Arikan S, Lozano-Chiu M, Paetznick V, Rex JH. In vitro synergy of caspofungin and amphotericin B against *Aspergillus* and *Fusarium* spp. Antimicrob Agents Chemother 2002; 46:245–247.
83. Stevens DA, Kan VL, Judson MA, et al. Practice guidelines for diseases caused by *Aspergillus*. Infectious Diseases Society of America. Clin Infect Dis 2000; 30:696–709.

84. Denning DW. Therapeutic outcome in invasive aspergillosis. Clin Infect Dis 1996; 23:608–615.
85. Aisner J, Wiernik PH, Schimpff SC. Treatment of invasive aspergillosis: relation of early diagnosis and treatment to response. Ann Intern Med 1977; 86:539–543.
86. Sugar AM. Mucormycosis. Clin Infect Dis 1992; 14(suppl. 1):s126–s129.
87. Morrison VA, McGlave PB. Mucormycosis in the BMT population. Bone Marrow Transplant 1993; 11:383–388.
88. Kontoyiannis DP, Wessel VC, Bodey GP, Rolston KVI. Zygomycosis in the 1990s in a tertiary-care cancer center. Clin Infect Dis 2000; 30:851–856.
89. Ribes JA, Vanover-Sams CL, Baker DJ. Zygomycetes in human disease. Clin Microbiol Rev 2000; 13:236–301.
90. Tedder M, Spratt JA, Anstadt MP, Hedge SS, Tedder SD, Lowe JE. Pulmonary mucormycosis: results of medical and surgical therapy. Ann Thorac Surg 1994; 57:1044–1050.
91. Hagensee ME, Bauwens JE, Kjos B, Bowden RA. Brain abscess following marrow transplantation: experience at the Fred Hutchinson Cancer Research Center, 1984–1992. Clin Infect Dis 1984; 19:402–408.
92. Migrino RQ, Hall GS, Longworth DL. Deep tissue infections caused by *Scopulariopsis brevicaulis*: report of a case of prosthetic valve endocarditis and review. Clin Infect Dis 1995; 21:672–674.
93. Aguilar C, Pujol I, Guarro J. In vitro antifungal susceptibilities of *Scopulariopsis* isolates. Antimicrob Agents Chemother 1999; 43:1520–1522.
94. Sellier P, Monsuez JJ, Lacroix C, et al. Recurrent subcutaneous infection due to *Scopulariopsis brevicaulis* in a liver transplant recipient. Clin Infect Dis 2000; 30: 820–833.
95. Gueho EM, Smith T, de Hoog GS, et al. Contributions to a revision of the genus *Trichosporon*. Antonie Van Leeuwenhoek 1992; 61:289–316.
96. Lussier N, Laverdiere M, Delorme J, Weiss K, Dandavino R. *Trichosporon beigelii* funguria in renal transplant recipients. Clin Infect Dis 2000; 31:1299–1301.
97. Ebright JR, Fairfax MR, Vazquez JA. *Trichosporon asahii*, a non-candida yeast that caused fatal septic shock in a patient without cancer or neutropenia. Clin Infect Dis 2001; 33:e28–e30.
98. Yoss BS, Sautter RL, Brenker HJ. *Trichosporon beigelii*, a new neonatal pathogen. Am J Perinatol 1997; 14:113–117.
99. Finkelstein R, Singer P, Lefler E. Catheter-related fungemia caused by *Trichosporon beigelii* in non-neutropenic patients. Am J Med 1989; 86:133.
100. Martinez-Lacasa J, Mana J, et al. Long-term survival of a patient with prosthetic valve endocarditis due to *Trichosporon beigelii*. Eur J Clin Microbiol Infect Dis 1991; 10: 756–758.
101. Keay S, Denning DW, Stevens DA. Endocarditis due to *Trichosporon beigelii*: in vitro susceptibility of isolates and review. Rev Infect Dis 1991; 13:383–386.
102. Walsh TJ, Melcher GP, Rinaldi MG, et al. *Trichosporon beigelii*, an emerging pathogen resistant to amphotericin B. J Clin Microbiol 1990; 28:1616–1622.
103. Kremery V, Krupova I, Denning DW. Invasive yeast infections other than *Candida* spp in acute leukaemia. J Hosp Infect 1999; 41:181–194.
104. Nahass GT, Rosenberg SP, Leonardi CL, Pennys NS. Disseminated infection with *Trichospororon beigelii*. Report of a case and review of the cutaneous and histologic manifestations. Arch Dermatol 1993; 129:1020–1023.
105. Meyer MH, Letscher-Bru V, Waller J, et al. Chronic disseminated *Trichosporon asahii* infection in a leukemic child. Clin Infect Dis 2002; 35:e22–e25.
106. McManus EJ, Jones JM. Detection of *Trichosporon beigelii* antigen cross-reactive with *Cryptococcus neoformans* capsular polysaccharide in serum from a patient with disseminated *Trichosporon* infection. J Clin Microbiol 1985; 21:681–685.

107. Tawara S, Ikeda F, Maki K, et al. In vitro activities of a new lipopeptide antifungal agent, FK463, against a variety of clinically important fungi. Antimicrob Agents Chemother 2000; 44:57–62.
108. McGinnis MR, Pasarell L, Sutton DA, et al. In vitro evaluation of voriconazole against some clinically important fungi. Antimicrob Agents Chemother 1997; 41:1832–1834.
109. Goodman D, Pamer E, Jakubowski A, Morris C, Sepkowitz K. Breakthrough trichosporonosis in a bone marrow transplant recipient receiving caspofungin acetate. Clin Infect Dis 2002; 35:e35–e36.
110. Erer B, Galimberti M, Lucarelli G, et al. *Trichosporon beigelii*: a life-threatening pathogen in immunocompromised hosts. Bone Marrow Transplant 2000; 25:745–749.
111. Walsh TJ, Lee JW, Melcher GP, et al. Experimental disseminated trichosporonosis in persistently granulocytopenic rabbits: implications for pathogenesis, diagnosis and treatment of an emerging pathogen. J Infect Dis 1992; 166:121–133.
112. Anaissie E, Gokoslan A, Hachem R, Rubin R. Azole therapy for trichosporoniasis: clinical evaluation of eight patients, experimental therapy for murine infection, and review. Clin Infect Dis 1992; 15:781–787.
113. Pfaller MA, Diekema DJ, Jones RN, et al. International surveillance of bloodstream infections due to *Candida* species: frequency of occurrence and in vitro susceptibilities to fluconazole, ravuconazole, and voriconazole of isolates collected from 1997 through 1999 in the SENTRY antimicrobial surveillance program. J Clin Microbiol 2001; 39:3254–3259.
114. Hazen KC. New and emerging yeast pathogens. Clin Microbiol Rev 1995; 8:462–478.
115. Dick JD, Rosengard BR, Merz WG, et al. Fatal disseminated candidiasis due to amphotericin-B-resistant *Candida guilliermondii*. Ann Intern Med 1985,102:67–68.
116. Pappagianis D, Collins MS, Hector R, Remington J. Development of resistance to amphotericin B in *Candida lusitaniae* infecting a human. Antimicrob Agents Chemother 1979; 16:123–126.
117. Barchiesi F, Tortorano AM, Di Francesco LF, et al. In-vitro activity of five antifungal agents against uncommon clinical isolates of *Candida* spp. J Antimicrob Chemother 1999; 43:295–299.
118. Favel A, Michel-Nguyen A, Chastin C, et al. In-vitro susceptibility pattern of *Candida lusitaniae* and evaluation of the Etest method. J Antimicrob Chemother 1997; 39: 591–596.
119. Rex JH, Walsh TJ, Sobel JD, et al. Practice guidelines for the treatment of candidiasis. Clin Infect Dis 2000; 30:662–678.
120. Wasan KM, Lopez-Berenstein G. Characteristics of lipid-based formulations that influence their biological behaviour in the plasma of patients. Clin Infect Dis 1996; 23:1126–1138.
121. Wong-Beringer A, Jacobs RA, Guglielmo BJ. Lipid formulations of amphotericin B: clinical efficacy and toxicity. Clin Infect Dis 1998; 27:603–618.
122. Hann IM, Prentice HG. Lipid-based amphotericin B: a review of the last 10 years of use. Int J Antimicrob Agents 2001; 17:161–169.
123. Bates DW, Su L, Yu DT, et al. Mortality and costs of acute renal failure associated with amphotericin B therapy. Clin Infect Dis 2001; 2:686–693.
124. Wingard JR, Kubilis P, Lee L, et al. Clinical significance of nephrotoxicity in patients treated with amphotericin B for suspected or proven aspergillosis. Clin Infect Dis 1999; 29:1402–1407.
125. Denning DW. Echinocandins and candins—a new antifungal class with a novel mode of action. J Antimicrob Chemother 1997; 40:611–614.
126. Sabo JA, Abdel-Rahman SM. Voriconazole: a new triazole antifungal. Ann Pharmacother 2000; 34:1032–1043.
127. Bennett JE, Dismukes WE, Duma RJ, et al. A comparison of amphotericin B alone and combined with flucytosine in the treatment of cryptococcal meningitis. N Engl J Med 1979; 301:126–131.

128. Larsen RA, Leal MA, Chan LS. Fluconazole compared with amphotericin B plus flucytosine for cryptococcal meningitis in AIDS. A randomized trial. Ann Intern Med 1990; 113:183–187.
129. Abele-Horn M, Kopp A, Sternberg U, et al. A randomized study comparing fluconazole with amphotericin B/5-flucytosine for the treatment of systemic *Candida* infections in intensive care patients. Infection 1996; 24:426–432.
130. Denning DW, Stevens DA. Antifungal and surgical treatment of invasive aspergillosis: review of 2,121 published cases. Rev Infect Dis 1990; 12:1147–1201.
131. Lewis RE, Kontoyiannis DP. Rationale for combination antifungal therapy. Pharmacotherapy 2001; 21:149s–164s.
132. Lewis RE, Lund BC, Klepser ME, Ernst EJ, Pfaller MA. Assessment of antifungal activities of fluconazole and amphotericin administered alone and in combination against a *C. albicans* using a dynamic in vitro mycotic infection model. Antimicrob Agents Chemother 1998; 42:1382–1386.
133. Scheven M, Schwegler F. Antagonistic interactions between azoles and AmB with yeasts depend on azole lipophilia for special test conditions in vitro. Antimicrob Agents Chemother 1995; 39:1779–1783.
134. Sanati H, Ramos CF, Bayer AS, Ghannoum MA. Combination therapy with amphotericin B and fluconazole against invasive candidiasis in neutropenic-mouse and infective-endocarditis rabbit models. Antimicrob Agents Chemother 1997; 41:1345–1348.
135. Le Monte, Washum KE, Smedema ML, Schnizlein-Bick C, Kohler SM, Wheat LJ. Amphotericin B combined with itraconazole or fluconazole for treatment of histoplasmosis. J Infect Dis 2000; 182:545–550.
136. Ghannoum MA, Elewski B. Successful treatment of fluconazole-resistant oropharyngeal candidiasis by a combination of fluconazole and terbinafine. Clin Diag Lab Immunol 1999; 6:921–923.
137. Balfour JA, Faulds D. Terbinafine: a review of its pharmacodynamic and pharmacokinetic properties and therapeutic potential in superficial mycoses. Drugs 1992; 43:259–284.
138. Jessup CJ, Ryder NS, Ghannoum MA. An evaluation of the in vitro activity of terbinafine. Med Mycol 2000; 38:155–159.
139. Hay R. Therapeutic potential of terbinafine in subcutaneous and systemic mycoses. Br J Dermatol 1999; 141(suppl. 56):36–40.
140. Romani L. Host immune reactivity and antifungal chemotherapy: the power of being together. J Chemother 2001; 13:347–353.
141. Mencaci A, Cenci E, Bacci A, Bistoni, Romani FL. Host immune reactivity determines the efficacy of combination immunotherapy and antifungal chemotherapy in candidiasis. J Infect Dis 2000; 181:686–694.
142. Gallin JI, Malech HL, Weening RS, et al. The International Chronic Granulomatous Disease Cooperative Study Group (1991). A controlled trial of interferon gamma to prevent infection in chronic granulomatous disease. N Engl J Med 1991; 324:509–516.
143. Van der Meer JWM, Vogels MTE, Netea MG, Kullberg BJ. Proinflammatory cytokines and treatment of disease. Ann N Y Acad Sci 1998; 856:243–251.
144. Poynton CH, Barnes RA, Rees J. Interferon gamma in the treatment of deep-seated fungal infection in acute leukemia. Clin Infect Dis 1998; 26:239–240.
145. Stevens DA, Walsh TJ, Bistoni F, et al. Cytokines and mycoses. Med Mycol 1998; (suppl. 36):174–182.
146. Natarajan U, Randhawa N, Brummer E, et al. Effect of granulocyte-macrophage colony-stimulating factor on candidacidal activity of neutrophils, monocytes or monocyte-derived macrophages and synergy with fluconazole. J Med Microbiol 1998; 47:359–363.
147. Hartung T, Docke W-D, Gantner F, et al. Effect of granulocyte colony-stimulating factor treatment on ex vivo blood cytokine response in human volunteers. Blood 1995; 85:2482–2489.

148. Volpi I, Perruccio K, Tosti A, et al. Postgrafting administration of granulocyte colony-stimulating factor impairs functional immune recovery in recipients of human leukocyte antigen haplotype-mismatched hematopoietic transplants. Blood 2001; 97:2514–2521.
149. Cenci E, Mencacci A, Del Sero G, Bistoni F, Romani L. Induction of protective Th1 responses to *Candida albicans* by antifungal therapy alone or in combination with an interleukin-4 antagonist. J Infect Dis 1997; 176:217–226.
150. Hubel K, Dale DC, Liles WC. Granulocyte transfusion therapy: update on potential clinical applications. Curr Opin Hematol 2001; 8:161–164.
151. Wong K, Waters CM, Walesby RK. Surgical management of invasive pulmonary aspergillosis in immunocompromised patients. Eur J Cardiothorac Surg 1992; 6:138–143.
152. Young VK, Maghur HA, Luke DA, et al. Operation for cavitating invasive pulmonary aspergillosis in immunocompromised patients. Ann Thorac Surg 1992; 53:621–624.
153. Robinson LA, Reed EC, Galbraith TA, et al. Pulmonary resection for invasive aspergillus infections in immunocompromised patients. J Thoracic Cardiovasc Surg 1995; 109: 1182–1197.
154. Caillot D, Casasnovas O, Bernard A, et al. Improved management of invasive pulmonary aspergillosis in neutropenic patients using early thoracic computed tomographic scan and surgery. J Clin Oncol 1997; 15:139–147.
155. Salerno CT, Ouyang DW, Pederson TS, et al. Surgical therapy for pulmonary aspergillosis in immunocompromised patients. Ann Thorac Surg 1998; 65:1415–1419.
156. Mencaci A, Cenci E, Bacci A, Bistoni F, Romani L. Host immune reactivity determines the efficacy of combination immunotherapy and antifungal chemotherapy in candidiasis. J Infect Dis 2001; 181; 686–694.
157. Rex JH, Pfaller MA Has antifungal susceptibility testing come of age? Clin Infect Dis 2002; 35:982–989.

18

Management of Multiple Drug-Resistant Malaria

Elizabeth Ashley and François Nosten

1. INTRODUCTION

Each year, malaria accounts for more deaths worldwide than any other parasitic disease, with mortality estimates of between 1.5 and 2.7 million *(1)*. Malaria not only is associated with huge morbidity and mortality, but also it hampers economic growth, trapping endemic countries in a cycle of poverty and disease *(2–4)*. The main disease burden is in Africa, and there is evidence that the incidence of malaria is increasing, as is childhood mortality. This may be directly attributed to the emergence and spread of chloroquine-resistant strains *(5)*. Faced with this disaster and the rapidly declining efficacy of sulfadoxine-pyrimethamine in East African countries, national malaria control programs are struggling with the decision of which treatment to recommend next *(6,7)*.

In Southeast Asia, this problem of multiple drug resistance of *Plasmodium falciparum* is not new. Chloroquine resistance was first documented in this region in the 1950s following the ill-fated chloroquine-medicated salt program sponsored by the World Health Organization (WHO). Resistance to subsequent drugs emerged even more quickly. The combination sulfadoxine-pyrimethamine was useful for only 5 yr, after which mefloquine was introduced. Mefloquine was initially deployed at a dose of 15 mg/kg body weight along the Thai-Burmese border in 1984 in combination with sulfadoxine-pyrimethamine. The efficacy of this regimen fell rapidly from 99 to 71% in 1990 *(8)*. The dose of mefloquine was then increased to 25 mg/kg body weight; again, initial high cure rates of 91% declined to only 60% within 4 yr *(9)*.

The consequences of resistance at an individual level include increased morbidity and mortality; at a population level, the consequences are increased transmission and the likelihood of epidemics, the effects of which can be devastating. In recent years, epidemics have occurred with increasing frequency in Asia and in Africa. The malaria epidemic in Burundi at the end of 2000 (for which chloroquine was used despite evidence of resistance) saw 720,000 registered cases in a single month and thousands of deaths *(7,10)*.

In this chapter, *multiple drug resistance* is defined as resistance to two or more antimalarial drugs with different mechanisms of action. At the moment, multiple drug resistance has been observed in falciparum malaria only. Chloroquine remains an effective treatment for nonfalciparum malaria in most areas of the world, although resistance has

From: *Management of Multiple Drug-Resistant Infections*
Edited by: S. H. Gillespie © Humana Press Inc., Totowa, NJ

been reported in areas of Papua New Guinea, Indonesia, the Indian subcontinent, and South America *(11,12)*. This chapter outlines the epidemiology and mechanisms of antimalarial drug resistance in *P. falciparum*; strategies of treatment and control, particularly the introduction of artemisinin combination chemotherapy (ACT); specific antimalarial treatment options for uncomplicated, hyperparasitemic, and severe infections; and the treatment of important subgroups of people affected, such as pregnant women and neonates.

2. EPIDEMIOLOGY AND MECHANISMS OF RESISTANCE

The factors influencing the development and spread of drug resistance can be summarized as follows:

Host: For instance, the level of natural or acquired immunity (or premunition) in a population, treatment-seeking behavior, prevalence of certain hemoglobinopathies (α-thalassemia, glucose-6-phosphate dehydrogenase [G6PD] deficiency) thought to confer some protection against parasite invasion of the red cell.

Parasite: The starting frequency of drug-resistant mutations and degree of genetic diversity within a parasite population, the parasite reproductive rate, and level of malaria transmission.

Drug: Pharmacokinetic/pharmacodynamic properties of individual drugs (e.g., terminal elimination half-life, speed and stage-specificity of action), as well as issues relating to drug policy, prescribing, and availability such as unregulated access to drugs, partial population coverage, incomplete treatment courses/nonadherence to therapy.

Environment: Population movement, deforestation, climate change.

Vector: Certain mosquito species have a greater propensity to carry malaria and bite at different times. This behavior may be linked to local agricultural practices. Also, in response to vector control efforts, mosquitoes have developed resistance to insecticides *(13)*.

Diagnosis: Or its absence, means that drugs are being misused, and this contributes to selection pressure, particularly with drugs that have a long half-life. Clinical signs are notoriously nonspecific and insensitive in the diagnosis of malaria *(14,15)*, and presumptive treatment with antimalarial drugs is a major factor driving resistance.

2.1. Reaction and Spread of Drug Resistance

Drug-resistant mutants occur naturally and are selected. The starting frequency of mutations is therefore one important determinant of the likelihood of selection; however, the most potent force selecting for drug resistance is drug pressure during the acute phase of illness *(16)*. Exposure of the parasites to drugs will depend partly on the level of malaria transmission and the age-dependent level of immunity in the population. This background premunition in the host influences the probability of having large parasite biomass in an individual: High parasitemias are more likely in children and in hosts with no or poorly effective premunition. It is these circumstances that are likely to generate resistant mutants *(17)*.

The discrepancy in the speed of the spread of drug resistance between some African and Asian countries illustrates this point. In malaria-endemic areas of Southeast Asia, transmission is more unstable (seasonal) and at a lower intensity, with an entomological inoculation rate of less than 10 infective bites per person per year. However, there are variations; for example, in Burma, certain zones are hyperendemic. Development of an effective immunity to the disease is uncommon compared to sub-Saharan African countries, where older children and adults are protected by a transient immune response, called *premunition*. As a result of this protection, individuals can be parasitemic with few or no symptoms and do not seek treatment.

Falciparum malaria infection in Southeast Asia is almost invariably symptomatic; consequently, it usually is treated. Patients with high parasite counts (>4% of parasitized red cells) are not uncommon in all age groups. This results in a higher proportion of the parasites exposed to antimalarial drugs and an increased chance of selecting drug-resistant mutants. This is even more likely if a treatment is inadequate (underdosage or insufficient duration of treatment). If the drug has a long terminal elimination half-life, such that the parasites are exposed to the drug for a prolonged period at subtherapeutic concentrations, resistant mutants inoculated during the elimination phase can be "filtered" and recrudesce, with resistant strains developing. It has also been observed that parasites show less genetic diversity in low transmission areas, another factor that will encourage the spread of resistance *(18)*. Recrudescent infections are more likely to carry gametocytes that will also increase transmission of resistant malaria *(19)*.

It is known that certain drugs have a greater propensity to select for resistance *de novo* than others; for example, the use of atovaquone as monotherapy in Thai clinical studies resulted in a 33% recrudescence rate regardless of the length of therapy *(20)*. Similarly, the earlier use of pyrimethamine in Southeast Asia was followed rapidly by the emergence of resistance strains *(21)*.

2.2. Molecular Basis for Drug Resistance

The genetic basis for drug resistance is still incompletely understood for a number of drugs.

2.2.1. Chloroquine

Resistant parasites show decreased accumulation of the drug chloroquine in the food vacuole. Resistance is linked to multiple mutations in PfCRT, a protein in the vacuole membrane thought to function as a transporter *(22–24)*. The *pfcrt* gene is on chromosome 7, and there are a number of polymorphisms in this gene that have been associated with chloroquine resistance *(25)*. The *pfmdr* genotype, implicated in mefloquine resistance, has also been associated with chloroquine resistance in some studies *(26)*.

2.2.2. Antifolate Drugs

The mechanism of resistance to antifolate drugs has been characterized in detail. Sulfadoxine-pyrimethamine (SP) is the antifolate drug in most widespread use for the treatment of malaria, and chlorproguanil-dapsone is a newer antifolate drug in the final stages of development. Sulfadoxine is a dihydropteroate synthase (DHPS) inhibitor, and pyrimethamine is a dihydrofolate reductase (DHFR) inhibitor. They act by preventing folate biosynthesis, essential for parasite replication and survival.

Resistance is the result of point mutations in the genes encoding for these two enzymes. The initial mutation conferring DHFR resistance is usually Ser →Asn at position 108 (S108N), and this appears to be the key mutation, increasing resistance to pyrimethamine by a factor of 100. There are three other point mutations, the presence of which results in even higher level resistance: N51I, C59R, and I164L. Similarly five point mutations conferring resistance to DHPS have been identified: S436A/F, A437G,

K540E, A581G, and A613S/T. Of these, the A437G mutation is found with the highest frequency in field isolates and so may be the key mutation for sulfonamide resistance *(27)*.

Unfortunately, there is a degree of cross-resistance between sulfadoxine-pyrimethamine and chlorproguanil-dapsone, which has important implications for where and how this new drug will be deployed *(28)*. The mutant strains do not seem to have a biological disadvantage: Most strains found on the Thai-Burma border carry the mutations despite the withdrawal of SP nearly 20 yr ago *(29)*.

2.2.3. *Mefloquine*

P-glycoprotein, an ATP-dependent membrane efflux pump is encoded by a small group of closely related genes called *MDR*. There are two *MDR* genes in the human genome, *mdr1* and *mdr2*. Two homologs of the *MDR* gene family have been identified in *P.falciparum*. Resistance to mefloquine may be mediated by the number of copies of the *pfmdr1* gene *(30,31)*.

2.2.4. *Quinine*

Like chloroquine, resistance to quinine is also associated with reduced drug uptake by the parasite, but the precise mechanism by which this occurs is unclear. Studies have suggested that quinine resistance also has a weak association with the *pfmdr* genotype *(32)*. However, resistance to quinine is probably the result of mutations in multiple genes.

2.2.5. *Atovaquone*

Atovaquone resistance, which develops rapidly (as described in Section 2.2.2.), is associated with single-point mutations in the cytochrome b gene of the parasite encoding the cytochrome BC1 complex (complex III) of the parasite's inner mitochondrial membrane *(33)*.

3. TREATMENT OF MULTIPLE DRUG-RESISTANT MALARIA

3.1. *Combination Therapy*

The strategy of using drug combinations has been employed for the treatment of malaria since the early 1980s, with the use of mefloquine plus sulfadoxine-pyrimethamine, quinine plus tetracycline, and more recently the artemisinin derivatives combined with another drug *(34)*. The rationale for this approach is that the starting frequency of mutant parasites resistant to two drugs will be substantially lower than that of parasites resistant to only one. By using two drugs, it is hoped that they will protect each other, with each drug able to kill any circulating parasites resistant to the partner drug. There is some evidence from rodent models to support the theory that drug combinations can delay selection of resistant parasites *(35,36)*.

There is increasing acceptance that, for malaria, a combination should not just be any two antimalarial drugs with independent modes of action, but that one of these drugs should always be an artemisinin derivative *(31,37–39)*.

3.1.1. *Artemisinin Combination Therapy*

The artemisinin derivatives, referred to as *quinghaosu* in China, their country of origin, are a class of antimalarial drug derived from the sweet wormwood plant *Artemisia annua*. Use of this plant as a febrifuge in traditional Chinese medicine dates to at least 300 AD, but the chemical structure of these compounds was only elucidated by Chinese scientists in the early 1970s *(40–42)*. They are sesquiterpene lactones with an endoperoxide bridge and have a unique mode of action, exerting their antimalarial effect by the production of carbon-centered free radicals that bind to parasite proteins.

These drugs are remarkably potent, capable of reducing the parasite biomass by a factor of 10^4 per asexual life cycle. This results in more rapid resolution of symptoms and parasite clearance than from any other class of antimalarial drug. In addition, the artemisinin derivatives lack toxicity, with mild side effects of nausea, vomiting, and anorexia in less than 30% of patients *(43,44)*. The neurotoxicity found in animal studies has not been reproduced in humans. Allergic reactions have been reported rarely *(45)*.

These drugs have a very short terminal elimination half-life of a matter of hours, which decreases the risk of selection for drug-resistant mutants, but means that longer courses of treatment are needed to treat malaria if used as monotherapy. However, they make an ideal partner in a multidrug combination. They will dramatically reduce the parasite burden and be cleared quickly from the circulation; the patient experiences rapid resolution of symptoms, and the second drug, with a slower mode of action, has a smaller residuum of parasites to clear from the body. Another advantageous property of these compounds is their broad stage specificity and gametocytocidal effect, leading to a reduction in transmission of malaria and potentially drug resistance. This property also makes them the drug of choice in the treatment of malaria epidemics.

Resistance to artemisinin compounds in vivo or in vitro has not been demonstrated. All of these advantageous characteristics have led to the recommendation that policymakers switch to artemisinin-containing combination therapies for the treatment of falciparum malaria. The success of this approach has been demonstrated in Thailand, where a 3-d regimen of mefloquine 25 mg/kg body weight plus artesunate 12 mg/kg body weight remains more than 95% efficacious almost 10 yr after it was originally deployed *(46,47)*. Concurrent in vitro monitoring of mefloquine resistance has shown a decrease in the IC_{50} (the antimalarial drug concentration resulting in 50% inhibition of parasite multiplication) for mefloquine (i.e., a reversal of drug resistance).

Choice of the second drug in an artemisinin-containing combination needs to take into account local patterns of resistance. Chloroquine resistance is spreading rapidly throughout Africa, and the efficacy of sulfadoxine-pyrimethamine is declining in East African countries. In the Indian subcontinent, there is widespread resistance to chloroquine, with pockets of sulfadoxine-pyrimethamine resistance, while in Southeast Asia and parts of South America, there is resistance to chloroquine, sulfadoxine-pyrimethamine, quinine, and mefloquine *(48)*.

The following are examples of ACT in use or being studied.

3.1.1.1. Artesunate Plus Mefloquine

Mefloquine is a fluorinated quinoline methanol compound. It was developed in the 1960s by the Walter Reed Army Institute of Research. There is no parenteral formulation. The terminal elimination half-life of mefloquine is 3 wk in healthy individuals and 2 wk in patients with malaria. It achieves *P. falciparum* parasite reductions of 100- to 1000-fold per asexual cycle *(49)*. The starting dosage at which mefloquine should be deployed should be 25 mg/kg body weight to delay the selection of resistance. A population pharmacokinetic model for mefloquine has been developed that showed that splitting the dose of 25 mg/kg body weight into 15 mg/kg body weight and 10 mg/kg body weight on consecutive days resulted in a 50% increase in oral bioavailability if used alone or a 20% increase in bioavailability when used in combination with artesunate *(50)*. The pharmacokinetic properties of this drug are relatively unaffected by demographic variables or disease severity. The main adverse effects are gastrointestinal and neuropsychiatric and seem to be influenced by age and race.

A 3 d regimen of these two drugs is the standard treatment for falciparum malaria in many parts of Thailand and in Cambodia and Burma. Plans are under way to manufacture this drug combination as a coformulation, which should improve adherence and reduce the risk of resistance emerging.

3.1.1.2. Artemether-Lumefantrine (Coartemether)

The combination of artemether-lumefantrine (coartemether) is manufactured as a coformulation. It is licensed in more than 30 countries. Lumefantrine was synthesized in China and belongs to the aryl amino alcohol group of antimalarials. It is a racemic 2,4,7,9-substituted fluorine derivative *(51)*. Lumefantrine is not available separately as monotherapy. A treatment course of coartemether is twice a day for 3 d. The reported adverse effects are remarkably few *(52–54)*.

Limitations of this therapy are the need for twice-daily dosing and the finding that oral bioavailability of the lumefantrine component varies greatly between individuals and is improved by coadministration with fat *(51,55)*.

3.1.1.3. Sulfadoxine-Pyrimethamine-Artesunate

The sulfadoxine-pyrimethamine-artesunate combination may be useful in African countries where antifolate resistance has not yet taken hold. It is relatively inexpensive, but there is a major disadvantage in that sulfadoxine-pyrimethamine is generally widely available as a monotherapy. A study in Gambia showed that the combination was more effective than SP monotherapy *(56)*.

Gametocyte carriage is increased by SP monotherapy; thus, malaria transmission may be enhanced by the use of this drug *(57–59)*.

3.1.1.4. Artesunate-Chlorproguanil Dapsone

Chlorproguanil-dapsone was developed in response to the emergence of chloroquine resistance in African countries. The terminal elimination half-life of both components is less than 1 d. A treatment course is 3 d in duration. Chlorproguanil is metabolized to chlorcycloguanil, a potent DHFR inhibitor eliminated more rapidly than sulfadoxine-pyrimethamine. It is effective against parasites with the triple DHFR resistance mutation, but not those with all four mutations. Following the rapid decline in efficacy of sulfadoxine-pyrimethamine, it was recognized that this drug may be vulnerable if deployed alone. A coformulation with artesunate is planned. For this reason, WHO is not recommending chlorproguanil-dapsone as monotherapy *(28)*.

3.1.1.5. Artesunate-Atovaquone-Proguanil

Malarone™ (GlaxoSmith Kline) is a fixed-dose combination of 250 mg of atovaquone and 100 mg of proguanil hydrochloride. Both compounds act on the ubiquinone metabolic pathway and can be shown to be synergistic in vitro. Used in combination with artesunate, it is a highly effective treatment for multidrug-resistant falciparum malaria *(60)*. Unfortunately, the cost of this treatment renders it unaffordable for routine use in malaria-endemic countries.

3.1.1.6. Artesunate Plus Amodiaquine

Trials have been conducted in Senegal, Kenya, and Gabon to study the efficacy of the combination of artesunate plus amodiaquine; cure rates of greater than 90% were observed at 14 d of follow-up. The main drawback to using this treatment is the availability of amodiaquine alone because development of increasing resistance to this drug would compromise the efficacy of the combination *(61–64)*. There are also concerns over the hematological toxicity of amodiaquine.

3.1.1.7. Artesunate-Chloroquine

The extent to which chloroquine resistance has taken hold means the combination of artesunate and chloroquine has little to offer for the treatment of drug-resistant falciparum malaria. There is an argument for using this combination for the treatment of nonfalciparum malaria to delay the emergence of chloroquine resistance.

Newer combination drugs that show great potential for the treatment of multidrug-resistant malaria are dihydroartemisinin plus piperaquine, which has already been registered in a number of Asian countries as Artekin® (HolleyKin Pharmaceutical); and artesunate-pyronaridine and dihydroartemisinin plus naphthoquine, which are under development. Piperaquine and naphthoquine are 4-aminoquinolines, and pyronaridine is a mannich base compound. All three drugs were developed in China, and piperaquine and pyronaridine are used there as monotherapy for the treatment of falciparum malaria.

3.1.2. Specific Treatment of Acute Multiple Drug-Resistant Malaria

This section assumes a diagnosis of falciparum malaria or mixed infection resistant to chloroquine and SP as confirmed microscopically or by rapid test. Tables 1–3 aim to provide as comprehensive a guide as possible for the treatment of multiple drug-resistant falciparum malaria. A number of alternative regimens are presented because it is recognized that not all regimens are available or practical in different treatment settings. Details are available at www.shoklo-unit.com.

3.1.2.1. Uncomplicated Multidrug-Resistant Falciparum Malaria

Suitable treatments for patients with uncomplicated malaria, that is, those not hyperparasitemic (less than 4% parasitized red blood cells), and with no clinical signs of severity include the following:

- Artesunate 4 mg/kg body weight per day for 3 d with mefloquine 25 mg/kg body weight (total dose), ideally given as a split dose of 15 mg/kg body weight on the second day of treatment and 10 mg/kg body weight on the final day. This approach enhances the oral bioavailability of the drug and improves tolerability *(50)*. Mefloquine should not be given if there is a history of psychiatric illness or epilepsy.

Or, if available,

- Artemether-lumefantrine (coartemether) twice daily for 3 d. Each tablet contains 20 mg artemether and 160 mg lumefantrine. The bioavailability of oral lumefantrine is significantly enhanced with coadministration of fat, and we would recommend giving a 200-mL carton of flavored milk with each dose. The sometimes-recommended four-dose regimen should be abandoned because it results in suboptimal levels of lumefantrine at d 7, the determinant factor of cure with this combination *(54)*.
- Artesunate-atovaquone-proguanil. The dose is artesunate 4 mg/kg body weight per day, atovaquone 20 mg/kg body weight per day, proguanil 8 mg/kg body weight per day for 3 d.

Table 1
Uncomplicated Multiple Drug Resistant Falciparum Malaria or Mixed Infection

Patient category	Treatment
Adult (Pregnancy excluded) or child 8 yr or older	Artesunate* 4 mg/kg body weight per day for 3 d plus Mefloquine†,a 25 mg/kg body weight given as 15 mg/kg body weight and 10 mg/kg body weight on the second and third days of treatment OR Artemether-lumefantrine†,b one dose twice daily for 3 d according to weight <15 kg, 1 tablet; 16–25 kg, 2 tablets; 26–36 kg, 3 tablets; >35 kg, 4 tablets OR Artesunate† 2 mg/kg body weight per day for 7 d plus Doxycycline 4 mg/kg body weight per day for 7 d OR Artesunate† 4 mg/kg body weight per day, atovaquone 20 mg/kg body weight per day, proguanil 8 mg/kg body weight per day for 3 d OR Quinine† 10 mg/kg body weight po three times a day for 7 d plus tetracycline 16 mg/kg body weight per day for 7 d given as three or four divided doses
Child younger than 8 yr	Artesunate* plus mefloquine as above OR Artemether-lumefantrine† as above OR Artesunate† 2 mg/kg body weight per day for 7 d OR Artesunate†, atovaquone, proguanil as above
Pregnant woman	Supervised quinine* 10 mg/kg body weight po three times a day for 7 d OR Artesunate† 2 mg/kg body weight per day po for 7 d OR Quinine† 10 mg/kg body weight po three times daily for 7 d plus Clindamycin 5 mg/kg body weight three times daily for 7 d OR Artesunate† 2 mg/kg body weight per day po for 7 d plus Clindamycin 5 mg/kg body weight three times daily for 7 d OR Artesunate† 2 mg/kg body weight per day po for 7 d plus Atovaquone† 20 mg/kg body weight per day, proguanil 8 mg/kg body weight per day for 3 d

(*continued*)

Table 1
Uncomplicated Multiple Drug Resistant Falciparum Malaria or Mixed Infection (*continued*)

Patient category	Treatment
Neonate (congenital malaria)	Quinine* 20 mg (salt)/kg body weight iv loading dose in 10% dextrose and water over 4 h, followed by 10 mg(salt)/kg body weight every 8 h or 10 mg (salt)/kg body weight im diluted with sterile water (50:50), followed by oral quinine 10 mg (salt)/kg body weight three times daily for 7 d OR Artesunate† 2 mg/kg body weight im on the first day of treatment, followed by 2 mg/kg body weight per day orally on the following 6 d
Returning traveler[c]	Artesunate* plus mefloquine as above OR Artemether-lumefantrine† as above OR Artesunate† plus atovaquone-proguanil as above OR Atovaquone† 20 mg/kg body weight per day, proguanil 8 mg/kg body weight per day for 3 d OR Quinine† plus tetracycline as above

The diagnosis is confirmed by a positive malaria smear/rapid test; there should be less than 4% red blood cells parasitized and no clinical signs of severity.

Artemether is an alternative to oral artesunate. The dose is the same.

*Denotes first-line treatment.

†Denotes alternative treatment regimen.

[a]Contraindications to mefloquine treatment include treatment with the drug in the previous 63 d, epilepsy or neuropsychiatric disorder, history of allergy.

[b]Each dose of artemether-lumefantrine should be given with food containing some fat (e.g., a carton of flavored milk).

[c]A returning traveler with mixed infection (i.e., falciparum and nonfalciparum species) should be given primaquine at a dose of 0.3 mg base/kg body weight daily (maximum dose 15 mg) for 14 d after excluding glucose-6-phosphate dehydrogenase deficiency to eradicate the dormant liver stage (hypnozoite) of nonfalciparum malaria.

If none of these options is available, the following, less-practical, regimens should be effective:

- Quinine-clindamycin. This is a 7-d treatment of quinine 10 mg (salt)/kg body weight plus clindamycin 5 mg/kg body weight (to the nearest 150 mg) three times daily.

or

- Quinine plus tetracycline (or doxycycline). Quinine 10 mg (salt)/kg body weight three times daily plus doxycycline 4 mg/kg body weight (to the nearest 100 mg) once daily or tetracycline 16 mg/kg body weight per day in three or four divided doses for 7 d. Tetracyclines are contraindicated in pregnancy and for children younger than 8 yr of age.

Table 2
Uncomplicated Multiple Drug-Resistant Hyperparasitemic Falciparum Malaria or Mixed Infection

Patient category	Treatment
Adult (pregnancy excluded) or child 8 yr or older	Artesunate* 4 mg/kg on the first day of treatment followed by 2 mg/kg body weight per day on the following 6 d plus mefloquine[a] 25 mg/kg body weight given as 15 mg/kg and 10 mg/kg on the 4th and 5th d of treatment OR Artesunate† 4 mg/kg body weight on the first day of treatment followed by 2 mg/kg body weight day on the following 6 d plus doxycycline 4 mg/kg body weight per day for 7 d OR Artesunate† 4 mg/kg body weight on the first day of treatment followed by 2 mg/kg body weight day on the following 6 days plus clindamycin 5 mg/kg body weight per day for 7 d OR Artesunate† 4mg/kg body weight on the first day of treatment followed by 2 mg/kg body weight per day on the following 6 d plus atovaquone 20 mg/kg body weight per day, proguanil 8 mg/kg body weight per day for 3 d
Child younger than 8 yr	Artesunate* plus mefloquine as above OR Artesunate† 4mg/kg body weight on the first day of treatment, followed by 2 mg/kg body weight per day on the following 6 d OR Artesunate† plus clindamycin as above OR Artesunate† plus atovaquone-proguanil as above
Pregnant woman	Artesunate* for 7 d, 4 mg/kg body weight on the first day followed by 2 mg/kg body weight on subsequent days (total dose16 mg/kg body weight) OR Artesunate† plus clindamycin as above OR Artesunate† plus atovaquone-proguanil as above

(continued)

3.1.2.2. Uncomplicated Hyperparasitemic Multidrug-Resistant Falciparum Malaria

On the Thai-Burmese border, a *P. falciparum* parasitemia of greater than or equal to 4% was associated with a 3% mortality, compared to a mortality rate of 0.15% for uncomplicated malaria cases with lower parasitemias *(65)*. This group of patients should receive inpatient treatment as these individuals are at increased risk of developing signs of severe malaria and anemia. As described in Section 2.1., patients with large parasite biomass are more likely to harbor resistant mutants. This large number of

Table 2
Uncomplicated Multiple Drug-Resistant Hyperparasitemic Falciparum Malaria or Mixed Infection *(continued)*

Patient category	Treatment
Neonate (congenital malaria)	Artesunate* for 7 d as above; it is advisable to give the first dose parenterally. OR Quinine† 20 mg (salt)/kg body weight iv loading dose in 10% dextrose and water over 4 h, followed by 10 mg (salt)/kg 8 hourly *or* 10 mg (salt)/kg body weight im diluted with sterile water (50:50), followed by oral quinine 10mg (salt) /kg body weight three times daily for 7 d.
Returning travelers[b]	As adults* OR As neonate† if artesunate not available

Hyperparasitemia on the Thai-Burma border is defined as a parasite count of 4% or greater (expressed as number of asexual forms per 1000 red blood cells).

*Denotes first-line treatment.

†Denotes alternative treatment regimen.

[a]Give mefloquine only if no contraindication (*see* Table 1).

[b]If artesunate is unavailable iv quinine should be used plus oral doxycycline as in the treatment of severe malaria (*see* Table 3).

parasites must be reduced quickly by a fast-acting drug, such as an artemisinin derivative, to reduce the risk of selection by the partner drug. Patients with higher parasitemia need a longer course of treatment to ensure cure. A 4% parasitemia equates to a parasite biomass greater than 10^{12}. A 7-d course of an artemisinin derivative will cover four asexual life cycles of the parasite and dramatically reduce the parasite biomass. Failure to do this will leave a larger residual number of parasites for the second, more slowly acting drug to eliminate, which increases the risk of selection for drug resistance. Options for treatment are shown in Table 2.

If the patient develops any clinical signs of severity, the protocol for severe malaria should be followed with parenteral therapy. In the presence of a rising parasitemia without clinical signs of severity, a single parenteral dose of 1.2 mg/kg body weight artesunate should be given.

3.1.2.3. Severe Multiple Drug-Resistant Falciparum Malaria

The priority of the immediate treatment of severe malaria is to save the patient's life. Initial treatment of severe malaria is always the same irrespective of the likelihood of a multidrug-resistant infection. The criteria for the definition of severe malaria have been described in detail elsewhere *(67)*.

The drugs used are parenteral artesunate, artemether, or quinine (*see* Table 3). An initial dose of 2.4 mg/kg body weight of intravenous artesunate is given, followed by 1.2 mg/kg body weight at 12 h and 24 h *(68)*. Thereafter, the patient is given 1.2 mg/kg body weight daily until oral medication is tolerated.

If artesunate is unavailable, intramuscular artemether may be used. There are unpublished data that suggest that this treatment is inferior to parenteral artesunate because a subgroup of patients absorb artemether poorly, and it will take considerably

Table 3
Severe Multiple Drug-Resistant Falciparum Malaria

Patient category	Treatment
Initial treatment	Artesunate* iv: Initial dose of 2.4mg/kg body weight followed by 1.2mg/kg at 12 h and 24 h; thereafter, give 1.2mg/kg body weight daily until patient can tolerate oral medication; total treatment duration 7 d OR Quinine† iv: Loading dose (LD[a]) 20 mg/kg given over 4 h, then 10mg given 8 h after the LD was started, followed by 10mg/kg every 8 h for 7d. *or* Quinine i.m: Loading dose (20 mg/kg) is given as 2 simultaneous injections in the anterior thigh after 50% dilution of the quinine in sterile water; the maintenance dose (10 mg/kg body weight) is given as one intramuscular injection every 8 h using the same dilution OR Artemether† im: Initial dose of 3.2mg/kg followed by 1.12 mg/kg body weight at 12 h and 24 h. Continue to give 1.6 mg/kg/body weight every 24 h until patient can tolerate oral medication; total treatment duration of 7 d. 1. Once the patient has recovered sufficiently to tolerate oral medication, a second drug should be added, such as doxycycline 4 mg/kg body weight for 7 d, clindamycin 5 mg/kg body weight three times daily for 7 d, or atovaquone 20 mg/kg body weight per day plus proguanil 8 mg/kg body weight per day for 3 d 2. The use of mefloquine for the treatment of severe malaria is relatively contraindicated because of the increased risk of postmalaria neurological syndrome.

Notes: Severe malaria was defined according to the World Health Organization criteria *(67)*.
Pregnant women receiving intravenous quinine are at very high risk of developing severe hypoglycemia.
*Denotes first-line treatment.
†Denotes alternative treatment regimen.
[a]Loading dose should always be given.

longer for therapeutic concentrations of the drug to be reached, which is likely to increase mortality in this severely ill group of patients (N. J. White; 2002, personal communication).

The dose of quinine is as follows: loading dose of 20 mg (salt)/kg body weight given intravenously over 4 h *(69,70)*. Eight hours after the start of treatment, give 10 mg/kg over 2 h and repeat this dose every 8 h (total daily dose 30 mg/kg body weight). When given by the intramuscular route, the loading dose (20 mg/kg body weight) is given in two simultaneous injections in the anterior thigh after 50% dilution of the quinine in sterile water. The maintenance dose (10 mg/kg body weight) is given in one intramuscular injection every 8 h using the same dilution. The parenteral treatment is discontinued only when the patient can eat and drink independently. Practically, there is no contraindication to the use of the loading dose. The main adverse effect of quinine in the acute phase is hypoglycemia. Failure to give a loading dose will result in suboptimal drug concentrations in some patients.

Studies to date have not clearly demonstrated an advantage in using the artemisinin derivatives over quinine in terms of mortality reduction except in adults with organ failure *(71,72)*.

One study looked at the effect of combining parenteral quinine and artesunate in the treatment of uncomplicated and severe malaria; no beneficial effect compared to use of the drugs alone was found *(73)*. Artemisinin suppositories have been used with success in the treatment of severe malaria and may be the best option for treatment in certain remote areas *(74–76)*.

These drugs will only be lifesaving if accompanied by good nursing care and supportive measures to manage the associated complications of this disease, such as coma, hypoglycemia, acidosis, pulmonary edema, convulsions, and concomitant bacterial infections *(67,77)*.

Routine anticonvulsant prophylaxis with phenobarbitone in cerebral malaria was previously recommended, but has been associated with an increase in deaths in children *(78,79)*.

Once the patient can eat and drink, a 7-d treatment course may be completed orally. A second drug should be added if possible (e.g., doxycycline 4 mg/kg body weight per day for 7 d). Mefloquine is contraindicated in severe malaria as there is an increased risk of developing neurological sequelae, the postmalaria neurological syndrome (PMNS) *(80)*.

If a patient develops a recrudescence of parasitemia, one of the alternative regimens in the tables may be used. Mefloquine should not be given again if the previous episode of malaria was in the 63 d before the second infection because of higher risk of severe central nervous system side effects. PCR genotyping is needed to reliably distinguish recrudescence from reinfection. This technique employs a population genetics approach using three polymorphic markers on three unlinked genes: merozoite surface proteins 1 and 2 (MSP-1 and MSP-2) and the glutamate-rich protein (GLURP). The method can reliably determine recrudescent infections with a probability of occurrence by chance of less than 0.05. This approach is suited to areas of low malaria transmission where multiple infections are uncommon and may not be appropriate for high-transmission areas, where it would be better to select a single highly polymorphic locus with less than 5% frequency of the most common allele *(18)*.

3.1.3. *Special Groups of Patients*

3.1.3.1. Treatment of Multiple Drug-Resistant Falciparum Malaria During Pregnancy

Consequences of multiple infections during pregnancy include severe anemia and low birth weight *(81)*. Quinine is the only drug recommended for use in the first trimester. There is a paucity of data on the safety of the newer antimalarials in pregnancy. In areas such as the Thai-Burma border, one in three episodes of falciparum malaria treated with a 7-d supervised course of quinine will not be cured *(82,83)*. Addition of clindamycin to the regimen will significantly improve efficacy, but is expensive *(84)*.

Mefloquine treatment during pregnancy was associated with an increased risk of stillbirth in a cohort of women in this area. Of 3587 pregnancies investigated, 208 (5.8%) were exposed to mefloquine, 656 (18.3%) to quinine only, and 909 (25.3%) to other antimalarials; 2470 (68.9%) had no documented malaria. There were 61 stillbirths and 313 abortions. Women who received mefloquine treatment during, but not before, pregnancy had a significantly greater risk of stillbirth than did women treated with quinine alone (odds ratio [OR] 4.72; 95% confidence interval [CI] 1.7–12.7), women exposed to other treatments (OR 5.10; 95% CI 2–13.1), and women who had no malaria (OR 3.50; 95% CI 1.6–7.6) ($p < 0.01$). This association remained after adjustment for all identified confounding factors. Mefloquine was not associated with abortion, low birth weight, neurological retardation, or congenital malformations *(85)*.

Artemisinin derivatives are not licensed for use during pregnancy; however, in areas of high-level drug resistance, there is no other option if quinine fails. The largest series of artemisinin treatments in pregnancy published found the artemisinins were well tolerated with no evidence of adverse effects. Birth outcomes did not differ significantly from community rates for abortion, stillbirth, congenital abnormality, and mean gestation at delivery *(86)*.

The added risks of malaria in pregnancy, even uncomplicated malaria, mean that every treatment in pregnant women should be supervised. Combinations for use in pregnancy, such as artesunate-sulfadoxine-pyrimethamine (which could be useful in African countries), should be studied as a matter of urgency.

Quinine should be used as the first-line treatment for uncomplicated infections in pregnancy. The normal dose is 10 mg/kg body weight three times a day for 7 d. Quinine-induced hypoglycemia is frequent in severe malaria and can occur in uncomplicated infections *(87)*.

Artesunate, 2 mg/kg body weight per day for 7 d, is the second-line drug of choice for multiple drug-resistant infections. For hyperparasitemic multidrug-resistant infections at any gestation of pregnancy, 7 d of artesunate should be given, with 4 mg/kg body weight given on the first day of treatment and 2 mg/kg body weight per day given on successive days.

The initial treatment of severe malaria is the same as for nonpregnant patients. The later addition of doxycycline in the recovery phase is contraindicated.

Particular complications of severe malaria in pregnancy are hypoglycemia, which will be further aggravated by quinine therapy, pulmonary edema, and premature labor.

Regarding lactation, quinine, chloroquine, and mefloquine are excreted in the breast milk, but the suckling neonate would receive only a few milligrams per day. Tetracyclines are thought to be safe during lactation because the drug binds to the calcium of the milk. There are no data on whether the newer antimalarials are excreted in breast milk.

3.1.3.2. Treatment of Falciparum Malaria in Very Young Children

Mefloquine and artesunate have been given to very young children (aged 3 mo; 4–5 kg). Artesunate was very well tolerated. Mefloquine gave fewer late side effects in children than in adults. The main problem was the very high incidence of vomiting during the first hour after mefloquine intake *(65,88,89)*. Some children do not tolerate mefloquine, and it is recommended that a dose not be repeated more than twice. In this situation, artesunate should be continued for a total of 7 d at a dose of 2 mg/kg body weight per day for 7 d.

Alternatives for use are artemether-lumefantrine (*see* Table 1) or artesunate 2 mg/kg body weight per day for 7 d. The initial treatment of severe malaria is as for adults, without the later addition of doxycycline.

3.1.3.3. Congenital Malaria

Vertical transmission of malaria can be diagnosed by finding parasites in the neonate within 7 d of birth. Evidence from most malarious parts of the world indicate that congenital malaria is uncommon despite the prevalence of placental infection *(90,91)*. Most cases of congenital malaria are asymptomatic, but there may be fever, irritability, feeding problems, hepatosplenomegaly, anemia, or jaundice. To exclude the diagnosis, every neonate born to a mother diagnosed with malaria at or close to delivery should have a malaria smear irrespective of the clinical picture. This should be done at birth and repeated at 7 d of age or sooner if the clinical condition of the neonate causes concern.

A neonate with malaria can deteriorate very quickly, and parenteral treatment with quinine or an artemisinin derivative is preferable initially. Quinine may be given intravenously in 10% dextrose and water, commencing with 20 mg (salt)/kg body weight over 4 h, followed by 10 mg (salt)/kg body weight every 8 h. Intravenous treatment is switched to oral quinine at 10 mg (salt)/kg body weight three times daily as soon as possible, with regular monitoring of blood glucose. Quinine may also be given by the intramuscular route: 10 mg (base)/kg salt immediately, followed by oral quinine 10 mg (salt)/kg three times daily for 7 d. Care must be taken with intramuscular quinine. It is necessary to dilute the dose of quinine by 50% with sterile water to reduce the risk of abscess formation. An alternative drug is artesunate 2 mg/kg body weight per day for 7 d. It is advisable to give the first dose parenterally.

The treatment of severe malaria is the same as for other patient groups without the addition of doxycycline. Maternal hypoglycemia, a common complication of malaria or its treatment with quinine, may cause marked fetal bradycardia and other signs of fetal distress. In all cases of congenital malaria, the mother, particularly if under quinine treatment, needs to be stimulated to take adequate amounts of glucose and fluids (3–5 L/d) to help breast milk production and to maintain the mother's and infant's blood sugar levels.

3.1.3.4. Travelers Returning from Areas Endemic With Multiple Drug-Resistant Malaria

The group of travelers returning from areas endemic with multiple drug-resistant malaria is relatively small, but important as it will include mainly nonimmune individuals returning to countries where there is no or limited access to the most effective drugs (i.e., the artemisinin derivatives). An accurate travel history is essential, and multiple drug resistance should be suspected in anyone with falciparum malaria who has been traveling in Southeast Asia. The best treatments for uncomplicated falciparum malaria or mixed infection in a returning traveler are those described in Section 3.1.2. (i.e., artesunate plus mefloquine or coartemether or artesunate plus doxycycline). If these drugs are unavailable, atovaquone-proguanil could be used or quinine plus tetracycline. Many clinicians would be reluctant to prescribe mefloquine in the light of the high level of public awareness of neuropsychiatric adverse events. Travelers with nonfalciparum malaria or mixed infection who move back to a nonendemic country should be given primaquine to ensure radical cure, providing there are no contraindications, such as G6PD deficiency.

4. STRATEGIES FOR PREVENTION AND CONTROL OF MULTIPLE DRUG-RESISTANT MALARIA

An effective malaria vaccine and a transgenic mosquito incapable of transmitting malaria remain distant prospects for prevention and control of multiple drug-resistant malaria *(92,93)*. The main strategies for prevention and control of malaria available now are early detection and treatment with an artemisinin-containing combination and established vector control measures. In practice, there are many obstacles to the successful implementation of a control program centered on the deployment of artemisinin-based combination therapy:

- Cost: As usual, cost is the main obstacle preventing effective control measures from getting to the areas that need them most. The Global Fund to Fight AIDS, Tuberculosis, and Malaria is one of a number of initiatives trying to keep malaria in the spotlight, but it remains to be seen whether sufficient funds can be made available for widespread deployment of ACT *(94)*.
- Inadequate diagnosis: The ability to provide a confirmed diagnosis of malaria is key to any effective control program. Presumptive clinical diagnosis of malaria has repeatedly been shown to be unreliable *(15)*. The development of rapid tests for diagnosis means confirmed diagnosis of malaria is now possible in areas where microscopy is not a feasible option. A control program is likely to fail without this, and giving a drug where the diagnosis is unconfirmed may even promote the spread of resistance.
- Inadequate population coverage: If ACT cannot be delivered to the population in sufficient numbers, then the use of this strategy as a method for delaying the spread of resistance will fail. It is hard to predict the minimum level of coverage required for a new combination treatment to delay the onset of resistance. High levels of population coverage may be difficult to achieve in countries where access to malaria treatment is dependent on ability to pay. Control programs may need to adopt novel social marketing initiatives in partnership with the private sector in places where this is the main source of diagnosis and treatment *(95)*. Ideally, any drugs to be used in combination that are also available as monotherapies would be removed from the marketplace. Quality assurance is another important issue, and it has been linked to the problem of counterfeit antimalarial drugs that have been found in many Asian countries *(96,97)*.
- Nonadherence to therapy: Nonadherence to all or part of a malaria treatment program is a fact of life now that the days of single-dose treatment are over. This may be minimized by prioritizing the development of short-course, once-daily, well-tolerated coformulations.
- Vector control measures: The vector control measures include residual spraying, insecticide-treated bednets, larva control, and personal protection. These measures need to be tailored to suit the epidemiology of the malaria in the areas where they are deployed *(98)*.

5. CONCLUSION

Multiple drug resistance to falciparum malaria is on the increase and looks set to sweep across Africa with devastating results unless action is taken quickly. While there are few drugs available to treat this disease, effective treatments do exist, particularly combinations containing artemisinin derivatives. Numerous advantages of these combinations were described, including delaying the development of drug resistance. It is often argued that these drugs are too expensive to be deployed; however, the ramifications of persistence with a policy of sequential monotherapies for malaria are far greater in terms of increased morbidity, mortality, and effect on already-struggling economies.

REFERENCES

1. Phillips RS. Current status of malaria and potential for control. Clin Microbiol Rev 2001; 14:208–226.
2. Sachs J, Malaney P. The economic and social burden of malaria. Nature 2002; 415:680–685.
3. Sachs JD, Mellinger AD, Gallup JL. The geography of poverty and wealth. Sci Am 2001; 284:70–75.
4. Gallup JL, Sachs JD. The economic burden of malaria. Am J Trop Med Hyg 2001; 64(1–2 suppl.):85–96.
5. Snow RW, Trape JF, Marsh K. The past, present and future of childhood malaria mortality in Africa. Trends Parasitol 2001; 17:593–597.
6. MacArthur J, Stennies GM, Macheso A, et al. Efficacy of mefloquine and sulfadoxine-pyrimethamine for the treatment of uncomplicated *Plasmodium falciparum* infection in Machinga District, Malawi, 1998. Am J Trop Med Hyg 2001; 65:679–684.
7. D'Alessandro U, Buttiens H. History and importance of antimalarial drug resistance. Trop Med Int Health 2001; 6:845–848.
8. Nosten F, ter Kuile F, Chongsuphajaisiddhi T, et al. Mefloquine-resistant falciparum malaria on the Thai-Burmese border. Lancet 1991; 337:1140–1143.
9. ter Kuile FO, Nosten F, Thieren M, et al. High-dose mefloquine in the treatment of multidrug-resistant falciparum malaria. J Infect Dis 1992; 166:1393–1400.
10. Etchegorry MG, Matthys F, Galinski M, White NJ, Nosten F. Malaria epidemic in Burundi. Lancet 2001; 357:1046–1047.
11. Maguire JD, Sumawinata IW, Masbar S, et al. Chloroquine-resistant *Plasmodium malariae* in south Sumatra, Indonesia. Lancet 2002; 360:58–60.
12. Singh RK. Emergence of chloroquine-resistant vivax malaria in south Bihar (India). Trans R Soc Trop Med Hyg 2000; 94:327.
13. Hemingway J, Field L, Vontas J. An overview of insecticide resistance. Science 2002; 298:96–97.
14. Faiz MA, Yunus EB, Rahman MR, et al. Failure of national guidelines to diagnose uncomplicated malaria in Bangladesh. Am J Trop Med Hyg 2002; 67:396–399.
15. Luxemburger C, Nosten F, Kyle DE, Kiricharoen L, Chongsuphajaisiddhi T, White NJ. Clinical features cannot predict a diagnosis of malaria or differentiate the infecting species in children living in an area of low transmission. Trans R Soc Trop Med Hyg 1998; 92:45–49.
16. Hastings IM. Modelling parasite drug resistance: lessons for management and control strategies. Trop Med Int Health 2001; 6:883–890.
17. White NJ, Pongtavornpinyo W. The de novo selection of drug resistant malaria parasites. Proc R Soc London B Biol Sci 2003; 270:545–554.
18. Brockman A, Paul RE, Anderson TJ, et al. Application of genetic markers to the identification of recrudescent *Plasmodium falciparum* infections on the northwestern border of Thailand. Am J Trop Med Hyg 1999; 60:14–21.
19. Price R, Nosten F, Simpson JA, et al. Risk factors for gametocyte carriage in uncomplicated falciparum malaria. Am J Trop Med Hyg 1999; 60:1019–1023.
20. Looareesuwan S, Viravan C, Webster HK, Kyle DE, Hutchinson DB, Canfied CJ. Clinical studies of atovaquone, alone or in combination with other antimalarial drugs, for treatment of acute uncomplicated malaria in Thailand. Am J Trop Med Hyg 1996; 54:62–66.
21. Verdrager J. Epidemiology of emergence and spread of drug-resistant falciparum malaria in Southeast Asia. Southeast Asian J Trop Med Public Health 1986; 17:111–118.
22. Wellems TE, Wootton JC, Fujioka H, et al. *P. falciparum* CG2, linked to chloroquine resistance, does not resemble Na+/H+ exchangers. Cell 1998; 94:285–286.
23. Wellems TE, Plowe CV. Chloroquine-resistant malaria. J Infect Dis 2001; 184:770–776.

24. Nomura T, Carlton JM, Baird JK, et al. Evidence for different mechanisms of chloroquine resistance in two *Plasmodium* species that cause human malaria. J Infect Dis 2001; 183: 1653–1661.
25. Djimde A, Doumbo OK, Cortese JF, et al. A molecular marker for chloroquine-resistant falciparum malaria. N Engl J Med 2001; 344:257–263.
26. Fidock DA, Nomura T, Talley AK, et al. Mutations in the *P. falciparum* digestive vacuole transmembrane protein PfCRT and evidence for their role in chloroquine resistance. Mol Cell 2000; 6:861–871.
27. Hopkins Sibley CH, Hyde JE, Sims PFG, et al. Pyrimethamine-sulfadoxine resistance in *Plasmodium falciparum*: what next? Trends Parasitol 2001; 17:582–588.
28. Winstanley P. Chlorproguanil-dapsone (LAPDAP) for uncomplicated falciparum malaria. Trop Med Int Health 2001; 6:952–954.
29. Nair S, Brockman A, Paiphun L, Nosten F, Anderson TJ. Rapid genotyping of loci involved in antifolate drug resistance in *Plasmodium falciparum* by primer extension. Int J Parasitol 2002; 32:852–858.
30. Price R, Robinson G, Brockman A, Cowman A, Krishna S. Assessment of pfmdr 1 gene copy number by tandem competitive polymerase chain reaction. Mol Biochem Parasitol 1997; 85:161–169.
31. White NJ. Preventing antimalarial drug resistance through combinations. Drug Res Updates 1998; 1:3–9.
32. Cowman AF. Mechanisms of drug resistance in malaria. Aust N Z J Med 1995; 25:837–844.
33. Vaidya AB, Mather MW. Atovaquone resistance in malaria parasites. Drug Resist Updat 2000; 3:283–287.
34. White NJ. Antimalarial drug resistance and combination chemotherapy. Phil Trans R Soc Lond B 1999; 354:739–749.
35. Peters W. The chemotherapy of rodent malaria. LVII. Drug combinations to impede the selection of drug resistance, Part 1: Which model is appropriate? Ann Trop Med Parasitol 1999; 93:569–587.
36. Peters W, Robinson BL, Stewart LB, Butcher GA. The chemotherapy of rodent malaria. LIX. Drug combinations to impede the selection of drug resistance, Part 3: Observations on cyproheptadine, an antihistaminic agent, with chloroquine. Ann Trop Med Parasitol 2000; 94:689–697.
37. Price RN, Nosten F. Drug resistant falciparum malaria: clinical consequences and strategies for prevention. Drug Resist Updat 2001; 4:187–196.
38. Nosten F, Brasseur P. Combination therapy for malaria. The way forward? Drugs 2002; 62:1315–1329.
39. World Health Organization. Antimalarial Drug Combination Therapy. Geneva, Switzerland: World Health Organization, 2001.
40. Chemical studies on *qinghaosu* (artemisinine). China Cooperative Research Group on qinghaosu and its derivatives as antimalarials. J Tradit Chin Med 1982; 2:3–8.
41. The chemistry and synthesis of *qinghaosu* derivatives. China Cooperative Research Group on qinghaosu and its derivatives as antimalarials. J Tradit Chin Med 1982; 2:9–16.
42. Clinical studies on the treatment of malaria with *qinghaosu* and its derivatives. China Cooperative Research Group on *qinghaosu* and its derivatives as antimalarials. J Tradit Chin Med 1982; 2:45–50.
43. Price RN. Artemisinin drugs: novel antimalarial agents. Expert Opin Investig Drugs 2000; 9:1815–1827.
44. Price R, van Vugt M, Phaipun L, et al. Adverse effects in patients with acute falciparum malaria treated with artemisinin derivatives. Am J Trop Med Hyg 1999; 60:547–555.
45. Leonardi E, Gilvary G, White NJ, Nosten F. Severe allergic reactions to oral artesunate: a report of two cases. Trans R Soc Trop Med Hyg 2001; 95:182–183.

46. Nosten F, van Vugt M, Price R, et al. Effects of artesunate-mefloquine combination on incidence of *Plasmodium falciparum* malaria and mefloquine resistance in western Thailand: a prospective study. Lancet 2000; 356:297–302.
47. Brockman A, Price RN, van Vugt M, et al. Plasmodium falciparum antimalarial drug susceptibility on the northwestern border of Thailand during 5 yr of extensive use of artesunate-mefloquine. Trans Roy Soc Trop Med Hyg 2000; 90:537–544.
48. White NJ, Nosten F, Looareesuwan S, et al. Averting a malaria disaster. Lancet 1999; 353: 1965–1967.
49. Simpson JA, Price R, ter Kuile F, et al. Population pharmacokinetics of mefloquine in patients with acute falciparum malaria. Clin Pharmacol Ther 1999; 66:472–484.
50. Price R, Simpson JA, Teja-Isavatharm P, et al. Pharmacokinetics of mefloquine combined with artesunate in children with acute falciparum malaria. Antimicrob Agents Chemother 1999; 43:341–346.
51. White NJ, van Vugt M, Ezzet F. Clinical pharmacokinetics and pharmacodynamics of artemether-lumefantrine. Clin Pharmacokinet 1999; 37:105–125.
52. van Vugt M, Brockman A, Gemperli B, et al. Randomized comparison of artemether-benflumetol and artesunate-mefloquine in treatment of multidrug-resistant falciparum malaria. Antimicrob Agents Chemother 1998; 42:135–139.
53. van Vugt M, Looareesuwan S, Wilairatana P, et al. Artemether-lumefantrine for the treatment of multidrug-resistant falciparum malaria. Trans R Soc Trop Med Hyg 2000; 94: 545–548.
54. van Vugt MV, Wilairatana P, Gemperli B, et al. Efficacy of six doses of artemether-lumefantrine (benflumetol) in multidrug-resistant *Plasmodium falciparum* malaria. Am J Trop Med Hyg 1999; 60:936–942.
55. Ezzet F, van Vugt M, Nosten F, Looareesuwan S, White NJ. Pharmacokinetics and pharmacodynamics of lumefantrine (benflumetol) in acute falciparum malaria. Antimicrob Agents Chemother 2000; 44:697–704.
56. von Seidlein L, Milligan P, Pinder M, et al. Efficacy of artesunate plus pyrimethamine-sulphadoxine for uncomplicated malaria in Gambian children: a double-blind, randomised, controlled trial. Lancet 2000; 355:352–357.
57. Robert V, Awono-Ambene HP, Le Hesran JY, Trape JF. Gametocytemia and infectivity to mosquitoes of patients with uncomplicated *Plasmodium falciparum* malaria attacks treated with chloroquine or sulfadoxine plus pyrimethamine. Am J Trop Med Hyg 2000; 62:210–216.
58. von Seidlein L, Jawara M, Coleman R, Doherty T, Walraven G, Targett G. Parasitaemia and gametocytaemia after treatment with chloroquine, pyrimethamine/sulfadoxine, and pyrimethamine/sulfadoxine combined with artesunate in young Gambians with uncomplicated malaria. Trop Med Int Health 2001; 6:92–98.
59. Mendez F, Munoz A, Carrasquilla G, et al. Determinants of treatment response to sulfadoxine-pyrimethamine and subsequent transmission potential in falciparum malaria. Am J Epidemiol 2002; 156:230–238.
60. van Vugt M, Leonardi E, Phaipun L, et al. Treatment of uncomplicated multidrug-resistant falciparum malaria with artesunate-atovaquone-proguanil. Clin Infect Dis 2002; 35:1498–1504.
61. Adjuik M, Agnamey P, Babiker A, et al. Amodiaquine-artesunate versus amodiaquine for uncomplicated *Plasmodium falciparum* malaria in African children: a randomised, multicentre trial. Lancet 2002; 359:1365–1372.
62. Olliaro P, Mussano P. Amodiaquine for treating malaria. Cochrane Database Syst Rev 2000; 2:CD000016.
63. Olliaro P, Nevill C, LeBras J, et al. Systematic review of amodiaquine treatment in uncomplicated malaria. Lancet 1996; 348:1196–1201.

64. Olliaro P, Taylor WR, Rigal J. Controlling malaria: challenges and solutions. Trop Med Int Health 2001; 6:922–927.
65. Luxemburger C, Nosten F, Raimond SD, Chongsuphajaisiddhi T, White NJ. Oral artesunate in the treatment of uncomplicated hyperparasitemic falciparum malaria. Am J Trop Med Hyg 1995; 53:522–525.
66. Price R, Luxemburger C, van Vugt M, et al. Artesunate and mefloquine in the treatment of uncomplicated multidrug-resistant hyperparasitaemic falciparum malaria. Trans Roy Soc Trop Med Hyg 1998; 92:207–211.
67. Severe falciparum malaria. World Health Organization, Communicable Diseases Cluster. Trans R Soc Trop Med Hyg 2000; 94(suppl. 1):S1–S90.
68. McIntosh HM, Olliaro P. Artemisinin derivatives for treating severe malaria. Cochrane Database Syst Rev 2000; 2:CD000527.
69. Lesi A and Meremikwu M. High first dose quinine regimen for treating severe malaria (Cochrane Review). Cochrane Database Syst Rev 2002; 3:CD003341.
70. White NJ, Looareesuwan S, Warrell DA, et al. Quinine loading dose in cerebral malaria. Am J Trop Med Hyg 1983; 32:1–5.
71. Pittler MH, Ernst E. Artemether for severe malaria: a meta-analysis of randomized clinical trials. Clin Infect Dis 1999; 28:597–601.
72. Artemether-Quinine Meta-Analysis Study Group. A meta-analysis using individual patient data of trials comparing artemether with quinine in the treatment of severe falciparum malaria. Trans R Soc Trop Med Hyg 2001; 95:637–650.
73. Newton PN, Chierakul W, Ruangveerayuth R, et al. A comparison of artesunate alone with combined artesunate and quinine in the parenteral treatment of acute falciparum malaria. Trans R Soc Trop Med Hyg 2001; 95:519–523.
74. Wilairatana P, Viriyavejakul P, Looareesuwan S, Chongsuphajaisiddhi T. Artesunate suppositories: an effective treatment for severe falciparum malaria in rural areas. Ann Trop Med Parasitol 1997; 91:891–896.
75. Cao XT, Bethell DB, Pham TP, et al. Comparison of artemisinin suppositories, intramuscular artesunate and intravenous quinine for the treatment of severe childhood malaria. Trans R Soc Trop Med Hyg 1997; 91:335–342.
76. Hien TT, Arnold K, Vinh H, et al. Comparison of artemisinin suppositories with intravenous artesunate and intravenous quinine in the treatment of cerebral malaria. Trans R Soc Trop Med Hyg 1992; 86:582–583.
77. White NJ. Pathophysiology of falciparum malaria. In: Strickland GT (ed.). Clinics in Tropical Medicine and Communicable Diseases I. London: Saunders, 1986, pp. 55–90.
78. Meremikwu M, Marson AG. Routine anticonvulsants for treating cerebral malaria (Cochrane Review). Cochrane Database Syst Rev 2002; 2:CD002152.
79. Crawley J, Waruiru C, Mithwani S, et al. Effect of phenobarbital on seizure frequency and mortality in childhood cerebral malaria: a randomised, controlled intervention study. Lancet 2000; 355:701–706.
80. Nguyen TH, Day NP, Ly VC, et al. Post-malaria neurological syndrome. Lancet 1996; 348:917–921.
81. Luxemburger C, McGready R, Kham A, et al. Effects of malaria during pregnancy on infant mortality in an area of low malaria transmission. Am J Epidemiol 2001; 154:459–465.
82. McGready R, Thwai KL, Cho T, et al. The effects of quinine and chloroquine antimalarial treatments in the first trimester of pregnancy. Trans R Soc Trop Med Hyg 2002; 96: 180–184.
83. McGready R, Cho T, Hkirijaroen L, et al. Quinine and mefloquine in the treatment of multidrug-resistant *Plasmodium falciparum* malaria in pregnancy. Ann Trop Med Parasitol 1998; 92:643–653.
84. McGready R, Cho T, Samuel, et al. Randomized comparison of quinine-clindamycin versus artesunate in the treatment of falciparum malaria in pregnancy. Trans R Soc Trop Med Hyg 2001; 95:651–656.

85. Nosten F, Vincenti M, Simpson J, et al. The effects of mefloquine treatment in pregnancy. Clin Infect Dis 1999; 28:808–815.
86. McGready R, Cho T, Keo NK, et al. Artemisinin antimalarials in pregnancy: a prospective treatment study of 539 episodes of multidrug-resistant *Plasmodium falciparum*. Clin Infect Dis 2001; 33:2009–2016.
87. Phillips RE, Looareesuwan S, White NJ, Silamut K, Kietinun S, Warrell DA. Quinine pharmacokinetics and toxicity in pregnant and lactating women with falciparum malaria. Br J Clin Pharmacol 1986; 21:677–683.
88. ter Kuile FO, Nosten F, Luxemburger C, et al. Mefloquine treatment of acute falciparum malaria: a prospective study of non-serious adverse effects in 3673 patients. Bull World Health Organ 1995; 73:631–642.
89. Luxemburger C, Price RN, Nosten F, Ter Kuile FO, Chongsuphajaisiddhi T, White NJ. Mefloquine in infants and young children. Ann Trop Paediatr 1996; 16:281–286.
90. Olowu JA, Sowunmi A, Abohweyere AE. Congenital malaria in a hyperendemic area: a revisit. Afr J Med Med Sci 2000; 29:211–213.
91. Ahmed A, Cerilli LA, Sanchez PJ. Congenital malaria in a preterm neonate: case report and review of the literature. Am J Perinatol 1998; 15:19–22.
92. Habeck M. Transgenic mosquitoes to control malaria. Lancet Infect Dis 2001; 1:210.
93. Richie TL, Saul A. Progress and challenges for malaria vaccines. Nature 2002; 415:694–701.
94. France T, Ooms G, Rivers B. The GFATM (Global Fund to Fight AIDS, Tuberculosis, and Malaria): which countries owe, and how much? IAPAC 2002; 8:138, 141.
95. Mills A, Brugha R, Hanson K, McPake B. What can be done about the private health sector in low-income countries? Bull World Health Organ 2002; 80:325–330.
96. Newton P, Proux S, Green M, et al. Fake artesunate in Southeast Asia. Lancet 2001; 357: 1948–1950.
97. Rozendaal J. Fake antimalaria drugs in Cambodia. Lancet 2001; 357:890.
98. Meek SR. Vector control in some countries in Southeast Asia: comparing the vectors and the strategies. Ann Trop Med Parasitol 1995; 89:135–147.

19

Schistosome Drug Resistance

Praziquantel

Michael J. Doenhoff and Katherine Wheatcroft-Francklow

1. INTRODUCTION

It is estimated that more than 200 million people in approx 70 countries in the developing world are infected with schistosomes, the parasites that cause the human disease schistosomiasis. Of those infected, 85% live in Africa *(1,2)*. Tourists and other visitors to endemic areas who do not take care to avoid infection are also at risk.

Schistosomes are digenetic trematode (flatworm) parasites that require two hosts for completion of their complex life cycles: aquatic or amphibious snails, restricted to freshwater bodies in the tropics and that serve as intermediate hosts in which asexual reproduction occurs, and vertebrate definitive hosts, which allow sexual reproduction.

Humans become infected when they contact water in which patently infected snails have recently released free-swimming larvae (cercariae). The cercariae penetrate and migrate through the skin; after 2–3 d, they enter the bloodstream via a capillary or the lymphatic system *(3)*. In 4–5 wk, the parasites mature into sexually differentiated adults that live in the blood of their hosts for the rest of their lives.

Humans are hosts to three main species of schistosome: *Schistosoma japonicum*, which was discovered in Japan and has been virtually eradicated from that country, but is still present in parts of China and some Pacific islands; *Schistosoma mansoni*, which is found in Africa, South America, and some Caribbean islands; and *Schistosoma haematobium*, which occurs very widely in Africa and also in some Middle Eastern countries. The adult male and female worms of *S. japonicum* and *S. mansoni* live in mesenteric capillaries, and their eggs leave the body in feces. *Schistosoma haematobium* worms live in blood vessels of the urinogenital system, and their eggs passed out of the body in urine. On contact with water, ciliated miracidia hatch from the eggs: They seek and penetrate a new host snail to reproduce asexually again and thus complete the life cycle.

Adult schistosome worms have been estimated to have half-lives of between 3 and 10 yr, but instances of worms surviving for three to four decades have been recorded. In many endemic areas, the heaviest infections are found in children and young adults. Infection intensities generally decline with increasing age thereafter, but prevalences

From: *Management of Multiple Drug-Resistant Infections*
Edited by: S. H. Gillespie © Humana Press Inc., Totowa, NJ

tend to remain high. Because of these patterns of intensity and prevalence, morbidity from schistosomiasis is most severe in younger age groups.

The burden of disease from schistosome infection is enormous: In sub-Saharan Africa, *S. haematobium* is estimated to cause hematuria in 70 million people, major bladder wall pathology in 18 million, and hydronephrosis in 10 million. Annually, 150,000 die from nonfunctioning kidneys because of *S. haematobium*, and 130,000 die from portal hypertension induced by *S. mansoni (4)*.

Attempts to control schistosomiasis have progressed through several stages. In the middle of the last century, emphasis was given to control of the snail hosts by chemical mollusciciding *(5)* and modification of their environment (e.g., concrete lining of water channels). Mollusciciding, however, was labor intensive, and the chemicals were expensive; transmission was controlled in some endemic foci, but complete eradication by this method never seemed likely.

There were high hopes that the molecular-biological revolution of the 1970s and early 1980s and exploitation of recombinant DNA technology would result in rapid development of a vaccine. Unfortunately, however, despite intense effort in many laboratories, no vaccine to prevent schistosomiasis has yet come to market.

Additional basic information on schistosomes and schistosomiasis can be found in refs. *6–8*.

2. CHEMOTHERAPY OF SCHISTOSOMIASIS

In 1912, antimony was found to be an effective treatment for schistosomiasis. Although this element and its organic derivatives were in extensive use for many years because of the absence of alternatives, they had the considerable disadvantages of having to be administered systemically and in repeated doses. From the 1950s, however, new compounds with schistosomicidal activity were found that were less toxic than the antimonials and effective after oral administration. Thus, developments that started in the 1970s have been described as a revolution in the treatment of this disease *(9)*.

The organophosphorous compound metrifonate was shown to have activity against *S. haematobium*, and by the 1970s, its effectiveness against this parasite in humans was established *(10)*. However, it is effective only against this human schistosome species.

Oxamniquine is one of a series of related drugs (including, for example, lucanthone and hycanthone) that was developed in Germany and the United Kingdom over a period of 30–40 yr from the 1940s. Oxamniquine, manufactured by Pfizer, was the only compound to get to market; the others had problems such as unacceptable toxicity or mutagenicity. Oxamniquine is effective only against *S. mansoni*, and it and hycanthone are unusual among schistosomicides in that their mechanism of action has been elucidated. They become active only after transformation by an esterifying enzyme; as a consequence, they can alkylate DNA (*see* ref. *11*, a review by Cioli et al. that is a very comprehensive description of all antischistosome drugs, including many not mentioned here, and covering the history of their development and their modes of action, toxicity, pharmacokinetics, and metabolism).

Early in the 1970s, it was decided to test the pyrazino-isoquinoline ring system, initially explored as a tranquilizer, for antihelminth activity *(12)*. More than 400 compounds were tested at Bayer *(13)*. One of the most effective was EMBAY 8440, now known as praziquantel (PZQ), which was initially marketed as a veterinary cestocide.

In 1977, it was shown to be effective against schistosomes in animals *(14)*. After satisfactory results from toxicological and pharmacological tests, clinical trials were set up jointly by the World Health Organization (WHO) and Bayer in Africa, Japan, the Philippines, and Brazil. The results of the trials were very positive, showing good efficiency and only mild side effects *(11)*.

PZQ is now the drug of choice for treatment of schistosomiasis. Three main factors have contributed to its current prime position. First, the loss of patent protection allowed several manufacturers to begin producing generic forms of PZQ, and the consequent market competition in the 1990s resulted in substantial price reductions and increasing consumption. The average cost of tablets required for a single adult treatment is now approximately US $0.40; in Egypt alone, it is estimated that 20 million treatments or 60 million tablets were administered in 1997–1999 *(15)*. Second, PZQ is effective against all three species of human schistosome. Oxamniquine and metrifonate are the only other schistosomicidal compounds possibly still obtainable for treatment of schistosomiasis, but oxamniquine has no effect against either *S. haematobium* or *S. japonicum*, and metrifonate is active only against *S. haematobium*. Any residual use of oxamniquine is in any case likely to be supplanted by PZQ because of the price differential. Third, PZQ is a safe drug: There are very few reports of toxic side effects. For example, WHO has recently decided that even infected pregnant and lactating women should be offered treatment if they are considered potentially at high risk from schistosomiasis *(16)*. These factors have thus placed PZQ at the center of plans to control schistosome-induced morbidity by chemotherapy *(17)*.

The prospect of having just one drug available to treat a disease affecting 200 million people is a cause for concern in the context of the development of resistance *(18)*. We are now in a period of some uncertainty as to whether any resistance or tolerance to PZQ exists, a situation that is perhaps not uncommon during the history of many antibiotics applied extensively. There is also some confusion in the literature over the use of the terms *resistance* and *tolerance*. For present purposes, both are assumed to be genetically inherited: resistance may be defined as an acquired reduction in drug sensitivity following therapy with the drug in question; tolerance is an innate insusceptibility to a drug to which the population has not previously been exposed. More extensive discussion and definition of these terms can be found elsewhere *(19–23)*.

The purpose of this chapter is to review the results of both field and laboratory studies indicating that drug-resistant schistosomiasis does indeed exist. The evidence for genetic, physiological, and morphological markers of that resistance is considered, as are some of the implications. We restrict the discussion almost entirely to PZQ because, for the foreseeable future, it is likely to be the only drug used to treat schistosomiasis. The topic has been the subject of several recent reviews, which provide additional information *(18,21,24–28)*. Discussion here is also restricted to schistosomiasis mansoni because of the virtual absence of any relevant published information on drug resistance in either *S. haematobium* or *S. japonicum*.

3. STUDIES INDICATING EXISTENCE OF PRAZIQUANTEL RESISTANCE

3.1. *Evidence of Praziquantel Resistance From the Field: Egypt and Senegal*

Reports of possible resistance of schistosomes to PZQ have come from Egypt and Senegal. In Egypt, Ismail et al. *(29)* treated 1607 patients living in the Nile delta region and infected with *S. mansoni* with 40 mg/kg body weight PZQ. After an additional two treatments, the last at 60 mg/kg body weight, 2.4% of the initially treated patients were still passing eggs. Miracidia from the eggs of several individuals who were not cured after PZQ treatment were passaged into snails and hence into mice. Worms from five of these isolates were "significantly more difficult to cure" when compared with an isolate obtained from a patient who was cured after only one treatment *(29)*. In this and a subsequent study, it was found that differences in cure rates after treatment of mice infected with Egyptian isolates identified as PZQ sensitive or resistant were not substantial, with the median effective doses (ED_{50}s) of the resistant isolates only up to five times higher *(29,30)* than those of the controls. Additional results from laboratory experiments on these isolates are considered in Section 3.3.

The outcome of treating *S. mansoni* infections in Senegal has also raised concerns about the efficacy of PZQ and the possible existence of drug-resistant or drug-tolerant schistosomes. Thus, in the early 1990s, the use of routine doses of PZQ to treat infected subjects in what was then a recently established focus of infection in northern Senegal resulted in cure rates of only 18–36% (instead of 70–90% as usually expected) and egg count reductions of 77–88% *(31)*. Increasing the dose of PZQ from 40 to 60 mg/kg body weight did not significantly improve cure rates *(32)*. Relatively low cure rates were again obtained in a more recent study in the same area *(33)*.

3.2. Are Poor Cure Rates With Praziquantel Because of Resistance?

The results from Senegal and from experiments performed on Senegalese schistosome isolates have been the subject of controversy. Several explanations, other than drug resistance, have been put forward to account for the apparently poor performance of PZQ in this area of West Africa.

First, *S. mansoni* was estimated to be transmitted at a very high rate in Senegal, with the possible consequence that many patients would harbor significant numbers of immature schistosome worms at the time of treatment and would also become reinfected between treatment and parasitological assessment. PZQ is relatively ineffective against immature *S. mansoni* infections in mice *(34)*; thus, young worms could also have survived in humans after administration of PZQ, which would account for continuation or early resumption of egg excretion after treatment.

Results from the application of a multiple-treatment protocol designed to kill any worms that matured after the first treatment *(35)* supported the idea that low cure rates in this area were because of maturation of prepatent infections after the first treatment and not the presence of drug-resistant schistosomes *(27)*. Also in support of this notion, Piquet et al. *(36)* showed that, although a relatively poor cure rate (42.5%) was obtained after a first treatment with PZQ, a second treatment given 40 d after the first gave a cure rate of 76.1%. (A cure rate of only 76% is nevertheless still somewhat lower than might be expected with this drug.)

Second, because infection intensities in northern Senegal were very high *(37)*, it has been suggested that, even if the drug was normally effective, more worms may have survived than after treatments of infections of lower intensity, thus resulting in seemingly lower cure rates *(27)*.

Finally, the schistosomicidal activity of PZQ in experimental animals is partially immune (antibody) dependent *(38,39)*. The infection focus in northern Senegal became established relatively recently, and antischistosome immunity may thus not have been fully developed in those given treatment. Van Lieshout et al. *(40)*, however, analyzed several host-related factors, including antibody levels to adult worm antigens, and found no significant differences between those cured and those not cured by PZQ.

In contrast to PZQ, the schistosomicidal drug oxamniquine performed satisfactorily in Senegal *(41)*. To explain this, Gryseels et al. *(27)* suggested that, in Senegal, oxamniquine may have had a stronger schistosomicidal effect than PZQ or that the former compound has a different mechanism of action, perhaps with respect to immune dependence.

There are, however, counterarguments to these suggestions. Oxamniquine seems not to be very different from PZQ with respect to lack of efficacy against immature *S. mansoni* infections *(34)* or immune dependence *(38)*. Furthermore, the superior efficacy of oxamniquine over PZQ is an assumption that would be hard to substantiate with the existing heterogeneous data from Africa; one study has indicated oxamniquine had low efficacy *(19)*, but others indicated that the two drugs are equally effective (e.g., refs. *42* and *43*).

In their comprehensive review of the evidence from Senegal, Gryseels et al. *(27)* concluded that there is no convincing evidence for PZQ resistance in this area. Mathematical modeling used in this analysis indicated that the results from Senegal were in fact compatible with those expected from settings with comparable prevalence and intensity of infection and for a drug showing 90 ± 5% efficacy. On the other hand, in meta-analysis comparing the data from Senegal with those from other areas, it was calculated that, even after accounting for intensity of infection and sensitivity of diagnosis, *S. mansoni* in Senegal remained atypical because it gave cure rates significantly lower than expected *(44)*. The authors of this study concluded that "the suspicion of tolerance or resistance to PZQ ... cannot be ruled out" *(44)*.

Furthermore, it is difficult to reconcile the conclusion that Senegalese *S. mansoni* responds to PZQ no differently from *S. mansoni* elsewhere in the world *(27)* with the differential efficacies of PZQ and oxamniquine in Senegal and the experimental observations that a Senegalese *S. mansoni* isolate transported to the United Kingdom in infected snails was less susceptible to PZQ in mice when compared with other control isolates at the disposal of the testing laboratory *(45,46)*.

Direct comparisons between field-collected isolates and those that have been in long-term laboratory culture are not ideal, however. Other human populations are being identified (e.g., *47*) with *S. mansoni* infections that are far from completely cured by standard PZQ treatment protocols, and these will provide an opportunity, as well as emphasize the need, for the "natural" range of susceptibility to PZQ in *S. mansoni* to be established by examination of a wider range of freshly collected isolates. Standardization and validation of the tests used to detect drug resistance are also required.

3.3. Laboratory Evidence for Resistance to Praziquantel

Fallon and Doenhoff *(48)* were the first to report success in selection for resistance to PZQ in laboratory-maintained *S. mansoni*. This was achieved after cercariae of four geographically different isolates that had already been laboratory maintained for many years were mixed and the resulting "hybrid" subjected to subcurative doses of PZQ during successive passages in mice. The drug treatments were given to the mice before or during early patency of the infections. The decreased sensitivity to PZQ of fully mature infections of this isolate has been independently confirmed in two different laboratories (*see* ref. *49*; L. Pica-Mattoccia and D. Cioli; 2002, personal communication); Pica-Mattoccia and Cioli observed a two- to threefold higher ED_{50} after in vivo treatment of the selected drug-resistant line compared with controls. Selection for resistance to PZQ did not result in resistance to oxamniquine and vice versa *(48)*.

In vitro studies provided further confirmation that selection for PZQ resistance in this line had been successful. Thus, when adult worms were exposed to PZQ overnight, washed, and subsequently cultured in normal medium, those of the selected line survived for longer after subjection to higher drug concentrations than cultured worms of unselected controls (L. Pica-Mattoccia and D. Cioli, personal communication).

Ismail et al. *(29)* established life cycles of *S. mansoni* in mice from eggs that were excreted by their Egyptian patients who had not been cured by several treatments of PZQ; experiments on these laboratory cultures has helped to shed light on the question whether host- or parasite-related factors account for apparent insusceptibility of the parasite to PZQ. First, when changes in muscle tension of individual worms were measured in response to drug administered in vitro, the isolates established from uncured patients showed a strong correlation between degree of resistance of the infections in mice and the diminished muscle responses of the respective adult worms to the drug in vitro *(30)*. It was also found that adult worms of two ostensibly drug-resistant isolates suffered less tegumental damage than worms of a control susceptible isolate after in vitro exposure to PZQ *(50,51)*. Because the schistosomicidal action of PZQ is immune dependent *(38,39,52)*, it was suggested *(50)* that, after drug treatment, the antigenic targets of the antibodies that act synergistically with PZQ *(52,53)* could be less exposed on resistant worms than on susceptible worms.

Three of the *S. mansoni* lines that were isolated from uncured Senegalese patients in the mid-1990s and subsequently passaged in laboratory mice without drug pressure for approx 5–6 yr have also been tested for susceptibility to PZQ; they were found to be less susceptible than several control isolates *(49)*. Thus, in tests of dose responsiveness in vitro, different life-cycle stages of the *S. mansoni* isolates from Senegal withstood the toxic effects of PZQ at higher concentrations or for longer periods than other *S. mansoni* isolates used as controls: the parameters measured included drug-induced tail loss by cercariae, adult worm death, inhibition of egg hatching, and change of shape by miracidia *(49)*. Some of these parameters may be found useful in assaying for drug-resistant parasites in endemic areas.

4. MARKERS AND MECHANISMS OF PRAZIQUANTEL RESISTANCE

There is at present no generally accepted explanation for the mode of action of PZQ. The laboratory-selected PZQ-resistant isolate, as well as putatively resistant isolates from Senegal and Egypt, have been used to begin identifying genetic and physiological differences that may relate to the drug-resistant phenotype. The results from these studies may in turn indicate how the drug exerts its schistosomicidal effect.

Analysis using a subtractive polymerase chain reaction (PCR) indicated that adult worms of the laboratory-selected resistant line were expressing subunit 1 of the mitochondrial enzyme cytochrome-c oxidase at a 5- to 10-fold higher rate than worms of the parental hybrid isolate from which the former was derived *(54)*. However, actual activity of the respective enzyme was 4-fold lower in the resistant worms.

Use of a random amplified polymorphic DNA (RAPD) PCR showed that there was differential amplification of at least two major DNA nucleotide sequences between an Egyptian PZQ-resistant isolate and several PZQ-sensitive isolates from the same endemic area *(55)*.

It is important to note that only a relatively limited number of putatively resistant and susceptible schistosome isolates were compared with each other in the above studies, and that ratification of these early results will require similar comparative studies to be performed on a larger scale.

Although the schistosomicidal mode of action of PZQ has not yet been precisely elucidated, the profound effect this and other drugs have on parasite calcium ion flux are well known. Recent results indicating that components of calcium ion channels are the molecular target of PZQ *(56)* are therefore of considerable interest. The β-subunits of the Ca^{++} channels of schistosomes were found to have different structural motifs from those of other known β-subunits. Nonschistosome cell lines, which PZQ had no effect on, were rendered highly sensitive to the drug after they had been transfected with gene coding for the schistosome β-subunit *(56)*. Comparisons of the sequences of the β-subunits and other constituents of the calcium ion channels of PZQ-resistant and -susceptible schistosomes are awaited with interest.

The genetic basis of resistance to PZQ is thus not yet at all clear. It seems likely, however, that it will be shown to be because of a multiplicity of genes and thus different from that of oxamniquine resistance, which has been unequivocally demonstrated in humans *(57)* and is because of the loss of a single drug-activating enzyme *(11)*.

5. DRUG RESISTANCE, BIOLOGICAL FITNESS, AND REFUGIA

Six of the isolates established from uncured Egyptian patients have been studied through multiple successive passages in mice over a period of 5 yr *(58)*. In the absence of drug pressure, three of these retained their initial levels of insusceptibility to PZQ, and two reverted to drug sensitivity that was no different from controls. The three isolates that retained decreased sensitivity to PZQ showed some evidence of decreased cercarial production by infected snails *(58)*, thus indicating there may be a cost of biological fitness in PZQ resistance.

Similar to the Egyptian isolates that remained resistant despite laboratory passage *(58)*, recently performed tests on the three Senegalese isolates established in the early 1990s from treated but uncured patients showed that they shed fewer cercariae per snail than other nonresistant non-Senegalese isolates, although the snails infected with the former survived longer *(59)*. Mice infected with these three Senegalese isolates also had more eggs in their tissues and excreted more eggs in their feces *(59)*.

Clearly, further studies on different parameters of the host–parasite relationship in both intermediate and definitive hosts, and more extensive comparisons between different schistosome isolates, are required to determine whether there is a cost in biological fitness associated with PZQ resistance.

The contribution that surviving drug-pressured, and therefore potentially more drug-resistant, stock will make to the genetic constitution of an endemic population of schistosomes will also greatly depend on the overall relative sizes of the parasite's "refugia." This is a concept that has become important in analysis of the dynamics of drug resistance in helminths of sheep and cattle *(60–62)* and that has potential relevance to human infectious diseases and schistosomiasis in particular.

Provided refugia populations remain large relative to the number of incoming offspring of drug-treated and uncured schistosomes, the impact of the latter on the genetic constitution of the population as a whole will be small. Large refugia are likely to be found in human populations living in areas of high infection intensity and prevalence and subjected to chemotherapy only randomly or selectively. Similarly, infested environments in which intense transmission is occurring without interference from measures intended to control it (e.g., mollusciciding) are likely to provide relatively large refugia.

Human populations subjected to mass chemotherapy or endemic areas with low transmission rates will provide smaller refugia. Scenarios that could enhance the impact of genetically drug-resistant organisms on the schistosome population as a whole can thus be envisaged, for example, provision of mass chemotherapy at a time when an intermediate host snail population was re-establishing itself and was therefore largely uninfested, as might occur soon after flooding or an application of molluscicide.

6. CONCLUSION

Results of in vivo and in vitro tests on several isolates of *S. mansoni* obtained from Egypt and Senegal and one that was derived by selection in the laboratory leave little room for doubt that a degree of resistance to PZQ can occur in this parasite. Fortunately, however, the level of PZQ resistance exhibited by the isolates so far examined is relatively low: None of them had a drug ED_{50} that was greater than five to six times those of the drug-susceptible isolates used as controls in the different laboratories. This can be compared with *S. mansoni* resistance to hycanthone and oxamniquine, which can rise to very high levels (i.e., almost 1000-fold differences) *(63)*.

Although the levels of PZQ resistance that have so far been perceived may not pose an obvious or immediate threat to its usefulness for the treatment of schistosomiasis, complacency and a failure to monitor developments may have serious consequences in the longer term. PZQ is now the only drug available for treating schistosomiasis, and particularly because of the recent very marked reductions in price *(15,64)*, the rate of usage can be expected to increase rapidly in the near future when programs using it to control schistosome-induced morbidity throughout sub-Saharan Africa are under way *(17,65)*.

These initiatives will build on the experience of PZQ usage gained in Egypt *(66)* and Senegal *(27)* during the last decade. The work program in Egyptian villages that included regular drug treatment of school children was clearly successful in reducing disease prevalence and intensity *(66)*, but it is not yet clear whether there has been a concomitant reduction in the potential of the parasite for transmission in the areas subjected to control by chemotherapy. Furthermore, despite novel antibody responses and other signs of humoral immunity generated because of PZQ treatment, cured individuals do not uniformly become resistant to reinfection because of the changes in antibody profile *(67,68)*. Chemotherapy may therefore need to be continued on a regular basis for as long as the risk of high transmission persists.

In Egypt, the proportion of overtly uncured patients detected in the treated populations seems fortunately to have remained relatively small, and there is so far no evidence that the program of regularly treating children during the last decade has caused the endemic schistosome population to shift genetically to a more drug-resistant state. However, there seems little doubt that offspring of schistosomes that have survived PZQ treatment have entered the environment in Egypt and other areas where the drug has been used with an ostensibly normal outcome. This is because post-treatment parasitological analyses have rarely, if ever, demonstrated cure rates of 100% (i.e., complete absence of eggs in the excreta of treated patients), and all the cure rates that have been recorded using post-treatment egg counts are in any case likely to be overestimates because of the relative insensitivity of diagnostic parasitology *(69)*.

Both a field-collected Senegalese isolate that was relatively resistant to PZQ *(46)* and the laboratory-maintained *S. mansoni* that was selectively bred to be PZQ resistant *(48)* remained susceptible to oxamniquine, which performed more satisfactorily than PZQ in infected Senegalese patients *(41)*. Oxamniquine is thus an obvious choice for use as an alternative to, or in combination with PZQ, but it is perhaps unrealistic to expect that it will be easy to adopt it in cases of PZQ failure because the price of oxamniquine has remained high, and its continued commercial availability is uncertain.

Much of the debate so far has been concerned with whether PZQ-resistant schistosomes now exist, thus largely obfuscating the fact that, when this drug was used according to recommended schedules in Senegal, it produced cure rates of less than 50% *(31,37)*. One obvious remedial strategy—increasing the dose—unfortunately did not appear to improve cure rates *(32)*. Adoption of protocols involving two successive closely spaced treatments with the same drug *(27,35)* or treatment of initial therapeutic failures with a different drug *(70)* may be effective, although adoption of such strategies of course will be more expensive. In any event, situations now unquestionably exist for which treatment of schistosomiasis with PZQ is not completely effective; this is most likely in part because of the intrinsic limitations of the drug when dealing with recent infections. In other words, in spite of its enormous usefulness, PZQ is not *the* perfect antischistosomal drug.

ACKNOWLEDGMENTS

K. F. is financially supported by the INCO-II Programme of the European Commission (contract ICA4-CT-2001-10079). Both authors are members of a European Commission (INCO-DC) Concerted Action on the Pattern of Praziquantel Usage and Monitoring of Possible Resistance in Africa.

We are grateful to Donato Cioli and Livia Pica-Mattoccia for permission to refer to their unpublished results and to members of Concerted Action and other colleagues for continuing helpful discussion and advice.

REFERENCES

1. Chitsulo L, Engels D, Montresor A, Savioli L. The global status of schistosomiasis and its control. Acta Tropica 2000; 77:41–51.
2. Engels D, Chitsulo L, Montresor A, Savioli L. The global epidemic of schistosomiasis and new approaches to control. Acta Tropica 2002; 82:139–146.
3. Curwen RS, Wilson RA. Invasion of skin by schistosome cercariae: some neglected facts. Trends Parasitol 2003; 19:63–66.
4. Van der Werf MJ, de Vlas SJ, Brooker S, et al. Quantification of clinical morbidity associated with schistosome infection in sub-Saharan Africa. Acta Tropica 2003; 86:125–139.

5. Sturrock RF. Schistosomiasis epidemiology and control: how did we get here and where should we go? Mem Inst Oswaldo Cruz 2001; 96(suppl.):17–27.
6. Mahmoud AF. Schistosomiasis. London: Imperial College Press, 2001.
7. Davis A. Schistosomiasis. In: Cook GC, Zumla A (eds.). Manson's Tropical Diseases. 21st ed. New York: Saunders/Elsevier Science, 2002, pp. 1431–1469.
8. Muller R. Worms and Human Disease. 2nd ed. New York: CABI, 2001.
9. Davis A. Recent advances in schistosomiasis. Q J Med 1986; 58:95–110.
10. Davis A, Bailey DR. Metrifonate in urinary schistosomiasis. Bull WHO 1969; 41:209–224.
11. Cioli D, Pica-Mattoccia L, Archer S. Antischistosomal drugs: past, present ... and future. Pharm Ther 1995; 68:35–85.
12. Groll E. Praziquantel. Adv Pharmacol Chemother 1984; 20:219–238.
13. Seubert J, Pohlke R, Loebich F. Synthesis and properties of praziquantel, a novel broad spectrum anthelminthic with excellent activity against schistosomes and cestodes. Experientia 1977; 33:1036–1037.
14. Gönnert R, Andrews P. Praziquantel, a new broad-spectrum anti-schistosomal agent. Zeit Parasitenk 1977; 52:129–150.
15. Doenhoff MJ, Kimani G, Cioli D. Praziquantel and the control of schistosomiasis. Parasitol Today 2000; 16:364–366.
16. Allen HE, Crompton DWT, de Silva N, LoVerde PT, Olds GR. New policies for using anthelmintics in high risk groups. Trends Parasitol 2002; 18:381–382
17. Savioli L, Stansfield S, Bundy DAP, et al. Schistosomiasis and soil-transmitted helminth infections: forging control efforts. Trans R Soc Trop Med Hyg 2003; 96:577–579.
18. Cioli D. Praziquantel: is there real resistance and are there alternatives? Curr Opin Infect Dis 2000; 13:659–663.
19. Coles GC, Mutahi WT, Kinoti GK, Bruce JI, Katz N. Tolerance of Kenyan *Schistosoma mansoni* to oxamniquine. Trans R Soc Trop Med Hyg 1987; 81:782–785.
20. Cioli D, Pica-Mattoccia L, Archer S. Drug-resistance in schistosomes. Parasitol Today 1993; 9:162–166.
21. Fallon PG, Tao LF, Ismail MM, Bennett JL. Schistosome resistance to praziquantel: fact or artifact. Parasitol Today 1996; 12:316–320.
22. Coles GC, Kinoti GK. Defining resistance in *Schistosoma*. Parasitol Today 1997; 13: 157–158.
23. Coles GC. Drug resistance or tolerance in schistosomes? Trends Parasitol 2002; 18:294.
24. Bennett JL, Day T, Liang FT, Ismail M, Farghaly A. The development of resistance to anthelmintics: a perspective with an emphasis on the antischistosomal drug praziquantel. Exp Parasitol 1997; 87:260–267.
25. Cioli D. Chemotherapy of schistosomiasis: an update. Parasitol Today 1998; 14:418–422.
26. Geerts S, Gryseels B. Drug resistance in human helminths: current situation and lessons from livestock. Clin Microbiol Rev 2000; 13:207–222.
27. Gryseels B, Mbaye A, De Vlas SJ, et al. Are poor responses to praziquantel for the treatment of *Schistosoma mansoni* infections in Senegal due to resistance? An overview of the evidence. Trop Med Int Health 2001; 6:864–873.
28. Doenhoff MJ, Kusel JR, Coles GC, Cioli D. Resistance of *Schistosoma mansoni* to praziquantel: is there a problem. Trans R Soc Trop Med Hyg 2002; 96:465–469.
29. Ismail M, Metwally A, Farghally A, Bruce J, Tao LF, Bennett JL. Characterization of isolates of *Schistosoma mansoni* from Egyptian villagers that tolerate high doses of praziquantel. Am J Trop Med Hyg 1996; 55:214–218.
30. Ismail M, Botros S, Metwally A, et al. Resistance to praziquantel: direct evidence from *Schistosoma mansoni* isolated from Egyptian villagers. Am J Trop Med Hyg 1999; 60: 932–935.
31. Stelma FF, Talla A, Sow S, et al. Efficacy and side-effects of praziquantel in an epidemic focus of *Schistosoma mansoni*. Am J Trop Med Hyg 1995; 53:167–170.

32. Guisse F, Polman K, Stelma FF, et al. Therapeutic evaluation of two different dose regimens of praziquantel in a recent *Schistosoma mansoni* focus in northern Senegal. Am J Trop Med Hyg 1997; 56:511–524.
33. Tchuem-Tchuente LA, Southgate VR, Mbaye A, Engels D, Gryseels B. The efficacy of praziquantel against *Schistosoma mansoni* infection in Ndombo, northern Senegal. Trans R Soc Trop Med Hyg 2001; 95:65–66.
34. Sabah AA, Fletcher C, Webbe G, Doenhoff MJ. *Schistosoma mansoni*—chemotherapy of infections of different ages. Exp Parasitol 1986; 61:294–303.
35. Renganathan E, Cioli D. An international initiative on praziquantel use. Parasitol Today 1998; 14:390–391.
36. Piquet M, Vercruysse J, Shaw DJ, Diop M, Ly A. Efficacy of praziquantel against *Schistosoma mansoni* in northern Senegal. Trans R Soc Trop Med Hyg 1998; 92:90–93.
37. Gryseels B, Stelma FF, Talla I, et al. Epidemiology, immunology and chemotherapy of *Schistosoma mansoni* infections in a recently exposed community in Senegal. Trop Geogr Med 1994; 46:209–219.
38. Sabah AA, Fletcher C, Webbe G, Doenhoff MJ. *Schistosoma mansoni*—reduced efficacy of chemotherapy in infected T-cell-deprived mice. Exp Parasitol 1985; 60:348–354.
39. Doenhoff MJ, Sabah AA, Fletcher C, Webbe G, Bain J. Evidence of an immune-dependent action of praziquantel on *Schistosoma mansoni* in mice. Trans R Soc Trop Med Hyg 1987; 81:947–951.
40. Van Lieshout L, Stelma FF, Guisse F, et al. The contribution of host-related factors to low cure rates of praziquantel for treatment of *Schistosoma mansoni* in Senegal. Am J Trop Med Hyg 1999; 61:760–765.
41. Stelma FF, Sall S, Daff B, Sow S, Niang M, Gryseels B. Oxamniquine cures *Schistosoma mansoni* in a focus in which cure rates with praziquantel are unusually low. J Infect Dis 1997; 176:304–307.
42. Polderman AM, Gryseels B, Decaluwe P. Cure rates and egg reduction in treatment of intestinal schistosomiasis with oxamniquine and praziquantel in Maniema, Zaire. Trans R Soc Trop Med Hyg 1988; 82:115–116.
43. Butterworth AE, Sturrock RF, Ouma JH, et al. Comparison of different chemotherapy strategies against *Schistosoma mansoni* in Machakos District, Kenya—effects on human infection and morbidity. Parasitology 1991; 103:339–355.
44. Dansio-Appiah A, De Vlas SJ. The interpretation of low praziquantel cure rates in population treatment of *Schistosoma mansoni* infection. Trends Parasitol 2002; 18:125–129.
45. Fallon PG, Sturrock RF, Niang CM, Doenhoff MJ. Short report—diminished susceptibility to praziquantel in a Senegal isolate of *Schistosoma mansoni*. Am J Trop Med Hyg 1995; 53:61–62.
46. Fallon PG, Mubarak JS, Fookes RE, et al. *Schistosoma mansoni*: maturation rate and drug susceptibility of different geographic isolates. Exp Parasitol 1997; 86:29–36.
47. Utzinger J, N'Goran EK, N'Dri A, Lengeler C, Tanner M. Efficacy of praziquantel against *Schistosoma mansoni* with particular consideration for intensity of infection. Trop Med Int Health 2000; 5:771–778.
48. Fallon PG, Doenhoff MJ. Drug-resistant schistosomiasis: resistance to praziquantel and oxamniquine induced in *Schistosoma mansoni* in mice is drug-specific. Am J Trop Med Hyg 1994; 51:83–88.
49. Liang Y-S, Coles GC, Doenhoff MJ, Southgate VR. In vitro responses of praziquantel-resistant and -susceptible *Schistosoma mansoni* to praziquantel. Int J Parasitol 2001; 31:1227–1235.
50. William S, Botros S, Ismail M, Farghally A, Day TA, Bennett JL. Praziquantel-induced tegumental damage is diminished in schistosomes derived from praziquantel-resistant infections. Parasitology 2001; 122:63–66.
51. Liang Y-S, Coles GC, Dai J-R, Zhu Y-C, Doenhoff MJ. Adult worm tegumental damage

and egg-granulomas in praziquantel-resistant and -susceptible *Schistosoma mansoni* treated in vivo. J Helminthol 2002; 76:327–333.
52. Brindley PJ, Sher A. The chemotherapeutic effect of praziquantel against *Schistosoma mansoni* is dependent on host antibody response. J Immunol 1987; 139:215–220.
53. Doenhoff MJ, Modha J, Lambertucci JR. Anti-schistosome chemotherapy enhanced by antibodies specific for a parasite esterase. Immunology 1988; 65:507–510.
54. Pereira C, Fallon PG, Cornette JC, Capron A, Doenhoff MJ, Pierce RJ. Alterations in cytochrome-c oxidase expression between praziquantel-resistant and susceptible strains of *Schistosoma mansoni*. Parasitology 1998; 117:63–73.
55. Tsai M-H, Marx KA, Ismail MM, Tao L-F. Randomly-amplified polymorphic DNA (RAPD) polymerase chain reaction assay for determination of *Schistosoma mansoni* strains sensitive or tolerant to anti-schistosomal drugs. J Parasitol 2000; 86:146–149.
56. Kohn AB, Anderson PAV, Roberts-Misterly JM, Greenberg RM. Schistosome calcium channel β subunits: unusual modulatory effects and potential role in the action of the antischistosomal drug praziquantel. J Biol Chem 2001; 276:36,873–36,876.
57. Katz N, Dias EP, Araujo N, Souza CP. Estudo de una cepa humana de *Schistosoma mansoni* resistente a agentes esquistossomicidas. Rev Soc Bras Med Trop 1973; 7:381–387.
58. William S, Sabra A, Ramzy F, et al. Stability and reproductive fitness of *Schistosoma mansoni* isolates with decreased sensitivity to praziquantel. Int J Parasitol 2001; 31:1093–1100.
59. Liang Y-S, Coles GC, Dai J-R, Zhu Y-C, Doenhoff MJ. Biological characteristics of praziquantel-resistant and -susceptible isolates of *Schistosoma mansoni*. Ann Trop Med Parasitol 2001; 95:715–723.
60. Martin PJ, Le Jambre LF, Claxton JH. The impact of refugia on the development of thiabendazole resistance in *Haemonchus contortus*. Int J Parasitol 1981; 11:35–41.
61. Van Wyk JA. Refugia—overlooked as perhaps the most potent factor concerning development of anthelmintic resistance. Onderstepoort J Vet Res 2001; 68:55–67.
62. Coles GC. The sustainable use of anthelmintics in grazing animals. Vet Rec 2002; 151: 165–169.
63. Pica-Mattoccia L, de Souza Dias LC, Moroni R, Cioli D. *Schistosoma mansoni*: genetic complementation analysis shows that two independent hycanthone/oxamniquine-resistant strains are mutated in the same gene. Exp Parasitol 1993; 77:445–449.
64. Kusel J, Hagan P. Praziquantel—its use, cost and possible development of resistance. Parasitol Today 1999; 15:352–354.
65. Appleton CC, Mbaye A. Praziquantel—quality, dosages and markers of resistance. Trends Parasitol 2001; 17:356–357.
66. El Khoby T, Galal N, Fenwick A. The USAID Government of Egypt's Schistosomiasis Research Project (SRP). Parasitol Today 1998; 14:92–96.
67. Correa-Oliveira R, Caldas IR, Gazzinelli G. Natural versus drug-induced resistance in *Schistosoma mansoni* infection. Parasitol Today 2000; 16:397–399.
68. Mutapi F. Heterogeneities in anti-schistosome humoral responses following chemotherapy. Trends Parasitol 2001; 17:518–524.
69. Doenhoff MJ. Is schistosomicidal chemotherapy sub-curative? Implications for drug resistance. Parasitol Today 1998; 14:434–435.
70. Katz N, Rocha RS, de Souza CP, et al. Efficacy of alternating therapy with oxamniquine and praziquantel to treat *Schistosoma mansoni* in children following failure of first treatment. Am J Trop Med Hyg 1991; 44:509–512.

V

Viral Infections

20

Management of HIV Drug-Resistant Infections

Deenan Pillay

1. INTRODUCTION

More than 16 drugs are currently licensed for therapy of human immunodeficiency virus (HIV) infection, categorized as nucleoside reverse transcriptase inhibitors (NRTIs), non-nucleoside reverse transcriptase inhibitors (nNRTIs), protease inhibitors (PIs), and most recently, fusion inhibitors. These are listed in Table 1. Virological resistance has been documented against all these drugs, both in vitro and in vivo, and the topic of this chapter is the implications of such resistance for clinical management.

Antiviral drug resistance is defined by reduced drug susceptibility of a viral isolate with a phenotypic assay and is therefore a quantitative measurement that is expressed either as an IC_{50} (concentration of drug required to inhibit virus replication by 50%) or a specific-fold decrease in susceptibility. This phenotype is determined by the presence of specific mutations within the HIV genome, described as the *genotype*. In some cases, such as for the nNRTIs and PIs, many of these amino acid changes directly affect the binding of drug to the target enzyme *(1,2)*. Recent structural studies of HIV-1 reverse transcriptase (RT) resistant to zidovudine (ZDV) also allow an appreciation of how nucleoside analog resistance mutations that appear distant to the active site may still impinge on the RT aspartyl active site. A causal relationship between specific mutations and reduced drug susceptibility must be confirmed by mutagenesis experiments. When such in vitro experiments have not been undertaken, genetic changes should be referred to as resistance-associated mutations.

Following the first demonstration in 1989 of phenotypic HIV drug resistance to ZDV *(3)*, a large body of literature has developed documenting genotypic correlates of reduced drug susceptibility in vitro and virological failure in vivo. However, before such data are crudely utilized to interpret resistance data from the clinic, caution should be applied. Many of these data are derived from monotherapy studies, which do not reflect more recent clinical practice. Thus, mutations leading to reduced susceptibility to one drug may attenuate or even reverse resistance to another drug. Other mutations appear not to have an impact on drug susceptibility *per se*, but rather compensate for the reduced growth characteristics generated by an initial resistance mutation.

Against the background of more than 16 antiretroviral drugs available for clinical use, it is difficult to assess the precise impact of specific mutations within the context of all possible drug combinations. Further, some regions of the HIV genome are highly

From: *Management of Multiple Drug-Resistant Infections*
Edited by: S. H. Gillespie © Humana Press Inc., Totowa, NJ

Table 1
Clinically Observed Drug Resistance Mutations for Licensed Antiretroviral Drugs

Drug	Key genotypic changes
Nucleoside/nucleotide reverse transcriptase inhibitors	
Zidovudine (ZDV)	M41L, D67N, K70R, L210W, T215Y/F, K219Q/E
Didanosine (ddI)	K65R, L74V
Zalcitabine (ddC)	K65R, T69D, L74V
Stavudine (d4T)	M41L, D67N, K70R, L210W, T215Y/F, K219Q/E
Lamivudine (3TC)	E44D, V118I, M184V/I
Abacavir (ABC)	K65R, L74V, Y115F, M184V
Tenofovir (TDF)	K65R
Multi-nRTI resistance:	M41L, E44D, D67N, K70R, V118I, L210W, T215 Y/F, K219 Q/E + 69 insertions
	+A62/V, V75I, F77L, F116Y, Q151M
Non-nucleoside reverse transcriptase inhibitors	
Nevirapine (NVP)	L100I, K103N, V106 A/M, V108I, Y181 C/I, Y188 C/L/H, G190A
Efavirenz (EFV)	L100I, K103N, V106M, V108I, Y181C/I, Y188/L, G190 S/A, P225/M
Protease inhibitors	
Indinavir (IDV)	M46 I/L, V82 A/F/T, I84V
Saquinavir (SQV)	G48V, L90M
Nelfinavir (NFV)	D30N, L90M
Amprenavir (APV)	I50V, I84V
Lopinavir/ritonavir (LPV/RTV)	L10 F/I/R/V, K20M/R, L24I, V32I, L33F, M46 I/L, I47V, 150V, F53L, I54 V/L, L63P, A71 V/T, G73S, V82 A/F/T/S, I84V, L90M (more than 7/8 of above)
Atazanavir (ATZ)	I50L
Fusion inhibitors	
T-20	G35D/S, V38A/M, Q40H, N42T, N43D/K/S, L44M, L45M

Reverse transcriptase inhibitor mutations refer to amino acid positions in the reverse transcriptase gene.
Protease inhibitor mutations refer to amino acid positions in the protease gene.
Fusion inhibitor mutations refer to amino acid positions in the gp41 gene.

variable, even within virus subtypes, which are genetic variants of the main (M) group of HIV-1, generally distributed on a geographical basis worldwide. For instance, 50% of the protease amino acids may vary in the absence of PIs, including changes previously associated with drug resistance *(4)*. As for nonclade B viruses, some of the well-recognized nNRTI resistance mutations can often be found as natural polymorphisms *(5)*. The impact of this variability on response to antiretroviral drugs remains unclear.

These issues highlight the importance of assimilating resistance data into prospective clinical trials of antiretroviral agents to determine the genotypic correlates of drug failure.

2. BIOLOGICAL BASIS OF DRUG RESISTANCE

HIV exists as a quasi species within each infected individual, consequent on the high replication rate and error-prone RT enzymatic activity. On average, one mutation will be incorporated into each newly synthesized virion. Therefore, viruses requiring only one mutation to generate high-level resistance will be represented within the prevailing quasi species. If more than one mutation is required, there is a reduced chance of these being generated spontaneously in any single replication cycle, and thus the risk of their pre-existence will be lower *(6)*.

By definition, the fittest virus within the quasi species will become the majority species; because many viruses with reduced drug susceptibilities are also relatively replication deficient (*see* Section 5.4.), they remain a small proportion until such time that the relevant drug selective pressure is imposed, when they become the majority species. The fate of newly produced replication-competent HIV virions is one of three options: They may infect an activated T cell, which will subsequently produce large quantities of virus prior to rapid cell death; they may infect macrophages, which then persistently produce virus with a slower cell turnover rate; finally, the virally infected T cell may become a resting memory cell, in which case the latent proviral DNA may become long lasting, compromising attempts to eradicate HIV infection.

Nevertheless, the success of maintaining such a state of viral latency depends on continuing suppression of viral replication *(7)*. If this viral DNA encodes drug resistance, then it may emerge at any time in the future, following cell activation. Clearly, under a suitable drug selective pressure, these species will predominate. Therefore, the absence of particular mutations within plasma HIV RNA does not preclude their existence within infected cells. This must be borne in mind when considering the apparent disappearance of drug resistance mutation from plasma virus following cessation of drug therapy *(8)*.

This consideration of antiretroviral drug resistance leads to two conclusions. First, it is to be expected that any potent anti-HIV drug will lead to the emergence of drug-resistant virus species because of the selective pressure imposed. Second, the best strategy to prevent emergence of antiviral drug resistance is the suppression of viral replication. This provides the rationale for current guidelines on the use of highly active antiretroviral therapy (HAART).

3. HIV RESISTANCE TESTING

Genotypic and phenotypic measurement of drug resistance in plasma virus can be undertaken. Because routine propagation of HIV from peripheral blood mononuclear cells for drug susceptibility assays is time consuming and costly, recombinant virus assays have been developed by which homologous recombination between relevant polymerase chain reaction (PCR) products from the patient's plasma virus and a modified HIV-1 vector is undertaken, creating a virus incorporating the drug resistance mutations of note. This virus can be rapidly screened for drug susceptibility. However, routine provision of this assay remains generally in the realm of commercial companies, and the assay has previously been limited by problems of interpretation.

Thus, the original cutoff values by which viruses were designated as drug sensitive or resistant were based on assay variability, such that a 2.5- or 4-fold cutoff was used by the two commercial companies providing such assays. It then became clear that biological cutoff values, which take into account the biological variability of fold susceptibility for any particular drug, were more appropriate. These cutoffs may vary from 1.5-fold to 10-fold, depending on the drug in question. A third tier of value, the clinical cutoff, is based on a prediction of clinical response to a particular drug. At the time of writing, such cutoffs have only been generated for a few drugs, such as the RT inhibitors abacavir (ABC) *(9)* and tenofovir (TDF) *(10)*.

By contrast, genotypic assays involve the sequencing of the relevant genes from plasma HIV-1 to identify specific mutations (compared to wild-type virus sequence) associated with drug resistance. The major problem with these methods is in the interpretation of single or groups of mutations as described in Section 2. A discussion of the utility of these assays is undertaken in Section 6.

4. REASONS FOR ANTIRETROVIRAL FAILURE

Long-term inhibition of viral replication by HAART is predicted by initial suppression of viral load (VL) to less than 50 copies/mL following initiation of therapy *(11)*. Nevertheless, despite tremendous advances in the control of HIV infection by HAART, up to 20% or more of patients initiating triple therapy are likely to fail virologically within the first year.

4.1. *Potency*

Historically, one of the most common reasons for virological failure has been the inadequate potency of antiretroviral drugs, particularly in the era of mono- and double therapy. Triple-therapy regimens demonstrate far superior potency. Nevertheless, the efficacy of some triple combinations appears suboptimal in patients with high baseline VLs (>100,000 copies/mL), which may reflect a lack of potency. As VL assays become even more sensitive, it is to be expected that inadequate suppression of replication will be more frequently revealed. As discussed in Section 2, continual virus replication in the presence of antiviral selective pressure will lead to the emergence of drug resistance; therefore, these patients have an increased risk of failing their regimen in the presence of resistance.

4.2. *Compliance*

More complex antiretroviral regimens require an almost obsessional commitment by patients to adhere fully to therapy. Up to 30 tablets/d may be required, which has an impact on the ability to lead a normal life. Prospective studies have demonstrated a direct link between the degree of adherence and the suppression of VL *(12)*. Thus, increasing effort is being made to ensure good compliance by provision of pretherapy counseling, ongoing community support of those on therapy, and rationalization and simplification of drug regimens. This includes twice daily, or even once daily, dosing and the combination of more than one compound within a single tablet.

4.3. *Pharmacological*

It is important that adequate drug levels are maintained throughout the dosing period. This not only relates to drug compliance, but also to individual patient differences in pharmacodynamics. Suboptimal levels of active compound are likely to increase the risk of emergence of resistance, as demonstrated for ritonavir (RTV) therapy *(13)*. In a randomized study of the utility of resistance assays (Viradapt), plasma drug levels were found to be an independent predictor of VL suppression *(14)*. Therefore, therapeutic drug monitoring (TDM) may be an important tool for preventing the virological failure and emergence of drug resistance in the future.

4.4. Compartmentalization

With the introduction of plasma VL measurements as a key surrogate of HIV disease progression, it must be remembered that HIV RNA within this blood compartment does not necessarily reflect viral replication in other anatomical or cellular sites within the body. For instance, virus evolution within the central nervous system or genital tract appears different from that in blood *(15,16)*, suggesting that the selective pressures determining virus evolution vary between these compartments. As for antiretroviral therapy, it is now apparent that differential drug penetration into these sites may occur, providing one explanation for the discordance observed in drug resistance mutations between sites *(17,18)*. It follows that suppression of blood VL by HAART may not necessarily be matched by suppression of replication in other tissues, which may lead to a reservoir of virus capable of reinfecting susceptible cells. This may lead to subsequent treatment failure, although such a scenario has not been formally demonstrated.

4.5. Drug Resistance Emerging During Therapy

It is therefore apparent that many factors lead to antiretroviral failure. Any increase in viral replication in the presence of a drug selective pressure can lead to the emergence of drug resistance; therefore, drug failure is often associated with resistance. In addition, the presence of virus with reduced drug susceptibility may itself directly cause failure of VL suppression or VL rebound. The emergence of high-level resistance to some drugs, such as PIs, requires a number of mutations within the protease gene *(19)*, whereas only one mutation is necessary to confer high-level resistance to drugs such as lamivudine (3TC) *(20)* or the nNRTIs *(21)*.

Because single mutants are more likely to pre-exist, some have argued that emergence of resistance will be delayed for drugs with a high "genetic barrier" (multiple mutations required for high-level resistance) because of the requirement for further evolution of the virus. This is no doubt true in monotherapy regimens, as has been observed in trials of nevirapine (NVP) therapy *(21)*. However, in the context of combination therapy, the situation is more complex. Initial drug failure will often be associated with emergence of resistance to those drugs within the combination that have a low genetic barrier for resistance. However, the overall risk of failure is more likely to be determined by the potency of the regimen rather than the number of drugs contained in the regimen with such a low genetic barrier.

Most data on prevalence of resistance derives from clinical trial data or highly biased patient populations. By contrast, little structured surveillance has been undertaken. In such a pilot study in the United Kingdom during the period 1998–2000, my group demonstrated that most treated patients with detectable VL had resistance to drugs within a least one class of antiretroviral drugs, and that the introduction of the nNRTI class of agent in 1999 led to the rapid emergence of resistance to these drugs *(22)*.

4.6. Transmission of Drug Resistance

There is good epidemiological evidence to demonstrate the transmission of drug-resistant HIV. These surveillance studies fall into two categories: those that assess the prevalence of resistance in drug-naive patients and those that assess patients with primary infection. There is a wide variation in prevalence of resistance among studies, up to 25% *(23,24)*. This variation can be explained by differences in the period of study, geographical differences, risk groups tested, methodologies used, and definitions of drug resistance. For instance, the inclusion of secondary PI resistance mutations in a definition of PI resistance dramatically increases the apparent prevalence of transmitted drug resistance. However, there is little evidence that these mutations alone confer resistance, and they are well recognized as natural polymorphisms.

Evidence has been presented that transmission of resistant strains is associated with suboptimal response to antiviral therapy *(23,25,26)*. This provides the rationale for undertaking resistance testing in patients at the time of first diagnosis or prior to initiating therapy.

5. RESISTANCE TO NUCLEOSIDE ANALOGS

The acquisition of high-level ZDV resistance requires several changes in the RT, including at amino acid positions 41, 67, 70, 215, and 219 *(27)*. Resistance emerges after 6–12 mo of monotherapy. Large surveillance studies of nucleoside analog–experienced patients identified T215Y as the most prevalent drug resistance mutation *(28)*. This is unsurprising in view of the time period for which ZDV has been available. An analysis of the ACTG 116B/117 trial, comparing continued ZDV therapy with switching ZDV monotherapy to didanosine (ddI) monotherapy, demonstrated that the presence of high-level phenotypic resistance to ZDV and the presence of mutations at positions 41 and 215 within RT were independent risk factors for disease progression and death *(29,30)*.

In an attempt to assess the possible impact of a number of RT mutations rather than the T215Y mutation alone, Leigh-Brown et al. *(31)* classified ZDV-experienced patients at baseline according to mutations at 13 loci of RT (positions 41, 44, 60, 69, 70, 104h, 135, 202, 207, 210, 211, 215, 219) and demonstrated that such clusters were better predictors of a 48-week response to new therapy (ACTG 241; ZDV/ddI vs. ZDV/ddI/NVP) compared to changes at the 215 position alone. Nevertheless, classification of mutations into these clusters still only explained up to 30% of the variance observed in virological response at week 48 of the study.

Thus, in the era of HAART, it is increasingly difficult to assess the precise impact of specific mutations because of the confounding influence of VL suppression consequent on new potent antiviral agents. In addition, interactions between mutations are increasingly evident, such as the attenuating effect of M184V (3TC resistance), L74V (ddI resistance), and Y181C (NVP resistance) on the phenotype of viruses containing ZDV resistance mutations *(32–34)*.

Long-term stavudine (d4T) therapy has been associated with the emergence of ZDV resistance *(35)*, and a poor response to d4T has been associated with the presence of ZDV resistance mutations *(36)*. In addition, the presence of the T215Y/F/Q mutation predicted a poor short-term response to a d4T/3TC combination in ZDV-experienced patients *(37)*. Although the phenotypic fold-resistance to d4T conferred by such mutations is relatively modest, it may be that small shifts in susceptibility are sufficient for this drug to lose efficacy.

High-level 3TC resistance is generated by the M184V mutation within RT and occurs within weeks on monotherapy *(38)*. It is also commonly observed as the initial mutation emerging following failure of a 3TC-containing triple regimen, suggesting that the loss of control of this drug drives the evolution of resistance against other components of the regimen. Nevertheless, some lines of evidence call into question the precise impact of this mutation. Virologic analysis of the NUCA 3001 study in drug-naïve patients demonstrated that 3TC with ZDV effected greater VL suppression over 24 wk compared to ZDV alone, despite the virtually universal emergence of M184V in the double therapy arm *(39)*. A longer term follow-up on a similar 3TC/ZDV patient cohort showed phenotypic resistance to ZDV, but not 3TC, as the only independent risk factor for virological failure *(40)*. Similar results have been presented from other clinical trials with a 3TC-containing arm.

A number of explanations of these observations have been put forward. The fitness of the M184V mutant may be reduced, thus contributing to a reduced virological rebound following emergence of 3TC resistance *(41)*. It has also been proposed that this mutation enhances RT fidelity, which in turn would reduce the rate at which new mutants (including drug-resistant mutants) are generated *(42)*. Third, the presence of M184V partially reverses the ZDV resistance phenotype in the presence of ZDV resistance mutations *(43)*. Finally, pyrophosphorylysis (the reverse step of nucleoside triphosphate incorporation) appears to be diminished within an M184V containing RT, thus enhancing the chain termination effect of the nucleoside analogs *(44)*.

All these mechanisms have been demonstrated within in vitro systems, often with purified RT, and may not be applicable in vivo. Indeed, there is conflicting evidence that reduced fitness or increased fidelity of the M184V mutant is a significant factor with infected individuals *(45–48)*. In addition, long-term therapy with ZDV and 3TC leads to the emergence of novel mutations, such as at positions 43, 44, R211K, L214F, and G333E/D *(49,50)*, suggesting routes to 3TC resistance that may bypass M184V.

ABC is the most recent antiretroviral nucleoside analog licensed. A more extensive analysis of the success of ABC use in salvage therapy demonstrates that ABC failure is associated with the presence of three or more ZDV resistance-associated mutations at baseline *(51)*. Nevertheless, even in heavily pretreated patients, the reduced susceptibility to ABC observed in phenotypic assays is often rather modest (less than eightfold resistant) *(51a)*. More data are required regarding failure of ABC therapy.

5.1. New Nucleoside Analogs With Potential Activity Against Resistant Viruses

Nucleoside analog drugs have been the mainstay of HIV therapy since ZDV was first licensed in 1988, and it is not surprising that resistance to this class of drugs is most common at a population level. Despite some specific signature mutations for individual nucleoside analogs, as discussed in Section 5.1., there increasing evidence for cross-resistance between certain drugs, such as ZDV and d4T, as well as the emergence of mutations conferring broad cross-resistance, such as the 69 insertions, and the Q151M constellation of mutations within RT. Interesting data have been presented for alovudine, a thymidine analog previously shown to have considerable toxicity in the clinic. Now reassessed at lower doses, activity was observed in patients with ZDV/d4T resistance (up to five thymidine analog resistance-associated mutations, TAMS), although antagonism between these thymidine analogs was observed when used in combination *(52,53)*. More data are awaited for this rejuvenated compound.

Amdoxovir (DAPD) is a new nucleoside analog prodrug; its oral administration leads to a rapid in vivo conversion to (–)-β-D-dioxalane guanosine (DXG). Resistance to this drug in the laboratory appears to involve the K65R and L74V mutations, similar to those observed for ABC (although ABC failure is rarely associated with these mutations in the clinic) *(54)*. Phase 1 and 2 studies demonstrated reasonable activity of this drug against nucleoside analog–resistant viruses, although more data are needed before clarifying its potential role *(55)*.

The drug attracting much interest at present is the recently approved nucleotide analog TDF, which appears to be unencumbered by the toxicity problems of its cousin adefovir. As for many other drugs, the HIV mutations in RT associated with reduced activity in the clinic are not necessarily those selected by TDF in the laboratory (K65R). This is because the drug has been most widely tested in drug-experienced patients in whom resistant virus already existed, and predictors of poor response could be identified. Thus, common nucleoside analog resistance mutations such as M41L, L210W (possibly a key marker in this respect), and T215Y appear to reduce, although not negate, clinical efficacy; nevertheless, the widespread use of TDF in salvage therapy and promising first-line treatment trial data suggest that it represents an important addition to our antiviral armory *(56–58)*.

5.2. Resistance to Non-Nucleoside Reverse Transcriptase Inhibitors

The nNRTIs are a structurally diverse group of compounds, of which NVP, efavirenz (EFV), and delavirdine (DLV) have been approved for clinical use. Despite this diversity, the current drugs all bind within the same RT pocket, occupied by the side chains of amino acids at positions 181 and 188, and the 103 residue is close to the entry to this site. In vitro selection experiments demonstrated the rapid acquisition of high-level resistance. The mutations associated with resistance may vary between drugs, with variable levels of phenotypic cross-resistance. However, wide cross-resistance appears evident in clinical practice.

Failure of nNRTIs is often caused by a single mutation; it is likely that these variants therefore pre-exist within the viral swarm, such as for the 3TC resistance mutation, and can quickly emerge if viral replication is maintained on therapy *(21)*. Indeed, the Y181C mutant has been detected in nNRTI-naïve patients *(59)*, and modeling of the rate of emergence of this mutation on NVP suggested its pre-existence at frequencies of 10–100 per 10,000 virus copies *(60)*.

Failure of EFV-containing triple regimens is associated with the K103N mutation in up to 90% of cases *(61)*, producing phenotypic cross-resistance to NVP and DLV. Other mutations, such as G190S/A/E, Y188L, and L100I, may also be observed, and they may be acquired sequentially *(61)*. This suggests that the emergence of high-level resistance with K103N does not preclude further selective pressure. The low genetic barrier to emergence of nNRTI resistance reaffirms the importance of maintaining optimal suppression of viral replication in those receiving this class of drugs.

The rapid emergence of resistance to NVP in monotherapy studies during the early 1990s led to a halt in further clinical development of this compound. More recently, efficacy of this drug has been demonstrated in the context of combination regimens. The genetic pathway to resistance is dependent on cotherapies. Thus, resistance to single therapy is usually caused by the Y181C mutation *(62)*. By contrast, in the presence of ZDV, other mutations, such as the K103N mutation, are the preferred route *(63)*. This may be explained by the in vitro observation that the Y181C mutation suppresses the emergence of ZDV resistance *(64)*. Thus, there may be an evolutionary bias against the emergence of the 181 mutation in such cotreated patients. Other interactions between nucleoside and non-nucleoside inhibitor resistance mutations have been observed, such as the emergence of 74 and 75 mutations (associated with ddI and d4T resistance) to compensate for the loss of fitness consequent on the G190E mutation (associated with resistance to the experimental compound HBY 097) *(65)*.

Phenotypic analyses of viruses containing nNRTI resistance mutations demonstrated variable cross-resistance between the three drugs discussed above. The K103N mutation leads to cross-resistance *(66)*, whereas laboratory strains of virus altered to contain the Y181C virus retains in vitro activity against EFV. However, this clear distinction does not appear to hold with clinical isolates. Thus, one study demonstrated that only 29% of isolates with the Y181C as the sole nNRTI mutation were sensitive to EFV *(66)*. This difference is likely to reflect the polymorphic background of the virus in question. The more important clinical question is whether second-line nNRTI therapy can be successful following emergence of resistance to an initial nNRTI. This has not been formally studied; however, in one retrospective survey, 6/7 patients failing a regimen containing NVP with the 181 mutation did not respond to a subsequent EFV-containing regimen *(67)*. It is unlikely that sequential therapy with existing nNRTIs would be a successful strategy.

Finally, it is noteworthy that "naturally" occurring resistance to nNRTIs has been observed in type O HIV-1 strains, as well as HIV-2 and simian immunodeficiency virus (SIV) *(68–71)*. In addition, many nonclade B subtypes of HIV-1 contain polymorphisms at RT positions that may have an impact on nNRTI susceptibility, such as 98, 101, and 179 *(72)*. More work is required to delineate the precise impact of these polymorphisms and whether they influence the genetic route to high-level nNRTI resistance.

5.2.1. New Non-Nucleoside Reverse Transcriptase Inhibitors With Potential Activity Against Resistant Viruses

Two new compounds, TMC 125 and TMC120, appear to have activity against existing nNRTI-resistant viruses both in vitro and in vivo *(73,74)*. Another compound (capravirine) demonstrated activity against a virus bearing the K103N, V106A, or L100I single mutation, although high-level resistance to this drug was reported in the presence of mutations at codon 181 *(75)*. It appears not so much that different patterns of resistance mutations are observed with these new nNRTIs drugs, but rather that emergence of resistance is much slower than for existing nNRTIs—note that single-dose NVP in pregnancy is sufficient to select for resistant mutants—and that the well-recognized nNRTI mutations have a marginal, and possibly clinically irrelevant, impact on fold susceptibility. It is argued that these properties are a function of the unique structures of these second-generation nNRTIs, in the context of binding to the RT enzyme. More extensive clinical trial data for both these drugs is anticipated.

5.3. Resistance to Protease Inhibitors

The development of HIV-1 PIs followed rapidly on from the publication of the crystal structure of HIV-1 protease in 1988. The enzyme itself is small, comprising a homodimer with 99 amino acids in each strand. Because the functional expression of protease (PR) is essential for virus replication, it was initially thought that emergence of drug resistance mutations within such a small gene would be limited. Not only has this proven incorrect, but also an extensive polymorphism of this gene has been demonstrated in viruses from PI-naïve patients, such that up to 50% of the amino acids may vary within clade B viruses *(4)*. This diversity widens if other HIV-1 subtypes are considered. Nevertheless, these variants do not appear to compromise in vitro or in vivo responses to PIs.

A large number of mutations associated with PI resistance have now been described. Not surprisingly, in view of the small size of protease, many of these lead to a virus with reduced replicative ability. This was first demonstrated by Ho et al. *(76)* through the in vitro selection of HIV-1 resistant to the A-77003 prototype PI, with mutations R8Q and M46I. The position 8 mutation conferred reduced drug susceptibility, whereas the 46 mutation compensated for the loss of replicative fitness consequent on the R8Q. This early observation allowed an appreciation of the multiple roles played by the array of PI resistance-associated mutations that have now been documented.

Saquinavir (SQV) was the first PI approved for clinical use, and many of the studies described here utilize regimens that will strike the reader as suboptimal. Further, the formulation of SQV initially used has now been replaced by a more bioavailable preparation, with corresponding increased potency within the clinic. Nevertheless, important data on the emergence of PI resistance in vivo was gleaned from these studies. Failure of monotherapy within clinical trials was commonly associated with the L90M mutation and rarely with the G48V, mutations that together severely reduce the catalytic efficiency of the enzyme. Although the residue 48 is in an important flap loop of the enzyme, the 90 residue appears distant to the active site and may lead to conformational effects on inhibitor binding *(77)*.

Early dose-ranging studies of indinavir (IDV) monotherapy generated detailed information on resistance-associated mutations for this drug. Sequential acquisition of mutations was observed, with changes at positions 10, 24, 46, 54, 71, 82, 84, and 90 significantly correlated with phenotypic resistance. Nevertheless, the V82A/F/T mutation is recognized as the best predictor of reduced IDV susceptibility occurring early in drug failure, with or without M46I/L/V (although not in themselves leading to significantly reduced susceptibilities). These changes are followed by a series of other more variable changes that confer increasing resistance and compensate for reduced fitness *(78)*. A significant advance in our understanding of PI resistance was made with the demonstration of mutations outside the protease gene, within the gag protease cleavage sites, in conjunction with protease mutations following failure of IDV therapy. Changes at the gag p7/p1 site are most commonly observed, and mutagenesis experiments suggested that their major role is to compensate for partial replication deficiency caused by the 82 or 46 mutations *(79)*. Similarly, some of the additional (secondary) mutations acquired within the protease gene may also be compensatory.

The more precise contribution of IDV resistance to failure of IDV-containing HAART regimens has been explored within an analysis of ACTG 343. This was a randomized study of switching patients receiving ZDV/3TC/IDV initial therapy to a maintenance regimen of IDV monotherapy or ZDV/3TC double therapy or continuing triple therapy in those with undetectable VL on the induction regimen. Of patients in the first two arms, 23% had early maintenance failure, compared to 3% in the triple maintenance arm. However, in none of the 26 failures tested (9 receiving IDV monotherapy and 17 receiving triple therapy) was phenotypic resistance to IDV apparent, and primary IDV resistance mutations (at 46 or 82) were present in only 1 patient. Plasma IDV levels were lower in patients with failure, providing one explanation for this observation. However, other possible factors leading to rebound with IDV-sensitive strains include impaired fitness of virus with 46/82 mutations and host–parasite changes, such that an increase in uninfected permissive cells provides more "space" for residual virus to replicate *(80)*. This observation is clinically important because it raises the possibility that some drugs within a failing regimen could be selected for continuation based on resistance assay results. However, the presence of resistant virus below the level of detection may compromise further treatment with the same drug, and such a hypothesis requires testing within clinical trials.

Failure of RTV monotherapy is associated with the stepwise acquisition of mutations, starting with V82A/T/F and followed by one or more changes at positions 10, 20, 33, 36, 46, 54, 63, 71, 84, 90, and 93. As is the case for IDV resistance, the 82 mutation alone does not confer significantly reduced susceptibility. This depends on the emergence of additional mutations, some of which are compensatory *(13)*. Resulting isolates also appear resistant to IDV, as would be expected from this mutational pattern, and SQV cross-resistance has been documented *(81)*. In vitro selection of RTV-resistant isolates also demonstrated the presence of gag cleavage site mutations at p1/p6 and p7/p1 *(82)*. However, RTV is now used as a pharmacological boosting mechanism at doses thought to be too low to generate resistance.

Lopinavir (LPV) is more potent than RTV and was developed to be active against viral isolates with the key resistance mutation at position 82 *(83)*. In vitro selection experiments identified LPV resistance-associated mutations at 84, 10, 46, 91, 32, and 47 *(84)*. However, it appears increasingly likely that the clinical benefit of this drug, coadministered with RTV, is because of the high plasma levels achieved, which may overcome reduced drug susceptibility *(85)*, rather than lack of cross-resistance patterns *per se*. This drug appears to be highly effective when used as first- or second-line PI therapy, and few data are yet available on the mutations that emerge during therapy to lead to drug failure.

Initial monotherapy studies with nelfinavir (NFV) identified a unique mutation, D30N, as responsible for reduced drug susceptibility without corresponding cross-resistance to other PIs *(86,87)*. It is now apparent that failure of NFV-containing triple regimens is associated with either the D30N or the L90M mutation *(88,89)*. The 30 mutation may be associated with N88D and A71T/V, whereas the 90 mutation emerges together with changes at one or more of positions 10, 20, 46, 60, 73, and 74. The constellation of mutations around L90M confer cross-resistance to SQV and possibly other PIs; therefore, the route taken for NFV resistance may determine the success of subsequent PI therapies. There is some limited data to support this hypothesis *(88)*.

In vitro selection of virus resistant to amprenavir (APV) identified I50V as a key resistance mutation, together with other secondary mutations *(90)*. However, cross-resistance of isolates from PI-experienced patients to APV can be predicted by the presence of M46I/L, I54L/V, I84V, and L90M. Thus, an algorithm of I84V or any two of the three mutations 46/54/90 allowed prediction of high-level resistance with a sensitivity of 88% and specificity of 79% *(91)*. In view of the poor pharmokinetics and high pill burden of APV, a prodrug, fos-amprenavir has recently been developed, and clinical trial data are awaited. Of note, the plasma drug levels achieved with APV appear to determine genetic route of emergence, with the I54V/L mutation more frequent at lower drug levels than the I50V mutation.

Regarding primary drug resistance, mutations identified through in vitro and early clinical studies, there appear to be some key differences among the currently approved PIs. Thus, SQV-resistant isolates containing mutations at positions 48 and 90 may retain susceptibility to other PIs *(92)*. NFV-resistant isolates containing the 30 mutation are more likely to be susceptible to other PIs compared to those bearing the 90 mutation *(87)*. In contrast, reduced susceptibility to IDV confers a greater degree of cross-resistance to other PIs, especially for viruses containing more than four of the primary and secondary mutations associated with IDV resistance *(78)*.

How do such patterns translate into clinical practice when PIs are used sequentially? It appears that second-line PI therapy after SQV failure is less successful than may be predicted from the in vitro data. Of interest, the array of mutations that evolve in the presence of IDV following SQV failure with the L90M change do not necessarily comprise the classical IDV resistance mutations, suggesting that SQV failure may "prime" the rapid emergence of resistance to other PIs. In contrast, when SQV failure is associated with the G48V mutation, the addition of V82A (the primary IDV resistance mutation) is observed whether these patients were switched to IDV or NFV or even continued to receive SQV *(93,94)*. The success of IDV therapy following NFV as the first-line PI is predicted by the presence of D30N as the NFV resistance mutation rather than L90M *(89)*, again suggesting that a constellation of mutations including L90M may generate more cross-class resistance than previously appreciated. Although many PI resistant virus isolates appear to retain susceptibility to APV, few data on the success of APV after prior PI failure are available.

Double PIs are increasingly used in antiretroviral therapy, especially in salvage regimens. RTV is commonly utilized at low doses to increase plasma levels of the coadministered PI (such as SQV, IDV, or APV), with associated increase in potency. Such a strategy is often successful at suppressing VL despite previous PI therapy. Indeed, susceptibility to these drugs at baseline may predict such success *(95)*. Nevertheless, the benefit of such a strategy may also be determined by the achievement of drug levels high enough to overcome a modest level of drug resistance. This may be the major mechanism by which LPV administered with RTV achieves its clinical benefit in PI-experienced patients despite virus isolates with reduced susceptibility to this compound *(85)*. It is likely that pharmacokinetics together with drug resistance determinants will have to be considered together in guiding optimal use of PIs in the future.

5.3.1. New Protease Inhibitors With Potential Activity Against Resistant Viruses

Issues of resistance and cross-resistance are particularly pertinent to the PI class of drugs. Many claims have been made on the apparent uniqueness of resistance patterns for specific drugs; these claims were based on in vitro data, which do not then translate into clinical benefit for that drug in PI-experienced patients. Two new PIs have now undergone initial clinical evaluation. Atazanavir (ATZ), soon to be available within an expanded access program, demonstrated different resistance profiles when used in PI naïve- or PI-experienced patients. In the former group, resistance emerged with the

I50L and A71V mutations *(96)*. This is a unique combination because APV resistance mutations include a different amino acid change at position 50 (namely, I50V), although the A71V mutation is a polymorphism (frequently observed in the absence of PI therapy). In contrast, in PI-experienced patients, some level of cross-resistance between ATZ and other PIs was apparent *(97)*. Because the 50,71 mutation combination does not appear to reduce susceptibility to other PIs, there may be advantage, from a resistance perspective, for using ATZ as a first-line PI; however, data are required on the actual efficacy of PI treatment after ATZ failure to fully assess the importance of the "unique resistance pattern."

Clinical data have also been presented for tipranavir, which shows potency against viruses containing a large variety of PI resistance mutants in vitro *(98)*. Clinical activity was indeed observed in PI-experienced patients, with a suggestion that many PI resistance mutations were required to compromise activity *(99)*. More work is required to clarify further such "clinical cutoffs" by which clinicians can be guided on the likely effect of this new drug in a patient with existing PI-resistant virus.

5.4. *New Classes of Drugs*

Data are now emerging from the trials of T-20 (enfuvirtide), the first fusion inhibitor to enter the clinic. Because the phase 3 trials were undertaken in heavily pretreated patients, it is not surprising that failure rates (lack of full suppression) were relatively high overall; however, this affords the opportunity to characterize the emergence of resistance *(100,101)*. Data from phase 2 studies demonstrated that the majority of such patients with failure had mutations in the gp41 region targeted by the drug, namely, between amino acids 36 and 45, which indeed confirmed that activity of the drug is mediated through the proposed mechanism *(102)*. Because variation in this region is very rare in T-20-naïve patients, including those infected with non-subtype B viruses, it can be assumed that prior RT inhibitor and PI therapy will not compromise T-20 activity *per se (103)*. The key issue with use of T-20 in salvage therapy will therefore be the choice of other active drugs to combine with it. Of interest, the second-generation fusion inhibitor T-1249 appears to be active against most T-20 resistance mutants, although this is based on in vitro evidence alone *(104)*.

Other new classes of antiretroviral agents include integrase inhibitors and CXCR4 (HIV-1 coreceptor) inhibitors, which show in vitro promise, but have yet to be investigated extensively in the clinic.

6. USE OF RESISTANCE TESTING TO GUIDE THERAPY

Many HIV therapy guidelines now suggest that resistance testing of plasma virus be undertaken at time of drug failure to optimize subsequent antiretroviral regimens. Such testing is expensive, and to assess which patients benefit most from such testing, prospective, randomized studies have been performed to address the use of resistance testing in drug-experienced patients (Table 2) *(105–110)*. The general structure of these studies is that patients are enrolled at the time of antiretroviral failure and then randomly selected to receive resistance testing or no resistance testing (standard of care, SOC). Different types of resistance assays have been used; end points of these studies represent virological suppression at 3–6 mo following randomization. However, the complexity of the study populations and different criteria used make generalizations

Table 2
Prospective Studies of HIV Drug Resistance Testing

Trial (*n*)	Randomization	Duration (weeks)	Outcome	Results	*p* value	Reference
VIRADAPT (108)	Geno vs. SOC	24	%VL < 200	Geno 32%, SOC 14%	0.07	*105*
GART (153)	Geno + EA vs. SOC	12	%VL < 500	Geno + EA 34%, SOC 22%	0.1	*106*
Havana (326)	Geno + EA vs. SOC ± EA	24	%VL < 400	Geno 48%, SOC 36%, EA 59%, No EA 41%	<0.05	*107*
ARGENTA (174)	Geno vs. SOC	24	%VL < 500	Geno 21%, SOC 17%	0.47	*108*
VIRA 3001 (272)	Pheno vs. SOC	16	%VL < 400	Pheno 40%, SOC 34%	0.08	*110*
CCTG 575 (256)	Pheno vs. SOC	48	%VL < 400	Pheno 48%, SOC 48%	Ns	*111*
NARVAL (541)	Geno vs. Pheno vs. SOC	12	%VL < 200	Pheno 35%, SOC 36%, Geno 44%, SOC 30%	0.92 0.02	*112*
VIHIRES (137)	Geno vs. Pheno	12	%VL < 200	Pheno 41%, Geno 39%	Ns	*113*
CERT (450)	Geno vs. Pheno vs. SOC		Time to failure	Pheno 521d, Geno 574d, SOC 478d	Geno/Pheno vs SOC 0.0004	*114*

Abbr: Geno, genotypic test; *n*, number of patients enrolled; pheno, phenotypic test; VL, viral load (copies HIV-1 RNA/mL plasma); vpheno, = virtual phenotype; SOC, standard of care; EA, expert opinion; NS, not significant.

about study results difficult, and the data require more detailed description. Below, the findings from the key studies are briefly described.

The VIRADAPT *(105)*, GART *(106)*, HAVANA *(107)*, and ARGENTA *(108)* trials assessed the use of a genotypic resistance test (G) against SOC. These trials individually showed that genotypic testing has a positive impact on virological response compared to SOC. However, all these trials reported a very limited proportion of patients who achieved undetectable VLs (approx 30%), and in the majority of cases, the sustained response was short-lived.

For VIRADAPT, NRTI- and PI-experienced patients were enrolled *(13)*. At 3 mo, a higher proportion of those allocated to the G arm demonstrated at least a 0.5 $\log_{10}$ decrease in VL and undetectable VL (<200 copies/mL) compared to SOC. This proportion remained essentially unchanged at 6 and 12 mo (although the statistical significance was now lost). The lack of significance has raised questions regarding a sustained response. It is disappointing that only approx 30% of patients achieved full VL suppression. The trial ended at 6 mo to allow the SOC group to receive a resistance test, and the proportion of patients in this group subsequently achieving undetectable VL increased from 14 to 26%, implying that, even after a delay in treatment, a resistance test can confer benefit *(109)*. Although no expert advice (EA) was formally used in the trial, patients who had failed a second or third regimen were discussed with two or more study physicians. An analysis of drug trough concentrations showed that patients in the G arm with optimal levels had the greatest reduction in VL (1.39 $\log_{10}$), implying that active drug levels are important.

The GART (CPCRA 046) *(106)* study enrolled patients who had received at least one PI and two NRTIs. Although the significant reduction in VL in the G arm was maintained at 12 wk, the proportion of patients with undetectable VL was not. This again encouraged questions pertaining to a lack of sustained response. However, in this trial, 83% of patients in the G arm did not receive the therapy recommended by the experts (54% had therapy altered by one drug, and 42% had all the drugs altered).

The Havana *(107)* trial, which enrolled many highly drug-experienced patients, showed that genotype was important; it was the first trial to establish the independent utility of EA (multivariate analysis for EA vs. no EA, odds ratio [OR] 2.13, $p = 0.003$; G vs. SOC, OR 1.92, $p = 0.01$). The expert advisory panel consisted of four clinicians and two virologists, each with more than 10 yr of experience in the management of HIV-infected patients. In addition, the EA was followed in 81% of patients. This trial, compared to the earlier GART and VIRADAPT trials *(99)*, produced higher proportions of patients achieving VL suppression in all groups, presumably because of an improved knowledge base regarding drug resistance management.

In contrast to the studies described in this section, patients enrolled in the ARGENTA *(108)* study were highly nNRTI experienced. The availability of a new class of drug for use at time of failure was a major determinant of success of the regimen and must be borne in mind when comparing these studies of drug resistance tests. At 3 mo, the G arm was equated with a greater proportion of patients with undetectable VL; however, this difference with the SOC arm was not sustained at 6 mo. Although 83% of the EA was acted on, the large proportion of previous nNRTI use may have precluded the use of a further nNRTI because of cross-resistance, thus yielding a lower success rate in both arms.

The VIRA3001 *(110)* and CCTG575 *(111)* trials compared the value of phenotyping (P) in relation to SOC. Both these trials had problems regarding the phenotypic cutoff interpretation for d4T and ddI. For VIRA3001, patients were enrolled after previous therapy with one PI and two NRTIs. Although analysis by intention-to-treat-observed (ITTO) criteria showed that a significantly greater proportion of patients achieved undetectable VL in the P arm compared to the SOC, statistical significance was not attained in the more rigorous intention-to-treat (ITT) analysis. The CCTG575 study showed no difference between the two arms according to either reduction in VL or undetectable virus. Entry requirements initially were at least one previous PI failure, but this was changed to two during the trial.

The NARVAL *(112)*, VIHRES *(113)*, and CERT *(114)* trials were developed to compare the value of genotyping versus phenotyping for choosing antiretroviral therapy. The NARVAL patient cohort was heavily drug experienced. The trial showed no value in the P arm over SOC. However, in the G arm (although significance was not reached), there appeared to be value in its use over SOC. A multivariate analysis showed that randomization to the G arm gave an OR of 2.13 *(115)*. There is concern that the lack of use of phenotyping may have been because the IC_{50}-fold changes were not optimal for the NRTIs.

The VIHRES trial enrolled only highly experienced patients and had no SOC arm. Both types of resistance tests helped the patient outcome (again with no difference between the arms), but again disappointing VL suppression data at 24 wk were achieved (50% in the G arm vs. 40% in the P arm), even with the assistance of EA.

CERT utilized patients failing at least one PI or nNRTI, and the outcome measure was days to virological failure. Both P and G arms showed a significantly higher number of days to failure than the SOC arm, with no significant difference between the P and G arms. However, the G arm interpretation system was changed during the study to the virtual phenotype, which impinges on how this trial should be assessed.

A meta-analysis of the VIRADAPT, GART, Havana, ARGENTA, NARVAL, and VIRA3001 was undertaken *(116)*. The proportion of patients with undetectable VL was assessed in all trials at 3 mo and in four trials at 6 mo. At 3 mo, results were 42.6% in the G arm and 33.2% in SOC (OR 1.7); at 6 mo, they were 38.8% in the G arm and 28.7% in the SOC arm (OR 1.6). When EA optimized the genotypic data, there was a higher rate of viral suppression, 50.7 versus 35.8% in the SOC arm (OR 2.4). At 3 mo, the P arm result was 37.5%, compared to 33.8% in the SOC arm (OR 1.1). These results support the use of genotypic, but not phenotypic, resistance tests and showed that EA can increase the virological response.

The variable impact of resistance testing in prospective studies as described in this section is not surprising. In the context of ongoing viral replication, with the ebb and flow of an increasing number of viral variants (including those with resistance), an assessment of the majority virus population in plasma at a single time point is unlikely to contain all the virological information necessary to predict response to therapy. Further, it increasingly appears that interpretation of resistance results, whether for sets of mutations or clinical cutoffs for phenotypic assays, is a key cause of the differing results observed. Nevertheless, resistance testing has now become SOC in many countries (according to national and international guidelines), and randomized studies (incorporating a no-resistance test arm) will be more difficult to undertake. The challenge is how to use large databases of resistance results and virological outcome to identify the clinical scenarios in which such testing will most beneficial. One of the greatest threats is that resistance data and interpretation become a proprietary product for which fee for service becomes the rule.

6.1. Inhibitory Quotients

Pharmacodynamic considerations may have an impact on antiviral responses and the concept of inhibiting quotient has been discussed in this context. In particular, the C_{trough} within the dosing period is thought to be the most important parameter in this regard. Thus, if the plasma drug levels fall below levels conferring maximal antiviral effect, then bursts of viral replication may occur, ultimately leading to emergence of resistance and failure. The logic of boosted PI regimens is to increase this C_{trough}, thus avoiding such viral breakthrough. The "optimal" level of drug is clearly a compromise between antiviral effect and potential for toxicities, and consensus panels are addressing this issue.

In the context of drug resistance, the concept of drug levels has even more significance. Phenotypic assessments of drug susceptibility provide a quantitative fold resistance, and this allows for the generation of a recommended inhibitory quotient (IQ) required for optimal inhibition by a particular drug. This is defined as the C_{trough}/IC_{50}. Thus, for a resistant virus, the level of drug required to remain inhibitory can be determined. The clinical reliance and predictability of the IQ is now being assessed in prospective studies. Of course, this is only a relevant concept for the PIs and nNRTIs, which do not require further intracellular metabolism for activity. In contrast, the relationship between plasma concentration of the NRTIs and the intracellular (active) drug triphosphate is highly variable; therefore, IQ cannot be used for this class of drug.

7. NOVEL APPROACHES TO MANAGEMENT OF MULTIRESISTANT VIRUS INFECTION

A number of new strategies have been suggested as means to deal with multiresistant HIV-1. Some of these strategies have been subject to pilot studies.

7.1. Treatment Interruption

Because wild-type (nonresistant) virus regrows as the majority species when treatment is stopped, it has been proposed that such a strategy will allow resensitization of the virus to treatment. A number of additional reasons have been given for the potential advantage of such an approach, such as provision of immune stimulation; however, there is little evidence that this provides any lasting benefit in subsequent response to therapy.

7.2. GIGA-HAART

A pilot study has been undertaken of treatment interruption in patients with low CD4 counts, followed by the use of up to eight and nine drugs, termed GIGA (or MEGA) HAART. Of interest, this provided some benefit *(117)*.

7.3. Continuing Therapy

Drug resistant viruses may have deficiencies in viral replicative capacity (fitness). This has led some to propose that continuing therapy to maintain the presence of drug resistance mutations may be beneficial compared to stopping therapy *(118)*. An alternative examination of these pathodata is that resistance is not all or nothing, and that drugs may maintain some residual activity.

8. CONCLUSION

Despite the undoubted success of antiretroviral therapy, clinical management of virological failure remains an important and difficult issue for physicians who treat patients with HIV. Because such patients often have drug-resistant virus, the choice of new combinations is often based, at least to some extent, on knowledge of resistance characteristics of available drugs. Although prospective studies of resistance testing have not provided overwhelming evidence for clinical utility, this probably reflects the complex heterogeneity of patients failing therapy and parameters other than resistance, such as adherence, toxicities and pharmacology must be considered absolute. After some years of promising in vitro data, these drugs have demonstrated promise in clinical trials, with particular interest focused on unique resistance patterns or the slow development of resistance.

As further clinical trial data are presented for new drugs, it is important for physicians who treat patients with HIV to ask two specific questions. First, what are the resistance patterns at baseline that define success or failure of this new drug in antiretroviral-experienced patients? Second, what are the resistance correlates of failure when used as a first-line drug? Answers to these questions will contribute to identifying the optimal role of these promising new drugs in routine clinical practice.

REFERENCES

1. Sardana VV, Emini EA, Gotlib L, et al. Functional analysis of HIV-1 reverse transcriptase amino acids involved in resistance to multiple non-nucleoside inhibitors. J Biol Chem 1992; 267; 17,526–17,530.
2. Erickson JW, Burt SK. Structural mechanisms of HIV drug resistance. Ann Rev Pharmacol Toxicol 1996; 36:545–571.
3. Larder BA, Darby G, Richman DD. HIV with reduced sensitivity to zidovudine (AZT) isolated during prolonged therapy. Science 1989; 243:1731–1734.
4. Kozal MJ, Shah N, Shen N, et al. Extensive polymorphisms observed in HIV-1 clade B protease gene using high-density oligonucleotide arrays. Nat Med 1996; 2:753–758.
5. Descamps D, Collin G, Letourneur F, et al. Susceptibility of human immunodeficiency virus type 1 group O isolates to antiretroviral agents: in vitro phenotypic and genotypic analyses. J Virol 1997; 71:8893–8898.
6. Bonhoeffer S, Nowak MA. Pre-existence and emergence of drug resistance in HIV-1 infection. Proc R Soc Lond B 1997; 264:631–637.
7. Ramratnam B, Mittler JE, Zhang L, et al. The decay of the latent reservoir of replication-competent HIV-1 is inversely correlated with the extent of residual viral replication during prolonged antiretroviral therapy. Nat Med 2000; 6:82–85.
8. Devereux HL, Youle M, Johnson MA, Loveday C. Rapid decline in detectability of HIV-1 drug resistance mutations after stopping therapy. AIDS 1999; 13:F123–F127.
9. Lanier ER, Scott J, Ait-Khaled M, et al. Predicting abacavir antiviral activity using HIV-1 reverse transcriptase genotype: a comparison of 12 algorithms. Antiviral Ther 2001; 6(suppl.):103.
10. Lu B, Hellmann NS, Bates M, Dawson K, Rooney J, Miller MD. Determination of clinical cut-offs for reduced response to tenofovir DF therapy in antiretroviral experienced patients. Antiviral Ther 2002; 7(suppl.):S137.
11. Raboud JM, Montaner SG, Conway B, et al. Suppression of plasma viral load below 20 copies/mL is required to achieve a long-term response to therapy. AIDS 1998; 12:1619–1624.
12. Paterson D, Swindells S, Mohr J, et al. Adherence to protease inhibitor therapy and outcomes in patients with HIV infection. Ann Intern Med 2000; 133(1):21–30.
13. Molla A, Korneyeva M, Gao Q, et al. Ordered accumulation of mutations in HIV protease confers resistance to ritonavir. Nat Med 1996; 2:760–766.
14. Garraffo R, Durant J, Clevenbergh P, et al. Relevance of protease inhibitor plasma levels in patients treated with genotypic adapted therapy: pharmacological data from the Viradapt study. Antivir Ther 1999; 4(suppl. 1):75.
15. Wong JK, Ignacio CC, Torriani F, et al. In vivo compartmentalisation of human immunodeficiency virus: evidence from the examination of *pol* sequences from autopsy tissues. J Virol 1997; 71:2059–2071.
16. Kiessling AA, Fitzgerald LM, Zhang D, et al. Human immunodeficiency virus in semen arises from a genetically distinct virus reservoir. AIDS Res Hum Retroviruses 1998; 14 (suppl. 1):S33–S41.
17. Taylor S, Back DJ, Workman J, et al. Poor penetration of the male genital tract by HIV-1 protease inhibitors. AIDS 1999; 13:859–860.

18. Kepler TB, Perelson AS. Drug concentration heterogeneity facilitates the evolution of drug resistance. Proc Natl Acad Sci 1998; 95:11,514–11,519.
19. Condra JH, Schleif WA, Blahy OM, et al. In vivo emergence of HIV-1 variants resistant to multiple protease inhibitors. Nature 1995; 374:569–571.
20. Schuurman R, Nijhuis M, van Leeuwen R, et al. Rapid changes in human immunodeficiency virus type 1 RNA load and appearance of drug-resistance virus populations in persons treated with lamivudine (3TC). J Infect Dis 1995; 171:1411–1419.
21. Richman DD, Havlir D, Corbeil J, et al. Nevirapine resistance mutations of human immunodeficiency virus type 1 selected during therapy. J Virol 1994; 68:1660–1666.
22. Scott P, Arnold E, Evans B, Shirley J, Cune P, Pillay D. Surveillance of HIV-1 drug resistance in the UK. Paper presented at: 10th Conference on Retroviruses and Opportunistic Infections, Boston, MA, 2003. Abstract 631.
23. Little SJ, Holte S, Routy JP, et al. Antiretroviral-drug resistance among patients recently infected with HIV. N Engl J Med 2002; 347:385–394.
24. UK Collaborative Group on Monitoring the Transmission of HIV Drug Resistance. Analysis of prevalence of HIV-1 drug resistance in primary infections in the United Kingdom. BMJ 2001; 322:1087–1088.
25. Grant RM, Hecht FM, Warmerdam M, et al. Time trends in primary HIV-1 drug resistance among recent infected persons. JAMA 2002; 288:181–188.
26. Riva C, Violin M, Cozzi-Lepri A, et al. Transmitted virus with substitutions at position 215 and risk of virological failure in anti-retroviral naive patients starting highly antiretroviral therapy. Antiviral Ther 2002; 7(suppl. 1):S103.
27. Larder BA. Interactions between drug resistance mutations in human immunodeficiency virus type 1 reverse transcriptase. J Gen Virol 1994; 75:951–957.
28. Yahi N, Tamalet C, Tourres C, et al. Mutation patterns of the reverse transcriptase and protease genes in human immunodeficiency virus type 1-infected patients undergoing combination therapy: survey of 787 sequences. J Clin Microbiol 1999; 37:4099–4106.
29. Japour AJ, Welles S, D'Aquila RT, et al. Prevalence and clinical significance of zidovudine resistance mutations in human immunodeficiency virus isolated from patients after long-term zidovudine treatment. J Infect Dis 1995; 171:1172–1179.
30. D'Aquila RT, Johnson VA, Welles SL, et al. Zidovudine resistance and HIV-1 disease progression during antiretroviral therapy. Ann Intern Med 1995; 122:401–408.
31. Leigh-Brown AJ, Günthard HF, Wong JK, et al. Sequence clusters in human immunodeficiency virus type 1 reverse transcriptase are associated with subsequent virological response to antiretroviral therapy. J Infect Dis 1999; 180:1043–1049.
32. Kuritzkes DR, Serin A, Young B, et al. Effect of zidovudine resistance mutations on virologic response to treatment with zidovudine-lamivudine-ritonavir: genotypic analysis of human immunodeficiency virus type 1 isolates from Aids Clinical Trials Group Protocol 315. J Infect Dis 2000; 181:491–497.
33. Gulick RM, Mellors JW, Havlir D, et al. Simultaneous versus sequential initiation of therapy with indinavir, zidovudine, and lamivudine for HIV-1 infection: 100-week follow-up. JAMA 1998; 280:35–41.
34. Larder BA. 3'-Azido-3'-deoxythymidine resistance suppressed by a mutation conferring human immunodeficiency virus type 1 resistance to non-nucleoside reverse transcriptase inhibitors. Antimicrob Agents Chemother 1992; 36:2664–2669.
35. Pellegrin I, Izopet J, Reynes J, et al. Emergence of zidovudine and multidrug-resistance mutations in the HIV-1 reverse transcriptase gene in therapy-naïve patients receiving stavudine plus didanosine combination therapy. STADI Group. AIDS 1999; 13:1705–1709.
36. Izopet J, Bicart-See A, Pasquier C, et al. Mutations conferring resistance to zidovudine diminish the antiviral effect of stavudine plus didanosine. J Med Virol 1999; 59:507–511.
37. Montaner JSG, Mo T, Raboud JM, et al. Human immunodeficiency virus-infected persons with mutations conferring resistance to zidovudine show reduced virologic responses to hydroxyurea and stavudine-lamivudine. J Infect Dis 2000; 181:729–732.

38. Wainberg MA, Hsu M, Gu Z, Borkow G, Parniak MA. Effectiveness of 3TC in HIV clinical trials may be due in part to the M184V substitution in 3TC-resistance HIV-1 reverse transcriptase. AIDS 1996; 10(suppl. 5):S3–S10.
39. Kuritzkes DR, Quinn JB, Benoit SL, et al. Drug resistance and virologic response in NUCA 3001, a randomised trial of lamivudine (3TC) versus zidovudine (ZDV) versus ZDV plus 3TC in previously untreated patients. AIDS 1996; 10:975–981.
40. Miller V, Phillips A, Rottmann C, et al. Dual resistance to zidovudine and lamivudine in patients treated with zidovudine-lamivudine combination therapy: association with therapy failure. J Infect Dis 1998; 177:1521–1532.
41. Back NK, Nijhuis M, Keulen W, et al. Reduced replication of 3TC-resistant HIV-1 variants in primary cells due to a processivity defect of the reverse transcriptase enzyme. EMBO J 1996; 15:4040–4049.
42. Wainberg MA, Drosopoulos WC, Salomon H, et al. Enhanced fidelity of 3TC-selected mutant HIV-1 reverse transcriptase. Science 1996; 271:1282–1285.
43. Larder BA, Kemp SD, Harrigan PR. Potential mechanism for sustained antiretroviral efficacy of AZT-3TC combination therapy. Science 1995; 269:696–699.
44. Gotte M, Arion D, Parniak MA, Wainberg MA. Mechanisms of HIV-1 resistance to zidovudine and lamivudine. Antivir Ther 1999; 4(suppl. 1):18.
45. Schmit JC, Cogniaux J, Hermans P, et al. Multiple drug resistance to nucleoside analogues and non-nucleoside reverse transcriptase inhibitors in an efficiently replicating human immunodeficiency virus type 1 patient strain. J Infect Dis 1996; 174:962–968.
46. Keulen W, van Wijk A, Schuurman R, Berkhout B, Boucher CA. Increased polymerase fidelity of lamivudine-resistance HIV-1 variants does not limit their evolutionary potential. AIDS 1999; 13:1343–1349.
47. Preston BD. Reverse transcriptase fidelity and HIV-1 variation. Science 1997; 275: 228–230.
48. Balzarini J, Petemans H, De Clercq E, Karlsson A, Kleim JP. Reverse transcriptase fidelity and HIV-1 variation. Science 1997; 275:230.
49. Kemp SD, Shi C, Bloor S, Harrigan PR, Mellors JW, Larder BA. A novel polymorphism at codon 333 of human immunodeficiency virus type 1 reverse transcriptase can facilitate dual resistance to zidovudine and L-2',3'-dideoxy-3'-thiacytidine. J Virol 1998; 72: 5093–5098.
50. Bloor S, Hertogs K, De Vroey V, Miller V, Sturmer M, Larder BA. Lamivudine-resistant HIV-1 clinical isolates lacking the Met184val mutation have novel polymorphisms in RT. Antivir Ther 1999; 4(suppl. 1):19.
51. Lanier R, Zhao H, Ait-Khaled M, et al. Analysis of possible predictors of response to abacavir (ABC) in antiretroviral-experienced adults; comparison of viral genotype, viral phenotype and patient treatment history. Paper presented at: Sixth Conference on Retroviruses and Opportunistic Infections, Chicago, IL, 1999. Abstract 134.
51a. Falloon J, Ait-Khaled M, Thomas DA, et al. HIV-1 genotype and phenotype correlate with virological response to abacavir, amprenavir and efavirenz in treatment experienced patients. AIDS 2002;16(3):387–396.
52. Calvez V, Tubiana R, Ghosen J, et al. MIC-310 reduced markedly viral load in patients with virological failure despite multiple drug therapy: result from a 4-week phase II study. Antivir Ther 2002; 7(suppl. 1):S5.
53. Vang L, Zhang H, Palmer S, et al. In vitro effects of MIV-310 (alovudine,3'-fluorodeoxythymidine, FLT) against HIV mutants. Antivir Ther 2002; 7(suppl. 1):S25.
54. Mewshaw J, Myrick FT, Wakefield DA, et al. Dioxolane guanosine, the active form of the prodrug diaminopurine dioxolane, is a potent inhibitor of drug-resistant HIV-1 isolates from patients for whom standard nucleoside therapy fails. J Acquir Immune Defic Syndr 2002 1; 29:11–20.

55. Eron J, Kessler H, Thompson M, et al. Clinical HIV suppression after short-term monotherapy with DAPD. Paper presented at: 40th Interscience Conference on Antimicrobial Agents and Chemotherapy, Toronto, Ontario, Canada, 2000. Abstract 690.
56. Squires K, Pierone G, Berger D, et al. Tenofovir DF: a 48-week final analysis from a phase III randomised, double blind placebo controlled study in antiretroviral experienced patients. Paper presented at: Ninth Conference on Retroviruses and Opportunistic Infections, Seattle, WA, 2002. Abstract P 413-W.
57. Staszewski S, Gallant J, Pozniak A, et al. Efficacy and safety of tenofovir disoproxil fumarate (TDF) versus stavudine (d4T) when used in combination with lamivudine (3TC) and efavirenz (EFV) in HIV-1 infected patients naive to antiretroviral therapy (ART): 48-week interim results. Paper presented at: 14th International AIDS Conference, Barcelona, Spain, 2002. Abstract 17.
58. Miller MD, Margot NA, Cheng AK, et al. Expanded response analysis of tenofovir DF therapy by base line resistance genotype and phenotype. Paper presented at: 14th International AIDS Conference, Barcelona, Spain, 2002. Abstract Th Or B1390.
59. Najera I, Holguin A, Quinones-Mateu ME, et al. Pol gene quasispecies of human immunodeficiency virus: mutations associated with drug resistance in virus for patients undergoing no drug therapy. J Virol 1995; 69:23–31.
60. Havlir DV, Eastman S, Gamst A, Richman DD. Nevirapine-resistant human immunodeficiency virus: kinetics of replication and estimated prevalence in untreated patients. J Virol 1996; 70:7894–7899.
61. Bacheler LT, George H, Abremski K, et al. Mutations associated with viral load rebound in patients treated with the HIV-1 non-nucleoside reverse transcriptase inhibitor DMP266 in combination with the HIV-1 protease inhibitor crixivan. Paper presented at: Interscience Conference on Antimicrobial Agents and Chemotherapy, Toronto, Ontario, Canada, September 1997. Abstract I-172.
62. Richman D, Shih C-K, Lowy I, et al. Human immunodeficiency virus type 1 mutants resistant to non-nucleoside inhibitors of reverse transcriptase arise in tissue culture. Proc Natl Acad Sci U S A 1991; 88:11,241–11,245.
63. MacArthur RD, Kosmyvia JM, Crane LR, Koran L. The presence or absence of zidovudine in a nevirapine-containing antiretroviral regimen determines which of two nevirapine-limiting mutations occur as virologic failure. Paper presented at: 39th Interscience Conference on Antimicrobial Agents and Chemotherapy, San Francisco, CA, 1999. Abstract 1171.
64. Larder BA. 3'Azido-3'-deoxythymidine resistance suppressed by a mutation conferring human immunodeficiency virus type 1 resistance to non-nucleoside reverse transcriptase inhibitors. Antimicrob Agents Chemother 1992; 36:2664–2669.
65. Boyer PI, Gao H-Q, Hughes SH. A mutation at position 190 of human immunodeficiency virus type 1 reverse transcriptase interacts with mutations at positions 74 and 75 via the template primer. Antimicrob Agents Chemother 1998; 42:447–452.
66. Casado JL, Hertogs K, Ruiz L, et al. Non-nucleoside reverse transcriptase inhibitor resistance among patients failing a nevirapine plus protease inhibitor-containing regimen. AIDS 2000; 14:F1–F7.
67. MacArthur RD, Kosmyna JM, Crane LR, et al. Sequencing of non-nucleoside reverse transcriptase inhibitors based on specific mutational patterns fails to lower plasma HIV-RNA levels in persons extensively pre-treated with antiretrovirals who are failing virologically on nevirapine-containing antiretroviral regimens. Paper presented at: Seventh European Conference on Clinical Aspects and Treatment of HIV-Infection, Lisbon, Portugal, 1999. Abstract 208.
68. Bacolla A, Shih CK, Rose JM, et al. Amino acid substitutions in HIV-1 reverse transcriptase with corresponding residues from HIV-2. Effect on kinetic constants and inhibition by non-nucleoside analogs. J Biol Chem 1993; 268:16,571–16,577.

69. Quinones-Mateu ME, Soriano V, Domingo E, Menendez-Arias L. Characterisation of the new reverse transcriptase of a human immunodeficiency virus type 1 group O isolate. Virology 1997; 236:364–373.
70. Descamps D, Collin G, Loussert-Ajaka I, et al. HIV-1 group O sensitivity to antiretroviral drugs. AIDS 1995; 9:977–978.
71. Descamps D, Collin G. Letourneur F, et al. Susceptibility of human immunodeficiency virus type 1 group O isolates to antiretroviral agents: in vitro phenotypic and genotypic analyses. J Virol 1997; 71:8893–8898.
72. Shafer RW, Stevenson D, Chan B. Human immunodeficiency virus reverse transcriptase and protease sequence database. Nucleic Acids Res 1999; 27:348–352.
73. Gruzdev B, Rakhmanova A, Van t'Klooster G, et al. One week of monotherapy with TMC-125, a novel highly potent nNRTI, produces a mean 2 log reduction in viral load in antiretroviral naïve HIV-1 infected volunteers. Paper presented at: Eighth European Conference on Clinical Aspects and Treatment of HIV Infection, Athens, Greece, 2001. Abstract 09.
74. Gazzard B, Pozniak A, Arasteh K, et al. TMC125, a next-generation nNRTI, demonstrates high potency after 7 days therapy in treatment-experienced HIV-1-infected individuals with phenotypic nNRTI resistance. Paper presented at: Ninth Conference on Retroviruses and Opportunistic Infections, Seattle, WA, 2002. Abstract 5.
75. Potts KE, Fujiwara T, Sato A, et al. Antiviral activity and resistance profile of AG-1549, a novel HIV-1 non-nucleoside reverses transcriptase inhibitor. Paper presented at: Sixth Conference on Retroviruses and Opportunistic Infections, Chicago, IL, 1999. Abstract 12.
76. Ho DD, Toyoshima T, Mo H, et al. Characterisation of human immunodeficiency virus type 1 variants with increased resistance to a C_2-symmetric protease inhibitor. J Virol 1994; 68:2016–2020.
77. Maschera B, Darby G, Palu G, et al. Mutations in the viral protease that confer resistance to saquinavir increase the dissociation rate constant of the protease-saquinavir complex. J Biol Chem 1996; 271:33,231–33,235.
78. Condra JH, Holder DJ, Schleif WA, et al. Genetic correlates of in vivo viral resistance to indinavir, a human immunodeficiency virus type 1 protease inhibitor. J Virol 1996; 70: 8270–8276.
79. ZhangY-M, Imamichi H, Imamichi T, et al. Drug resistance during indinavir therapy is caused by mutations in the protease gene and in its gag substrate cleavage sites. J Virol 1997; 71:6662–6670.
80. Havlir DV, Hellmann NS, Petropoulos CJ, et al. Drug susceptibility in HIV infection after viral rebound in patients receiving indinavir-containing regimens. JAMA 2000; 283: 229–234.
81. Eastman PS, Mittler J, Kelso R, et al. Genotypic changes in human immunodeficiency virus type 1 associated with loss of suppression of plasma viral RNA levels in subjects treated with ritonavir (Norvir) monotherapy. J Virol 1998; 72:5154–5164.
82. Carrillo A, Stewart KD, Sham HL, et al. In vitro selection and characterisation of human immunodeficiency virus type 1 variants with increased resistance to ABT-378, a novel protease inhibitor. J Virol 1998; 72:7532–7541.
83. Sham HL, Kempf DJ, Molla A, et al. ABT-378, a highly potent inhibitor of the human immunodeficiency virus protease. Antimicrob Agents Chemother 1998; 42:3218–3224.
84. Mo H, Lu L, Chernyavskiy T, et al. Characterisation of HIV-1 variants in response to in vitro passage with ABT-378/ritonavir. Antivir Ther 1999; 4(suppl. 1):63.
85. Kempf D, Xu Y, Brun S, et al. Baseline genotype and phenotype do not predict response to ABT-378/ritonavir in PI-experienced patients at 24 and 48 weeks. Paper presented at: Seventh Conference on Retroviruses and Opportunistic Infections, San Francisco, CA, 2000. Abstract 731.

86. Markowitz M, Conant M, Hurley A, et al. A preliminary evaluation of nelfinavir mesylate, an inhibitor of human immunodeficiency virus (HIV-1) protease, to treat HIV infection. J Infect Dis 1998; 177:1533–1540.
87. Patick AK, Duran M, Cao Y, et al. Genotypic and phenotypic characterisation of human immunodeficiency virus type 1 variants isolated from patients treated with the protease inhibitor nelfinavir. Antimicrob Agents Chemother 1998; 42:2637–2644.
88. Condra JH, Holder DJ, Schleif WA, et al. Genetic correlates of virological response to an indinavir-containing salvage regimen in patients with nelfinavir failure. Antivir Ther 1999; 4(suppl. 1):44.
89. Dronda F, Casado JL, Moreno S, et al. Cross-resistance to nelfinavir can be predicted by previous antiretroviral exposure in the absence of D30N mutation. Paper presented at: Seventh Conference on Retroviruses and Opportunistic Infections, San Francisco, CA, 2000. Abstract 729.
90. Partaledis JA, Yamaguchi K, Tisdale M, et al. In vitro selection and characterisation of human immunodeficiency virus type 1 (HIV-1) isolates with reduced sensitivity to hydroxyethylamino sulfonamide inhibitors of HIV-1 aspartyl protease. J Virol 1995; 69: 5228–5235.
91. Schmidt B. Cross-resistance to amprenavir in PI-treated patients. Paper presented at: Seventh Conference on Retroviruses and Opportunistic Infections, San Francisco, CA, 2000. Abstract 726.
92. Craig C, Race E, Sheldon J, et al. HIV protease genotype and viral sensitivity to HIV protease inhibitors following saquinavir therapy. AIDS 1998; 12:1611–1618.
93. Winters MA, Shapiro JM, Lawrence J, Merigan TC. Human immunodeficiency virus type 1 protease genotypes and in vitro protease inhibitor susceptibilities of isolates from individuals who were switched to other protease inhibitors after long-term saquinavir treatment. J Virol 1998; 72:5303–5306.
94. Dulioust A, Paulous S, Guillemot L, Delaville A-M, Boué F, Clavel F. Constrained evolution of human immunodeficiency virus type 1 protease during sequential therapy with two distinct protease inhibitors. J Virol 1999; 73:850–854.
95. Zolopa AR, Hertogs K, Shafer R, et al. A comparison of phenotypic, genotypic and clinical/treatment history predictors of virological response to saquinavir/ritonavir salvage therapy in a clinic-based cohort. Antivir Ther 1999; 4(suppl. 1):47.
96. Colonno RI, Friborg J, Rose RE, et al. Identification of amino acid substitutions correlated with atazanavir susceptibility in patients treated with atazanavir-containing regimens. Antivir Ther 2002; 7(suppl. 1):S56.
97. Robinson B, Riccardi K, Gong Y, et al. BMS-232632, a highly potent human immunodeficiency virus protease inhibitor that can be used in combination with other available antiretroviral agents. Antimicrob Agents Chemother 2000; 44:2093–2099.
98. Larder BA, Hertogs K, Bloor S. Tipranavir inhibits broadly protease inhibitor-resistant HIV-1 clinical samples. AIDS 2000; 14:1943–1948.
99. Schwartz R, Kazanjian P, Slater L, et al. Resistance to tipranavir is uncommon in a randomized trial of tipranavir/ritonavir (TPV/RTV) in multiple-PI-failure patients (BI 1182.2). Paper presented at: Ninth Conference on Retroviruses and Opportunistic Infections, Seattle, WA, 2002. Abstract 562.
100. Henry K, Lalezari J, Ohearn M, et al. Enfuvirtide (T-20) in combination with an optimized background (OB) regimen versus OB alone in patients with prior experience or resistance to each of the three classes of approved antiretrovirals in North America and Brazil (TORO 1). Paper presented at: 14th International AIDS Conference, Barcelona, Spain, 2002. Abstract LbOr19B.
101. Clotet B, Lazzarin A, Cooper D, et al. Enfuvirtide (T-20) in combination with an optimized background (OB) regimen versus OB alone in patients with prior experience or

resistance to each of the three classes of approved antiretrovirals in Europe and Australia (TORO 2). Paper presented at: 14th International AIDS Conference, Barcelona, Spain, 2002. Abstract LbOr19A.
102. Greenberg ML, Sista P, Miralles GD, et al. Characterization of baseline and treatment-emergent resistance to T-20 (enfuvirtide) observed in Phase II clinical trials: substitutions in gp41 amino acids 36-45 and enfuvirtide susceptibility of virus isolates. Antivir Ther 2002; 7(suppl. 1):S16.
103. Xu L, Hue S, Taylor S. Minimal variation in T-20 binding domain of different HIV-1 subtypes from antiretroviral naïve and experienced patients. AIDS 2002; 16:1684–1686.
104. Greenberg ML, Davison D, Jin L, et al. In vitro antiviral activity of T-1249: a second generation fusion inhibitor. Antivir Ther 2002; 7(suppl. 1):S10.
105. Durant J, Clevenbergh P, Halfon P, et al Drug-resistance genotyping in HIV-1 therapy: the VIRADAPT randomised controlled trial. Lancet 1999; 353:2195–2199.
106. Baxter JD, Mayers DL, Wentworth DN, et al. A randomised study of antiretroviral management based on plasma genotypic antiretroviral resistance testing in patients failing therapy. AIDS 2000; 14:F83–F93.
107. Tural C, Ruiz L, Holtzer C, et al Clinical utility of HIV-1 genotyping and expert advice: the Havana trial. AIDS 2002; 16:209–218.
108. Cingolani A, Antinori A, Rizzo MG, et al. Usefulness of monitoring HIV drug resistance and adherence in individuals failing highly active antiretroviral therapy: a randomised study (ARGENTA). AIDS 2002; 16:369–379.
109. Clevenbergh P, Durant J, Halfon P, et al. Persisting long term benefit of antiretroviral genotypic guided treatment for HIV-infected patients failing HAART: the VIRADAPT study, week 48 follow-up. Antivir Ther 1999; 4:42.
110. Cohen CJ, Hunt S, Sension M, et al. A randomised trial assessing the impact of phenotypic resistance testing on antiretroviral therapy. AIDS 2002; 16:579–588.
111. Haubrich RH, Keiser PH, Kemper CA, et al. CCTG 575: a randomised, prospective study of phenotype testing versus standard of care for patients failing antiretroviral therapy. Antivir Ther 2001; 6:63.
112. Meynard JL, Vray M, Morand-Joubert L, et al. Phenotypic or genotypic resistance testing for choosing antiretroviral therapy after treatment failure: a randomised trial. AIDS 2002; 16:727–736.
113. Blanco JL, Valdecillos G, Arroyo JR, et al A prospective randomised study on the usefulness of genotypic resistance tests versus real phenotypic resistance tests in heavily pretreated patients with virological failure (VIHRES study). Paper presented at: 14th International AIDS Conference, Barcelona, Spain, 2002. Abstract TuPeB4624.
114. Wegner SA, Wallace M, Aronson N, et al. Long-term clinical efficacy of resistance testing: results of the CERT trial. Paper presented at: 14th International AIDS Conference, Barcelona, Spain, 2002. Abstract ThOrB1389. Antivir Ther 2002; 7:S129.
115. Vray M, Meynard JL, Dalban C, et al. Multivariate logistic regression analysis of factors predictive of the virological response in the NARVAL trial. Paper presented at: 14th International AIDS Conference, Barcelona, Spain, 2002. Abstract ThOrB1387.
116. Torre D, Tambini R. Antiretroviral drug resistance testing in patients with HIV-1 infection: a meta-analysis study. HIV Clin Trials 2002; 3:1–8.
117. Katlama C, Dominguez S, Duvivier C, et al. Long term benefit of treatment interruption in Salvage therapy (GIGHAART ANRS 97). Paper presented at: 10th Conference on Retroviruses and Opportunistic Infection, Boston, MA, 2003. Abstract 68.
118. Deeks SG. When to switch antiretroviral therapy. Paper presented at: 10th Conference on Retroviruses and Opportunistic Infection, Boston, MA, 2003. Abstract 188.

21
Multidrug Resistance in Human Cytomegalovirus

Vincent C. Emery, Mohammad Raza Naqvee, and Anuradha Chawla

1. INTRODUCTION

Human cytomegalovirus (HCMV) is a member of the Herpesviridae family and infects the majority of the human population. In developed countries, seroprevalance rates are approx 60%; in developing countries, seroprevalance increases to between 90 and 100%. In common with other members of the herpesvirus family, following initial infection, the virus can remain latent within the human host and be subject to reactivations under appropriate conditions *(1,2)*. In the immunocompetent host, HCMV rarely causes significant problems, although primary infection has been associated with hepatitis and a mononucleosislike syndrome. However, in the individual whose immune system is immature, such as the neonate or the patient receiving immunosuppressive drugs (e.g., as a transplant recipient or for human immunodeficiency virus [HIV] infection), the virus can assert its full pathogenic potential. Thus, in the neonate, congenital CMV infection is a major cause of mental retardation and sensory-neural hearing loss. In the individual with HIV, HCMV causes retinitis, gastrointestinal tract disease, and central and peripheral nervous system disorders (encephalitis and polyradiculopathy, respectively). In the transplant recipient, the virus can cause a number of symptoms, including pneumonitis, hepatitis, gastrointestinal tract disease, or prolonged pyrexial debilitating disease. Infection has been associated with organ rejection *(3,4)*.

As a consequence of the importance of HCMV in the diseases summarized above, antiviral chemotherapy aimed at reducing viral replication has become a major method of combatting the pathological consequences of infection. There have been a number of recent comprehensive reviews on HCMV drug resistance *(5–7)*. In this chapter, we briefly focus on the current knowledge of HCMV replication and the host immune response to HCMV in the immunocompetent and the immunocompromised host; then, we summarize the current antiviral chemotherapeutic measures used to combat infection. Finally, we consider the issue of multidrug resistance in HCMV and its relevance in the context of new antiviral drugs that may become available for the treatment of this serious infection.

From: *Management of Multiple Drug-Resistant Infections*
Edited by: S. H. Gillespie © Humana Press Inc., Totowa, NJ

2. REPLICATION IN THE HUMAN HOST

With the advent of sensitive quantitative measures of viral replication such as quantitative polymerase chain reaction (PCR), an improved appreciation of the replication dynamics of HCMV in the human host has been obtained. Contrary to the results using established cell culture methods, the virus can replicate rapidly in the human host, with a doubling time/half-life of the infected cell of approx 1 d *(8)*. As a consequence of this rapid replication, at the peak of a viremic episode (typically 10^4 to 10^6 genomes per milliliter of blood), a large number of virions will be produced and destroyed each day, so the capacity to introduce mutations into the genome is high. These data have relevance for both the rapid diagnosis of HCMV infection in individuals at risk of disease and in the generation of drug resistance mutations within key genes (*see* Section 6). Many groups have shown that viral load is an important factor in determining pathogenesis, such that symptomatic individuals frequently have higher viral loads than asymptomatic individuals, and that the rate of increase in viral load in the early stages of infection has been used to identify individuals at risk of future HCMV disease *(9–19)*.

The peak virus load and the rate at which virus load increases is dependent on many factors, including the immunosuppressive state of the individual concerned and whether the individual has been previously exposed to HCMV (i.e., if they have some element of immune memory). In the context of solid organ transplant recipients, seropositive recipients of a seropositive organ will limit both the rate of HCMV replication and the peak of virus load attained following transplantation compared to patients who are seronegative recipients of a seropositive organ *(20)*. As a consequence, individuals with the D+R+ combination are at a significantly reduced risk of HCMV disease when compared to the those of the D+R– group, where D is the donor, R is the recipient, + indicates previously infected, and – indicates previously uninfected.

3. IMMUNE CONTROL OF CYTOMEGALOVIRUS REPLICATION

Significant progress has been made in understanding the host immune response against HCMV. The work of many groups has provided a detailed account of the flux and phenotype of CD8 T cells in immunocompetent individuals undergoing primary infection, and many have contributed to the understanding of the immune control of HCMV in the immunocompromised host *(21)*.

Taken together, these studies illustrate that, despite the complexity of the HCMV genome, the majority T-cell response of the immune system is directed against one or two proteins in the virus, mainly ppUL83 (pp65)*(22–25)* and IE2 (ppUl123)*(26,27)*, while the majority B-cell response is elicited by the surface glycoproteins: glycoprotein B (gpUL55)*(28)*, glycoprotein H (gpUL75)*(29)*, and the glycoprotein M/N complex *(30,31)*. In the context of T-helper responses, the data suggest that these responses are directed predominantly against the sites selected for CD8 T-cell responses and for B-cell responses, namely, ppUL83 and gpUL55. A number of studies have shown the importance of maintaining CD4 and CD8 T-cell responses post-transplantation for the control of HCMV replication and hence disease *(32)*. Indeed, the successful control of HCMV replication and the disease through adaptive immunotherapy requires the presence of both CD4 and CD8 T cells expanded against HCMV *(33)*.

4. ANTIVIRAL CHEMOTHERAPY

In the past, deployment of antiviral chemotherapy for HCMV was initiated after the onset of symptoms. However, with the advent of rapid diagnostic methods such as shell vial assays, antigenemia, and qualitative and quantitative PCR methods, the ability to detect the virus at much earlier stages of infection and to identify patients at much higher risk of future disease has enabled development of other strategies. At the time of writing, there are two main strategies in place for the prevention of CMV disease through the deployment of chemotherapy. The first approach relies on the administration of prophylaxis with anti-HCMV drugs in high-risk individuals, such as D+R– solid organ transplant recipients, to suppress replication in the critical first 3 mo of transplantation. An alternative approach is the use of laboratory markers such as antigenemia positivity or persistent PCR positivity to trigger antiviral therapeutic initiation. The latter approach is known as pre-emptive therapy. Reasoned arguments supporting both approaches are available *(34,35)*. Prophylaxis and pre-emptive therapy have proven clinical benefit, but it is clear that prolonged exposure to antiviral agents, especially when given at lower doses, can provide an environment in which drug resistance can emerge. It is therefore not surprising that the majority of drug resistance has been observed in patients requiring long-term therapy to control their HCMV infection/disease or when suboptimal dosing schedules have been adopted (*see* Section 6).

5. DRUG ACTIVATION—CONTRIBUTIONS OF THE VIRUS

The mainstay of therapy of HCMV in recent years has been ganciclovir (GCV), a nucleoside analogue that requires triphosphorylation to become a competitive inhibitor of dGTP in the DNA polymerization catalyzed by the viral DNA polymerase (UL54). GCV is activated to the monophosphate moiety via the HCMV UL97 protein kinase *(36,37)*. This gene product will also activate aciclovir to its monophosphate *(38)*. Subsequent phosphorylation to the triphosphate moiety is achieved through cellular kinases, and when fully activated, GCV triphosphate and aciclovir triphosphate act as competitive inhibitors of dGTP. Cidofovir, a phosphonate derivative already carries a pseudomonophosphate group; hence, cellular kinases activate it to the cidofovir diphosphate, at which stage it acts as a competitive inhibitor of the HCMV DNA polymerase *(39)*. Foscarnet (phosphonoformic acid), a pyrophosphate analogue, acts as a product inhibitor of the HCMV DNA polymerase and does not require any activation by viral or cellular enzymes *(40)*.

Two drugs have been used predominantly in prophylaxis against HCMV. These are aciclovir (and, more recently, valaciclovir) and GCV, initially as an intravenous formulation, then as an oral formulation, and more recently as the prodrug valganciclovir. Information on a number of double-blind controlled trials is available in the literature, attesting to the utility of these compounds in suppressing HCMV replication and hence preventing HCMV disease during the period of prophylaxis or maintenance suppressive therapy for acquired immunodeficiency syndrome (AIDS) retinitis (*see* Table 1).

In addition, the trial of valaciclovir in renal transplant recipients showed that, in the D+R– group, acute graft rejection was reduced by approx 50%, arguing that HCMV contributes to acute graft rejection in the renal transplant setting *(41)*. In the era preceding the availability of highly active antiretroviral therapy (HAART), HCMV retinitis

Table 1
Emergence of Clinical Drug Resistance for Human Cytomegalovirus

Study	Title	Article type/ patient group	Resistance against	No. of patients
1	Ganciclovir-resistant cytomegalovirus encephalitis in a bone marrow transplant recipient *(61)*	Case report/bone marrow transplant	Ganciclovir	1
2	Clinical characteristics of 13 solid organ transplant recipients with ganciclovir-resistant cytomegalovirus infection *(62)*	Review of individual cases/solid organ	Ganciclovir	13
3	Emergence of ganciclovir-resistant cytomegalovirus in lung transplant recipients *(63)*	Retrospective analysis/ lung transplant	Ganciclovir	212
4	Emergence of late cytomegalovirus central nervous system disease in hematopoietic stem cell transplant recipients *(64)*	Case report/ haploidentical HSC transplantation	Ganciclovir	2
5	Case study: rapid emergence of a cytomegalovirus UL97 mutant in a heart transplant recipient on pre-emptive ganciclovir therapy *(65)*	Case report/heart transplant	Ganciclovir	1
6	Cytomegalovirus ventriculoencephalitis in a bone marrow transplant recipient receiving antiviral maintenance: clinical and molecular evidence of drug resistance *(66)*	Case report/bone marrow transplant	Ganciclovir or foscarnet	1
7	Progressive retinitis-encephalitis due to ganciclovir-resistant cytomegalovirus associated with aplastic anemia *(67)*	Case report/aplastic anemia	Ganciclovir	1
8	Ganciclovir-resistant cytomegalovirus infection: two cases with different clinical impact *(68)*	Case report/bone marrow transplant and HIV	Ganciclovir	2
9	Treatment of ganciclovir-resistant cytomegalovirus with foscarnet: a report of two cases occurring after bone marrow transplantation *(69)*	Case report/bone marrow transplant	Ganciclovir	2
10	A 42-yr-old lung transplant patient with ganciclovir-resistant cytomegalovirus (CMV) infection *(70)*	Case report/lung transplant	Ganciclovir	1
11	Ganciclovir resistance in a heart transplant recipient infected by cytomegalovirus *(71)*	Case report/heart transplant	Ganciclovir	1
12	Ganciclovir-resistant cytomegalovirus disease after allogeneic stem cell transplantation: pitfalls of phenotypic diagnosis by in vitro selection of an UL97 mutant strain *(72)*	Case report/allogenic stem cell transplant	Ganciclovir	1

(*continued*)

Table 1 (*continued*)

Study	Title	Article type/ patient group	Resistance against	No. of patients
13	Comparison of cytomegalovirus (CMV) UL97 gene sequences in the blood and vitreous of patients with acquired immunodeficiency syndrome and CMV retinitis *(73)*	Retrospective analysis/AIDS	Ganciclovir	87
14	Resistance to ganciclovir and clinical outcomes of patients with cytomegalovirus retinitis. Cytomegalovirus *(74)*	Prospective cohort study	Ganciclovir	197
15	Cytomegalovirus drug resistance and clinical implications *(6)*	Review/solid organ transplant	Ganciclovir	
16	Sequence analysis of UL54 and UL97 genes and evaluation of antiviral susceptibility of human cytomegalovirus isolates obtained from kidney allograft recipients before and after treatment *(75)*	Renal transplant patients	Ganciclovir	24
17	High incidence of ganciclovir-resistant cytomegalovirus infection among lung transplant recipients receiving preemptive therapy *(76)*	Lung transplant patients	Ganciclovir	45
18	Discordant phenotypes and genotypes of cytomegalovirus (CMV) in patients with AIDS and relapsing CMV retinitis *(77)*	AIDS	Ganciclovir	4

was a major pathological consequence experienced by HIV-infected individuals *(42)*. As a consequence, a number of treatment modalities were developed, including the use of GCV, foscarnet and cidofovir, and combinations of GCV and foscarnet *(43,44)*. The nature of HCMV retinitis required the drug to be given at a high concentration for an induction period (usually 3 wk) in the case of intravenous GCV, followed by lower levels of maintenance therapy, usually 1 g three times daily with oral GCV. To date, the major database of knowledge in the context of drug resistance has been derived from these cohorts of individuals (*see* Section 6).

6. DRUG RESISTANCE—MONOTHERAPY

Cytomegalovirus produces low-level drug resistance via the evolution of mutations within the UL97 protein kinase. These mutations have been mapped to a number of key amino acids within the protein and consist of point mutations or in-frame deletions that affect substrate binding or ATP-binding sites, but do not affect normal function of this gene in HCMV replication (*see* Fig. 1). Indeed, attempts to produce UL97 null mutants of HCMV have been unsuccessful, arguing that this gene is essential for HCMV replication *(45)*.

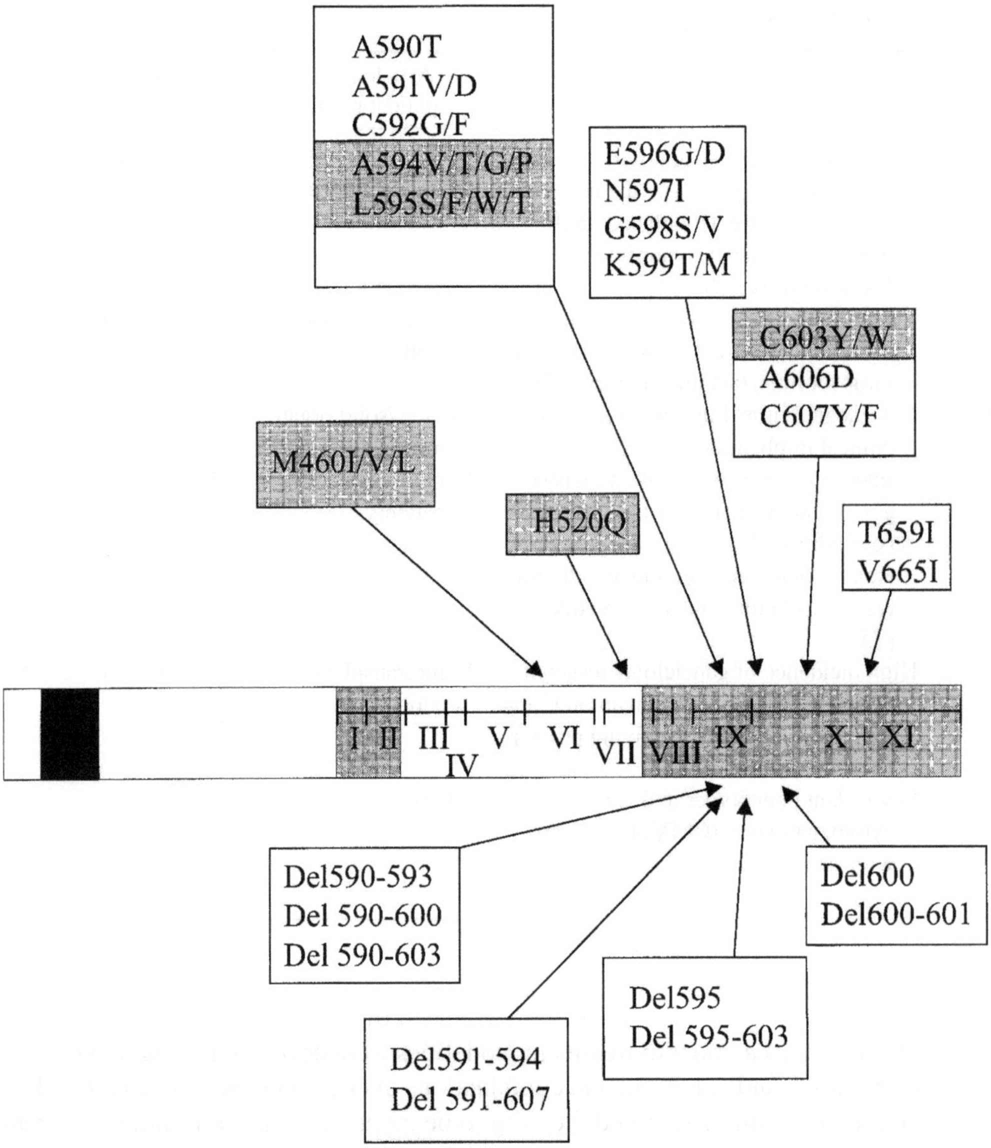

Fig. 1. Distribution of mutations identified in clinical strains of HCMV resistant to ganciclovir. Mutations associated with the majority of drug resistance (approx 85%) are shown as shaded boxes.

The mutations frequently observed in the clinical setting are at amino acids 460, 520, 594, 595, and 603. Mutations within UL97 give rise to low-level resistance to GCV (approximately fivefold), and viruses carrying these mutations are marginally debilitated in their replication competence when compared to wild-type strains of virus *(46)*. However, in the presence of prolonged exposure to GCV, high-level resistance can develop. This resistance pattern involves mutations within UL97 in addition to mutations developing within the HCMV DNA polymerase *(47)*. Unlike the situation with UL97, the mutations within UL54 that have been identified in clinically derived

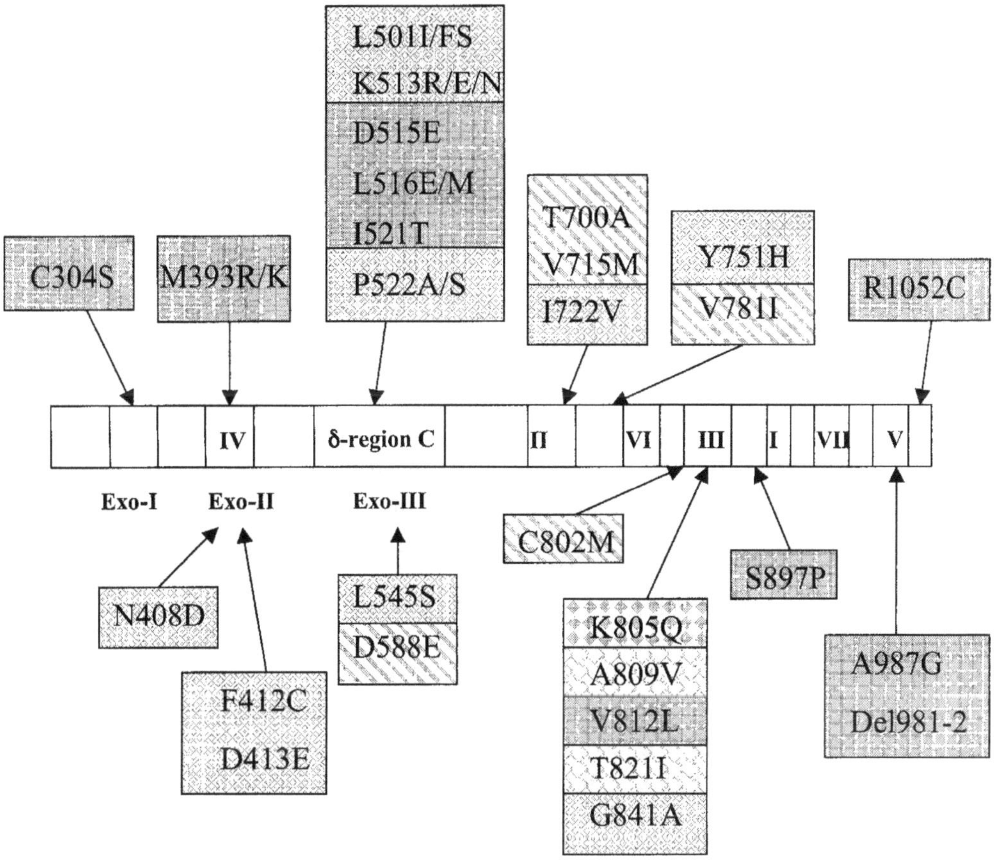

Fig. 2. Distribution of mutations identified in clinical strains of HCMV resistant to ganciclovir/foscarnet/cidofovir. The cross-resistance profile is shown for each mutation. Gray box, GCV^r CDV^r FOS^r; dotted background, GCV^r CDV^r FOS^s; diagonal striped background, GCV^s CDV^s FOS^r; wavy background, GCV^r CDV^s FOS^r; diamond background, GCV^s CDV^r FOS^{hs} where s = drug sensitive, r = drug resistant, and hs = hypersensitive to drug.

virus strains are widely distributed across the gene (*see* Fig. 2), although the majority lie within the domains shared between different polymerases, while natural polymorphisms lie outside these conserved domains *(48)*. A number of these mutations are associated with cross-resistance to other anti-HCMV agents (*see* Section 7).

In the context of transplant recipients, HCMV drug resistance has been observed in a number of case reports, usually when HCMV replication has been insufficiently suppressed with antiviral chemotherapy, so the patient requires a further course of therapy, followed by therapy at a lower level to control CMV replication. As observed in the HIV-infected group, prolonged treatment with lower levels of GCV such as that achieved with 1 g oral GCV three times daily is insufficient to inhibit CMV replication completely; hence, replication occurs in the context of selective advantage from mutants that may be generated. It is therefore not surprising that these approaches have been associated with generation of CMV resistance in the clinic *(49)*.

In patients requiring higher levels of immunosuppressive therapy, GCV resistance is more likely. For example, in lung transplant recipients, Limaye showed that 27% of

CMV-seronegative recipients of a lung from HCMV-seropositive donors exposed to GCV therapy for a median of 100 d were excreting GCV-resistant virus, compared to only 3% in patients who were already CMV seropositive *(50)*.

In patients with AIDS, using either phenotypic or genotypic methods, the incidence of resistant virus in patients who had never been exposed to GCV was low *(51–55)*, consistent with the fitness loss of mutant viruses relative to wild-type drug-sensitive viruses *(46)*. In the context of the temporal appearance of resistance, Boivin and colleagues *(51)* showed that, in patients receiving valganciclovir (900 mg once a day), resistance at mo 3, 6, 12, and 18 after initiation of maintenance therapy was 2, 7, 13, and 15%, respectively. In contrast, in patients given oral GCV (1 g three times daily) maintenance therapy (which achieves plasma levels of GCV approximately half of those achieved with valganciclovir), the incidence of GCV resistance was higher in two reports: 28% at 9 mo using a phenotypic assay *(55)* and 22% after 3 mo using a genotypic assay *(56)*. In patients exposed to foscarnet therapy, a similar picture emerged, with estimates of 37% resistance after 9 mo of therapy *(57)*.

7. CROSS-RESISTANCE AND MULTIDRUG RESISTANCE

Because of the relative paucity of compounds available for the treatment of HCMV and because of the side effect profile of these compounds, there have been relatively few examples of the use of combination chemotherapy. A notable exception is the combination of GCV and foscarnet, which has been assessed in HIV-infected and transplant recipients, with each drug given at half the normal dose *(43)*. Because the UL97 gene product activates both GCV and aciclovir, a UL97-resistant mutation generated as a consequence of GCV exposure would be expected to be resistant against acyclovir *(58)*. However, aciclovir and valaciclovir have been predominantly used for prophylaxis in the transplant setting, so it is not clear whether sufficient drug pressure was generated in this setting to facilitate the evolution and persistence of a large UL97 mutant virus population.

There are no cases in the literature to our knowledge for which a patient has been proved to develop an HCMV UL97-resistant mutant in the presence of aciclovir that was then refractile to therapy with GCV. This could partially reflect that the UL97 strains of HCMV are only marginally less sensitive to GCV such that on achieving an appropriate dose (e.g., using 5 mg/kg body weight iv GCV), the UL97 mutant strains are still inhibited *(46)*.

A number of in vitro studies have shown that the mutation patterns observed in the HCMV DNA polymerase can frequently give rise to cross-resistance to other compounds used in the treatment of HCMV. These data are summarized in Fig. 2 and clearly show that a number of mutations produce cross-resistance to GCV, cidofovir, and foscarnet, whereas other mutations yield cross-resistance to GCV and cidofovir, but the virus remains sensitive to foscarnet. In one case (K805Q), the virus is resistant to both GCV and cidofovir, but hypersensitive to foscarnet.

It is important to realize that, although these UL54 mutants have been derived from patients, the cross-resistance studies have been predominantly performed in vitro. Consequently, it is difficult to extrapolate the true consequences of these mutations with respect to clinical multidrug resistance. Nevertheless, there are sufficient data to suggest that such multidrug-resistant strains can be generated under the selective pressure of a single agent such as GCV. Indeed, there have been reports for the evolution of multidrug resistance in vivo, with patients treated with more than one compound unsuccessfully because of the cross-resistance profile.

There are a number of new drugs in development for HCMV, although none at the time of writing is currently undergoing extensive phase II/III clinical trials *(59)*. A number of other nucleoside analogues are undergoing development together with drugs such as benzimidivir (maribavir), a benzimadazole compound that selectively targets the HCMV UL97 protein kinase. Drug resistance against this compound has been generated in vitro and has mapped to amino acid 397 of the UL97 protein kinase, a mutation that has never been observed in patients treated with GCV. At present, the effect of this mutation in the background of GCV resistance on auto- (phosphorylation of UL97 itself) and transphosphorylation (phosphorylation of other proteins besides UL97) and on GCV kinase action is not known, but will be important to determine before the deployment of this agent in the clinic. Interestingly, maribavir has also been shown to provide additive inhibition when used in combination with existing anti-HCMV agents such as GCV, foscarnet, and cidofovir illustrating the potential for combination therapy for HCMV *(60)*.

8. CONCLUSIONS

At present, the limited availability of compounds to inhibit HCMV in the clinical setting has resulted in the relatively infrequent occurrence of HCMV drug resistance and a relatively low frequency of strains showing multiple resistance phenotypes. It is clear that inappropriate duration and level of drug therapy for HCMV promotes an environment in which drug-resistant strains can develop; with the availability of newer orally bioavailable formulations for existing compounds such as GCV, it is possible that issues relating to drug resistance may increase. Consequently, it is important that physicians and virologists involved in the management of patients at risk of HCMV infection and disease actively investigate patients for the presence of drug resistance to single agents and assess the likely impact that these resistant mutations will have in the context of other antiviral drugs that may be used to control HCMV replication.

REFERENCES

1. Griffiths PD, Emery VC. Cytomegalovirus. Clinical Virology. 2nd ed. 2002.
2. Fish KN, et al. Cytomegalovirus persistence in macrophages and endothelial cells. Scand J Infect Dis Suppl 1995; 99:34–40.
3. Rubin RH. Infection, antimicrobial resistance, and newly emerging pathogens: the growing role of fungi. Transpl Infect Dis 2001; 3:187–188.
4. Soderberg-Naucler C, Emery VC. Viral infections and their impact on chronic renal allograft dysfunction. Transplantation 2001; 71:SS24–SS30.
5. Drew WL, Paya CV, Emery V. Cytomegalovirus (CMV) resistance to antivirals. Am J Transplant 2001; 1:307–312.
6. Chou SW. Cytomegalovirus drug resistance and clinical implications. Transpl Infect Dis 2001; 3(suppl. 2):20–24.
7. Gilbert C, Bestman-Smith J, Boivin G. Resistance of herpesviruses to antiviral drugs: clinical impacts and molecular mechanisms. Drug Resist Updat 2002; 5:88–114.
8. Emery VC, et al. The dynamics of human cytomegalovirus replication in vivo. J Exp Med 1999; 190:177–182.
9. Cope AV, et al. Interrelationships among quantity of human cytomegalovirus (HCMV) DNA in blood, donor-recipient serostatus, and administration of methylprednisolone as risk factors for HCMV disease following liver transplantation. J Infect Dis 1997; 176:1484–1490.

10. Gor D, et al. Longitudinal fluctuations in cytomegalovirus load in bone marrow transplant patients: relationship between peak virus load, donor/recipient serostatus, acute GVHD and CMV disease. Bone Marrow Transplant 1998; 21:597–605.
11. Emery VC, et al. Application of viral-load kinetics to identify patients who develop cytomegalovirus disease after transplantation. Lancet 2000; 355:2032–2036.
12. Boivin G, et al. Virological features and clinical manifestations associated with human metapneumovirus: a new paramyxovirus responsible for acute respiratory-tract infections in all age groups. J Infect Dis 2002; 186:1330–1334.
13. Bowen EF, et al. Cytomegalovirus retinitis in AIDS patients: influence of cytomegaloviral load on response to ganciclovir, time to recurrence and survival. AIDS 1996; 10:1515–1520.
14. Bowen EF, et al. Cytomegalovirus (CMV) viraemia detected by polymerase chain reaction identifies a group of HIV-positive patients at high risk of CMV disease. AIDS 1997; 11:889–893.
15. Boeckh M, et al. Late cytomegalovirus disease and mortality in recipients of allogeneic hematopoietic stem cell transplants: importance of viral load and T-cell immunity. Blood 2003; 101:407–414.
16. Spector SA, et al. Plasma cytomegalovirus (CMV) DNA load predicts CMV disease and survival in AIDS patients. J Clin Invest 1998; 101:497–502.
17. Spector SA, et al. Cytomegalovirus (CMV) DNA load is an independent predictor of CMV disease and survival in advanced AIDS. J Virol 1999; 73:7027–7030.
18. Sia IG, et al. Cytomegalovirus (CMV) DNA load predicts relapsing CMV infection after solid organ transplantation. J Infect Dis 2000; 181:717–720.
19. Humar A, et al. Cytomegalovirus (CMV) virus load kinetics to predict recurrent disease in solid-organ transplant patients with CMV disease. J Infect Dis 2002; 186:829–833.
20. Emery VC, et al. Human cytomegalovirus (HCMV) replication dynamics in HCMV-naive and -experienced immunocompromised hosts. J Infect Dis 2002; 185:1723–1728.
21. Reddehase MJ. The immunogenicity of human and murine cytomegaloviruses. Curr Opin Immunol 2000; 12:390–396.
22. Gillespie GM, et al. Functional heterogeneity and high frequencies of cytomegalovirus-specific CD8(+) T lymphocytes in healthy seropositive donors. J Virol 2000; 74:8140–8150.
23. Wills MR, et al. Human virus-specific CD8+ CTL clones revert from CD45ROhigh to CD45RAhigh in vivo: CD45RAhighCD8+ T cells comprise both naive and memory cells. J Immunol 1999; 162:7080–7087.
24. Kern F, et al. Cytomegalovirus (CMV) phosphoprotein 65 makes a large contribution to shaping the T cell repertoire in CMV-exposed individuals. J Infect Dis 2002; 185:1709–1716.
25. McLaughlin-Taylor E, et al. Identification of the major late human cytomegalovirus matrix protein pp65 as a target antigen for CD8+ virus-specific cytotoxic T lymphocytes. J Med Virol 1994; 43:103–110.
26. Frankenberg N, et al. Identification of a conserved HLA-A2-restricted decapeptide from the IE1 protein (pUL123) of human cytomegalovirus. Virology 2002; 295:208–216.
27. Khan N, et al. Comparative analysis of CD8+ T cell responses against human cytomegalovirus proteins pp65 and immediate early 1 shows similarities in precursor frequency, oligoclonality, and phenotype. J Infect Dis 2002; 185:1025–1034.
28. Utz U, et al. Identification of a neutralizing epitope on glycoprotein gp58 of human cytomegalovirus. J Virol 1989; 63:1995–2001.
29. Urban M, et al. Glycoprotein H of human cytomegalovirus is a major antigen for the neutralizing humoral immune response. J Gen Virol 1996; 77(pt. 7):1537–1547.
30. Pignatelli S, et al. Human cytomegalovirus glycoprotein N (gpUL73-gN) genomic variants: identification of a novel subgroup, geographical distribution and evidence of positive selective pressure. J Gen Virol 2003; 84:647–655.

31. Mach M, et al. Complex formation by human cytomegalovirus glycoproteins M (gpUL100) and N (gpUL73). J Virol 2000; 74:11,881–11,892.
32. Reusser P, et al. Cytomegalovirus-specific T-cell immunity in recipients of autologous peripheral blood stem cell or bone marrow transplants. Blood 1997; 89:3873–3879.
33. Riddell SR, Greenberg PD. T cell therapy of human CMV and EBV infection in immunocompromised hosts. Rev Med Virol 1997; 7:181–192.
34. Emery VC. Prophylaxis for CMV should not now replace pre-emptive therapy in solid organ transplantation. Rev Med Virol 2001; 11:83–86.
35. Hart GD, Paya CV. Prophylaxis for CMV should now replace pre-emptive therapy in solid organ transplantation. Rev Med Virol 2001; 11:73–81.
36. Littler E, Stuart AD, Chee MS. Human cytomegalovirus UL97 open reading frame encodes a protein that phosphorylates the antiviral nucleoside analogue ganciclovir. Nature 1992; 358:160–162.
37. Sullivan V, et al. A protein kinase homologue controls phosphorylation of ganciclovir in human cytomegalovirus-infected cells. Nature 1992; 358:162–164.
38. Talarico CL, et al. Acyclovir is phosphorylated by the human cytomegalovirus UL97 protein. Antimicrob Agents Chemother 1999; 43:1941–1946.
39. De Clercq E. What can be expected from non-nucleoside reverse transcriptase inhibitors (NNRTIs) in the treatment of human immunodeficiency virus type 1 (HIV-1) infections? Rev Med Virol 1996; 6:97–117.
40. Chrisp P, Clissold SP. Foscarnet. A review of its antiviral activity, pharmacokinetic properties and therapeutic use in immunocompromised patients with cytomegalovirus retinitis. Drugs 1991; 41:104–129.
41. Lowance D, et al. Valacyclovir for the prevention of cytomegalovirus disease after renal transplantation. International Valacyclovir Cytomegalovirus Prophylaxis Transplantation Study Group. N Engl J Med 1999; 340:1462–1470.
42. Dunn JP, Jabs DA. Cytomegalovirus retinitis in AIDS: natural history, diagnosis, and treatment. AIDS Clin Rev 1995; 99–129.
43. Combination foscarnet and ganciclovir therapy versus monotherapy for the treatment of relapsed cytomegalovirus retinitis in patients with AIDS. The Cytomegalovirus Retreatment Trial. The Studies of Ocular Complications of AIDS Research Group in Collaboration with the AIDS Clinical Trials Group. Arch Ophthalmol 1996; 114:23–33.
44. Lalezari JP, et al. Intravenous cidofovir for peripheral cytomegalovirus retinitis in patients with AIDS. A randomized, controlled trial. Ann Intern Med 1997; 126:257–263.
45. Prichard MN, et al. A recombinant human cytomegalovirus with a large deletion in UL97 has a severe replication deficiency. J Virol 1999; 73:5663–5670.
46. Emery VC, Griffiths PD. Prediction of cytomegalovirus load and resistance patterns after antiviral chemotherapy. Proc Natl Acad Sci U S A 2000; 97:8039–8044.
47. Smith IL, et al. High-level resistance of cytomegalovirus to ganciclovir is associated with alterations in both the UL97 and DNA polymerase genes. J Infect Dis 1997; 176:69–77.
48. Chou S, et al. Interstrain variation in the human cytomegalovirus DNA polymerase sequence and its effect on genotypic diagnosis of antiviral drug resistance. Adult AIDS Clinical Trials Group CMV Laboratories. Antimicrob Agents Chemother 1999; 43:1500–1502.
49. Limaye AP, et al. Emergence of ganciclovir-resistant cytomegalovirus disease among recipients of solid-organ transplants. Lancet 2000; 356:645–649.
50. Limaye AP. Ganciclovir-resistant cytomegalovirus in organ transplant recipients. Clin Infect Dis 2002; 35:866–872.
51. Boivin G, et al. Rate of emergence of cytomegalovirus (CMV) mutations in leukocytes of patients with acquired immunodeficiency syndrome who are receiving valganciclovir as induction and maintenance therapy for CMV retinitis. J Infect Dis 2001; 184:1598–1602.
52. Drew WL, et al. Cytomegalovirus (CMV) resistance in patients with CMV retinitis and AIDS treated with oral or intravenous ganciclovir. J Infect Dis 1999; 179:1352–1355.

53. Jabs DA, et al. Cytomegalovirus retinitis and viral resistance. Prevalence of resistance at diagnosis, 1994. Cytomegalovirus Retinitis and Viral Resistance Study Group. Arch Ophthalmol 1996; 114:809–814.
54. Jabs DA, et al. Cytomegalovirus retinitis and viral resistance: ganciclovir resistance. CMV Retinitis and Viral Resistance Study Group. J Infect Dis 1998; 177:770–773.
55. Jabs DA, et al. Mutations conferring ganciclovir resistance in a cohort of patients with acquired immunodeficiency syndrome and cytomegalovirus retinitis. J Infect Dis 2001; 183:333–337.
56. Bowen EF, et al. Cytomegalovirus polymerase chain reaction viraemia in patients receiving ganciclovir maintenance therapy for retinitis. AIDS 1998; 12:605–611.
57. Jabs DA, et al. Incidence of foscarnet resistance and cidofovir resistance in patients treated for cytomegalovirus retinitis. The Cytomegalovirus Retinitis and Viral Resistance Study Group. Antimicrob Agents Chemother 1998; 42:2240–2244.
58. Michel D, et al. Aciclovir selects for ganciclovir-cross-resistance of human cytomegalovirus in vitro that is only in part explained by known mutations in the UL97 protein. J Med Virol 2001; 65:70–76.
59. Emery VC, Hassan-Walker AF. Focus on new drugs in development against human cytomegalovirus. Drugs 2002; 62:1853–1858.
60. Selleseth DW, et al. Interactions of 1263W94 with other antiviral agents in inhibition of human cytomegalovirus replication. Antimicrob Agents Chemother 2003; 47:1468–1471.
61. Julin JE, et al. Ganciclovir-resistant cytomegalovirus encephalitis in a bone marrow transplant recipient. Transpl Infect Dis 2002; 4:201–206.
62. Isada CM, et al. Clinical characteristics of 13 solid organ transplant recipients with ganciclovir-resistant cytomegalovirus infection. Transpl Infect Dis 2002; 4:189–194.
63. Bhorade SM, et al. Emergence of ganciclovir-resistant cytomegalovirus in lung transplant recipients. J Heart Lung Transplant 2002; 21:1274–1282.
64. Wolf DG, et al. Emergence of late cytomegalovirus central nervous system disease in hematopoietic stem cell transplant recipients. Blood 2003; 101:463–465.
65. Gilbert C, LeBlanc MH, Boivin G. Case study: rapid emergence of a cytomegalovirus UL97 mutant in a heart-transplant recipient on pre-emptive ganciclovir therapy. Herpes 2001; 8:80–82.
66. Seo SK, et al. Cytomegalovirus ventriculoencephalitis in a bone marrow transplant recipient receiving antiviral maintenance: clinical and molecular evidence of drug resistance. Clin Infect Dis 2001; 33:e105–e108.
67. Sasaki T, et al. Progressive retinitis-encephalitis due to ganciclovir-resistant cytomegalovirus associated with aplastic anemia. Intern Med 1997; 36:375–379.
68. Reusser P, Hostettler B, Attehbofer R. Ganciclovir-resistant cytomegalovirus infection: 2 cases with different clinical impact. [German] Schweiz Med Wochenschr 1996; 126:1779–1784.
69. Razis E, et al. Treatment of gancyclovir resistant cytomegalovirus with foscarnet: a report of two cases occurring after bone marrow transplantation. Leuk Lymphoma 1994; 12: 477–480.
70. Basgoz N. A 42-year-old lung transplant patient with ganciclovir-resistant cytomegalovirus (CMV) infection. Transpl Infect Dis 1999; 1:218–225.
71. Manso JV, et al. Ganciclovir resistance in a heart transplant recipient infected by cytomegalovirus. Int J Cardiol 1999; 71:97–98.
72. Hamprecht K, et al. Ganciclovir-resistant cytomegalovirus disease after allogeneic stem cell transplantation: pitfalls of phenotypic diagnosis by in vitro selection of an UL97 mutant strain. J Infect Dis 2003; 187:139–143.
73. Hu H, et al. Comparison of cytomegalovirus (CMV) UL97 gene sequences in the blood and vitreous of patients with acquired immunodeficiency syndrome and CMV retinitis. J Infect Dis 2002; 185:861–867.

74. Jabs DA, et al. Cytomegalovirus resistance to ganciclovir and clinical outcomes of patients with cytomegalovirus retinitis. Am J Ophthalmol 2003; 135:26–34.
75. Mousavi-Jazi M, et al. Sequence analysis of UL54 and UL97 genes and evaluation of antiviral susceptibility of human cytomegalovirus isolates obtained from kidney allograft recipients before and after treatment. Transpl Infect Dis 2001; 3:195–202.
76. Limaye AP, et al. High incidence of ganciclovir-resistant cytomegalovirus infection among lung transplant recipients receiving preemptive therapy. J Infect Dis 2002; 185:20–27.
77. Gilbert C, Boivin G. Discordant phenotypes and genotypes of cytomegalovirus (CMV) in patients with AIDS and relapsing CMV retinitis. AIDS 2003; 17:337–341.

Index

A

Abacavir, 356, 358
Aciclovir, 381
Acinetobacter spp.
  Acinetobacter baumannii
    bacteremia, 121–124
    clinical features, 122
    epidemiology, 119,120
    infection control, 130–131
    mechanisms of resistance, 124–127
    meningitis, 122,128
    mortality, 121,122
    nosocomial pneumonia, 121,122,128
    soft tissue infection, 123
    taxonomy, 118,119
    urinary tract infection, 121,122
    ventilator acquired pneumonia, 122
  Acinetobacter calcoaceticus, 118
  Acinetobacter haemolyticus, 118
  Acinetobacter johnsonii, 119
  Acinetobacter junii, 118
  Acinetobacter lwoffii, 117–119
  Acinetobacter radioresistens, 118–119
  Acinetobacter schindleri, 118
  Acinetobacter urinigii, 118
  Acinetobacter venetianus, 118
Activated protein C, 215
Alveolar epithelial lining fluid, 12,13
Alveolar macrophages, 12
Amdoxovir, 362
Amikacin,
  in the treatment of *Acinetobacter* infections, 127,128
  in the treatment of tuberculosis, 248
  in the treatment of *M. avium-intracellulare* infections
Aminoglycoside modifying enzymes, 126
Amoxicillin, 9–11, 21
  in the treatment of *Helicobacter* infections, 144
  in the treatment of *Salmonella* infections, 196–198
  in the treatment of Vancomycin resistant Enterococcal infections, 95
Amoxicillin-clavulanate, 5,8,11
  in the treatment of *Bacillus circulans* infection, 95
  in the treatment of *Burkholderia pseudomallei* infection, 213–214
  in the treatment of urinary tract infection, 177
Amphotericin B
  combination therapy, 307–308
  in the treatment of *Aspergillus* infections, 302–303
  in the treatment of *Fusarium* infections, 301
  in the treatment of non-albicans *Candida*, 276
  in the treatment of refractory oropharyngeal candidiasis, 281–282
  in the treatment of refractory vulvovaginal candidiasis, 287
  in the treatment of urinary tract infections, 183

liposomal and other lipid preparations, 298,302,306
mechanism of action, 271–2, 297–298
mechanism of resistance, 273
recommended dose, 285
Ampicillin
in the treatment of *Salmonella* infections, 198
in the treatment of urinary tract infections, 176–178
in the treatment of Vancomycin resistant Enterococci, 95
Ampicillin and sublactam, 20
Anidulofungin, 272
Arbekacin, 83
Arcanobacterium haemolyticum, 93
Artemesinin
combinations
with amodiaquine, 325
with atovoquone proguanil, 324–325
with chloroquine, 325
with chlorproguanil dapsone, 324
with lumefantrine, 324–325,332
with Mefloquine, 323
in the treatment of MDR falciparum malaria, 330–333
in the treatment of congenital malaria, 333
in the treatment of malaria, 323
origin, 322
pharmacokinetics, 323
Aspergillus fumigatus, 301
Aspergillus flavus, 297–298, 301
Aspergillus nidulans, 301
Aspergillus niger, 301
Aspergillus terreus, 297–298,301–302
Atazanavir, 356–366
Atovaquone,
mechanism of resistance, 322
Azithromycin,
in the treatment of *Burkholderia pseudomallei* infection, 216
in the treatment of *Neisseria gonorrhoeae* infection, 164
in the treatment of *Salmonella* infections, 196–197
in the treatment of *Streptococcus pneumoniae* infections, 9, 11–13,20
in the treatment of tuberculosis, 249
Azoles, Fluconazole, itraconazole, voriconazole

B

Bacillus circulans, 93,94
Benzimidir, 387
β-lactamases
Amp-C, 124–125,193
extended spectrum, 124–125,193
in *Burkholderia pseudomallei*, 212
in *Helicobacter pylori*, 144
in *Neisseria gonorrhoeae*, 162–163
nitrocefin detection, 165–166
OXA, 124–125
SHV-9, 193
Burkholderia mallei, 209–210
Burkholderia pseudomallei
adjunctive therapy, 214–215
antimicrobial susceptibility, 210–211
β-lactam allergy, 214
clinical features of infection, 209–210
diagnosis of infection, 210–211
maintenance therapy, 215–216
mortality, 211–214
treatment of relapse cases, 215

C

Candida albicans
adjunctive therapy, 289,307
chronic disseminated candidaemia, 287
definition of resistance, 274
infection control, 289–290
in HIV, 272

recurrent vulvovaginal candidiasis, 287–289
refractory oropharyngeal candidiasis, 280–281
resistance candidaemia, 282
urinary tract infection, 183
Candida dubliniensis, 278,280
Candida glabrata, 272–273,277–278,280,282–284,286,288,305,307
Candida guiliermondii, 275,277,280,286,305
Candida krusei, 272–273,276–278,280,283,286
Candida lusitaniae, 275,278,286,298,305,307
Candida parapsilosis, 277–278,280,283,286,305
Candida tropicalis, 276,278,280,286,305
Capravirin, 363
Capreomycin, 248
Carbapenems
in the treatment of *Acinetobacter* infections, 126
in the treatment of *Burkholderia pseudomallei*, 211
pharmacodynamic properties, 8
Caspofungin
antifungal activity, 286,306
in the treatment of refractory oropharyngeal candidiasis
mechanism of action, 272,306
resistance testing, 275
Cefalosporins
in the treatment of *Acinetobacter* infections, 127
in the treatment of *Neisseria gonorrhoeae* infections, 163
in the treatment of urinary tract infections, 176–180
pharmacodynamic properties, 8
resistance, 38,40–41
Cefaclor, 10
Cefapime, 129
Cefdinir, 10
Cefditoren, 10
Cefixime, 5,178,196–197
Cefotaxime, 7–11,20,36–42,180, 196–197,211
Cefpirome, 129,213
Cefpodoxime, 10
Cefprozil, 10
Ceftazidime, 211–214
Ceftriaxone, 5,8,–11,20,36, 38–40,180,196–197,211
Cefuroxime, 5,10–11,20
Chlamydia trachomatis, 161
Chloramphenicol
in the treatment of *Acinetobacter* infections, 127
in the treatment of *Burkholderia pseudomallei* infection, 211–214,216
in the treatment of *Salmonella* infections, 196–197
in the treatment of *Streptococcus pneumoniae* pneumonia, 4
in the treatment of *Streptococcus pneumoniae* meningitis, 35–36,38,41
Chronic obstructive pulmonary diseases, 14–16,18
Clarithromycin
in the treatment of *Helicobacter pylori* infection, 142, 144
in the treatment of *Mycobacterium avium* infection, 263
in the treatment of *Mycobacterium kansasii* infection, 260
in the treatment of rapidly growing mycobacteria, 264–265
in the treatment of *Streptococcus pneumoniae* infection, 9, 11–13,20
in the treatment of tuberculosis, 260
mechanism of resistance, 142,148
Chloroquine, 319–320
Clindamycin, 4,11–12,52
Cidofovir, 381

Ciprofloxacin, 14–20,65,67, 127–128,160,196,248,260,263,282
Colistin, 128
Community acquired pneumonia, 3–4,8–9,14–21,51
Computed Tomography, 33–34
CSF
  antibiotic penetration, 37,41
    cefotaxime, 38–42
    rifampin, 39–40
    vancomycin, 38–40,42
  antigen detection, 34
  culture, 40–42
  Gram stain, 34,37,42
  inflammation, 32,37
  pressure, 33
Cycloserine, 249
Cytomegalovirus, (CMV)
  clinical features, 379–390
  drug resistance mechanisms, 383–384, 386
  immunological control of infection, 380
  management of resistant infection, 383–386

D

DNA gyrase
  in *Neisseria gonorrhoeae*, 164
  in *Salmonella*, 192
  in *Staphylococcus aureus*, 126
  in *Streptococcus pneumoniae*, 15,61,64–65,69,72
Dalbavancin, 86
Daptomycin
  in the treatment of resistant *Staphylococcus aureus* infections, 85
  in the treatment of Vancomycin resistant Enterococcal infections, 96
  mechanism of action, 85
Dexamethazone, 34–35,37,39
Didanosine, 356,360
Doxycycline
  in the treatment of *Acinetobacter* infections, 128
  in the treatment of *Burkholderia pseudomallei* infections, 216–217
  in the treatment of malaria, 331–332
  in the treatment of urinary tract infections, 175
  in the treatment of Vancomycin resistant Enterococcal infections, 95

E

Echinocandins *see* Caspofungin
Economic modelling
  in MRSA control, 110
Efavirenz, 356, 362–363
Efflux pump
  for azoles, 272
  for fluoroquinolones, 16,126
  for macrolides, 10–11,165
Enterococcus casseliflavus, 9, 95
Enterococcus faecalis, 81,91,93,95–96
Enterococcus faecicum, 91, 93, 96
Enterococcus gallinarum, 91,95
Epidemiological modelling
  MRSA infection, 102
Erythromycin, 10,13,20
Escherichia coli,
  in prostatitis, 182
  in urinary tract infections, 179
Etest
  for β-lactams resistance testing, 41
  for detection of heteroresistance
  for fungal resistance testing, 274–275,305
  for glyopeptide resistance testing, 81
  for *Helicobacter pylori* resistance testing, 145–146
  for *Neisseria gonorrhoeae* resistance testing, 166
Ethambutol
  in *Mycobacterium avium-intracellulare* infections, 262,264
  in *Mycobacterium kansasii* infections, 260–262
  in *Mycobacterium xenopi* infections, 261

in tuberculosis, 229,248,252
mechanism of resistance, 243
prophylaxis of tuberculosis, 251
Ethionamide, 249
Extended spectrum β-lactamases
in *Acinetobacter* infections, 124
in *Salmonella* infections, 193, 200

F

Fluconazole
definition of resistance, 274
epidemiology of resistant strains, 277–278
in treatment of non-albicans *Candida*, 283–285
in treatment of refractory oropharyngeal candidiasis, 280–281
in treatment of refractory vulvo-vaginal candidiasis, 287–289
mechanism of action, 272
mechanism of resistance, 272
Flucytosine
combination therapy, 307
definition of resistance, 274
mechanism of activity, 272
recommended dose, 285
resistance testing, 275
Fluoroquinolones
epidemiology of resistance, 62–64
in *Acinetobacter* infections, 126–128
in *Burkholderia pseudomallei* infections, 211,214–215
in *Helicobacter pylori* infections, 145
in *Mycobacterium avium-intracellulare* infections, 264
in *Mycobacterium kansasii* infections, 240
in *Mycobacterium malmoense* infections, 261
in *Neisseria gonorrhoeae* infections, 160,164
in prostatitis, 182–183
in *Salmonella* infections, 196–199
in tuberculosis, 248–249,252
in urinary tract infections, 176,178,180
mechanism of action, 61,64
mechanism of resistance, 15,67
molecular structure, 59,61
treatment of meningitis, 42–43
treatment of resistant *Staphylococcus aureus*, 85
treatment of rapidly growing mycobacteria, 264
Fusarium sp., 297–298, 300

G

Ganciclovir, 381, 383–387
Gatifloxacin, 14–20,65,67,71–72,128
Gentamicin
in *Acinetobacter* infections, 128
in staphylococcal endocarditis, 80
in urinary tract infection treatment, 178,180
Guidelines
American Association of Pediatrics urinary tract infection, 177
American Thoracic Society Community acquired pneumonia, 14, 19–20
Canadian Infectious Diseases Society community acquired pneumoniae, 14, 19–20, 174
Infectious Diseases Society of America antifungal treatment, 281,302
Infectious Diseases Society of America Community acquired pneumonia, 19–20
in HIV treatment, 368–370
Neisseria gonorrhoeae treatment, 160–161

H

Haemophilus influenzae ,31,33,35,163
Helicobacter pylori
epidemiology of resistance, 142
susceptibility testing, 145–149
therapy of resistant cases, 148–149
Heteroresistance, 81
Human immunodeficiency virus (HIV)

antifungal drug resistance, 275
antiretroviral resistance, 355–372
Candida spp., 271
Candida krusei, 276
Candida tropicalis, 276
Cytomegalovirus infection, 381
filamentous fungal infection, 300
GIGA HAART, 351
nontuberculosis mycobacterial infection, 259,261
Mycobacterium avium-intracellulare, 262–264
oropharyngeal candidiasis, 279–281
quasispecies, 357
resistance mutations, 356,360–362
resistance testing, 357,359
Salmonella infection, 191
vancomycin resistant *Streptococcus bovis*, 94
viral load, 358

I

Imipenem
in *Acinetobacter* infections, 127
in *Burkholderia pseudomallei* infection, 213
in *Streptococcus pneumoniae* meningitis therapy, 42
in urinary tract infection therapy, 180
Indinavir, 356,362–366
Intensive Care Unit (ICU)
Acinetobacter infection, 117–132
Intrinsically vancomycin resistance non-enterococcal infections, 93
MRSA, 104
Intrinsically vancomycin resistance enterococci
see Enterococcus casseliflavus
see Enterococcus flavescens
see Enterococcus gallinarum
Intrinsically vancomycin resistant non-enterococcal species, 92
Isoniazid
in *Mycobacterium kansasii* infections, 260
in prophylaxis of tuberculosis, 251
in treatment of tuberculosis, 229,248,252
in treatment of rapidly growing mycobacteria, 264
management of resistant infections, 243
mechanism of resistance, 229–230, 235
Itraconazole
definition of resistance, 274
in the treatment of *Trichosporon* infection, 304
maintenance therapy of refractory vulvo-vaginal candidiasis, 288–289
recommended dose, 285

K

Kanamycin, 212
Ketoconazole, 272, 288
Ketolide, 11
Kirby Bauer method, 41
Klebsiella pneumoniae
acquisition of carriage in an ICU, 119
source of β-lactamase, 164
in urinary tract infections, 179

L

Lamivudine, 356
Levofloxacin, 14–20,43,65,67,71–72
Lexipafant, 215
Linezolid,
resistance mechanism, 96
in *Staphylococcus aureus* infections, 83–84,87
in *Streptococcus pneumoniae* meningitis, 43
in tuberculosis, 250
in vancomycin resistant enterococcal infections, 96
Listeria monocytogenes, 33
Lopinovir, 356,364–366
Lymphadenitis, 254,263

Lysostaphin, 86

M

Macrolide resistance mechanisms, 10–13
Mannitol, 34–34
Mathematical modelling
  in MRSA infection control, 108
Methicillin resistant *Staphylococcus aureus* (MRSA)
  complications, 80
  epidemic MRSA, 79
  epidemiology, 79,81
  infection control, 80,86–87,101–112
  mecA, 81,83
  mortality, 80
  treatment of MRSA infection, 80
Meropenem, 42
Metrifonate, 343
Metronidazole
  in *Helicobacter pylori* infection, 142–144
  mechanisms of resistance, 142–144
Mefloquine
  combination therapy, 323–324
  in pediatric infections, 332
  in multiple drug resistant infection in pregnant women, 331
  resistance mechanisms, 322
Minocycline, 128
Micafungin, 272
Molecular susceptibility tests
  clarithromycin
    in *Helicobacter pylori*, 147
    in *Neisseria gonorrhoeae*, 166–167
  metronidazole, 147
Mouse models
  Helicobacter pylori, 143
  Staphylococcus aureus, 86
  Streptococcus pneumoniae, 8
Moxifloxacin, 14–20,65,67,71–72,128
Mupiricin, 101
Mutant prevention concentration, 65–72
Mutation
  fluoroquinolone resistance, 15–9,64–68,72,192,229–230
  in CMV, 383–386
  in HIV, 360–367
  in *Neisseria gonorrhoeae*, 162, 164–165
  in *Mycobacterium tuberculosis*, 229–231
  in *Salmonella*, 192,195
  metronidazole resistance, 143
  rate, 66–69
  rpoB, 54,229,235–236
  sulfodoxime-pyrimethamine, 321
Mycobacterium abscessus, 264–265
Mycobacterium avium-intracellulare,
  clinical features, 259
  diagnosis, 258
  pulmonary disease, 262–264
Mycobacterium fortuitum, 264–265
Mycobacterium genevense, 259
Mycobacterium kansasii, 258, 260–261
Mycobacterium malmoense, 258–259,261
Mycobacterium marinum, 269
Mycobacterium tuberculosis
  clinical features, 244–248
  control of resistant infection, 251–253
  costs of resistant infection, 251
  diagnosis, 228
  DOTS, 252
  epidemiology, 225,227–228,231,233–234,243–244,257
  fitness of resistant strains, 235
  latency, 234
  molecular mechanisms of resistance, 229–231,246
  mortality of resistant infection, 244
  resistance, 229–233
  surgery for resistant infection, 249–250
  virulence, 234
Mycobacterium ulcerans, 259
Mycobacterium vaccae, 251
Mycobacterium xenopi, 258–259, 261–262

Mycoplasma hominis, 175

N

National Committee for Clinical Laboratory Standards
  fungal susceptibility tests, 274,286,298,305
  Neisseria gonorrhoeae susceptibility tests, 166
  Streptococcus pneumoniae susceptibility tests, 6, 8–9,13,53,66
  Vancomycin resistant *Staphylococcus aureus* definition, 81
Nelfinavir, 356,364–366
Nevirapine, 356, 359
Neisseria gonorrhoeae, 159–168
Neisseria meningitidis, 33, 122
Nitrofurantoin
  in the treatment of urinary tract infections, 176–177,180,183
  in the treatment of vancomycin resistant enterococcus, 95
Non nucleoside reverse transcriptase inhibitors (nNRTI), 355–356, 362–363

O

Ofloxacin, 160,196,248
Oritavancin, 85,96
Otitis media, 33
Oxaminquine, 342,343,345

P

Penicillin
  in *Neisseria gonorrhoeae* infections, 162
  in *Staphylococcus aureus* infections, 80
  in *Streptococcus pneumoniae* meningitis, 41–42
  in *Streptococcus pneumoniae* pneumonia, 5,9,15
  resistance, 3,15,20,35–6,41–42, 51–52
Penicillin binding proteins
  in *Helicobacter pylori*, 144
  in *Neisseria gonorrhoeae*, 162
  in *Streptococcus pneumoniae*, 3,15,30,35
Pharmacodynamics, 7–8,11–13, 16,21,71,83,358
Pharmacokinetics, 167
Piperacillin, 211,213
Plasmodium falciparum
  acute disease management, 325–334
  congenital malaria, 333
  combination therapy, 322–332
  epidemiology of resistance, 320
  management of resistant infections, 329–334
  management of infection in travellers, 333
  prevention of disease, 334
  treatment of severe MDR disease, 329
Polycationic peptides, 129
Posoconazole, 300, 304
Praziquantel
  mechanism of action, 342,346
  resistance, 345–346
  use 343
Probiotics, 183
Prostatitis
  diagnosis, 181–182
  therapy, 181–182
Protease inhibitors, 355–356,363–365
Prothionamide, 249,260
Pseudoallescheria boydii, see Scedospoium
Pseudomonas aeruginosa
  urinary tract infection, 180,183
Pyrazinamide
  mechanism of resistance, 229–230
  prophylaxis of tuberculosis, 251

Q

Quinine
  mechanism of resistance, 322
  use in therapy, 329–331
Quinolone resistance determining region

in *Salmonella*, 192
in *Streptococcus pneumoniae*, 64,66
Quinupristin-dalfopristin
in *Staphylococcus aureus* infections, 83–85
in vancomycin resistant Enterococcal infections, 95

R

Rabbit model
Staphylococcus aureus endocarditis, 83
Streptococcus pneumoniae meningitis, 40,58
Reverse transcriptase inhibitors (RTI), 255–256
Ribosomal subunit
23S, 10,144,165
50S, 10,84
Rifabutin
in *Helicobacter pylori* infections, 145
in *Mycobacterium avium-intracellulare* infections, 263–264
resistance mechanism, 145
Rifampin
in *Acinetobacter* infections, 129
in *Bacillus circulans* infections, 95
in MRSA infections, 83
in *Mycobacterium avium-intracellulare* infections, 260,262
in *Mycobacterium kansasii* infections, 260
in *Mycobacterium malmoense* infections, 261
in *Mycobacterium xenopi* infections, 261
in rapidly growing mycobacterial infections, 264
in tuberculosis
in *Streptococcus pneumoniae* infections, 39–40,42,55–56.
in Vancomycin resistant *Staphylococcus aureus* infections, 83
mechanism of action, 54

S

Salmonella
antibiotic resistance mechanism, 196
classification, 189
clinical features, 190,197,199
epidemiology, 189–193,195
in children, 197
in pregnancy ,198
mortality, 190,197,199
relapse, 198
treatment, 195–198
Saquinavir, 356, 364–366
Scedosporium apispermum, 304
Scedosporium prolificans, 297–301
Schistosoma spp.
Schistosoma haematobium, 198, 341–349
Schistosoma mansoni, 341–349
Schistosoma japonicum, 341–349
Selective digestive decontamination, 131
Spectinomycin, 162,164
Staphylococcus aureus
clinical presentation, 79–80
glycopeptide intermediate susceptibility, 79
penicillinase production, 79
treatment, 80
Staphylococcus epidermidis
in urinary tract infection, 179
Stavudine, 356
Streptococcus bovis
vancomycin resistance, 94
Streptococcus gallolyticus
vancomycin resistance, 94
Streptococcus mitis
vancomycin resistance, 94–95
Streptococcus pneumoniae
amoxicillin, 8–10
amoxicillin-clavulanate, 5,8
bacteremia, 3,13,33,20
β-lactams, 4–9,52
chloramphenicol, 4,35–36
clindamycin, 4,52
fluoroquinolone resistance, 4, 14–19,21,64–72

ketolide, 11
macrolide resistance, 4,9–14,53
meningitis, 31–42
mortality, 3,7,12,31,33–35
multiple drug resistance, 3–9,15,19–21
penicillin resistance, 3,15,20,35–36,41–42,51–53
rifampin resistance, 54,56
risk factors for resistance, 4,15
tetracycline, 3,4,52
trimethoprim sulphamethoxazole, 3,4,52
vaccination, 21,43
vancomycin resistance, 57
Streptomycin, 248,252,260,262
Sublactam, 128
Sulfadoxine-pyrimethamine, 319,321

T

T-20, 356,367
TMC-120, 363
TMC-125, 363

Teicoplanin
in *Bacillus circulans* infections, 95
in Enterococcus infections, 90,93
in *Staphylococcus aureus* infections, 80–81
Telithromycin, 11
Tenofovir, 356, 358
Terbinafine, 308
Tetracycline
in *Burkholderia pseudomallei* infection, 212–214
in *Helicobacteri pylori* infections, 145
in *Neisseria gonorrhoeae* infections, 160, 165
Tigecycline
in *Acinetobacter* infections, 129
in *Staphylococcus aureus* infections, 86
in vancomycin resistant Enterococcus, 96
Topoisomerase IV, 15,61,64–6,69,72,126,164,192–193.
Trichosporon spp, 299,303
Trimethoprim, 176
Trimethoprim-sulfamethoxazole
in *Burkholderia pseudomallei* infections, 211–216
in *Neisseria gonorrhoeae*, 165
in *Salmonella* infections, 196–198
in *Straphylococcus aureus* infections, 83
in urinary tract infections, 176–178
in vancomycin resistant Enterococcus infections, 95
Typing
Acinetobacter, 120
Mycobacterium tuberculosis, 225–236
Salmonella, 195

U

Ureaplasma urealyticum, 175
Urethral syndrome, 175–176
Urinary tract infection
complicated, 180
diagnosis, 174–176
definition ,173–175
in pregnancy, 177
prophylactic treatment, 181
suppressive treatment, 181
vaccines, 183

V

Valaciclovir, 381
Van genes
VanA, 81–82,92–94
VanB, 92–95
VanC, 91,95
VanE, 93
VanR, 91
Vancomycin
in the treatment of urinary tract infections, 180
intrathecal therapy, 41
mechanism of action, 55–56
pneumococcal meningitis, 35,37–42
resistance in *Staphylococcus aureus*, 80,83

resistance in *Streptococcus mitis*, 95
resistance in *Streptococcus pneumoniae*, 20
Vancomycin resistant Enterococcus, 56,91–92
Vancomycin resistant *Staphylococcus aureus*,
definition, 81
epidemiology, 81
mechanism of resistance, 56,81–82
mortality, 82
therapy, 83–86
Vancomycin resistant *Streptococcus pneumoniae*, 57–60,95
Voriconazole
in *Apsergillus* infections, 352
in *Fusarium* infections, 301
in *Trichosporon* infections, 304
recommended dose, 283
use against resistant and non-albicans *Candida*, 285

Z

Zalcitabine, 356
Zidovudine, 356,360
Zygomyces, 299,303

MIX
Papier aus verantwortungsvollen Quellen
Paper from responsible sources
FSC® C105338

If you have any concerns about our products,
you can contact us on
ProductSafety@springernature.com

In case Publisher is established outside the EU,
the EU authorized representative is:
Springer Nature Customer Service Center GmbH
Europaplatz 3, 69115 Heidelberg, Germany

Printed by Libri Plureos GmbH
in Hamburg, Germany